Principles and Practice of Critical Care Toxicology

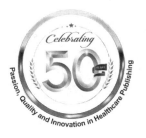

Principles and Practice
of
Critical Care Toxicology

Principles and Practice of Critical Care Toxicology

Editors

Omender Singh MD FCCM
Director
Institute of Critical Care Medicine
Max Superspecialty Hospital
Saket, New Delhi, India

Deven Juneja DNB FNB EDIC FCCP FICCM FCCM
Associate Director
Institute of Critical Care Medicine
Max Superspecialty Hospital
Saket, New Delhi, India

Foreword

Farhad N Kapadia

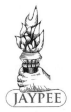

JAYPEE BROTHERS MEDICAL PUBLISHERS
The Health Sciences Publisher
New Delhi | London | Panama

Jaypee Brothers Medical Publishers (P) Ltd

Headquarters
Jaypee Brothers Medical Publishers (P) Ltd
4838/24, Ansari Road, Daryaganj
New Delhi 110 002, India
Phone: +91-11-43574357
Fax: +91-11-43574314
Email: jaypee@jaypeebrothers.com

Overseas Offices

J.P. Medical Ltd
83 Victoria Street, London
SW1H 0HW (UK)
Phone: +44 20 3170 8910
Fax: +44 (0)20 3008 6180
Email: info@jpmedpub.com

Jaypee-Highlights Medical Publishers Inc
City of Knowledge, Bld. 235, 2nd Floor
Clayton, Panama City, Panama
Phone: +1 507-301-0496
Fax: +1 507-301-0499
Email: cservice@jphmedical.com

Jaypee Brothers Medical Publishers (P) Ltd
Bhotahity, Kathmandu, Nepal
Phone: +977-9741283608
Email: kathmandu@jaypeebrothers.com

Website: www.jaypeebrothers.com
Website: www.jaypeedigital.com

© 2019, Jaypee Brothers Medical Publishers

The views and opinions expressed in this book are solely those of the original contributor(s)/author(s) and do not necessarily represent those of editor(s) of the book.

All rights reserved. No part of this publication may be reproduced, stored or transmitted in any form or by any means, electronic, mechanical, photocopying, recording or otherwise, without the prior permission in writing of the publishers.

All brand names and product names used in this book are trade names, service marks, trademarks or registered trademarks of their respective owners. The publisher is not associated with any product or vendor mentioned in this book.

Medical knowledge and practice change constantly. This book is designed to provide accurate, authoritative information about the subject matter in question. However, readers are advised to check the most current information available on procedures included and check information from the manufacturer of each product to be administered, to verify the recommended dose, formula, method and duration of administration, adverse effects and contraindications. It is the responsibility of the practitioner to take all appropriate safety precautions. Neither the publisher nor the author(s)/editor(s) assume any liability for any injury and/or damage to persons or property arising from or related to use of material in this book.

This book is sold on the understanding that the publisher is not engaged in providing professional medical services. If such advice or services are required, the services of a competent medical professional should be sought.

Every effort has been made where necessary to contact holders of copyright to obtain permission to reproduce copyright material. If any have been inadvertently overlooked, the publisher will be pleased to make the necessary arrangements at the first opportunity. The **CD/DVD-ROM** (if any) provided in the sealed envelope with this book is complimentary and free of cost. **Not meant for sale**.

Inquiries for bulk sales may be solicited at: jaypee@jaypeebrothers.com

Principles and Practice of Critical Care Toxicology

First Edition: **2019**

ISBN: 978-93-5270-674-7

Printed at Rajkamal Electric Press, Plot No. 2, Phase-IV, Kundli, Haryana.

Dedicated to

Our lovely and enthusiastic colleagues
for their motivation and support throughout this endeavor.
Our organizations of practice
for providing us state of the art infrastructure and resources,
and above all we extend profound gratefulness
to our patients for their faith in us.

Contributors

Akhilesh Singh MD
Senior Consultant
Institute of Critical Care Medicine
Max Superspecialty Hospital
Saket, New Delhi, India

Amit Goel MD EDIC
Senior Consultant
Institute of Critical Care Medicine
Max Superspecialty Hospital
Saket, New Delhi, India

Anish Gupta MD FNB EDIC
Senior Consultant
Institute of Critical Care Medicine
Max Superspecialty Hospital
Saket, New Delhi, India

Anjali Chaudhari MD
Fellow Critical Care
Institute of Critical Care Medicine
Max Superspecialty Hospital
Saket, New Delhi, India

Anna L Condella MD
Consultant
Harvard Affiliated Emergency Medicine Residency
Brigham and Women's Hospital/Massachusetts
General Hospital
Boston, Massachusetts, USA

Aruna Dewan MD
Director
CEARCH (Centre for Education, Awareness and Research
on Chemicals and Health)
Head, Toxicology Division
Unipath Specialty Laboratory Ltd
Ahmedabad, Gujarat, India

Arvinth Soundarrajan MBBS MEM
Registrar
Department of Emergency Medicine
Meenakshi Mission Hospital and Research Center
Madurai, Tamil Nadu, India

Ashish Bhalla MD FICCM
Additional Professor
Department of Internal Medicine, Postgraduate Institute of
Medical Education and Research (PGIMER)
Chandigarh, India

Ashwinkumar Patel MSC
Consultant, Unipath Specialty Laboratory Ltd
Ahmedabad, Gujarat, India

Bharat Jagiasi MD IDCCM
Head
Critical Care, Terna Specialty Hospital
and Research Center
Mumbai, Maharashtra, India

Desh Deepak MD FNB EDIC
In-Charge Critical Care
Medeor Hospital, VPS Healthcare
Dubai, UAE

Deven Juneja DNB FNB EDIC FCCP FICCM FCCM
Associate Director
Institute of Critical Care Medicine
Max Superspecialty Hospital
Saket, New Delhi, India

Dinesh Chaudhari MD
Associate Consultant
Department of Neurosciences
Indraprastha Apollo Hospital
New Delhi, India

Dinesh Khullar MBBS MD DM
Professor and Head
Department of Nephrology
Max Superspecialty Hospital
Saket, New Delhi, India

Edward W Boyer MD PhD
Director of Academic Development
Department of Emergency Medicine
Brigham and Women's Hospital
Associate Professor
Harvard Medical School
Boston, Massachusetts, USA

Farah Dadabhoy MD
Consultant, Harvard Affiliated
Emergency Medicine Residency Program
Boston, Massachusetts, USA

Gunjan Chanchalani MD FNB IDCCM IFCCM EDIC
Chief Intensivist
Nanavati Superspecialty Hospital
Mumbai, Maharashtra, India

Ipe Jacob PGDIP FAM MED CTCCM
Fellow, Department of Intensive Care
Columbia Asia Referral Hospital
Bengaluru, Karnataka, India

Jamshed Nayer MD
Assistant Professor
Department of Emergency Medicine
All India Institute of Medical Sciences (AIIMS)
New Delhi, India

Jeetendra Sharma MD IFCCM
Director and Head, Critical Care
Artemis Hospital
Gurugram, Haryana, India

Jitendra Shukla MD DNB
Resident, Department of Medicine
Maulana Azad Medical College
and associated Hospitals
New Delhi, India

JV Peter MD DNB MAMS FRACP FJFICM FCICM FICCM
Professor
Department of Critical Care
Medical Intensive Care Unit
Christian Medical College
Vellore, Tamil Nadu, India

Lalit Kumar MBBS
Resident, Department of Medicine
Maulana Azad Medical College and associated Hospitals
New Delhi, India

Michael E Nelson MD MS
Consultant, Department of Emergency Medicine
Division of Toxicology
Cook County Hospital
Chicago, Illinois, USA

Mohit Mathur MD IDCCM EDIC
Principal Consultant
Department of Critical Care Medicine
Max Hospital
Gurugram, Haryana, India

Mradul Kumar Daga MD FRCP FCCP
Director Professor
Department of Medicine and
Intensive Care Medical ICU
Maulana Azad Medical College and associated Hospitals
New Delhi, India

Neha Sharma MD
Senior Resident
Department of Forensic Medicine and Toxicology
All India Institute of Medical Sciences (AIIMS)
New Delhi, India

Nipun Verma MD DM
Assistant Professor
Department of Hepatology
PGI, Chandigarh, India

Omender Singh MD FCCM
Director
Institute of Critical Care Medicine
Max Superspecialty Hospital
Saket, New Delhi, India

Ponniah Thirumalai Kolundu Subramanian MD
Head
Department of Internal Medicine
Chennai Medical College Hospital and Research Center
Trichy, Tamil Nadu, India

Pradeep Rangappa
DNB FJFICM EDIC FCICM PGDIPECHO MBA FICCM PGDMLE
Consultant Intensivist
Department of Intensive Care
Columbia Asia Referral Hospital
Bengaluru, Karnataka, India

Prakash K Khernar MD IDCCM IFCCM
Consultant
Critical Care
Metro Hospital
Faridabad, Haryana, India

Prashant Nasa MD FNB EDIC
Specialist, Critical Care Medicine
Head Prevention and Control of Infection
Department of Critical Care Medicine
NMC Specialty Hospital, Dubai, UAE

Prashant Singh MD
Associate Consultant
Institute of Critical Care Medicine
Max Superspecialty Hospital
Saket, New Delhi, India

Pravin Amin MD FCCM
Consultant, Critical Care
Bombay Hospital
Mumbai, Maharashtra, India

Rajesh Chawla MD FICCM FCCM
Senior Consultant
Department of Pulmonary Medicine and Critical Care
Indraprastha Apollo Hospital
New Delhi, India

Ravi Jain MD FNB
Associate Consultant
Department of Critical Care Medicine
Max Hospital
Gurugram, Haryana, India

Rohit Yadav DA IDCCM
Senior Consultant
Institute of Critical Care Medicine
Max Superspecialty Hospital
Saket, New Delhi, India

Sahil Bagai MD DM
Associate Consultant
Department of Nephrology
Max Superspecialty Hospital
Saket, New Delhi, India

Sanjay V Patne MD
Director and In-Charge of Critical Care Unit
JJ Plus Hospital
Aurangabad, Maharashtra, India

Saswati Sinha MD EDIC
Consultant, Critical Care and
Emergency Department
Advanced Medicare and
Research Institute (AMRI) Hospitals
Kolkata, West Bengal, India

Shivakumar Mutnal MD IDCCM IFCCM
Registrar
Department of Intensive Care
Columbia Asia Referral Hospital
Bengaluru, Karnataka, India

Shivangi Khanna MD
Fellow, Critical Care Medicine
Artemis Hospital
Gurugram, Haryana, India

Shreya Singh MD
Assistant Professor
Department of Medical Microbiology
Postgraduate Institute
Chandigarh, India

Shweta Gupta DA DNB MNAMS FCCP
Specialist and In-Charge of Pulmonology
Dr Baba Saheb Ambedkar Hospital
New Delhi, India

Subhash Kumar Todi MD MRCP
Head
Critical Care and Emergency Department
Advanced Medicare and
Research Institute (AMRI) Hospitals
Kolkata, West Bengal, India

Subramanian Senthilkumaran
MD DIP A&E FCCM MSC PHD
Head, Department of Emergency and Critical Care
Manian Medical Center
Erode, Tamil Nadu, India

Sudhir K Gupta MBBS (Gold Medalist) MD DNB MNAMS
Professor and Head
Department of Forensic Medicine and Toxicology
All India Institute of Medical Sciences (AIIMS)
New Delhi, India

Suneel Kumar Garg MD FNB EDIC FCCP
Senior Consultant, Institute of Critical Care Medicine
Max Superspecialty Hospital
Saket, New Delhi, India

Supradip Ghosh DNB EDIC
Director
Department of Critical Care Medicine
Fortis-Escorts Hospital
Faridabad, Haryana, India

Timothy B Erickson MD
Associate Professor
Division of Medical Toxicology
Department of Emergency Medicine
Brigham and Women's Hospital
Harvard Medical School
Harvard Humanitarian Initiative
Boston, Massachusetts, USA

Vijay Kumar Agarwal MD IDCCM IFCCM
Director
Critical Care Medicine and Academic Programs
Senior Consultant
Pulmonology and Sleep Medicine
Metro Hospital, Faridabad, Haryana, India

Vikas Suri MD
Associate Professor
Department of Internal Medicine
Postgraduate Institute of Medical
Education and Research (PGIMER)
Chandigarh, India

Vinay Amin MBBS
Mumbai, Maharashtra, India

Yash Javeri DA IDCCM
Director
Apex Healthcare Consortium
New Delhi, India

Foreword

It gives me great pleasure to review this book *Principles and Practice of Critical Care Toxicology* by Dr Omender Singh and colleagues. I have been following his work and his presentations on the critical care aspects of toxicology for more than 10–15 years and it is befitting that he has brought out this book with like-minded and vastly experienced colleagues. The authors include international and national experts in the field of toxicology, and the content and depth of the material in each subject only confirm the expertise of the authors and editors.

The material is presented in a format, which is easy to read and digest. Despite having a fair bit of basic sciences, this is ultimately a practical bedside book. Readers will easily pick-up the salient aspects of each specific poisoning syndrome and clinicians and ICU residents will be able to use it as a manual to follow when dealing with these patients. I also personally found some of the material novel, specifically the use of Lipid Emulsion Therapy (LET) and the role of Extracorporeal Membrane Oxygenation (ECMO) in acute toxicity. Readers like me, who do a lot of critical care, but only deal infreqeuntly with poisonings, will find this a very useful update on recent advances in the field.

The book includes poisoning management ranging from common household poisons to drug overdose, industrial, agricultural, chemical warfare and nerve agent poisonings, from ABC of poisoning to extracorporeal and emerging treatment modalities (LET). I recommend this book be part of each ICU, library and emergency room. The staff of these departments will find it a comprehensive, pragmatic and useful resource.

Farhad N Kapadia
MD MRCP DA (UK) EDIC (European Diploma of Intensive Care
European Society of Intensive Care Medicine)
FRCP (Royal College of Physicians, Edinburgh)
Consultant Physician and Intensivist
PD Hinduja Hospital
Mumbai, Maharashtra, India

Preface

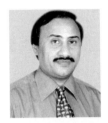
Omender Singh

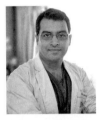
Deven Juneja

From the beginning of written history, poisons and their effects have been well described. Paracelsus (1493–1541) correctly noted that "All substances are poisons; there is none which is not a poison. The right dose differentiates a poison…" As life in the modern era has become more complex, so has the study of poisons and their treatments.

Critical care toxicology is a field of medicine dedicated to the evaluation and treatment of poisoned and envenomated patients. This book to us is about our zeal to practice critical care toxicology and improve outcomes of poisoned patients in the era of complex poisonings with almost negligible evidence-based guidelines in the field of medical toxicology.

Over the past decade, the field of Medical Toxicology has grown in conjunction with the emergence of new pharmaceuticals, new drugs of abuse, chemicals within the workplace, environmental toxins and agents of terrorism. The clinical outcome of patients poisoned by a specific agent depends largely on the quality of care delivered within the first few hours in the emergency and critical care setting. This book will highlight the nuances of clinical toxicology with in-depth and most recent management of poisoning. It will serve physicians working in the fields of critical care medicine, emergency medicine, internal medicine and other allied specialties involved in the management of critically-ill poisoned patients.

We have made a conscious effort to incorporate the expertise and experience of clinical toxicologists from diverse specialties from across the globe, to author relevant chapters. We commend the authors for providing a single resource that covers a broad spectrum of toxicologic emergencies in a succinct, clinically relevant, and cutting-edge manner.

We are confident that this book will be a useful resource for clinicians, leading to improved outcomes of critically-ill poisoned patients.

We wish to thank Jaypee Brothers Medical Publishers, New Delhi, India, to bring our skills and ideas to a wide audience, and we are thankful for their collaboration.

Editors

Acknowledgments

I owe an enormous gratitude towards many individuals; some of them deserve a special mention. Especially my parents Late Sh. Surendra Pal Singh and my mother Smt. Singari Devi, my wife Rimple Singh and my lovely children Sofiya and Nikshay for allowing me to spend time for this book, which was rightfully theirs. My teacher Dr Farhad Kapadia, and my inspirational mentors Dr Pervez Ahmed and Dr NK Pandey for their guidance and support. I would also like to extend my gratitude to Ms Poonam Joshi for her unconditional support.

Omender Singh

To my parents, Dr BK Juneja and Mrs Kumud Juneja, for being my source of inspiration and encouragement. To my wonderful wife, Payal and my lovely daughters Aanya and Arayna for being my support and tolerating me and my career.

Deven Juneja

xviii   Principles and Practice of Critical Care Toxicology

Section 2 *Drugs of Abuse*

7. Central Nervous System Depressants: Overdose and Management 77
Mradul Kumar Daga, Lalit Kumar, Jitendra Shukla

Common Central Nervous System Depressants: Mechanism of Action and Uses **77**
Central Nervous System Depressant Overdose and its Management **78**   Management of
Sedative Hypnotic Overdose and Role of Flumazenil **79**   Opioid Overdose and its Management **80**
Cannabinoids Toxicity **80**   Gamma-Hydroxybutyric Acid Overdose **80**   Party Drugs **80**

8. Sympathomimetic Drugs 84
Anish Gupta, Omender Singh

Central Nervous System Stimulants **85**   Hallucinogens **87**
Dissociative Anesthetics **90**

9. Cocaine Intoxication 93
Omender Singh, Anish Gupta

Pathophysiology **93**   Clinical Features **93**   Diagnosis **95**
Management **95**   Prognosis **97**

10. Newer Drugs of Abuse 99
Omender Singh, Rajesh Chawla, Deven Juneja

Substituted Cathinones or "Bath Salts" **99**   Synthetic Cannabinoids **101**
Substituted Phenethylamines (2C Drugs) **102**   Piperazines **102**   Tryptamines **103**
Kratom **103**   Salvia **103**   Hawaiian Baby Woodrose **104**   Desomorphine **104**

Section 3 *CNS Toxins*

11. Toxins-induced Seizures 109
Dinesh Chaudhari, Anjali Chaudhari, Omender Singh

Toxin-induced Seizures **109**   Status Epilepticus **115**

12. Toxic Alcohols 118
Michael E Nelson, Farah Dadabhoy, Timothy B Erickson

Ethanol **118**   Methanol **120**   Ethylene Glycol **122**   Isopropyl Alcohol **123**

13. Botulism 128
Anjali Chaudhari, Deven Juneja

Epidemiology **128**   Classification **128**   Pathogenesis **129**   Clinical Presentation **129**
Differential Diagnosis **130**   Diagnosis **130**   Treatment **131**   Prognosis **131**
Prevention **131**

14. Anticonvulsant Overdose 133
Rohit Yadav, Deven Juneja

Classification **133**   Management of Antiepileptic Drugs Overdose Based on Mechanism of Action **134**
General Points to Remember in Management of Anticonvulsants Overdose **141**

Contents

Section 1 *General Management of Poisoning or Overdose*

1. Approach to a Poisoned Patient 1

Omender Singh, Prashant Nasa, Deven Juneja

Initial Resuscitation and Assessment **3**　　Disability and Decontamination **5**　　Toxidromes **9**
Laboratory Testing of Poisoning **14**　　Admission to Intensive Care Unit **15**　　Antidotes **15**
Advanced Life Support Considerations **16**

2. Laboratory Testing in Poisoning 19

Aruna Dewan, Ashwin Patel

Approach to Laboratory Tests in Acute Poisoning **19**　　Toxicology Tests at Centre for Education,
Awareness and Research on Chemicals and Health Laboratory (CEARCH, Ahmedabad) **21**

3. Acid-base Disorders in Poisoning 26

Pradeep Rangappa, Shivakumar Mutnal, Ipe Jacob

Acid-base Disturbances **26**　　Metabolic Acidosis **26**　　Osmolar Gap **28**　　Metabolic Alkalosis **29**
Acute Respiratory Acidosis **29**　　Acute Respiratory Alkalosis **29**

4. Antidotes 31

Omender Singh, Anish Gupta

N-Acetylcysteine **31**　　Atropine **33**　　Botulinum Antitoxin-Heptavalent **34**
Botulinum Immuno Globulin (Intravenous Human) (Babybig) **35**　　Bromocriptine **35**
Activated Charcoal **36**　　Calcium **37**　　Calcium Disodium EDTA (CaNa$_2$ EDTA) **37**
Dantrolene **38**　　Deferoxamine **39**　　Dimercaprol **39**　　Digoxin-specific Antibody Fragments **40**
Flumazenil **40**　　Fomepizole (4-Methylpyrazole) **41**　　Folic Acid (Vitamin B$_9$) **42**　　Glucagon **42**
High-dose Insulin Therapy **42**　　Hydroxocobalamin **43**　　Hyperbaric Oxygen **43**　　Methylene Blue **44**
Naloxone **44**　　Penicillamine **45**　　Physostigmine **46**　　Phytonadione (Vitamin K$_1$) **46**
Pralidoxime (2-Pam) **47**　　Protamine Sulfate **48**　　Pyridoxine (Vitamin B$_6$) **49**　　Sodium Nitrite **50**
Sodium Thiosulfate **51**　　Succimer [Dimercaptosuccinic Acid (DMSA)] **51**　　Silymarin **52**
Sodium Bicarbonate **52**　　Leucovorin (Folinic Acid) **53**　　Levocarnitine **54**　　Octreotide **54**
Thiamine (Vitamin B$_1$) **55**　　Potassium Iodide **55**　　Anti-Snake Venom (ASV) **56**

5. Lipid Emulsion Therapy 60

Omender Singh, Deven Juneja

Mechanism of Action **60**　　Lipid Preparations **61**　　Dose and Delivery **61**
Adverse Effects **62**　　Indications of Use **63**

6. Forensic Toxicology for the Critical Care Specialist 68

Sudhir K Gupta, Neha Sharma

Definitions **68**　　Laws Relating to Poisons **68**　　Legal Provisions Pertaining to
Poisoning **69**　　Circumstances of Poisoning **70**　　Duties of a Medical Practitioner in a Patient of
Suspected Poisoning **70**　　Evidence Collection and Preservation of Samples in a Patient of Suspected
Poisoning **71**　　Important Points for Dispatch of Sample for Chemical Analysis **72**　　Algorithm of
Management of a Patient with Suspected Poisoning **72**　　Toxidrome Approach **72**　　List of Common
Poisons and their Antidotes **72**　　Reason for Negative Chemical Analysis Report in a Patient with Positive
History of Poisoning **72**

Section 4 Pulmonary Toxins

15. Approach to Respiratory Failure 145
Suneel Kumar Garg, Shweta Gupta

Pathogenesis **145**   Approach to Respiratory Failure **146**   Specific Management **148**

16. Inhalational Poisoning 151
Suneel Kumar Garg, Shweta Gupta

Classification **151**   Epidemiology **152**   Pathogenesis **152**   Agents Causing Direct Pulmonary
Injury **153**   Agents Causing Systemic Toxicity **154**   Combination Agents **157**   Chemical Warfare
and Riot Control Agents **158**

17. Carbon Monoxide Poisoning 162
Ashish Bhalla, Vikas Suri, Jamshed Nayer

Sources of Carbon Monoxide **162**   Mechanism of Carbon Monoxide Toxicity **162**
Clinical Features **162**   Diagnosis **163**   Treatment **163**

Section 5 Cardiac Toxins

18. Poisoning Induced Circulatory Failure 167
Omender Singh, Desh Deepak

Epidemiology **167**   Pathophysiology **167**   Management **168**   Future Therapies **171**

19. Aluminum Phosphide Poisoning 174
Ashish Bhalla

Pathophysiology and Toxicodynamics **174**   Clinical Presentation **175**   Diagnosis **175**
Laboratory Workup **175**   Treatment **175**   Prognosis **176**

20. Beta-blocker and Calcium Channel Blocker Overdose 178
Saswati Sinha, Subhash Kumar Todi

Pharmacology **178**   Clinical Features **178**   Management Principles **179**

21. Sodium Channel Blockers 185
Deven Juneja, Omender Singh

Tricyclic Antidepressants **185**   Antihistamine (Diphenhydramine) **190**

22. Digoxin and Other Cardiac Glycosides 194
Supradip Ghosh

Cardiac Glycosides: Pharmacology **194**   Clinical Features **195**
Management **195**

Section 6 Gastrointestinal and Liver Toxins

23. Acetaminophen (Paracetamol) Poisoning 203
Anish Gupta, Deven Juneja

Introduction/Epidemiology **203**   Pharmacology **203**   Toxicology **203**   Clinical Features **204**
Diagnosis **205**   Management **206**   Special Cases **208**   Prognosis/Outcome **208**

Principles and Practice of Critical Care Toxicology

24. NSAID Overdose **210**
Anish Gupta, Omender Singh

Pharmacology **210** Classification **210** Toxic Doses **210** Toxic Features **211** Diagnosis **211**
Management **211** Salicylates **212**

25. Corrosive Ingestion: Acids and Alkalis **218**
Desh Deepak

Epidemiology **218** Causative Agents **218** Common Corrosive Agents **222**

Section 7 *Hematological Toxins*

26. Warfarin and Superwarfarin Toxicity **227**
Mohit Mathur

Brief History of Warfarin and Superwarfarins **227** Mechanism of Action **228** Epidemiology **228**
Approach Considerations **229** Clinical Presentation and Evaluation **229**
Laboratory Investigations **230** Treatment **230**

27. Overdose of Newer Anticoagulants **236**
Pravin Amin, Vinay Amin

Therapeutic Role and Monitoring of DOACS **236** Bleeding with DOACS **237**
Management of Severe Bleeding with DOACS **238** Agent-specific Interventions for Reversals **239**

28. Dyshemoglobinemias **242**
Jeetendra Sharma, Shivangi Khanna

Carboxyhemoglobinemia **242** Methemoglobinemia **247** Cyanide Toxicity **250**
Sulfhemoglobinemia **251**

Section 8 *Renal Toxins and Extracorporeal Therapies*

29. Approach to Toxin Induced Acute Renal Failure **257**
Sahil Bagai, Dinesh Khullar

Clinical Features **257** Mechanisms of Injury **258** Agents Causing Acute Kidney Injury **258**
Heavy Metal Poisoning and AKI **259** Envenomation and Bites Causing AKI **260**
Approach to AKI with Poisoning **261** General Management of AKI **261**
Prognosis of Patients who had AKI **262**

30. Extracorporeal Therapies: General Principles **264**
Deven Juneja, Omender Singh

Factors Affecting Dialyzability **264** Types of Extracorporeal Toxin Removal **265**
Issues with Extracorporeal Toxin Removal **269**

31. Extracorporeal Therapies: Specific Poisons **274**
Deven Juneja, Omender Singh

Acetaminophen **274** Barbiturates **275** Carbamezapine **276** Lithium **277**
Metformin **277** Methanol **278** Phenytoin **279** Salicylic Acid **280** Thallium **281**
Theophylline **282** Valproic Acid **283**

Contents | xxi

32. Extracorporeal Membrane Oxygenation 288
Anna L Condella, Edward W Boyer

Brief History **288**   Mechanics of Extracorporeal Membrane Oxygenation **289**
Indications for Extracorporeal Membrane Oxygenation **289**   Pharmaceutical Overdoses **290**
Nonpharmaceutical Poisoning **290**   Pediatric Considerations **291**

Section 9 *Pesticides and Rodenticides*

33. Organophosphorus 295
JV Peter

Clinical Presentation **295**   Determinants of Toxicity of Organophosphate
Compounds **295**   Management of Poisoning **296**

34. Carbamates and Newer Insecticides 303
Vijay Kumar Agarwal, Prakash K Khernar, Amit Goel

Carbamates **303**   Pyrethroids **307**   Organophosphate-Pyrethroid
Combination **309**

35. Herbicides Poisoning: Paraquat and Diquat 312
Amit Goel, Omender Singh

Chemistry **312**   Mechanism of Toxicity **312**   Clinical Presentation **314**
Management **315**   Outcome **317**

36. Organochlorines 320
Ravi Jain, Omender Singh

Pharmacology **320**   Pathophysiology and Mechanism of Toxicity **322**   Approach to Patient **323**
Biochemical Effects of Toxins **323**   Differential Diagnosis **324**   Treatment of Organochlorine
Pesticide Poisoning **325**

37. Rodenticides 330
Sanjay V Patne, Subramanian Senthilkumaran

Classification of Rodenticides **330**   Biochemistry **330**
Pathophysiology **331**   Clinical Features **331**   Clinical Manifestations **332**
Workup **332**   Treatment **332**

Section 10 *Miscellaneous Toxicities*

38. Heavy Metal Poisoning 339
Prashant Nasa

Pathophysiology **340**   General Principles of Assessment and Management **340**
Specific Metals **342**

39. Envenomation: Snake, Scorpion, and Spider 348
Subramanian Senthilkumaran, Ponniah Thirumalai Kolundu Subramanian

Types of Snakes **348**   Toxic Effects of Snake Venom **348**   Pathophysiology **348**
Clinical Features **349**   Diagnosis **349**   Investigations **350**   Management of Snake Bite **350**
Indications for Antivenom **351**   Adverse Reaction to Antivenom **351**   Management in Special
Situations **352**   Scorpion Stings **352**   Hymenoptera Stings **354**

Principles and Practice of Critical Care Toxicology

40. Plant Poisonings 357

Arvinth Soundarrajan, Subramanian Senthilkumaran, Ponniah Thirumalai Kolundu Subramanian

Indian Poisonous Plants **357**

41. Mushroom Poisoning 367

Nipun Verma, Ashish Bhalla, Shreya Singh

Background **367**   Pathophysiology **367**   Epidemiology **368**   Clinical Presentation **369**
Differential Diagnoses **370**   Laboratory Studies **370**   Treatment of Mushroom Poisoning **371**
Prognosis **372**

42. Methotrexate and Other Chemotherapeutic Agents Toxicity 374

Akhilesh Singh, Omender Singh

Chemotherapeutic Drug-associated Toxicity **377**   Extravasation of
Chemotherapeutic Agents **382**

43. Metformin and Other Oral Hypoglycemic Agents 386

Prashant Singh, Omender Singh

Biguanides (Metformin) **387**   Sulfonylureas **388**   Meglitinides **390**
Alpha-Glucosidase Inhibitors **391**   Dipeptidyl Peptidase-4 Inhibitors **391**   Serum Glucose
Transporter-2 Inhibitors **391**

44. Chemical and Biological Warfare 395

Yash Javeri, Bharat Jagiasi, Gunjan Chanchalani

Chemical Warfare **396**   Biological Warfare **398**

Index 403

SECTION 1

General Management of Poisoning or Overdose

1. **Approach to a Poisoned Patient**
   Omender Singh, Prashant Nasa, Deven Juneja

2. **Laboratory Testing in Poisoning**
   Aruna Dewan, Ashwin Patel

3. **Acid-base Disorders in Poisoning**
   Pradeep Rangappa, Shivakumar Mutnal, Ipe Jacob

4. **Antidotes**
   Omender Singh, Anish Gupta

5. **Lipid Emulsion Therapy**
   Omender Singh, Deven Juneja

6. **Forensic Toxicology for the Critical Care Specialist**
   Sudhir K Gupta, Neha Sharma

1 CHAPTER

Approach to a Poisoned Patient

Omender Singh, Prashant Nasa, Deven Juneja

INTRODUCTION

The patients with suspected poisoning are commonly encountered by acute medicine and critical care physicians. The poisoning in these cases may be accidental or intentional (suicidal or homicidal). Any chemical available can be potentially toxic to humans, provided the quantity is large. The high index of suspicion is warranted to identify these patients early especially when direct history of intoxication is not available. The knowledge and recognition of a specific toxidrome is critical, but one has to be aware of pitfalls like symptoms either may be nonspecific or masked (e.g. intracranial hemorrhage in cocaine poisoning).

The physical examination should be focused in case of critical condition and comprehensives once the patient is stabilized. The vital signs and level of consciousness is paramount in assessing the degree of toxicity. Initial vitals assessment by emergency staff or other paramedic must include respiratory rate, heart rate, blood pressure, and temperature; are of utmost importance as clinical signs may change by treatment. The patient neurological state (level of consciousness), pupils size, reaction to light, and presence of seizures may provide clues regarding the identity of the ingested poison.

The management approach in these patients is based on rapid and early diagnosis, decontamination and prevent further exposure, appropriate specific treatment while providing multiorgan supportive care. We have divided this chapter into following sections:

A. Initial resuscitation and assessment
B. Toxidromes
C. Laboratory testing in poisoning
D. Advanced cardiac life support concerns in poisoning
E. Antidotes.

INITIAL RESUSCITATION AND ASSESSMENT

Most of the patients with poisoning respond well with early general intensive supportive measures with close watch on red flag signs. The supportive measures can be similar to any critically ill patient with "ABCD" approach (airway, breathing, circulation) however D in poisoning is different and means disability and decontamination. In case patient has an altered level of consciousness, the priority is airway management and cervical spine must be immobilized till it is clear of any injury. The initial resuscitation of patient is similar to any critical patient with systematic approach to evaluate and identify a life-threatening problem, and treat the problem before proceeding to next. The ABCD approach usually employed in critical care or emergency is useful.

Airway

Airway patency should be assessed in all cases unless a conscious-oriented patient without signs of upper airway obstruction. In case of altered sensorium or patient with stridor, hoarseness and other signs of upper airway

General Management of Poisoning or Overdose

obstruction, airway should be secured with maneuver like headtilt-chinlift or may need airway adjuncts. Endotracheal intubation may be required in these patients for airway protection and patency. The other indications are acute respiratory failure, high supplemental oxygen in case of carbon monoxide poisoning.[1] The urine or blood toxicology screening should be obtained before any sedatives or hypnotics are administered. Some toxins (acid or alkali ingestion) require special care during airway management and involve an expert help in such cases. Whenever endotracheal intubation is required in patients with unknown poisoning, rapid sequence induction (RSI) using short-acting sedatives and paralytics is generally preferred as time from last meal is either unknown or erroneous. The succinylcholine is the neuromuscular paralytic agent of choice; however, it should be avoided in suspected organophosphorus poisoning as duration may be prolonged in view of decreased acetylcholinesterase levels. The intubation is necessary for most patients with above indications, but if possible intubation in aspirin (difficult to attain hyperventilation) and gamma-hydroxybutyrate (rapid recovery) poisoning can be avoided or delayed unless the patients present with clinical or blood gas evidence of respiratory failure.[1]

Breathing

If breathing or respiratory effort is inadequate beside the endotracheal intubation, respiratory support is also required. Endotracheal intubation besides altered level of consciousness to protect airway is indicated in acute respiratory failure. The supplemental oxygen in case of poisoning like carbon monoxide poisoning is additional indication.

The patient's oxygen saturation (SpO_2) with standard bedside pulse oximetry can be misleading in poisoning with dyshemoglobinemias (e.g. carbon monoxide poisoning), where co-oximeter should be used to identify abnormal hemoglobins and true SpO_2. The target SpO_2 is 94–99% for most of the poisoning except in some poisoning where high SpO_2 is associated with oxygen-mediated toxicity, e.g. chlorine gas, paraquat and diquat.[2] In these patients lowest possible PaO_2 (~50–60 mm Hg) and SpO_2 (~90–93%) should be targeted essential to prevent tissue hypoxia and in order to avoid oxygen-mediated toxicity.[3]

If standard lung-protective invasive ventilation strategy is acceptable for most of the poisoning except in salicylates where any acidosis due to hypoventilation during intubation and/or lung protective ventilation may cause clinical deterioration.[4,5]

The patients where intubation may be required for correction of hypoxemia or other presentation of respiratory failure should be identified and managed early (Table 1).

Table 1: Drugs/poisons causing hypoxemia.

Aspiration pneumonia	• Poisons/drugs causing altered mental status
Bronchospasm	• β-blockers • Cocaine • Organophosphates • Drugs resulting in aspiration • Drugs associated with myocardial depression (cardiac asthma)
Cardiogenic pulmonary edema	• Antiarrhythmics β-blockers • Tricyclic antidepressants • Calcium channel blockers (Verapamil)
Cytopathic (cellular) hyoxia	• Hydrogen sulfide • Carbon monoxide • Cyanide • Methemoglobinemia
Hypoventilation	• Alcohols (ethanol, methanol, ethylene glycol) • Botulinum toxin • Barbiturates • Benzodiazepines • Opioids • Sedative/hypnotics • Snake bite • Neuromuscular blockade • Tricyclic antidepressants • Tetanus
Hemorrhage (Alveolar)	• Cocaine • Anticoagulants • Thrombolytics • Amiodarone • Nitrofurantoin • Penicillamine • Toluene
Noncardiogenic pulmonary edema	• Toxic inhalation gases (e.g. hydrocarbons, phosgene • Cocaine • Ethylene glycol • Opioids • Salicylates
Pneumothorax	• Cocaine • IV drug abuse • Kerosene
Gases (inert)	• Carbon dioxide • Methane • Nitrogen • Propane

Circulation

The patients with poisoning may present with hypotension or hypertension, brady- or tachyarrhythmias (Tables 2 and 3). The continuous monitoring of electrocardiogram along with blood preesure and heart is thus vital for all these patients.

Bradycardia and/or Hypotension: Bradycardia is mainly seen with β-blockers and calcium-channel blockers but sometimes significant enough to require temporary pacing especially if associated with hemodynamic instability (Table 3).

- *Hypotension/Bradycardia*—calcium-channel blockers, β-blockers, digoxin, aluminum phosphide (celphos) insecticide
- *Hypertension/Tachycardia*—Sympathomimetics, cocaine.

The cause of hypotension in a patient with poisoning can be multifactorial which includes hypovolemia, poison causing direct myocardial depression, arrhythmias,

and/or profound systemic vasodilation. The patients with intoxication of sympathomimetic drugs, anticholinergics, ergot derivatives, cocaine and withdrawal of nicotine, alcohol, and sedatives instead present with hypertension. The initial resuscitation must include peripheral venous access using two large bore cannula (16- or 18-gauge) with targeted fluid resuscitation and/or vasopressors or inotropes if required for correction of hypotension. The treatment of hypertension is goal-oriented and may depend on factors like inciting agent, severity and associated complications.[6]

DISABILITY AND DECONTAMINATION

The target-oriented neurological assessment in poisoned patients presenting with altered mental status is must (Box 1). In patients presenting with focal neurological deficit an imaging may be required to rule out any structural brain injury. There are simple bedside scores like Glasgow Coma Score or Alert/Verbal/Painful/ Unresponsive (AVPU) score which can be used to assess consciousness and need to protect the airways. However neither has been validated and found to predict prognosis of the poisoned patient.[3]

Seizure is common neurological finding along with pupillary abnormalities. The assessment of pupil may help to suspect some poison along with other systemic findings (Table 4).

Table 2: Agents causing hypotension and hypertension.

Hypotension (SCAR)	Hypertension (SCAN)
Sedative/hypnotics	**S**ympathomimetics
Calcium-channel blockers	**C**ocaine
Antidepressants, antihypertensives	**A**nticholinergics and amphetamines
Rodenticides (e.g. arsenic, cyanide)	**N**icotine

Table 3: Drugs causing bradycardia and tachycardia.

Bradycardia	Tachycardia
Calcium-channel blockers	Anticholinergics
β-blockers	Amphetamines
Class 1A and 1C antiarrhythmics	Antihistaminics
Tricyclic antidepressants	Carbon monoxide
Digoxin	Cyanide poisoning
Lithium	Clonidine
Metoclopramide	Cocaine
Opioids	Cyclic antidepressants
Organophosphates and carbamates	Hydralazine
Physostigmine	Methemoglobinemia
Quinidine	Phencyclidine, phenothiazines Pseudoephedrine
	Theophylline

Box 1: Poisoning present with altered level of unconsciousness (LETHARGIC).

L: metals like lead, lithium
E: Alcohol like ethanol, ethylene glycol
T: Tricyclic antidepressants, antipsychotics
H: Heroin, hydrogen sulfide, hypoglycemics
A: Arsenic, antidepressants, anticonvulsants, antihistamines
R: Rohypnol (sedative hypnotics), risperidone
G-GHB
I: Isoniazid, insulin
C: Carbon monoxide, cyanide, clonidine

Table 4: Agents causing pupillary abnormalities.

Miosis (SCOP)	Mydriasis (SAD)
Sedative-hypnotics	**S**ympathomimetics
Cholinergics,carbamates (organophosphates)	**A**nticholinergics
Opiates	**D**rug withdrawal
Phenothiazines (antipsychotics)	

General Management of Poisoning or Overdose

The "coma cocktail" traditionally included dextrose (1 ampule of D50% IV), oxygen (5–10 L/min), flumazenil (0.2 mg IV), naloxone (2 mg IV), and thiamine (100 mg IV) and was advocated in unknown poisoning with unconsciousness and coma. This is helpful in prehospital to avoid intubation and to treat common causes of altered level of consciousness. The later studies have found use of flumazenil in this cocktail was counterproductive.

The flumazenil was used for diagnosis of intentional benzodiazepine overdose. However empirical flumazenil can increase the risk of seizures and agitation by benzodiazepine withdrawal in chronic abuse.[7] It can also stimulate seizure, ventricular tachycardia in mixed overdose, e.g. amitriptyline, chloral hydrate.[7-10]

In a very large meta-analysis with more than 900 patients treated with flumazenil in emergency room, the number of patients needs to be treated for a very severe adverse events (e.g. arrhythmia and seizure) and for any adverse event (e.g. vomiting, agitation, and dysphoria) were 50 and 6.2 respectively.[11] The patients given flumazenil has higher risk of seizures especially those on chronic treatment or abusing benzodiazepines, pre-existing seizure disorder or traumatic head injury, and patients who have been co-overdosed with tricyclic antidepressants.[12] In light of available evidence on flumazenil epileptogenic effect, chances of precipitating an acute withdrawal, and some studies showed supportive management for benzodiazepine overdose is as effective; the use of empirical flumazenil is reduced in recent years and is currently recommended for highly selective subgroup of patients.[13,14]

The empirical naloxone can also precipitate opioid withdrawal or vomiting in nonopioid cause of coma. Fortunately with short half-life of naloxone, in case withdrawal is seen, symptoms wear off in 1–2 hours. However, the higher mortality of the opioids overdose over the benzodiazepines in view of respiratory depression still continue to recommend its use but dose titration should be to respiration rather to wakefulness.[14] The administration of empirical thiamine is considered with history or suspicion of chronic alcohol abuse and in patients with severe malnutrition. There is a small risk of severe anaphylaxis with intravenous thiamine. Oxygen should be target to SpO_2 95–99%. The "coma cocktail" can thus be revisited into more evidence based (Table 5).[14]

Decontamination

The evidence-based literature regarding proper decontamination methods are limited. There is paucity about the approved agents and there therapeutic indications and most of the principles have been taken from warfare fields and radiation accident protocols. Healthcare workers should use appropriate personal protective equipments (PPEs) like splash resistant goggles, gloves and gowns, while decontaminated patients with unknown poisoning to prevent any dermal or eye exposure. The decontamination is avoided in prehospital setting if adequate PPEs and other decontamination equipment are not available. The decontamination is effective only if done early and should not be delayed pending identification of the definitive offending agent.

Dermal and Eye Decontamination

In poisoning with possible dermal route, the patients' clothings should be removed and a mild soap, and copious amount of lukewarm water should be used for decontamination. The body temperature should be monitored to avoid hypothermia, strong detergents, or hot water however should be avoided. In case of eye contamination, decontamination should be done with copious irrigation of normal saline solution and periodic monitoring of pH under supervision of ophthalmologists.[3]

Table 5: Revised "coma cocktail".

Agents	Indications	Dosage recommended
Dextrose	Capillary blood glucose less than 50 mg/dL	50 mL of 50% dextrose IV
Oxygen	Pulse oximetry (SpO_2 less than 92–94%)	At 5–10 L/min
Naloxone	Bradypnea (± miosis)	40–200 µg IV bolus, repeat every 2–3 minutes till respiratory depression improves or maximum dose 10 mg whichever is earlier
Thaimine	In alcoholic or malnourished patients for prevention of precipitation of Wernicke encephalopathy	100 mg IV/IM

Gastrointestinal Decontamination

Gastrointestinal (GI) decontamination can be simply defined as measures to prevent or reduce the absorption of an ingested substance. The process of GI decontamination has evolved significantly over the last three decades and focus is now on minimally or less invasive techniques. This has happened partially because of recent research showed lack of benefit with many techniques of GI decontamination and in some cases serious complications with these procedures. There have been updation of many position statements by the American Academy of Clinical Toxicology (AACT) and the European Association of Poison Centers and Clinical Toxicologists (EAPCCT) on various techniques of GI decontamination.[15]

Cathartics: It can decrease the absorption of substances by its prokinetic effect and their rapid expulsion of poisons from the GI tract. There are broadly two types of osmotic cathartics: saccharide based (sorbitol) or saline based (magnesium citrate, magnesium sulfate and sodium sulfate). The mechanism of action is mainly useful for slowly absorbed poisons. Based on recent evidence, the current policy statement of AACT and EAPCCT on cathartics, there is no definite indication for them in poisoning. Besides there are contraindications such as corrosives, ileus or intestinal obstruction, recent abdominal trauma or surgery, and intestinal perforation. Magnesium cathartics is contraindications with renal failure, renal insufficiency, or heart block. Cathartics is to be avoided in elderly or the very young (<1 year of age) and hypotensive patients or electrolyte imbalances.[16]

Gastric lavage: It is used for removal of unabsorbed poison and to small extent decrease absorption of ingested substances for over 200 years. The technique has been described using a wide bore, orogastric tube (16–18 gauge) with patient position trendelenburg position (head down) and left lateral decubitus position. The lavage is then performed with approximately 250 mL (or around 10 mL/kg in pediatric patients) of water or saline followed by aspiration. The procedure is repeated until the aspirated solution is clear of any particulate matter.[3,6] The gastric lavage is associated with complications sunch as aspiration, esophageal perforation, epistaxis, hypothermia. It is not indicated in patients with nontoxic overdoses or combative and uncooperative patients and contraindicated in suspected corrosive substance or a volatile hydrocarbon poisoning (kerosene) as may cause aspiration associated lung injury.[3,6]

In recent policy statement of AACT and EAPCCT the evidence supporting for gastric lavage routinely in poisoned patients is weak. If physicians on their clinical judgment decide to use gastric lavage it should be done under supervision with preference for activated charcoal or only observation over gastric lavage.[17]

Ipecac syrup: Ipecac-induced emesis is less traumatic than gastric lavage, and is therefore being still used in prehospital settings or in pediatric patients. Ipecac is most useful if administered immediately after ingestion with effectiveness decreases rapidly to only 30–40% removal rate even 1 hour after ingestion. The Ipecac is contraindicated in unconscious patients; seizures, poisoning with corrosives, and petroleum products are absolute contraindications due to risk of aspiration and lung injury.[3,6] The Ipecac use is benign with complications relatively uncommon and easily treatable like diarrhea and/or vomiting. Serious complications are reported, e.g. Mallory–Weiss tears, pneumomediastinum, and aspiration pneumonia but are very rare.[3] In case of Ipecac use, the activated charcoal should only be given after 1–2 hours. The current policy statement of AACT and EAPCCT on Ipecac-induced emesis is insufficient evidence supporting its use after poison ingestion.[18] The Ipecac if considered should be administered early (within 60 minutes) in a patient who has consumed significant toxic dose and no altered consciousness.

Activated charcoal: This is an inert, nontoxic, powerful, and nonspecific substance which produces irreversible bonds to many intraluminal drugs and thus may interfere with their absorption. The process of activation includes steam heating and chemical treatment, where the surface area of charcoal is increased and available for adsorption. The activated charcoal can create a diffusion gradient between blood and gut, and can secondarily decreased serum drug levels of absorbed drug a process referred to as "GI dialysis" (Table 6). Charcoal can either be sole GI decontaminating agent or can be administered after both gastric lavage and Ipecac-induced emesis. The activated charcoal is generally well-tolerated with complications which are infrequent. The usual contraindications of all GI decontaminants like altered state of consciousness and/or unprotected airway, protracted vomiting, and intestinal obstruction or perforation too applies to

General Management of Poisoning or Overdose

Table 6: Recommendations for use of multiple doses of activated charcoal.

Indicated (supported by evidence)	Unclear (Neither supported or refuted by evidence)	Controversial (insufficient supporting evidence
Carbamazepine	Phenytoin	Salicylates
Dapsone	Disopyramide	
Phenobarbital	Amitriptyline	
Quinine	Dextropropoxyphene	
Theophylline	Digitoxin	
	Sotalolol	

activated charcoal. Few uncommon side effects like aspiration pneumonia bronchiolitis obliterans, ARDS, and death has been reported in literature.[3,7,19] The ideal dose should give a charcoal-to-drug ratio of 10:1. The dose required in children is 0.5–1 g/kg body weight, while in adults a fixed single dose of 50–100 g is indicated.[19,20] The charcoal can be administered with cathartics (magnesium sulfate, magnesium citrate) to avoid its constipation effect. There are few drugs where charcoal is not found effective (Box 2).

Single-dose charcoal: The routine administration of single-dose activated charcoal is not indicated in poisoned patient. It should be considered only in a patient with significant toxic dose and when presented within the first hour of the event.

Mutidose-activated charcoal: The multiple dose is initial dose of 50–100 g (pediatric 10–25 g) followed by repeated frequency of hourly, 2 hourly, or 4 hourly at equivalent dose of 12.5 g/h. This repeated dose is the main principle behind GI dialysis. The evidence for multiple doses of activated charcoal in decreased morbidity or mortality is lacking and therefore routine administration is not recommended in the poisoned patient.[20-22] Indications for administration of multi-dose activated charcoal (any of the following criteria):

- Intake of the poison exceeds the capacity to be adsorbed by a single dose.
- *Drugs with significant enterohepatic circulation*: To prevent the reabsorption by enterohepatic circulation of the active substance, metabolite, or drug conjugate.
- Intoxication by drugs with sustained release.
- Poisoning by drugs that decrease GI transit (anticholinergics, tricyclic antidepressants, opioids, and phenothiazine).

Box 2: Drugs not absorbed by activated charcoal.

Potassium, pesticides like organophosphates and carbamates
Hydrocarbons
Alcohol, acids
Iron
Lithium
Solvents

Whole bowel irrigation (WBI): The WBI works on the principle of preventing absorption of ingested matter by inducing a liquid stool through use of an osmotically balanced solvent [e.g. polyethylene glycol electrolyte solution (PEG-ES)].[19] In current policy statement by AACT and EAPCTT, in view of lack of sufficient evidence, WBI was not recommended as a routine GI decontamination method and can be considered only in certain situations.[23]

Indications where WBI can be considered:[19]

- Sustained release products, medicines (like potassium chloride)
- Body Stuffers/Packers
- Drugs where activated charcoal does not work (heavy metals—iron, lithium or lead foreign body)
- Ingestion whole transdermal patches like fentanyl, clonidine, etc.

Contraindications for WBI:

- Bowel perforations
- Bowel obstruction, ileus
- Significant GI bleeding
- Unprotected airway
- Hypotensive patient
- Protracted vomiting
- Signs of leakage of illicit drug packets.

Renal elimination: Forced diuresis and urine alkalanization are the most used methods of renal elimination.[3,19]

Forced diuresis: The factors which decide renal excretion of a substance are glomerular filtration rate (GFR), tubular secretion if any and passive tubular reabsorption. The GFR depends on molecular weight, protein-binding and volume of distribution of a substance inside the body. The substance with larger volume of distribution, high degree of protein binding and/or higher molecular weight will have only a small fraction available for filtration and, therefore, forced diuresis will not be helpful. The efficacy of this technique has not been found in limited number of toxins (Table 7).

Approach to a Poisoned Patient

Table 7: Toxins which can be removed through renal elimination.

Forced diuresis	Urine alkalinization
Cyclophosphamide	2,4-Dichlorophenoxyacetic acid
Thallium	Chloropropamide
Isoniazid	Diflunisal
Meprobamate	Fluoride
5-fluorouracil, cisplatin	Methotrexate
Fluoride, iodide, bromides	Phenobarbital
Barium, chromium	Salicylates
Ethylene glycol	Sulfonamides
Salicylates	Lithium

Box 3: The various techniques of extracorporeal toxin removal.

Intermittent hemodialysis (IHD)
Sustained low-efficiency dialysis (SLED)
Intermittent hemofiltration (IHF) and hemodiafiltration (IHDF)
Continuous renal replacement therapy (CRRT)
Hemoperfusion (HP)
Therapeutic plasma exchange (TPE)
Exchange transfusion
Peritoneal dialysis (PD)
Albumin dialysis
Cerebrospinal fluid exchange
Extracorporeal membrane oxygenation (ECMO)
Emergency cardiopulmonary bypass

Urine alkalinization: It works on the principle of increased elimination of substance in urine by altering urine pH to cause increased ionized form of active substance and which decreases its tubular reabsorption. The drug should have mainly renal elimination, high volume of distribution, and high protein-binding. The alkalnization is done using 20–35 mEq/L of bicarbonate diluted in 5% dextrose with half-normal saline with target of urine output at 3–6 mL/kg/h and urine pH 7.5–8.5. Hypokalemia is the most common complication and tetany because of alkalosis and intracellular calcium shift is reported very rarely. The most definitive indication is for salicylate poisoning is that it can be used for other poisioning (Table 7), the evidence supporting its use in them is insufficient.[24]

Urine acidification: Urine acidification in weak bases toxicity was tried for their enhanced renal excretion. The ammonium chloride or ascorbic acid can be used for acidification and is tried for poisoning like amantadine, amphetamine, quinidine, or phencyclidine poisoning. The procedure is now obsolete because of only moderate elimination and significant complications (metabolic acidosis).[24]

Extracorporeal elimination of toxins: Extracorporeal treatments encompass heterogeneous modalities of treatments for either endogenous or exogenous poisons. The various techniques have been used for extracorporeal elimination of toxins (Box 3).

Principles for Selection of Extracorporeal Therapy

Screening of patients: After the initial stabilization of a poisoned patient, a detailed assessment is required to determine the need and modality of extracorporeal therapy (ECTR). There is lack of randomized controlled trials comparing ECTR to conservative conventional management because of various issues like ethical, cost, unbiased randomization and infrastructure. Even the observation studies are uncommon and very heterogeneous. In absence of evidence-based medicine, the need of ECTR is to be decided by crude measures like dose of poison, availability of any antidote, condition of the finally whether availability and expertise of ECTR is present in the hospital. Time bound decisions is critical too as most studies show effectiveness of ECTR when initiated early. In cases where risk of mortality (aluminum phosphide, paraquat, salicylates) or irreversible injury (blindness with methanol poisoning) is high, the decision tilts in favor of ECTR based on cost-effectiveness ratio (Tables 8 and 9). In other scenarios where either effective antidotes are available or morbidity is not much severe (e.g. methanol poisoning without acidosis), decision of ECTR should be taken case-by-case basis.[25]

Toxicokinetic considerations: There are four critical determinants which can be used to identify the success of ECTR in enhance poison removal: (1) molecular weight, (2) degree of protein binding, (3) any endogenous clearance, and (4) poison extracellular volume of distribution.

TOXIDROMES

The detailed and targeted history from patients or accompanying attendants is essential to understand

General Management of Poisoning or Overdose

Table 8: Critical toxicokinetic considerations for various modalities of ECTR.

	HD	HF	HP	Albumin dialysis	PD	ET	TPE
Principle mechanics	Diffusion	Convection	Adsorption on	Diffusion/ Convection	Diffusion	Separation	Centrifugation/ Separation/ Convection
Molecular Weight (cut off)	Low-flux: 1000 Da High-flux: 11,000 Da	40,000 Da	5,000–10,000 Da	MARS/SPAD: 60,000 Da, Prometheus: %100,000 D	<500 Da	No restriction	1,300,000 Da
Degree of protein binding	<80%	<80%	<90%	Likely high	Likely low	No restriction	No restriction
V_D	Low					Very low	

(ET: exchange transfusion; HD: hemodialysis; HF: hemofiltration; HP: hemoperfusion; MARS: molecular adsorbent recirculating system; PD: peritoneal dialysis; SPAD: single pass albumin dialysis; TPE: therapeutic plasma exchange; VD: volume of distribution)

Table 9: Indications of dialysis and hemoperfusion.

Hemodialysis	Hemoperfusion	Plasmapheresis	ECMO
Methanol	Theophylline	Tricyclic antidepressants	Amiodarone
Ethylene glycol	Phenobarbital	Thyroxine	β-blocker
Boric acid	Phenytoin	Heavy metals	Calcium-channel blockers
Salicylates	Carbamazepine	Theophylline	Opioids
Lithium	Paraquat	Ethyl dibromide	Organophosphorous
	Glutethimide		Paraquat
			Tricyclic antidepressants

(ECMO: extracorporeal membrane oxygenation)

the timeline of symptoms and/or withdrawal state. The history should not be limited to but also include the amount of substance consumed, time since the last exposure (acute versus chronic), amount taken, and route of administration (i.e. ingestion, intravenous, and inhalation). The history must include prescription and nonprescription drugs, nonallopathic like herbal, ayurvedic products and empty bottles/containers if any found. The vial "pill count" to ascertain the number of consumed pills can be helpful to assess the amount. The history from the patient and/or attendant may not always be reliable. The medical record of any previous medical exposure before admission, and data from emergency medical staff is vital and should be registered. Initial vital signs, presenting state, neurological assessment (autonomic excitability, peripheral reflexes, and cognition affection) should be noted, along with previous medication history. The subsequent change in vital signs during the hospital course should be included in decision making about diagnosis of either a new toxin or effect of

treatment process and/or withdrawal from chronic used substances.

The different clinical and laboratory features can be used for a clinical diagnosis of suspected group of poisoning or a particular toxidrome. The toxidrome is a constellation of symptoms and signs, laboratory results and/or ECG changes which can guide to a specific class of poisons and thus subsequent management.[3,19,26]

The common toxidromes encountered based on clinical settings and their associated class of poisons are discussed in Table 10. The specific toxicologic syndromes, or toxidromes, are helpful in narrowing the wide-list of differential diagnosis to a specific class of poisons and guide subsequent management. They may not be useful for a diagnosis of individual drug but can guide immediate class specific management.

While toxidromes are useful in emergency after initial resuscitation to identify possible class of drug, it is important to understand their limitations.[19,26] Firstly, the toxidromes can have several overlapping feature,

Approach to a Poisoned Patient

Table 10: Toxidromes on basis of clinical features.

Toxidrome	Drugs	Clinical features
Anticholinergics	Belladona alkaloids and synthetic congeners (Atropine, ipratropium, scopolamine, homatropine, tropicamide), antihistamines, antispasmodics, tricyclic antidepressants, phenothiazines, antiparkinsonian agents, psychedelic mushroom	"Hot as a hare (hyperpyrexia), blind as a bat (mydriasis), dry as a bone (dry skin, eyes and mucosa), red as a beet (flushed face), mad as a wet hen (delirium)" Hyperthermia, mydriasis, dry skin and mucous membrane, altered mental status, delirium, hallucinations, tachycardia, anhidrosis, decrease bowel sounds, and urinary retention
Sympathomimetics	Beta-adrenergic agonists, monoamine oxidase inhibitors (MAOIs), amphetamines, decongestants (pseudoephedrine, ephedrine), phenylephrine cocaine	Nausea, vomiting, abdominal pain, agitation, hallucinations, mydriasis, tachycardia, hypertension, arrhythmias, hyperthermia, and diaphoresis
Cholinergics	Organophosphates, carbamate insecticides, cholinesterase inhibitors	SLUDGE: HyperSalivation, **L**acrimation, **U**rinary incontinence, **D**iarrhea, **G**astrointestinal cramps, **E**mesis (SLUDGE), bradycardia, diaphoresis, miosis, bronchorrhea, pulmonary edema, bronchospasm, weakness, muscle fasciculations, paralysis
Opioids	Hydromorphone, fentanyl, morphine, propoxyphene, codeine, heroin	Sedation, miosis, decreased bowel sounds, respiratory depression, bradycardia, hypothermia (mild)
Sedatives/hypnotics	Benzodiazepines, nonbenzodiazepine GABA agonists, barbiturates, ethanol, chloral hydrate, ethchlorvynol, meprobamate	CNS depression, hyporeflexia, respiratory depression, hypothermia, hypotension, and bradycardia (mild)
Neuroleptics	Chlorpromazine, promethazine, prochlorperazine, fluphenazine, perphenazine, haloperidol, olanzapine, quetiapine	Hypotension, arrhythmias, oculogyric crisis, trismus, dystonia, ataxia, parkinsonism, neuroleptic malignant syndrome, anticholinergic manifestations
Serotonergics	Selective serotonin reuptake inhibitors, tricyclic antidepressants, MAOIs, buspirone, tramadol, fentanyl, synthetic stimulants	Akathisia, tremor, agitation, hyperthermia, hypertension, diaphoresis, hyper-reflexia, clonus, lower extremity muscular hypertonicity, and diarrhea

(CNS: central nervous system; GABA: gamma-aminobutyric acid)

i.e. the sympathomimetic agents can have findings similar to anticholinergic baring few exception like sympathomimetic agents produce diaphoresis, on the other hand warm, dry, and flushed skin is seen with anticholinergics. Secondly, the findings seen in individual toxidromes may not be all present and can be altered by inter-individual variability, comorbid conditions, and coingestants or polypharmacy. Thirdly, the individual agents in a class may not have one or more toxidrome findings, i.e. pethidine produces mydriasis instead of miosis seen with other opiates.

Laboratory Toxidromes

Osmolol gap

The serum osmole gap (OG) can be used as an important bedside laboratory test in evaluating poisoned patients.

Serum osmolality (mOsm/kg) or osmolarity (mOsm/L) can be measured (Osm_{mae}) using osmometer, which works on principle of freezing point depression and calculated (Osm_{cal}) using sodium, blood urea nitrogen (serum urea) and glucose.

$$Osm_{cal}: 2(sodium) + (urea\ nitrogen)/2.8\ or\ blood\ urea/6 + (glucose)/18$$

Osmotically active substances that are reported in milligrams per deciliter (e.g. urea nitrogen and glucose), are converted using a conversion factor. The conversion factor for urea nitrogen is 2.8 and for glucose 18. In case of unusual osmotically active substances like ethanol and toxical alcohol, the equation will be:

$$Osm_{cal}: 2(sodium) + (urea\ nitrogen)/2.8 + (glucose)/18 + (ethanol)/4.6 + (methanol)/3.2 + (ethylene\ glycol)/6.2 + (isopropanol)/6.0.$$

General Management of Poisoning or Overdose

The serum OG can then be calculated using Osm_{mae} and Osm_{cal}. The Osm_{mae} is in units of osmolality (milliosmoles per kilogram) and the calculated form is in units of osmolarity (milliosmoles per liter), however for clinical purpose this is considered insignificant and OG can be written in any unit.

$$OG = Osm_{mae} - Osm_{cal}$$

An increase in the OG is a marker of presence of an osmotically active substance in the blood. There are however limitations dependent on the baseline OG and time when test was done in relation to substance ingestion. An OG of 10 has been conventionally defined as normal. Many studies have debated that this so-called normal value has revealed a wide range from –9 to +20 mOsmol/kg. The OG helps in identification of poisoning with abnormal osmotic active substance, however there is wide variation in acceptable normal (Table 11). The patient with OG of 9 mOsm/kg—near-normal value (10 mOsm/kg), but if this patient had ingested a toxic alcohol and had baseline (preingestion) OG of –5 mOsm/kg, the patient's OG has to be raised by 14 mOsm/kg to reach 9 mOsm/kg, which in certain poisoning like ethylene glycol is equivalent to a toxic level of 86.8 mg/dL. In other patients where there is delay in testing of OG, the poison is already metabolized where metabolites will not influence the OG because being anions they will displace bicarbonate and will double the serum sodium. Finally, the contribution of OG is dependent on molecular weight of active compound. Compounds with larger molecular weights contribute less to the osmolal gap and hence less significant OG (e.g. ethylene glycol).[26-29]

The OG interpretation should be done with above limitations and is used as an adjunct to clinical decision making. The positive value has significance and leads to further investigation; however, a "normal" osmole gap should be interpreted with caution, appropriate therapy should be initiated on suspicion pending confirmation of serum levels of suspected poison.

Anion Gap

The basic electrolytes (sodium, potassium, chloride and bicarbonate) should be done in all patients with poisoning. Whenever metabolic acidosis or low serum bicarbonate is seen an anion gap must be calculated using the equation:

$$\text{Anion gap (AG)} = Na^+ - (Cl^- + HCO_3^-)$$

Table 11: Agents with high Osmolol gap.

Methanol	Methanol, mannitol
Ethylene glycol	Uremia
Diabetic ketoacidosis, diuretics	Diabetic ketoacidosis
Isopropyl alcohol	Propylene glycol, propranolol
Ethanol	Ischemia, isopropanolol
	Lactic acidosis
	Ethylene glycol, ethanol
	Salicylates, starvation ketoacidosis, shock

Essentially the AG is a difference of major cations and major known anions in body. In case of poisoning multiple substance acting as anions (e.g. sulfate, phosphate, or organic anions) cannot be measured and may contribute to AG. The anion gap thus helps in measuring or suspecting these "unmeasured" ions. The normal range for the anion gap is 8–16 mEq/L.[19,26] The unmeasured anions may be endogenous (e.g. lactate) or exogenous (e.g. salicylate) and a common cause have been enumerated (Table 12).

The increased anion gap metabolic acidosis should identify the individual cause as hypoperfusion and resultant lactic acidosis may cause elevation of AG. This AG, however, may improve after adequate initial resuscitation and supportive care including hydration and oxygenation. If, AG metabolic acidosis worsen or does not improve despite adequate initial supportive care, the other causes of high AG metabolic acidosis should be checked especially toxic alcohols (Table 12).

Electrocardiogram Toxidromes

There are wide varieties of electrocardiogram (ECG) changes that can be seen in a poisoned patient. However, many of them are either nonsignificant or multiple unrelated drugs overdose may have common ECG effects. The ECG changes can be broadly divided into two toxidromes (depending on predominant mechanism of channel blockade): QT prolongation (cardiac potassium channel blockade) and QRS prolongation (sodium channel blockade).

QT prolongation: This is a relative common finding in drug overdoses (around 3% of all noncardiac prescriptions may cause QT prolongation). The primary mechanism is efflux potassium channel blockade causing prolongation

Approach to a Poisoned Patient

Table 12: Causes of anion gap metabolic acidosis (Mnemonic: METAL ACID GAP or MUDPILES)

Anion gap metabolic acidosis (Mnemonic: METAL ACID GAP or MUDPILES)		Decreased anion gap
Methanol, metformin, massive overdoses	**M**ethanol	Increased unmeasured cation (potassium, calcium, magnesium)
Ethylene glycol	**U**remia	Acute lithium intoxication
Toluene	**D**iabetic ketoacidosis	Elevated IgG (myeloma in alcoholic; cationic paraprotein)
Alcoholic ketoacidosis	**P**araldehyde, phenformin	Unmeasured decreased anion (bromide, iodide, lithium)
Lactic acidosis	**I**ron, inhalants (i.e. carbon monoxide, cyanide, toluene), isoniazid, ibuprofen	Hypoalbuminemia
Acetaminophen (large overdoses)	**L**actic acidosis	Drugs (Polymyxin B)
Cyanide, carbon monoxide, colchicine	**E**thylene glycol, ethanol (alcoholic) ketoacidosis	Analytical artifact (Hypernatremia, hyperlipidemia)
Isoniazid, iron, ibuprofen	**S**alicylates, starvation ketoacidosis, sympathomimetics	
Diabetic ketoacidosis		
Generalized seizure-producing toxins		
Acetylsalicylic acid or other salicylates		
Paraldehyde, phenformin		

of repolarization manifesting on ECG as QT prolongation and T or U wave abnormalities. The abnormal prolonged repolarization actually produces inward depolarization current (early after depolarization) which may promote an auto-trigging causing re-entry phenomenon and hence malignant polymorphic ventricular tachycardia (torsades de pointes variant) (Table 13). QT prolongation is independently associated with higher mortality.[27]

QT interval is calculated from the Q wave of the QRS complex, till to the end of the T wave. QT interval is influenced by many factors including patient's age, sex, and heart rate. The calculation of the QT interval should include patient's heart rate which is known as corrected QT interval (QTc) using the Bazett formula (QTc = QT/ $RR^{1/2}$). Significant QT prolongation is considered when the QTc interval is greater than 440 milliseconds (msec) in men and 460 msec in women with torsades seen mostly with values greater than 500 msec. There is not only inter-drug but also inter-individual variation for arrhythmia for a given QT interval. The drugs commonly associated with QT prolongation are mentioned in (Table 13).

QRS prolongation: Cardiac sodium channels are usually present in the cell membrane and involved in cellular depolarization. The drugs which may block

Table 13: Drugs causing QT prolongation.

Cardiac drugs	Class 1A, IC and III antiarrhythmics. (Amiodarone, sotalol, disopyramide, dofetilide, procainamide, quinidine)
Antidepressants	Tricyclic antidepressants, selective serotonin reuptake inhibitors, lithium
Antipsychotics	Haloperidol, quetiapine, chlorpromazine, thioridazine, risperidone, droperidol
Antihistaminics	Loratadine, terfenadine, diphenhydramine, astemizole
Antimicrobials	Clarithromycin, erythromycin, fluoroquinolones, fluconazole, voriconazole, pentamidine, quinine, chloroquine
Others	Arsenic, hydroxychloroquine, tacrolimus, methadone, halofantrine

sodium channel basically bind to the transmembrane side and decrease the availability of number of channels for depolarization. This effect is considered traditionally as membrane stabilizing effect, but in toxic concentrations, it may cause slowing of upslope of depolarization and manifesting as wide QRS complex on ECG. Due to progressive QRS prolongation, the difference of ventricular and supraventricular rhythms

General Management of Poisoning or Overdose

Table 14: Drugs causing QRS prolongation on electrocardiogram.

Cardiac drugs	Class 1A and 1C antiarrhythmics (Quinidine, disopyramide, procainamide, flecainide, propafenone), propranolol, verapamil, diltiazem
Antipsychotics	Citalopram, phenothiazines
Antidepressants	Tricyclic antidepressants
Anticonvulsants	Carbamazepine
Others	Chloroquine, quinine, cocaine, amantadine

becomes difficult; and finally, produces a sine wave pattern or, even asystole. The sodium channel blockers can also produce various conduction blocks, or a re-entry causing ventricular tachycardia or ventricular fibrillation. Bradyarrhythmias are also rarely seen in clinical practice because of associated anticholinergic or sympathomimetic properties of some drugs. The drugs causing QRS prolongation may cause blockade of other channels like calcium influx or potassium efflux channels (Table 14). The prominent R' wave in lead aVR as well as the deep S wave in lead I is pathognomonic of tricyclic antidepressants cardiotoxicity.[19,26]

These drugs are however one common management, the administration of hypertonic saline or sodium bicarbonate in case of QRS prolongation of more than 120 msec. The patients with prolonged QRS interval and hemodynamic stability can be treated empirically with 1–2 mEq/kg of sodium bicarbonate.

LABORATORY TESTING OF POISONING

A basic laboratory panel of investigations should be obtained in all poisoned patients:

- Complete blood count
- Serum electrolytes
- Blood urea nitrogen and creatinine
- Blood glucose and bicarbonate level
- Liver functions test
- Arterial blood gases
- ECG
- A pregnancy test in a female of child-bearing age, unless proven otherwise
- The anion gap, serum osmolality, and osmolality gap
- Chest and plain abdominal X-ray

- The gastric content testing is controversial and has no effect on clinical decision making; is required only for regulatory requirements and/or medicolegal considerations.

Specific Investigations

Sample for urine toxicology screening for common drugs must be taken before giving any sort of sedation to these patients. Common urine test available in hospital.

- Cocaine
- Opiates
- Barbiturates
- Amphetamines
- Propoxyphene
- Phencyclidine (PCP)
- Tricyclic antidepressants.

In general, urine toxicology screens are mere screening tests and have low clinical utility than do serum assays. The urine toxicology has poor correlation to clinical signs and symptoms, also has low sensitivity and specificity for clinical diagnosis. There are many point-of-care urine assays (with the exception of that for the cocaine metabolite) available which have poor specificity with high false positive rate and require clinical interpretation. There are also assays which have principle of antibody binding to drug metabolites. The assays are however influenced by time of ingestion, fat solubility of poison, and associated drugs consumed. There are some drugs in which urine assays may be positive many days after use and can be unrelated to current clinical picture. The review of current drug usage is important. The routine urine drug testing has been proved of little impact of on patient management and should be discouraged.[30-33]

On the other hand, few drugs of abuse are not detected on routine urine drug screen, e.g. gamma-hydroxybutyrate (GHB), fentanyl, and ketamine. There are many false positive and false negatives seen in some urine assays [EMIT (DuPont Medical Products, Wilmington, DE, USA) and TDx (Abbott Laboratories, North Chicago, IL, USA) urine immunoassays], e.g. false positive benzodiazepine in patients who have ingested nonsteroidal anti-inflammatory drug like oxaprozin.[26,34]

The urine assays results are thus to be used with clinical judgment and other suggestive laboratory, and other investigations like ECG but not in isolation. The serum toxicology assays are more specific to drug intoxication and to be sent in case of high index of suspicion/history of drug overdose or abuse (Table 15).

Approach to a Poisoned Patient

Chapter 1

Table 15: Drugs/toxins which can be measured by serum levels.	
Drugs	Toxins
Salicylate	Iron
Lithium	Arsenic
Theophylline	Lead
Valproic acid	Ethyl alcohol
Carbamazepine	Methyl alcohol
Digoxin	Aluminum
Phenobarbital (if urine barbiturates are positive)	
Phenytoin	
Acetaminophen (paracetamol)	
Digitalis	

- *The cholinesterase level for organophosphorus poisoning*: Specific levels of cholinesterase can guide treatment
- *Oxygen saturation gap (SaO$_2$ – SpO$_2$)*: An oxygen saturation gap is diagnosed when more than a 5% difference between arterial blood gas (SaO$_2$) saturation and saturation measured by CO-oximetry (SpO$_2$). An elevated oxygen saturation gap is commonly found in carbon monoxide, methemoglobinemia, cyanide, and hydrogen sulfide poisoning.

ADMISSION TO INTENSIVE CARE UNIT

The indication to intensive care unit (ICU) admission includes any of the following:[19,26]
- Respiratory depression (PaCO$_2$ > 45 mm Hg)
- Emergency intubation
- Seizures
- Cardiac arrhythmia (QT prolongation, preferably corrected QTc)
- QRS duration more than 0.12 ms
- Second- or third-degree atrioventricular block
- Systolic BP less than 80 mm Hg
- Unresponsiveness to verbal stimuli
- Glasgow Coma Scale score less than 12
- Need for emergency dialysis, hemoperfusion, or extracorporeal membrane oxygenation
- Increasing metabolic acidosis
- Pulmonary edema induced by toxins (including inhalation) or drugs

- Tricyclic or phenothiazine overdose manifesting anticholinergic signs, neurologic abnormalities, QRS duration more than 0.12 s, or QT more than 0.5 s
- Administration of pralidoxime in organophosphate toxicity
- Antivenom administration in envenomation
- Need for continuous infusion of naloxone.

ANTIDOTES

Most poisoned patients require intensive supportive care and have an uneventful recovery but in some cases an antidote can change the outcome. Antidotes are substances which either may antagonize the toxic effect or minimize the effect by competitive or noncompetitive action to primary drug. They can have their own toxicity and are indicated only in specific clinical circumstances. With the exception of naloxone, the role of other antidotes in unknown poisoning is very limited. The clinician should be familiar with the types of antidotes, their indications, and the availability with adequate stocking case of emergency (Table 16). Although antidotes can be "life-saving" but their use is very limited in bedside toxicology and in a minority of poisonings.[35,36]

Those that should be immediately available within ICU/emergency department:[3,5,12]

Table 16: Drugs/poisons and their antidotes.	
Agent	Antidote
Benzodiazepines	Flumazenil
Beta-blockers	Glucagon, high-dose insulin
Bupivacaine	Intralipid
Cyanide	Cyanocobalamin/sodium thiosulfate
Digoxin	Fab
Ethylene glycol	Ethyl alcohol, fomepizole
Isoniazid	Pyridoxine
Methanol	Ethyl alcohol, fomepizole
Methemoglobinemia	Methylene blue, vitamin C (ascorbic acid)
Organophosphate	Atropine, pralidoxime
Opiates	Naloxone
Lead	Dimercaprol, BAL
Valproate	Carnitine
Iron	Desferrioxamine
Heparin	Protamine
Warfarin	Vitamin K

General Management of Poisoning or Overdose

- Acetylcysteine
- Activated charcoal
- Atropine
- Pralidoxime
- Calcium gluconate/calcium chloride
- Hydroxocobalamin
- Diazepam
- Flumazenil
- Glucagon
- Glyceryl trinitrate
- Methylene blue
- Naloxone
- Sodium bicarbonate
- Sodium nitrite
- Sodium thiosulfate.

ADVANCED LIFE SUPPORT CONSIDERATIONS

Advanced life support is an important terminal event in a critically ill-poisoned patient. The patient may develop cardiac arrest on initial presentation, or may have out of hospital cardiac arrest and admitted after or with ongoing resuscitation.

The focused assessment along with standard resuscitation as per American Heart Association guidelines is important. The resuscitation must include consideration of poisoning and events preceding to cardiac arrest which may help in identifying the precipitating cause and specific management. There are antidotes or toxin-specific interventions that are recommended besides standard resuscitation during resuscitation from cardiac arrest.[19,26,36,37]

A simple mnemonic for special consideration to poisoning can be:

R—Resuscitation and risk assessment
I—Investigations
D—Decontamination
E—Enhanced elimination
A—Antidotes if indicated.

Resuscitation

- The airway obstruction or drugs/poisons with inhalation toxicity should be considered and when hypoxia is the precipitating cause—early intubation and ventilation with 100% oxygen should be considered

- 100% oxygen is recommended for certain poisoning like cyanide, carbon monoxide
- Hyperventilation is to be avoided in resuscitation, however, may be considered in cases with salicylate and cyanide poisoning.
- 100% oxygen and hydroxocobalamin, with or without sodium thiosulfate, is recommended for cyanide poisoning
- Cardiac toxicity by certain drugs will need specific management, e.g. high-dose insulin therapy, IV glucagon, calcium for refractory shock with β-blocker and/or calcium-channel blocker toxicity. Digoxin-specific antibodies for digoxin toxicity causing bradyarrhythmia and cardiac arrest
- Sodium bicarbonate can be considered in case of cardiac arrest due to tricyclic antidepressant overdose
- No role of naloxone and standard life support should be followed in case of in opioid overdose causing cardiac arrest
- Atropine consideration and (at higher doses) for organophosphorous poisoning
- Role of prolonged cardiopulmonary resuscitation (CPR) and extracorporeal membrane oxygenation (ECMO) for poisoning patient with cardiac arrest also need to mention and have been evidenced as salvage measure in few case reports.

Intravenous fat emulsion (IFE) has been suggested as a probably beneficial therapy in the management of local anesthetic overdose. It has also been tried in several other poisoning with varied results. The exact mechanism of action of IFE in poisoning is unknown, it is postulated to mediate antidote activity or act by compartmentalization of the offending xenobiotic into lipid phase, and hence moving it away from its target receptors (Table 17). As per one strategy, 20% emulsion is given in bolus at 1.5 mL/kg, and can be repeated 1–2 more times in case of persistent cardiac arrest. This can be followed by an infusion at 0.25 mL/kg/min for 30–60 minutes.[19,38,39]

CONCLUSION

An approach to unknown poisoning is based on standard principles of management in Intensive care like securing airway, breathing and circulation. The approach may be general but a index of suspicion and knowledge of toxidromes may be helpful in diagnosis. The lack of availability of antidotes for all poisoning, and lack of clear recommendations on reduction of absorption and enhanced eliminations make the management difficult.

Approach to a Poisoned Patient

Table 17: Drugs which may benefit by use of intravenous fat emulsion.

Probable benefit (stronger evidence)	Possible benefit (weak evidence)
Local anesthetics: Bupivacaine, mepivacaine, ropivacaine, levobupivacaine, prilocaine, lignocaine, lidocaine	*Anti-epileptics*: Carbamazepine, lamotrigine
	Anti-psychotics: Chlorpromazine, haloperidol, olanzapine, quetiapine
	Anti-histamine: Diphenhydramine
	Barbiturates: Pentobarbital, phenobarbital, thiopental
	Beta-blockers: Atenolol, carvedilol, metoprolol, nebivolol, propranolol
	Calcium-channel blockers: Amlodipine, diltiazem, felodipine, nifedipine, verapamil
	Disease-modifying anti-rheumatic drug: Hydroxychloroquine
	Tricyclic antidepressants: Amitriptyline, clomipramine, dosulepin, dothiepin, doxepin, imipramine
	Other anti-depressants: Bupropion, venlafaxine
	Others: Baclofen, cocaine, endosulfan, flecainide, propanone

There is increasing trends of poisoning with multiple substances and chronic drug abuse which should be considered while using general and specific therapies.

KEY POINTS

- Keep a high index of suspicion for intoxication
- Initiate initial resuscitation based on ABCDE approach
- Gastric lavage and aspiration if required should be done within 1 hour
- Obtaining a detailed history is vital in diagnosing poisoning
- General supportive measures and measures to reduce absorption and enhance elimination should be instituted immediately
- Apart from routine investigations, an ABG and specific investigations like drug levels should be sent, as per the suspected poisoning
- Specific therapy or antidotes, if available, should be started early
- Most of these patients would require ICU care and monitoring.

REFERENCES

1. Lopes AT, Manso C. Paraquat and diquat: mechanisms of toxicity. Acta Med Port. 1989;2(1):35-9.
2. Gawarammana IB, Buckley NA. Medical management of paraquat ingestion. Br J Clin Pharmacol. 2011;72(5):745-57.
3. Erickson TB, Thompson TM, Lu JJ. The approach to the patient with an unknown overdose. Emerg Med Clin North Am. 2007;25(2):249-81.
4. Bora K, Aaron C. Pitfalls in salicylate toxicity. Am J Emerg Med. 2010;28(3):383-4.
5. Boyle JS, Bechtel LK, Holstege CP. Management of the critically poisoned patient. Scand J Trauma, Resuscit Emerg Med. 2009;17:29.
6. Mokhlesi B, Leiken JB, Murray P, et al. Adult toxicology in critical care: part I: general approach to the intoxicated patient. Chest. 2003;123(2):577-92.
7. Ngo AS, Anthony CR, Samuel M, et al. Should a benzodiazepine antagonist be used in unconscious patients presenting to the emergency department? Resuscitation. 2007;74:27-37.
8. Marchant B, Wray R, Leach A, et al. Flumazenil causing convulsions and ventricular tachycardia. BMJ (Clinical research ed.). 1989;299:860.
9. Burr W, Sandham P, Judd A. Death after flumazenil. BMJ (Clinical research ed.). 1989;298:1713.
10. Short TG, Maling T, Galletly DC. Ventricular arrhythmia precipitated by flumazenil. BMJ (Clinical research ed.) 1988;296:1070-71.
11. Penninga EI, Graudal N, Ladekarl MB, et al. Adverse events associated with flumazenil treatment for the management of suspected benzodiazepine intoxication: A systematic review with meta-analyses of randomised trials. Basic Clin Pharmacol Toxicol. 2016;118(1): 37-44.
12. Dart RC, Borron SW, Caravati EM, et al. Expert consensus guidelines for stocking of antidotes in hospitals that provide emergency care. Ann Emerg Med. 2009;54: 386-94.
13. Seger DL. Flumazenil–Treatment or toxin. J Toxicol–Clin Toxicol. 2004;42:209-16.

14. Sivilotti ML. Flumazenil, naloxone and the 'coma cocktail'. Br J Clin Pharmacol. 2016;81(3):428-36.
15. Caravati EM, Mégarbane B. Update of position papers on gastrointestinal decontamination for acute overdose. Clin Toxicol. 2013;51(3):127.
16. American Academy of Clinical Toxicology and European Association of Poisons Centres and Clinical Toxicologists, Position Paper: Cathartics. J Toxicol: Clin Toxicol. 2004;42(3):243-53.
17. Benson BE, Hoppu K, Troutman WG, et al. Position paper update: gastric lavage for gastrointestinal decontamination. Clin Toxicol (Philadelphia). 2013;51(3):140-6.
18. Höjer J, Troutman WG, Hoppu K, et al. Position paper update: ipecac syrup for gastrointestinal decontamination. Clin Toxicol (Phila). 2013;51(3):134-9.
19. Thompson TM, Theobald J, Lu J, et al. The general approach to the poisoned patient. Dis Mon. 2014;60(11):509-24.
20. Chyka PA, Seger D, Krenzelok EP, et al. Position paper: Single-dose activated charcoal. Clin Toxicol (Phila). 2005;43(2):61-87.
21. Tenenbein M. Multiple doses of activated charcoal: time for reappraisal II. Ann Emerg Med. 2003;42(4):597-8.
22. Bonilla-Velez J, Marin-Cuero DJ. The Use of Activated Charcoal for Acute Poisonings. Int J Med Students. 2017;5(1):45-52.
23. Thanacoody R, Caravati EM, Troutman B, et al. Position paper update: whole bowel irrigation for gastrointestinal decontamination of overdose patients. Clin Toxicol (Phila). 2015;53(1):5-12.
24. Ghannoum M, Gosselin S. Enhanced poison elimination in critical care. Adv Chronic Kidney Dis. 2013;20(1):94-101.
25. Ghannoum M, Roberts DM, Hoffman RS, et al. A stepwise approach for the management of poisoning with extracorporeal treatments. Semin dial. 2014;27(4):362-70.
26. Holstege CP, Borek HA. Toxidromes. Crit Care Clin. 2012;28(4):479-98.
27. Glaser DS. Utility of the serum osmol gap in the diagnosis of methanol or ethylene glycol ingestion. Ann Emerg Med. 1996;27(3):343-6.
28. Eder AF, McGrath CM, Dowdy YG, et al. Ethylene glycol poisoning: toxicokinetic and analytical factors affecting laboratory diagnosis. Clin Chem. 1998;44(1):168-77.
29. Haviv YS, Rubinger D, Zamir E, et al. Pseudo-normal osmolal and anion gaps following simultaneous ethanol and methanol ingestion. Am J Nephrol. 1998;18(5):436-8.
30. Schade Hansen C, Pottegård A, Ekelund U, et al. Association between QTc prolongation and mortality in patients with suspected poisoning in the emergency department: a transnational propensity score matched cohort study. BMJ Open. 2018;8(7):e020036.
31. Kellermann AL, Fihn SD, LoGerfo JP, et al. Impact of drug screening in suspected overdose. Ann Emerg Med. 1987;16(11):1206-16.
32. Brett A. Toxicologic analysis in patients with drug overdose. Arch Intern Med. 1988;148(9):2077.
33. Bast RP, Helmer SD, Henson SR, et al. Limited utility of routine drug screening in trauma patients. South Med J. 2000;93(4):397-9.
34. Camara PD, Audette L, Velletri K, et al. False-positive immunoassay results for urine benzodiazepine in patients receiving oxaprozin (Daypro). Clin Chem. 1995;41(1): 115-6.
35. Smollin CG. Toxicology: pearls and pitfalls in the use of antidotes. Emerg Med Clin North Am. 2010;28(1): 149-61.
36. Marraffa JM, Cohen V, Howland MA. Antidotes for toxicological emergencies: a practical review. Am J Health Syst Pharm. 2012;69(3):199-212.
37. Lavonas EJ, Drennan IR, Gabrielli A, et al. Part 10: Special Circumstances of Resuscitation: 2015 American Heart Association Guidelines Update for Cardiopulmonary Resuscitation and Emergency Cardiovascular Care. Circulation. 2015;132(18 Suppl 2):S501-18.
38. American College of Medical Toxicology. ACMT position statement: interim guidance for the use of lipid resuscitation therapy. J Med Toxicol. 2011;7:81-2.
39. Lam SH, Majlesi N, Vilke GM. Use of Intravenous Fat Emulsion in the Emergency Department for the Critically Ill Poisoned Patient. J Emerg Med. 2016;51(2):203-14.

2 CHAPTER

Laboratory Testing in Poisoning

Aruna Dewan, Ashwin Patel

INTRODUCTION

Poisoning, whether acute or chronic, is rampant in India.[1-4] Chronic poisonings may not be easy to recognize, but acute poisonings are seen and treated at every level of health-care facility. The reason for acute poisoning in adolescents and adults is mostly intentional (suicidal) and accidental poisoning is more common in children. Experienced physicians can often diagnose the type of poisoning from a brief clinical examination even when definite history is difficult to obtain. For confirmation, relatives can be asked to bring empty containers, drug strips or provide images of same on mobile applications.

Clinical laboratory investigations available in hospital emergency laboratories may offer useful leads toward the suspected toxic agent.[5] Marked and sustained hypoglycemia may be due to overdose of antidiabetic drugs. Respiratory acidosis and hypoxia often occurs with central nervous system (CNS) depressants. Elevated osmolar gap accompanied by anion gap acidosis suggests poisoning by methanol or ethylene glycol. To confirm the diagnosis and start a definite line of treatment, toxicology tests are needed.

APPROACH TO LABORATORY TESTS IN ACUTE POISONING

Toxicology tests will vary according to clinical suspicion and severity of poisoning. If a patient is not in acute distress, immediate toxicology testing may not be needed. But there are instances:

- When a young person is found unconscious and brought to emergency by unknown persons or police
- Clinical picture is of poisoning but relatives deny the same
- Poisoning is a differential diagnosis in a critically ill patient.

Such cases of "Unknown or Suspected Poisoning" pose a challenge and a dialog between the clinician and the analytical toxicologist (if available) becomes necessary to decide the appropriate plan of action.

One or more of the following tests may be carried out based on the clinical picture.

Qualitative Tests or Toxicology Screens

These tests can be done to detect the presence of some common pharmaceuticals, drugs of abuse, few chemicals or their metabolites. Tests are routinely carried out on urine samples and few can also be done on gastric lavage samples. Testing of gastric contents may be done when the treating doctor wants to confirm whether he is dealing with a harmless ingestion or a similar look-alike highly toxic substance [mercury tablets vs. aluminum phosphide (AIP tablet)].

Urine Drug Screens

These screens are often ordered for differential diagnosis when a patient presents with nonspecific clinical features, such as drowsiness, coma or convulsions.

As a routine, nine-drug panel cassettes are used which include: amphetamine, barbiturates, benzodiazepines, cocaine, opiates, marijuana [tetrahydrocannabinol (THC)], methamphetamine, phencyclidine and methadone.

Limitations of urine drug screens: These include:

- A negative screen does not rule out the possibility of poisoning
- Even therapeutic amounts of some drugs such as opioids and benzodiazepines, may be detected if they are within the cut-off limits
- False negatives may be seen with synthetic opioids like oxycodone and fentanyl in the opiate assay
- A positive urine drug screen should be interpreted very carefully and medication history should be available (Table 1).

A variety of multidrug test panels (Rapid Response™) are now becoming available. They offer customized combinations of any 2–12 drugs from those listed below for screening of urine samples. This can give a wider choice for emergency drug screens provided the manufacturer supplies information about cross-reacting drugs.

Drugs included: 6-monoacetylmorphine (6-MAM) (heroin metabolite), acetaminophen, alcohol, amphetamines, barbiturates, benzodiazepines, buprenorphine, cocaine, cotinine, ecstasy [3,4-methylenedioxy methamphetamine (MDMA)], 2-ethylidene-1,5-dimethyl-3,3-diphenylpyrrolidine [EDDP (methadone metabolite)], ethyl glucuronide (EtG) (ethanol metabolite), fentanyl, ketamine, lysergic acid diethylamide (LSD), marijuana (THC), methadone, methamphetamine, methaqualone, methylphenidate, methylphenidate metabolite, morphine, opiates, oxycodone, phencyclidine, propoxyphene, synthetic marijuana (K2), tramadol, tricyclic antidepressants and zolpidem.

Quantitative Tests

In these tests, level of a drug or its metabolite is measured in blood samples. Quantitative blood tests are needed only for those drugs for which blood levels will predict subsequent toxicity or guide specific therapy. At times, it is more practical to rely on other biomarkers of toxic effect such as cholinesterase (ChE) activity or coagulation profile, rather than on the concentration of the toxicant itself.

The National Academy of Clinical Biochemistry has prepared a set of guidelines for two tiers of laboratory tests that should be available for poisoning patients in emergency departments. These guidelines are based on the recommendations of an expert panel of analytical toxicologists and emergency physicians specializing in clinical toxicology.[9]

Stat Quantitative Serum Toxicology Assays Recommended to Support an Emergency Department (Tier I Tests)

- *Drugs*: Acetaminophen (paracetamol), lithium, salicylates, iron, theophylline, valproic acid, carbamazepine, digoxin, phenobarbital

Table 1: False positives in urine drug screens.[6-8]	
Drug	*Drugs which may give false-positive results*
Amphetamine/ methamphetamine	Chlorpromazine, fluoxetine, phentermine, phenylephrine, promethazine, propranolol/labetalol, pseudoephedrine, ranitidine, tricyclic antidepressants
Phencyclidine	Ibuprofen, imipramine, ketamine, lamotrigine, meperidine, tricyclic antidepressants, tramadol
Methadone	Chlorpromazine, quetiapine ,tricyclic antidepressants venlafaxine
Opiates	Loperamide, quinine, quinolones, rifampin, tricyclic antidepressants, verapamil
Benzodiazepines	Sertraline, verapamil
Marijuana (THC)	Ibuprofen, naproxen, pantoprazole/PPIs, promethazine
Barbiturates	Ibuprofen, naproxen, phenytoin
Cocaine	Fluconazole, ibuprofen, naproxen

(PPIs: proton-pump inhibitors; THC: tetrahydrocannabinol)

- *Ethanol, methanol, ethylene glycol*: In acute intoxications, a simple breath analyzer test may be appropriate for alcohol estimation. EtG, which is a metabolite of ethanol, can remain positive for 3–4 days in urine samples. Methanol and ethylene glycol are to be estimated by gas chromatography (GC)
- *Methemoglobin, carboxyhemoglobin*: Methemoglobin and carboxyhemoglobin can be easily determined by a CO-oximeter.

Some of the above mentioned drugs like lithium, carbamazepine, valproic acid and digoxin can be estimated on automated calibrated instruments used in laboratories which carry out routine investigations.

Since many developing countries do not have facilities for analytical toxicology, World Health Organization has published a manual entitled "Basic Analytical Toxicology".[10] This book has been compiled by a group of international experts and is available free on the web.[11] The purpose of this book is to provide practical guidelines for clinical laboratories to develop simple analytical tests. A variety of qualitative and quantitative tests for drugs and chemicals with detailed instructions are covered in this manual. Laboratory staff, with some training, can select and standardize tests which are relevant to their area to provide an analytical toxicology service to emergency physicians.

Advanced Toxicology Tests (Tier II Tests)

In situations where the patient is not improving and no definite agent has been identified, an experienced toxicologist (if available) should be consulted before a second tier of more advanced and costly tests is recommended.[9] Advanced methods such as GC with mass spectrometry (GC-MS) and liquid chromatography-tandem mass spectrometry (LC-MS-MS) can identify drugs and their metabolites and measure unknown substances at minuscule levels[12-17] in all types of biological samples. Their use in emergency toxicology is restricted because of high cost of the instruments and need for highly trained personnel and long turnaround time (TAT).

Most of the hospitals do not have laboratories which can do such tests and patient's specimens may be sent to different reference laboratories or a regional toxicology laboratory. Forensic toxicology laboratories are capable of general unknown screening (GUS) or systematic toxicological analysis (STA) and can be approached.

Analysis by GC is limited to apolar, volatile, and thermally stable compounds such as ethanol, methanol, ethylene glycol, etc. Gas chromatography–mass spectrometry (GC-MS) is an analytical method that combines the features of GC and MS to identify different substances within a test sample. It has built-in library of standardized spectra of a large number of drugs and chemicals which can be matched with unknown samples.[12,13] However, GC-MS cannot detect polar, thermally labile, and nonvolatile compounds. To overcome these limitations, high-performance liquid chromatography with diode array detector (HPLC-DAD) system has been found to be useful for screening a wide range of compounds including common drugs encountered in poisoning cases like benzodiazepines, hypnotics, analgesics, psychotropic and recreational drugs.[17]

It would be ideal to have a reliable technique for GUS to cover a broad spectrum of toxicologically relevant substances, in one analytical run.[18] The combinations of MS with suitable chromatographic procedures are the methods of choice. In recent years, such techniques are being applied for identification of novel psychoactive substances.

Toxicology Tests in Chronic Poisoning

Chronic poisoning is often seen due to environmental or occupational exposures to heavy metals like lead, arsenic, or mercury because these toxic metals bioaccumulate in the body. Source of lead exposure can be from leaded paint, lead mining and smelting operations, informal recycling activities, leaded water pipes, traditional medicines and cosmetics.[19] Blood lead is considered as the standard biomarker of lead exposure and toxicity.[20,21]

Large scale arsenic poisoning has occurred in Bangladesh and West Bengal due to high levels of arsenic in well water.[22,23] Metal elements can be measured by atomic absorption spectrophotometer (AAS) or ion coupled plasma atomic emission spectrometry (ICP-MS).

TOXICOLOGY TESTS AT CENTRE FOR EDUCATION, AWARENESS AND RESEARCH ON CHEMICALS AND HEALTH LABORATORY (CEARCH, AHMEDABAD)

Based on the type of poisonings prevalent in the area, Centre for Education, Awareness and Research

General Management of Poisoning or Overdose

on Chemicals and Health (CEARCH) Toxicology laboratory[24] has standardized some tests useful in clinical toxicology. Only those tests which are relevant, economical and have a quicker TAT, and those which make a difference in emergency management of poisoning, have been developed. They have been adapted from standard textbooks and peer-reviewed journals and standardized by employing techniques like thin-layer chromatography (TLC) or color tests for qualitative analysis and UV-Visible spectrophotometry/ HPLC for quantitative analysis.

The laboratory provides 24 × 7 service (excluding tests on HPLC) and carries out the tests after discussion with the clinician. Any significant results are conveyed by telephone so that physician can confidently start the specific treatment. Hard copies of the reports are sent at the earliest possible.

Qualitative Tests

Nine-drug Screen from Urine

Screening for nine drugs of abuse mentioned earlier is carried out on urine samples by using lateral flow immunoassay cassettes. Comments on cross-reactivity are mentioned in the report when any of the drugs is found positive.

Color Tests for Some Common Drugs from Urine

Tests mentioned below are described in detail in the book "Basic Analytical Toxicology".[10] They can be standardized in any laboratory with common equipment and easily available reagents. It is especially important to look for presence of paracetamol or salicylates in urine samples. These drugs are often present in the commonly available over-the-counter (OTC) preparations and can produce severe toxicity which can be treated if recognized early.

Paracetamol (o-cresol reagent): Hydrolysis of the urine sample is done by boiling with concentrated hydrochloric acid giving p-aminophenol, which is conjugated with o-cresol to form a strongly colored dye. A strong blue to blue-black color indicate positive result.

Salicylates (Trinder reagent): Violet color with Trinder reagent indicates the presence of salicylates.

Phenothiazines (FPN reagent): The test is based on the reaction of phenothiazine compounds with ferric ion under acidic conditions. Color ranging from red, orange, violet or blue indicates the presence of phenothiazines.

Imipramine and related compounds (Forrest reagent): Mixing Forrest Reagent with urine sample gives green-blue color. Yellow-to-green color deepening through dark green to blue indicates the presence of imipramine and related compounds.

A positive color test for paracetamol or salicylates in urine is followed by quantitative estimation of these drugs in blood using spectrophotometer.

Detection of paraquat: Paraquat is an extremely toxic herbicide. It can be detected from urine or gastric lavage samples with sodium dithionite reagent. If the test is strongly positive (blue or blue-black color) in a urine sample 4 hours after ingestion, it is indicative of sufficient absorption and a poor prognosis.

Differentiation between mercury tablets (grain preservative) and phosphides from gastric lavage sample: Silver nitrate test will give positive result with phosphide.

Clinical implication: Some clinicians utilize this test to increase their confidence in making diagnosis and to rule out toxic phosphide ingestion.

Elemental mercury is not absorbed orally and patient will be clinically normal whereas in aluminum phosphide poisoning, patient is often critically ill and in shock. Presence of mercury in lavage samples can also be confirmed by Reinsch test.

Detection of common steroids: Steroids (prednisolone, methylprednisolone, betamethasone, dexamethasone, etc.) in unknown drugs or powders are detected by TLC.

Quantitative Tests

These tests are done mainly on UV-Visible spectropho-tometer or HPLC.

Tests on UV-Visible Spectrophotometer

Each test needs 2–3 mL blood collected in ethylenedi-aminetetraacetic acid (EDTA) and brought to the laboratory in cold condition at the earliest. TAT for the tests is 1–2 hours.

Cholinesterase Levels

This test has been modified at CEARCH laboratory and therefore is being described in detail. Pesticide poisoning

Laboratory Testing in Poisoning

is the commonest poisoning in India and many South East Asian countries.[1,2] ChE activities in blood are the standard biochemical biomarker for diagnosis after potential exposure to organophosphorus (OP) or carbamate pesticides and nerve agents. Chlorpyrifos is an OP insecticide and is commonly used as household antitermite agent. Easy access to this pesticide makes it a very common agent for intentional poisoning.[24] Other OP pesticides such as monocrotophos, dimethoate, quinalphos, phorate, etc. are mostly used for destroying agricultural pests. The toxicity of OP and carbamate pesticides is due to inhibition of the enzyme acetylcholinesterase (AChE) which is present at central and peripheral nerve synapses.

Plasma/serum cholinesterase which is also referred to as butyrylcholinesterase (BChE) or pseudocholinesterase (EC 3.1.1.8) can be measured in clinical laboratories using easily available kits. A normal plasma ChE may be enough to rule out OP or carbamate exposure or poisoning. However, at times very-low plasma ChE levels may be seen without any clinical signs and symptoms typical of cholinergic poisoning. This has been specially observed in poisoning due to formulations containing 20% chlorpyrifos (personal observation). Even when plasma ChE levels are very low, there is no miosis, bradycardia, or increased secretions. In these patients, red blood cell (RBC) ChE levels are mostly in the normal range and thus correlate very well with the clinical picture.

Red blood cells cholinesterase also known as AChE or true ChE (EC 3.1.1.7.) is a better indicator of toxicity and severity of OP and carbamate pesticide poisoning. However, kits are not easily available for estimation of this enzyme.

Method Used at CEARCH Toxicology Laboratory for Estimation of Plasma and Red Blood Cell Cholinesterase

It is based on Ellman's method[25] and has been modified in CEARCH lab by one of the authors (Ashwin Patel). The principle of the method is to measure the rate of production of thiocholine using acetylthiocholine as the substrate. The enzyme activity is estimated by UV-VIS spectrophotometer measuring the increase of yellow color at 412 nm produced from thiocholine when it reacts with dithiobisnitrobenzoate (DTNB) ion. For plasma ChE, only one set of measurement is done from plasma. For RBC ChE, it involves the dilution of an aliquot of blood in normal saline and separation of supernatant by centrifugation. Cholinesterase levels are estimated in the whole blood and supernatant in two different steps using the above substrate. RBC ChE activity is derived from the difference between whole blood and the supernatant levels.

Both tests can be carried out from blood collected in EDTA. The results of tests carried out at CEARCH laboratory have been found to correlate very well with the diagnosis and severity of OP poisoning.

- Reference value for plasma ChE in blood: 2,900–5,800 U/L
- Reference value for RBC ChE in blood: 1,700–3,500 U/L.

The above reference values, in normal individuals, have been established by us at CEARCH laboratory.

Blood methemoglobin levels: Acute methemoglobinemia is commonly encountered in the industries which manufacture dyes and dye intermediates[26] or can be due to a number of drugs.[27]

Principle: Methemoglobin levels are estimated by spectrophotometry using sodium azide and potassium ferricyanide reagent. Methemoglobin reacts with sodium azide to convert methemoglobin to cyanmethemoglobin which is measured at 630 nm.

Serum salicylate levels:

Principle: Spectrophotometry using Trinder reagent—ferric ion of Trinder reagent reacts with the phenolic ring of salicylate to form blue-to-purple complex which is measured at 540 nm.

Serum paracetamol (acetaminophen) levels: Paracetamol is a widely used analgesic. Toxicity can occur due to miscalculation of dose in children or intentional overdose.[28] In many countries, acetaminophen toxicity has become the most common cause of acute liver failure.[29] Because of delayed toxicity, it is important to measure paracetamol level even in the absence of clinical symptoms.

Specimen requirement: About 3 mL blood, plain or anticoagulated with EDTA. Blood collection should be done at least 4 hours after ingestion.

Principle: Protein from serum is precipitated with trichloroacetic acid. To the protein free filtrate, HCl and sodium nitrite solution are added for diazotization then, excess nitrous acid is removed by ammonium sulfamate and absorbance of azo dye is measured at 570 nm in alkaline condition.

Interpretation of results: Blood level of paracetamol at specific times after the ingestion can be plotted on the Rumack-Matthew nomogram. If 4 hours after ingestion, paracetamol level is more than 150 μg/mL (150 mg/L), it is an indication of possible toxicity and need for *N*-acetylcysteine therapy (Fig. 1).[30]

Blood lead levels: (By using Lead-Care II Analyzer and lead test kits):

Technique: The Lead-Care II relies on electrochemistry (anodic stripping voltammetry) and a unique sensor to detect lead in whole blood. The blood is mixed with treatment reagent to lyse the red blood cells making the lead available for detection. This is applied on the sensor to display the result as μg/dL.

Reportable range: Lead, 3.3–65 μg/dL. This method can measure blood lead only up to 65 μg/dL. Levels above this need to be sent to reference laboratories to get the exact value using AAS or ICP-MS.

Tests Based on High-performance Liquid Chromatography

High-performance liquid chromatography is considered a highly sensitive and accurate technique for estimation of many drugs and toxic substances. It can be used in toxicology as well as for therapeutic drug monitoring (TDM).

Some of the HPLC techniques have been standardized and validated at CEARCH laboratory. These include estimation of blood levels of following drugs for TDM as well as some cases of overdose:

- *Antifungal drugs*: Voriconazole, posaconazole
- *Antiepileptic drugs or their metabolites*: Phenobarbitone, phenytoin, carbamazepine, and its epoxide, oxcarbazepine and its monohydroxy metabolite, levetiracetam
- *Antibiotic*: Vancomycin
- *Anticancer drug*: Methotrexate

Turnaround time: Six hours.

CONCLUSION

This chapter describes some of the relevant tests useful in poisoning cases in India and mentions advanced tests which can be developed. The CEARCH laboratory has made a beginning by providing dedicated toxicology services to local hospitals in Ahmedabad and surrounding areas. Method for RBC ChE estimation developed at CEARCH has proved very useful to determine the severity of OP poisoning.

KEY POINTS

- Laboratory tests can play a vital role in the diagnosis and management of poisoned patients
- Newly available drug screens for a large number of drugs may be tried for emergency cases
- Toxicology laboratories which can undertake STAT or Tier I investigations, should ideally be available in the emergency laboratory
- Emergency laboratories can use the manual available at http://www.who.int/ipcs/publications/training_poisons/basic_analytical_tox/en/index11.html for developing some common toxicology tests.

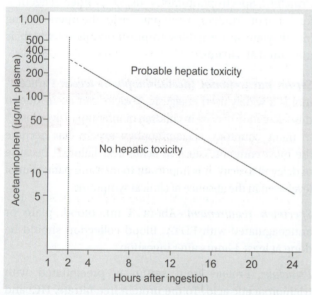

Fig. 1: Semilogarithmic plot of plasma acetaminophen levels versus time.
Source: Rumack BH, Matthew H. Acetaminophen poisoning and toxicity. Pediatrics. 1975;55:871-6.

REFERENCES

1. Murali R, Bhalla A, Singh D, et al. Acute pesticide poisoning: 15 years experience of a large North-West Indian hospital. Clin Toxicol (Phila). 2009;47:35-8.
2. Jesslin J, Adepu R, Churi S. Assessment of prevalence and mortality incidences due to poisoning in a South Indian tertiary care teaching hospital. Indian J Pharm Sci. 2010;72:587-91.
3. Indu TH, Raja D, Ponnusankar S. Toxicoepidemiology of acute poisoning cases in a secondary care hospital in

rural South India: A five-year analysis. J Postgrad Med. 2015;61:159-62.

4. Maharani B, Vijayakumari N. Profile of poisoning cases in a tertiary care Hospital, Tamil Nadu, India. J App Pharm Sci. 2013;3(1):91-4.

5. In: Olson KR, Anderson IB, Benowitz NL, Blanc PD, Clark RF, Kearny TE, Osterloh JD, (Eds). Poisoning and Drug Overdose, 5th edition. New York, NY: McGraw Hill Lange; 2007.

6. Moeller KE, Lee KC, Kissack JC. Review on urine drug screening: Practical Guide for Clinicians. Mayo Clinic Proceedings. 2008;83:66-76.

7. Saitman A, Park HD, Fitzgerald RL. False-positive interferences of common urine drug screen immunoassays: a review. J Anal Toxicol. 2014;38(7):387-96.

8. Mdaware. Urine drug screen false positive (Table). [online] Available from: http://mdaware.blogspot.com/2016/04/urine-drug-screen-false-positive-table.html.

9. Wu AH, McKay C, Broussard LA, et al. National Academy of Clinical Biochemistry Laboratory Medicine Practice guidelines: Recommendations for the use of laboratory tests to support poisoned patients who present to the emergency department. Clin Chem. 2003;49(3):357-79.

10. Flanagan RJ, Braithwaite RA, Brown SS, Widdop B, de Wolff FA (Eds). Basic Analytical Toxicology. Geneva: World Health Organization; 1995.

11. World Health Organization. Basic Analytical Toxicology. [online] Available from http://www.who.int/ipcs/publications/training_poisons/basic_analytical_tox/en/index11.html [Accessed October, 2018].

12. Moffat AC, Osselton MD, Widdop B, Watts JO (Eds). Clarke's Analysis of Drugs and Poisons, 4th edition, 1st volume. Chicago, London: Pharmaceutical Press; 2011.

13. Flanagan RJ, Taylor AA, Watson ID, Whelpton R, editors. Fundamentals of Analytical Toxicology. Chichester: John Wiley & Sons; 2008.

14. Meyer GM, Weber AA, Maurer HH. Development and validation of a fast and simple multi-analyte procedure for quantification of 40 drugs relevant to emergency toxicology using GC-MS and one-point calibration. Drug Test Anal. 2014;6(5):472-81.

15. Mueller DM, Duretz B, Espourteille FA, et al. Development of a fully automated toxicological LC-MS(n) screening system in urine using online extraction with turbulent flow chromatography. Anal Bioanal Chem. 2011;400(1):89-100.

16. Michely JA, Maurer HH. A multianalyte approach to help in assessing the severity of acute poisonings-Development and validation of a fast LC-MS/MS quantification approach for 45 drugs and their relevant metabolites with one-point calibration. Drug Test Anal. 2018;10:164-76.

17. Elliott SP, Hale KA. Applications of an HPLC-DAD drug-screening system based on retention indices and UV spectra. J Anal Toxicol. 1998;22:279-89.

18. Stefan S. A general unknown screening for drugs and toxic compounds in human serum. Thesis submitted to the Faculty of Natural Sciences of the University of Basel, Switzerland for a Ph. D. Degree, Basel, 2005;1-108.

19. Dargan PI, Gawarammana IB, Archer JRH, et al. Heavy metal poisoning from Ayurvedic traditional medicines: an emerging problem? Int J Environ Health. 2008;2(3/4):463-74.

20. Needleman H. Lead poisoning. Annu Rev Med. 2004;55:209-22.

21. Karri SK, Saper RB, Kales SN. Lead encephalopathy due to traditional medicines. Curr Drug Saf. 2008;3(1):54-9.

22. Guha Mazumder DN, Chakraborty AK, Ghosh A, et al. Chronic arsenic toxicity from drinking tube-well water in rural West Bengal. Bull World Health Organ. 1988;66:499-506.

23. Guha Mazumder DN, Ghosh A, Majumdar KK, et al. Arsenic contamination of ground water and its health impact on population of district of Nadia, West Bengal, India. Indian J Comm Med. 2010;35(2):331-8.

24. http://www.cearch.in

25. Ellman GL, Courtney KD, Andres V Jr, et al. A new and rapid colorimetric determination of acetylcholinesterase activity. Biochem Pharmacol. 1961;7:88-95.

26. Dewan A, Patel AB, Saiyed HN. Acute methemoglobinemia—A common occupational hazard in an industrial city in western India. J Occup Health. 2001;43:168-71.

27. D'sa SR, Victor P, Jagannati M, et al. Severe methemoglobinemia due to ingestion of toxicants. Clin Toxicol. 2014;52:897-900.

28. Woolley D, Woolley A (Eds). Practical Toxicology: Evaluation, Prediction, and Risk, 3rd edition. London: CRC Press; 2017. pp. 330.

29. Lee WM. Acute liver failure. Semin Respir Crit Care Med. 2012;33(1):36-45.

30. Rumack BH, Matthew H. Acetaminophen poisoning and toxicity. Pediatrics. 1975;55:871-6.

3 CHAPTER

Acid-base Disorders in Poisoning

Pradeep Rangappa, Shivakumar Mutnal, Ipe Jacob

INTRODUCTION

In most critically ill patients biochemical and metabolic abnormalities are common and acid-base status is an essential modality in monitoring these parameters.[1] In cases of poisoning, these abnormalities are seen either due to metabolic pathways that are directly affected by the poison or due to organ dysfunction. Blood gas derangement might be due to many drugs and toxins and should be ruled out in any patient presenting with abnormal blood gases to the hospital, failing which irreversible organ damage and death can occur.[2]

ACID-BASE DISTURBANCES

Blood gas disturbances may arise and fluctuate in short periods of time and need to be recognized and treated early, necessitating the facility for immediate blood gas analysis. Understanding a blood gas report is essential to prevent further impairment of intermediary cell metabolism and organ dysfunction.

METABOLIC ACIDOSIS

The algorithm for analysis of metabolic acidosis is described in Flowchart 1.

Etiology of Metabolic Acidosis

Metabolic acidosis may arise from one or more of the following mechanisms:[2,3]

- As a secondary response to respiratory alkalosis
- Addition of acid (e.g. HCl)
- Endogenous (e.g. lactate, ketones) or exogenous (e.g. salicylate, ethylene glycol, methanol) generation of H^+
- Excess hydrogen from dietary proteins remaining unexcreted by kidneys [types 1 and 4 renal tubular acidosis (RTA)]
- Gastrointestinal tract (diarrhea) or kidney (type 2 RTA) wasting of bicarbonates.

Analysis of Metabolic Acidosis

Calculating the anion gap is the first step in the analysis of metabolic acidosis and differentiates between the various causes. The normal anion gap ranges from 4 to 12. Metabolic acidosis with an anion gap in this range is defined as a normal anion gap metabolic acidosis. On the other hand, metabolic acidosis with an anion gap above 12 is defined as a high anion gap metabolic acidosis.[3]

High Anion Gap Metabolic Acidosis Secondary to Poisoning

The most common causes of metabolic acidosis with elevated anion gap can be kept in mind with the popular mnemonic "GOLDMARK".

- G—glycols (ethylene and propylene glycol)
- O—oxoproline
- L—lactate

Acid-base Disorders in Poisoning

Flowchart 1: Algorithm for analysis of metabolic acidosis.

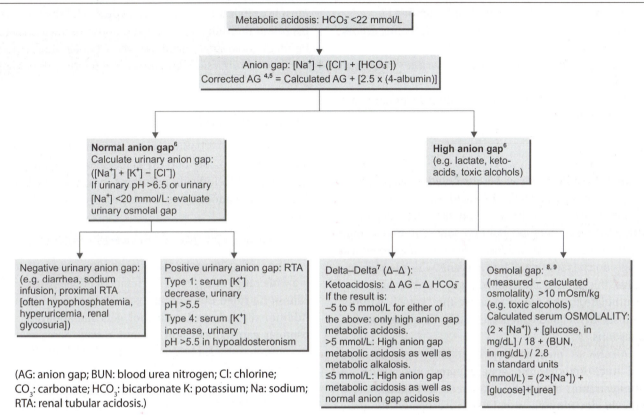

- D—D-lactate
- M—methanol
- A—aspirin
- R—renal failure (uremia)
- K—ketoacidosis.

Eliciting a good clinical history is important as this may point toward a specific cause. Lactic acidosis is seen in the majority of cases. Other common causes include ketoacidosis and uremia, although the latter is not seen unless serum creatinine rises to 5–6 mg/dL or above. After ruling out these causes by specific tests and history if it is inconclusive, then patient should be investigated for toxic alcohols (ethylene glycol and methanol). If suspected, either fomepizole (alcohol dehydrogenase inhibitor) or ethanol has to be administered without delay as the laboratory tests may take several days.

It should be noted that the above list does not include causes such as nonsteroidal anti-inflammatory drugs (NSAIDs), vasoactive drugs, numerous mitochondrial poisons and systemic toxins (aluminum phosphide).

Lactic Acidosis[10]

Metabolic acidosis with a high lactate may be divided into two types:

1. Type A (associated with hypoperfusion or hypoxemia) and
2. Type B (usually due to toxins, inborn errors of metabolism or underlying disease).

However, there may be instances of overlap where both type A and type B are seen, for example, when some toxins such as iron lead to tissue hypoxemia or hypoperfusion which in turn causes elevation of lactate. In this regard, the basal cause of an increased lactate should be investigated—either due to excess generation of lactate or the failure to clear it. Majority cases of lactic acidosis related to toxicology are secondary to increased production of lactate.

Toxicological Causes of Increased Serum Lactate

Increased serum lactate in toxicology scenarios can be attributed to any of the following mechanisms:

- *Toxins leading to seizures:* Isoniazid (INH), bupropion, camphor and theophylline
- *Toxins that increase oxygen demand above supply:* Iron, acetaminophen and β-agonists
- *Localized vasoconstriction and hypoperfusion leading to tissue hypoxemia:* Nucleoside reverse transcriptase

inhibitors, cyanide, hydrogen sulfide, carbon monoxide, cyanide, propofol and rotenone
- *Interference with oxygen utilization*: Cocaine, ergots, amphetamines and cathinones
- *Direct metabolism of a toxin to lactate:* Propylene glycol
- *Failure to excrete lactate*: Metformin/phenformin and ethanol.

Ketones[11]

In toxicology, ketosis can be attributed to isopropanol intoxication and alcoholic ketoacidosis (AKA). Ketosis is also caused by valproate and salicylate overdose. Amongst these, only alcohol and salicylate excess may result in a metabolic acidosis. Alcohol dehydrogenase breaks down isopropanol into acetone, which is a ketone body. This is not metabolized any further and may accumulate in the blood to cause the "ketosis without acidosis" associated with acute and isolated isopropanol ingestions.

Alcoholics may develop high anion gap acidosis and trace ketones and generally respond rapidly to administration of thiamine, dextrose and fluids. Those who do not improve should be investigated for toxic alcohol ingestion without receiving specific antidote or concurrent ethanol toxicity.

Toxic Alcohols[11]

Unexplained high anion gap metabolic acidosis without accompanying ketoacidosis, uremia or lactic acidosis bears consideration of poisonings by certain toxic alcohols. Such acidosis may be caused either metabolism of neutral compounds to strong acids or rarely by direct ingestion of acids. In methanol and ethylene glycol poisonings, the parent compound is oxidized to aldehyde and then acid by hepatic alcohol and aldehyde dehydrogenase, respectively. The acids thus formed are formic and glycolic acid and are nonmeasured anions, thus causing an increased anion gap. Formic acid may injure the retina and cause blindness. Ethylene glycol forms two metabolites—(1) glycolate, which leads to metabolic acidosis and (2) oxalate, which is nephrotoxic. In cases of late presentation after ingestion of the poison, findings of visual loss or renal failure may point towards diagnosis.

The clinical course in toxic alcohol poisoning is characterized by worsening metabolic acidosis. Serum levels of toxic alcohols should be obtained in such patients. However, these tests are usually outsourced by most hospitals and results may be delayed. When a clear history is unavailable, a decision about therapy should be made looking at corroborative evidence obtained at the time of admission like serum osmolality and ethanol levels.

OSMOLAR GAP[12]

The osmolar gap is defined as the difference between the measured osmolality and the calculated osmolality and may be used to indicate poisoning by various alcohols. Calculated osmolality is measured by the following formula:

$$Osm_{calc} = 2 \times (Na^+) + Glucose/18 + BUN/2.8$$

The normal osmolar gap ranges from –14 to 10. This is a wide range and glycol (methanol or ethylene) toxicity cannot be ruled out with an osmolar gap in this range. Additionally, when the alcohol gets metabolized, the osmolar gap reduces and the anion gap increases. On the other hand, a slightly increased osmolar gap does not imply poisoning by a toxic alcohol. Lactic acidosis and alcoholic ketoacidosis may lead to a very high osmolar gap. A very high osmolar gap (40–60 Osm) usually implies poisoning by a toxic alcohol.

Normal Anion Gap Metabolic Acidosis[11]

The mechanisms whereby a normal anion gap metabolic acidosis is generated are limited and include:
- RTA inducing toxins (Table 1)
- *Diarrhea-inducing toxins*: Cholestyramine, Erythromycin, metoclopramide, methotrexate, antineoplastics, magnesium citrate, lactose, mannitol and stimulant laxatives
- *Intake of an absorbable acid*: Hydrochloric acid
- *Carbonic anhydrase inhibitors*: Acetazolamide and topiramate
- Toluene and ethylene glycol
- Dilutional acidosis.

Overdoses with the drugs listed in Table 1 are not common. Only a prolonged usage of these drugs leads to metabolic acidosis. Carbonic anhydrase inhibitors like acetazolamide and some nephrotoxic drugs like amphotericin B, may cause RTA secondary to urinary bicarbonate loss. Volatile solvents, particularly toluene, may be abused, leading to renal injury and loss of potassium and bicarbonate, which presents with hypokalemic paralysis and acidosis.[13]

Acid-base Disorders in Poisoning

Table 1: Selected toxins causing renal tubular acidosis (RTA).

Type 1 (Distal)	Type 2 (Proximal)	Type 4 (Hypoaldesteronism)
Amphotericin B	Cadmium	Angiotensin-converting enzyme inhibitors
Ifosfamide	Antiretroviral therapy	Angiotensin receptor antagonists
Lithium carbonate	Lead	Eplerenone
Toluene	Ifosfamide	NSAIDs
Zoledronate		Pentamidine
		Spironolactone
		Trimethoprim

(NSAIDs: nonsteroidal anti-inflammatory drugs.)

In such scenarios, the underlying etiology of the acidosis must be treated. Treating acidosis by administering large boluses of sodium bicarbonate only gives a temporary benefit and may also lead to intracellular acidosis, extracellular fluid (ECF) overload and pulmonary edema.

METABOLIC ALKALOSIS[11]

There are a number of basic mechanisms that may lead to metabolic alkalosis:

- Secondary to respiratory acidosis
- Administration of bicarbonate
- Chloride loss
- Excess of mineralocorticoid due to therapeutic causes or pathological causes (renin/aldosterone-producing tumors, renal artery stenosis and Bartter syndrome).

These various causes may be differentiated by urinary chloride.

Metabolic alkalosis is indicated by blood gas analysis showing the following findings: pH >7.45 or $H^+ < 35$ nmol/liter with raised bicarbonate (>25 mmol/liter) and a base excess (> +2.3 mmol/liter). Usually bicarbonate in excess of 25 mmol/liter is excreted in the urine. A persistent metabolic alkalosis may result from renal retention of bicarbonate. This is seen in hyperaldosteronism in which there is continuous excretion of hydrogen ions from the renal tubules. This occurs most commonly due to ECF volume depletion, which in turn activates the renin angiotensin system (RAS) leading to secondary hyperaldosteronism resulting in increased proximal tubule reabsorption of sodium and bicarbonate and increased excretion of hydrogen and potassium from the distal tubule. This is referred to as a "saline-responsive" or "contraction" metabolic alkalosis,[14] where there is loss of water without loss of bicarbonate. Alkalosis results because the pCO_2 is kept within normal limits by ventilation. This alkalosis may be seen in poisonings resulting in dehydration (typically due to diuretics) and can be corrected by normal saline infusion.

Newer studies suggest that the saline-responsive metabolic alkalosis is caused by chloride depletion rather than volume loss. Hence this condition could be referred to as "chloride depletion alkalosis". Pendrin, a chloride/bicarbonate exchanger, is crucial to the development of this form of alkalosis. In both animal and human studies, acidosis caused by furosemide and dietary chloride restriction has been corrected by repletion of chloride even when there is volume loss and sodium depletion.[15]

ACUTE RESPIRATORY ACIDOSIS[11]

Acute respiratory acidosis [high pCO_2 (45 mm Hg) and normal standard bicarbonate] results from hypoventilation, the common toxicological causes of which are intoxication with sedative—hypnotics and opioids. Usually, well before respiratory acidosis shows up on an acid blood gas report, the underlying hypoventilation would have been noted clinically and rectified. However, it should be noted that hypoventilation may even occur when tidal volumes are inadequate, although the respiratory rate may be normal. In such conditions, there is decreased minute ventilation and proportionally more dead space ventilation, leading to type II respiratory failure.

Overdose of sedatives (opiates, tricyclic antidepressants and now uncommonly barbiturates) may lead to depressed brainstem respiratory reflexes and hypoventilation, resulting in a respiratory acidosis. This may also be seen when a mix of sedatives and alcohol is taken together.[16,17] There may be accompanying tissue hypoxia from poor gas exchange leading to metabolic acidosis and type A lactic acidosis.

In the field of chemical warfare, certain choking agents may be deployed. These are inhalational gases like chlorine, phosgene and nitrogen oxides which may cause pulmonary edema and military smokes which may lead to respiratory acidosis.[18] Associated hypoxemia with this again leads to type A lactic acidosis.

ACUTE RESPIRATORY ALKALOSIS[11]

Respiratory alkalosis is usually seen as a compensation for a metabolic acidosis, although the pH never rises above 7.40. It is seen in overdose of salicylates, aspirin and theophylline.

Salicylates are complicated metabolic toxins which may cause a characteristic acid-base abnormality that varies according to the delay in presentation. If they present early following an overdose, patients will generally exhibit a primary respiratory alkalosis. This is secondary to direct stimulation of the medulla, which will in turn cause increase in respiratory rate and tidal volume, as a compensation for impaired oxygenation from pulmonary toxins. This stage may be not be seen in children who lack the ventilatory reserve which is present in the adults. As toxicity progresses, patients may have metabolic alkalosis secondary to vomiting and metabolic acidosis, cause of which is generally multifactorial.

Similarly, aspirin and theophylline overdose may stimulate the respiratory center in central nervous system resulting in undue hyperventilation, respiratory alkalosis and hypocapnia.

Hyperventilation Secondary to Impaired Oxygenation

Several drugs may lead to pulmonary fibrosis or pulmonary edema causing impaired gas exchange.[18] There is a resulting tachypnea and hyperpnea. Severe impairment of oxygenation may also result in a concomitant lactic acidosis from anaerobic metabolism.

CONCLUSION

Acid-base analysis is essential in treating cases of poisoning. A handful of tests such as blood biochemistry, arterial blood gas analysis, lactate, ketones, serum osmolality, serum ethanol levels, blood ammonia and urinary electrolytes and pH can aid in narrowing down the differential diagnosis and help with a focused therapy. Acid-base status is reflective of the clinical pathophysiology of several toxicological processes and its better understanding implies a better understanding of the disease.

KEY POINTS

- Acid-base status and its analysis is essential in diagnosing and managing most of the critically ill patients
- Metabolic acidosis being the most common, having an algorithmic approach will help in narrowing down the diagnosis and treating them
- The most common causes of high anion gap acidosis like lactic acidosis, ketoacidosis and uremia are

excluded then poisoning by toxic alcohols should be given a priority
- A very high osmolar gap (40–60 osm) is almost always a poisoning by the toxic alcohol
- Acid-base status reflects pathophysiology of many diseases/toxicological processes and understanding it better entails a better understanding of the disease.

REFERENCES

1. Adrogue HJ, Madias NE. Management of life-threatening acid-base disorders. First of two parts. N Engl J Med. 1998;338(1):26-34.
2. Gluck SL. Acid-base. Lancet. 1998;352:474-9.
3. Berend K, de Varies AP, Gans RO. Physiological Approach to Assessment of Acid–Base Disturbances. N Engl J Med. 2014;371:1434-45.
4. Emmett M, Narins RG. Clinical use of the anion gap. Med Baltim. 1977;56:38-54.
5. Hatherill M, Waggie Z, Purves L, et al. Correction of the anion gap for albumin in order to detect occult tissue anions in shock. Arch Dis Child. 2002;87:526-9.
6. Enger E. Acidosis, gaps and poisonings. Acta Med Scand. 1982;212:1-3.
7. Rastegar A. Use of the DeltaAG/DeltaHCO3-ratio in the diagnosis of mixed acid-basedisorders. J Am Soc Nephrol. 2007;18:2429-31.
8. Lynd LD, Richardson KJ, Purssell RA, et al. An evaluation of the osmole gap as a screening test for toxic alcohol poisoning. BMC Emerg Med. 2008;8:5.
9. Krahn J, Khajuria A. Osmolality gaps: diagnostic accuracy and long-term variability. Clin Chem. 2006;52:737-9.
10. Kraut JA, Madias NE. Lactic Acidosis. N Engl J Med. 2014;371;24.
11. Wiener SW. Toxicologic Acid-Base Disorders. Emerg Med Clin N Am. 2014;32:149-65.
12. Hoffman RS, Smilkstein MJ, Howland MA, et al. Osmol gaps revisited: normal values and limitations. J Toxicol Clin Toxicol. 1993;31:81-93.
13. Jone CM, Wu AH. An unusual case of toluene-induced metabolic acidosis. Clin Chem. 1988;34:2596-9.
14. Garella S, Chang BS, Kahn SI. Dilution acidosis and contraction alkalosis: review of a concept. Kidney Int. 1975;8:279-83.
15. Luke RG, Galla JH. It is chloride depletion alkalosis, not contraction alkalosis. J Am Soc Nephrol. 2012;23: 204-7.
16. Takeda S, Eriksson LI, Yamamoto Y, et al. Opioid action on respiratory neuron activity of the isolated respiratory network in newborn rats. Anesthesiology. 2001;95: 740-9.
17. Mullen WH. Toxin-related noncardiogenic pulmonary edema. PCCSU article. Am Coll Chest Physicians. 2013.
18. Tenney SM, Miller RM. The respiratory and circulatory action of salicylate. Am J Med. 1955;19:498-508.

4
CHAPTER

Antidotes

Omender Singh, Anish Gupta

INTRODUCTION

Antidotes are substances which counteract and reverse the effects of poisons and toxins. Despite advances in medical science antidotes are available for a small number of toxins and poisons. However, whenever available they can be life-saving.

Antidotes act by various mechanisms to alleviate the effects of poisons (Table 1).

N-ACETYLCYSTEINE[1]

Specific antidote for paracetamol (acetaminophen) overdose/poisoning.

Mechanism of action:

- N-acetylcysteine (NAC) is a *glutathione* (GSH) precursor which increases GSH stores

- Directly binds to N-acetyl-p-benzoquinone imine (NAPQI)
- Increases metabolism of acetaminophen by sulfation pathway
- Antioxidant effect—reduces free radical generation and injury

Dose

Acute Paracetamol Poisoning

Both oral and intravenous routes can be used with no difference in efficacy. Both protocols are United States: the Food and Drug Administration (US-FDA) approved (Box 1).

Table 1: Mechanism of action of antidotes.	
Mechanism	*Examples*
Chelation Antidotes combine with the poison to form inert nontoxic complexes, thus preventing their absorption and adverse effects	Deferoxamine, D-penicillamine, sodium calcium edetate, digoxin specific antibody fragments, pralidoxime, protamine
Detoxification of poison Certain antidotes prevent conversion of the poison to its toxic metabolite and hence prevent adverse effects	Fomepizole, ethanol, N-acetyl cysteine, methylene blue, sodium thiosulfate
Compete with effective receptor sites	Oxygen, naloxone, phytomenadione
Block the receptors through which toxic effects are mediated	Oxygen, glucagon, atropine.
Increase elimination	

General Management of Poisoning or Overdose

Box 1: Dosage protocols of N-acetylcysteine (NAC) for acute acetaminophen poisoning.

Protocols for NAC
Oral protocol: • Loading dose: 140 mg/kg orally   • Maintenance doses: 70 mg/kg orally every 4 hours—Total 17 doses
IV protocol: 20-hour protocols (3 bag regimen and 2 bag regimen)
Traditional 3 bag regimen: • Loading dose of 150 mg/kg IV over 1 hour, followed by   • 50 mg/kg IV over the next 4 hours (12.5 mg/kg/h), followed by   • 100 mg/kg IV over the next 16 hours (6.25 mg/kg/h)   The dilution is in 5% dextrose
2 bag regimen:[2]   • 50 mg/kg/hour over 4 hours (total 200 mg/kg) followed by   • 6.25 mg/kg/hour for 16 hours (total 100 mg/kg over 16 hours)
12 hour protocol: • 50 mg/kg for 2 hours followed by   • 20 mg/kg/hour for 10 hours

When to Administer N-acetylcysteine?

The maximum benefit is when NAC is administered within 8 hours of acute acetaminophen ingestion but should be administered as soon as possible. It can be administered beyond 8 hours in cases of suspected poisoning, delayed presentation and ingestion of sustained release tablets.

Duration of Therapy

- Both the NAC protocols are time and fixed dose-based therapies.
- By convention, IV N-acetylcysteine is given for at least 20–21 hours and oral NAC is given for at least 72 hours.
- Extended duration of therapy may be needed in certain situations vis-à-vis:
  - ○ Hepatic failure
  - ○ Massive overdose, and
  - ○ Ingestion of extended or sustained release preparations.

In such cases, treatment is continued till patients show clinical improvement, aminotransferase levels show a declining trend, coagulation parameters show an improving trend and the serum acetaminophen level is falling or undetectable (<10 µg/mL).

Adverse Effects of N-acetylcysteine

Allergic Reactions

Seen in 10–50% cases. Most often witnessed with intravenous preparations. Patients present with rash and urticaria. Although uncommon, anaphylactoid reactions can occur and are life-threatening. Reactions are related to the rate of NAC administration and are more often seen in asthmatics and in patients with low serum acetaminophen levels. In case a reaction occurs, the drug should be stopped and an antihistaminic should be administered. H1 antihistamine such as diphenhydramine is given IV at a dose of 25–50 mg and can be repeated to a maximum of 400 mg in 24 hours. Once symptoms settle, the infusion can be restarted at half the rate for 30 minutes, followed by the normal rate of infusion in the absence of any allergic reaction. In case of severe reactions, management is as for anaphylactic shock. Airway, breathing and circulation are assessed and stabilized. Adrenaline (1 mg/mL) at a dose of 0.1 mg/kg is administered intramuscularly in the vastus lateralis muscle (lateral aspect of mid-thigh).

All patients on NAC therapy should be monitored, preferably in an intensive care unit for any adverse reactions.

Nausea and Vomiting

Oral NAC is not palatable and leads to nausea and vomiting. To counter this effect, it is usually given with juices or as a chilled solution. In case vomiting occurs within 1 hour, the dose should be repeated. In patients intolerant to oral NAC, intravenous therapy may be needed.

Special situations

Massive Overdose (>500 mg/kg or >30 g)

The intravenous dose of NAC is same as previously mentioned except that the dose of the final infusion is doubled from 100 mg/kg to 200 mg/kg and continued till hepatic transaminase levels start declining and patient shows clinical improvement.

Dialysis

N-acetylcysteine is dialyzable and serum levels are reduced with hemodialysis. There are no clear-cut guidelines but it is advisable to double to dose of NAC during HD.

Antidotes   33

Pregnancy/Breastfeeding

N-acetylcysteine is a pregnancy category B drug. It can be administered in pregnancy at usual doses as described for adults. It is not known if acetylcysteine is excreted in breast milk. Acetylcysteine is cleared off the body in about 30 hours. Nursing mothers can resume feeding 30 hours after the last dose.

ATROPINE[3]

It is an anticholinergic agent which inhibits the action of acetylcholine on parasympathetic sites and acts as a competitive antagonist of acetylcholine at muscarinic receptors. Atropine has no action on nicotine receptors. The indications of atropine are summarized in Table 2.

We will be discussing role of atropine in organophosphates poisoning.

Indications

Organophosphate and Carbamate Poisoning (OPC)[4]

These compounds bind to the enzyme acetylcholinesterase and inhibit its activity. As a result, there is excess acetylcholine (Ach) at the neuromuscular junction leading to cholinergic toxicity. Respiratory failure is the most common cause of death in OP poisoning and is secondary to muscarinic (bronchospasm, bronchorrhea, arrhythmias, and hypotension) and nicotinic effects (weakness and paralysis).

Atropine competitively inhibits the action of acetylcholine by competing with Ach for the muscarinic effects thus alleviating the cholinergic symptoms.

There is no standard dosing regimen of atropine for OP poisoning. The commonly followed dosing protocol is mentioned in the subsequent Box 2.

Other routes of administration: Atropine can be administered by intraosseous route or via endotracheal tube.

Intraosseous administration: The dose is 1:1 with IV dose.

Table 2: Indications of atropine.

General	Off-label
<ul><li>Bradycardia</li><li>Preanesthetic agent</li><li>Organophosphorus compounds poisoning</li><li>Nerve agent poisoning</li><li>Beta-blocker poisoning</li></ul>	<ul><li>Rapid sequence intubation</li><li>Stress echocardiography (chronotropic effect)</li><li>Mushroom poisoning (antimuscarinic effects)</li></ul>

Box 2: Dosing schedule for atropine in organophosphate (OP) poisoning.

Dose of Atropine

Adults
Loading dose:
Initial dose is 1–3 mg IV (depending on the severity)
Initial bolus dose can be 5 mg IV (in severe cases)
Double the dose every 3–5 minutes till atropinization is achieved
Continue bolus doses of atropine till the

- Heart rate > 80 beats/min
- Systolic blood pressure > 80 mm Hg and } Atropinization
- Chest is clear of secretions

Tachycardia and pupillary dilatation (mydriasis) are no longer considered appropriate markers for atropinization as they can be confounded by hypoxia, hypovolemia and sympathetic overactivity.

Maintenance dose:
- About 10–20% of the total loading dose is started as an infusion to be administered over 1 hour
- Monitor for inadequate or excessive atropine dosing. In cases with inadequate dosing the cholinergic signs and symptoms may re-emerge while in excessive dosing the patient may become confused, agitated, hyperpyrexic and develop constipation and urinary retention

In cases of atropine toxicity it is advisable to stop the infusion for about an hour and let the symptoms abate before restarting the infusion.

Children (<12 years)
Loading dose: 0.05 mg/kg IV
Maintenance dose: 10–20 % of total loading dose and is usually in the range of 0.02–0.05 mg/kg/hour
Monitoring for features of cholinergic toxicity (suboptimal dosing) or atropine toxicity (excessive dosing)

General Management of Poisoning or Overdose

Endotracheal tube (ETT) administration: The dose is 2–3 times the IV dose diluted with 5 mL of normal saline and administered via ET. This is followed by five positive pressure breaths.

Nerve Agent Poisoning

Atropine can be used for nerve agent poisoning. However, the total dose required is lesser as compared to that required for organophosphorus compounds and depends on the severity of clinical features.

Mild features: Dose is 0.05 mg/kg by IV, IM or IO route (maximum 2 mg/dose).

Moderate features: Dose is 0.05 mg/kg (maximum 4 mg/dose).

Repeat every 3–5 minutes with a target of decrease in bronchial secretions and bronchospasm. Pralidoxime is administered along with atropine and will be discussed elsewhere.

Severe features: Dose is 0.1 mg/kg by IM route only (maximum 6 mg/dose). Dose can be repeated and titrated as per clinical end points.

Cardiac Glycoside Poisoning

Atropine has a role in the management of symptomatic bradycardia and high-degree AV-block due to cardiac glycoside toxicity and has been used with moderate success. The dose of atropine used is as per the 2010 ALCS/PALS guidelines for symptomatic bradycardia.

Adults: A bolus of 0.5 mg IV. The dose can be repeated every 5 minutes to a maximum of 3 mg.

Children: Bolus dose 0.02 mg/kg IV (minimum 0.1 mg, maximum 0.5 mg), repeated up to maximum 0.04 mg/kg (not to exceed 3 mg).

Beta-blocker and Calcium Channel Blocker Poisoning

Atropine can be used for mild cases of β-blocker and calcium blocker induced bradycardia but is usually ineffective. The doses are similar to that mentioned for cardiac glycoside toxicity.

Pregnancy/Breastfeeding

Pregnancy category B/C. Atropine crosses the placenta. No adverse events reported in animal studies. Atropine may suppress lactation. Use with caution.

BOTULINUM ANTITOXIN-HEPTAVALENT

It is an equine-derived antitoxin which is effective against 7 *Clostridium botulinum* antitoxins namely A, B, C, D, E, F and G (hence the name heptavalent). The total volume in a vial varies from 10 mL to 20 mL. It is used for the treatment of botulism.

Botulism[5]

Dose

The dose is based on the age and weight of the patient.

For infants less than 1 year of age, 10% of a single vial is to be administered irrespective of weight.

For patients 1–17 years of age dose is calculated based on weight of patient and varies from 20% to 100% of the vial. A minimum of 20% is to be used. The following formulas are used for calculating the dose.

≤30 kg: Percentage (%) of adult dose to be administered
$$= Weight (kg) \times 2$$
>30 kg: Percentage (%) of adult dose to be administered
$$= Weight (kg) + 30$$

For patients more than 17 year of age one vial is administered.

There are no dose modifications in patients with renal or liver impairment.

Administration

The frozen antitoxin is thawed in a water bath at a temperature of 37°C. The vial should be inspected for any particulate matter, impurities and discoloration. Do not shake the vial and avoid any foaming. The antitoxin is diluted with normal saline (0.9%) to a ratio of 1:10. In some cases a premixed bag may be stored but should be used within 8–10 hours.

A hypersensitivity testing should be performed before starting the infusion. An intradermal test can be performed with 0.02 mL of 1:1,000 saline diluted antitoxin. A positive test is defined as a wheal with erythema of more than 3 mm than the control test with normal saline. The test is read at 15–20 minutes.

The antitoxin is administered by a slow IV infusion via an infusion pump at a dose of 0.5 mL/min for the first 30 minutes. In case there are no reactions the infusion is doubled every 30 minutes to a maximum of 2 mL/min. Epinephrine, antihistamines and crash cart should be kept available and accessible in case of dire emergencies.

Pediatric patients (1–17 years): Start the infusion at 0.01 mL/kg/min for the first 30 minutes. In case of no reactions, increase the rate by 0.01 mL/kg/min every 30 minutes to a maximum rate of 0.03 mL/kg/min.

Adverse Effects

The common adverse effects are headache, chills, rash, urticaria, pruritis, fever, nausea, and anaphylaxis.

Pregnancy/Breastfeeding

Not known if the toxin crosses the placenta or is excreted in breast milk. Nursing mothers may have to discontinue feeding during therapy.

BOTULINUM IMMUNO GLOBULIN (INTRAVENOUS HUMAN) (BABYBIG)[6]

It provides antibodies from immunized adults for use in infant botulism (<1 year of age) caused by toxin type A and B. The dosage schedule is discussed in Box 3.

Administration

- Preferably administer via an infusion pump with a low-volume tubing.
- Always infuse through a separate IV line.
- Do not administer if solution is turbid.
- No dose modifications in renal/hepatic impairment.

Adverse Effects

Exact frequency is not defined. All systems can be affected and are more related to infant botulism rather than the immunoglobulin.

For allergic reactions, anaphylaxis the infusion should be slowed or temporarily stopped. Keep epinephrine handy for severe acute allergic reactions.

Box 3: Dose of botulinum immunoglobulin.

- Single dose 50 mg/kg as intravenous infusion.
- Always verify dose with manufacturer's drug insert as the dose may vary with each manufactured lot.
- Start infusion at 25 mg/kg/hour for the first 15 minutes, *then*
- Increase the infusion to a maximum rate of 50 mg/kg/hour (if well tolerated).
- The infusion should be completed in about 4 hours (if no adverse reaction).

Contraindications

- Hypersensitivity or previous allergic reaction to immune globulin or any component of the formulation
- Selective IgA deficiency.

Pregnancy/Breastfeeding

Only for use in infants less than 1 year. Do not administer to pregnant and breastfeeding women.

BROMOCRIPTINE

It is an ergot alkaloid with dopamine D2 receptor agonist activity. It activates the postsynaptic dopamine receptors in the tuberoinfundibular and nigrostriatal pathways, thereby decreasing prolactin secretions and increasing coordinated motor control.

Uses

- Parkinson's disease
- Hyperprolactinemia
- Acromegaly
- Diabetes mellitus—not routine recommendation
- Neuroleptic malignant syndrome (off-label use)

Neuroleptic Malignant Syndrome[7]

- Used for moderate to severe cases. Evidence supporting its use is minimal
- Dose—2.5 mg via PO route 3–4 times per day. Maximum dose 45 mg/day
- Continue treatment till NMS is controlled. Pediatric dose is unknown
- Administer with food to alleviate gastrointestinal distress
- No renal/hepatic dose modifications.

Adverse Effects

Orthostatic hypotension and syncope are commonly seen during initiation and escalation of therapy.

Most adverse effects are seen after prolonged use. Cardiac valvular fibrosis, pleural/pericardial effusions and fibrosis (pleural, pulmonary and retroperitoneal) have been reported.

Increased risk for melanoma especially in patients with Parkinson's disease.

CNS depression, hallucinations and loss of impulse control have all been reported.

Use with caution in tasks requiring mental activity.

Discontinuation of therapy or dose reduction may be needed in some cases.

Pregnancy/Breastfeeding

- Pregnancy risk factor category B. It crosses placenta but data has not shown to increase the risk of birth defects. Preferable to discontinue bromocriptine once pregnancy is confirmed.
- Contraindicated during breastfeeding as it is known to inhibit lactation.

ACTIVATED CHARCOAL

It is commonly known as the "universal antidote". It is the most frequently used substance for gastrointestinal decontamination. It acts by the mechanism of adsorption wherein it binds various ingested drugs and toxins and prevents their systemic absorption. However, not all drugs/toxins can be adsorbed by charcoal and hence the term universal antidote may be a misnomer. It can be administered as both single-dose activated charcoal (SDAC) and multiple-dose activated charcoal (MDAC). MDAC is helpful for adsorbing toxins/drugs with high enterohepatic circulation. The efficacy of activated charcoal depends upon the lag time between toxin ingestion and AC administration. The more the lag time the lesser is the efficacy.

Dose

Previously, the recommended dosing was a ratio of 10:1 for charcoal: poison.[8] However, in most cases the amount of poison ingested is unknown making this approach challenging and impractical.[9]

The usual dose is 1 g/kg to a maximum for 50 g for a single dose.[9]

MDAC—the initial dose is up to 50 g followed by 25–50 g every 4 hours.

Administration

- Activated charcoal is unpalatable. Use flavoring or thickening agents (e.g. chocolate syrup, concentrated fruit juice, bentonite, carboxymethyl cellulose) to increase its palatability. However, these may reduce the ability of activated charcoal to adsorb poisons.
- Always check for the presence of bowel sounds before administration.

- Intravenous antiemetics may be required to reduce the risk of vomiting.
- Shake the activated charcoal container thoroughly before administration.
- Rinse the container with a small quantity of water to ensure that the patient has received all of the activated charcoal.[10]

Indications

Used in cases of poisoning wherein:
- Severe systemic toxicity is anticipated
- No effective antidote is available
- A modified release or extended release formulation is ingested
- Absence of contraindications (such as decreased mental status, poor airway reflexes precluding to an unprotected airway, uncooperative patient, ileus or intestinal obstruction).

It is important to note that AC is not effective in cases of poisoning with hydrocarbons, caustic acids and alkali, lithium and iron.

Administration of SDAC is not mandatory and decision is clinical and based on the risk: benefit ratio.

The maximal benefit of activated charcoal is when it is administered within 1 hour of poison ingestion.

Safety

Activated charcoal is considered safe as it has no systemic absorption. Risks include pulmonary aspiration, bezoar formation and intestinal obstruction.

Contraindications

As per the American Academy of Clinical Toxicology (AACT) and the European Association of Poisons Centers and Clinical Toxicologists (EAPCCT) the contraindications to the use of AC are:
- Intestinal obstruction
- Anatomically abnormal GI tract
- Risk of GI hemorrhage or perforation
- Unprotected airway (poor airway reflexes, depressed level of consciousness, Glasgow coma scale < 8).

Pregnancy and Breastfeeding

Activated charcoal has no systemic adsorption after oral administration. Hence, use during pregnancy and breastfeeding is not expected to result in significant fetal exposure. In general antidotes if clearly indicated should be administered to a pregnant woman and should not be withheld because of the fear of teratogenicity.[11]

CALCIUM

Calcium is mainly used in body for modulation of nerve and muscle function. It plays a role in various metabolic and chemical reactions in the body.

Indications

- Hypocalcemia
- Calcium blocker overdose/poisoning (off label use)
- Beta-blocker overdose/poisoning (off label use)
- Hydrofluoric acid exposure/burns (off label use).

Calcium Channel Blocker Poisoning (Off Label)[12]

Indications: Causing hypotension and conduction disturbances.

Shock not responding to standard therapy:
- Bolus
  - Calcium gluconate (10%): 0.6 mL/kg. Repeat as needed
  - Calcium chloride (10%): 0.2 mL/kg
- Infusion
  - Calcium gluconate (10%): 0.6–1.5 mL/kg/hour *or*
  - Calcium chloride (10%): 0.2–0.5 mL/kg/hour.

Titrate the infusion rate to achieve adequate hemodynamic response (i.e. improvement in blood pressure and cardiac contractility).

Monitor serum ionized calcium levels. Goal is to maintain ionized calcium at twice normal only in life-threatening situations. Avoid hypercalcemia. Infusions should be administered only via a central venous access.

Beta-blocker Poisoning (Off-label)

- Hypotension or conduction disturbances not responding to standard therapy
- Optimal dose has not been established.
- The bolus dose and infusion are same as mentioned above for calcium channel blocker (CCB) poisoning.

Hydrofluoric Acid Burns/Exposure

Calcium gluconate provides calcium ions which complex with free fluoride ions and thus prevent or reduce toxicity and correct fluoride-induced hypocalcemia.

Used as various formulations:
- *Topical treatment*: Calcium gluconate gel (2.5%) to be applied within 3 hours of exposure.
- *Subcutaneous dose*: 0.5 mL/cm² of 5–10% calcium gluconate to be infiltrated 0.5 cm away from the margin of the injured tissue. Endpoint of therapy is relief of pain. Never use calcium chloride for subcutaneous injection.
- *Intra-arterial*: To be performed only by an expert accustomed with the technique. A clinical toxicologist should be consulted prior to administration. Meticulous care needs to be taken to prevent extravasation.

  Dilute 10–20 mL of 10% calcium gluconate in 50 mL of normal saline or 5% dextrose and infuse into the artery supplying the affected area. Give the infusion slowly over 4 hours.
- *Inhalation*: A 2.5% nebulization solution is used for nebulization. Mix 1.5 mL of 10% calcium gluconate solution with 4.5 mL NS.

Note: Ocular exposure is treated with saline or sterile water irrigation. Calcium is not used in the irrigation fluid for cleaning eyes.

CALCIUM DISODIUM EDTA (CaNa$_2$EDTA)[13,14]

It is a chelating agent used in the treatment of lead poisoning and cadmium poisoning (off label). The heavy metal ions displace calcium and form calcium as nonionizing soluble complexes. These complexes are readily excreted in urine.

Indications

Lead Poisoning

Adults

Therapy recommended when blood lead levels > 50 µg/dL with symptoms *or* Blood levels > 100 µg/dL with or without symptoms Repeat doses may be required but should be administered after 2–3 days depending on blood lead levels. The dosing regimens are mentioned in Table 3.

General Management of Poisoning or Overdose

Table 3: Dosing regimen of edetate calcium disodium (CaNa$_2$EDTA).

Blood lead levels and symptoms	Dose
<70 µg/dL + asymptomatic	1000 m^2/day for 5 days (IV, IM)
>70 µg/dL + symptomatic	Treat with both CaNa$_2$EDTA and dimercaprol Begin treatment with CaNa$_2$EDTA followed by dimercaprol IM, IV: 1,000 mg/m^2/day or 25–50 mg/kg/day for 5 days; a maximum dose of 3,000 mg has been suggested
Lead encephalopathy	Dimercaprol added to treatment regimen Begin treatment with CaNa$_2$EDTA with the second dimercaprol dose 1,500 mg/m^2/day or 50–75 mg/kg/day for 5 days (maximum dose—3,000 mg)
Lead nephropathy	Modify dosing regimen due to decrease in creatinine clearance Regimen may need to be repeated monthly till lead levels are reduced to an acceptable level Creatinine: 2–3 mg/dL: 500 mg/m^2 every 24 hours x 5 days Creatinine: 3–4 mg/dL: 500 mg/m^2 every 48 hours for 3 doses Creatinine: >4 mg/dL: 500 mg/m^2 once weekly

Administration: Both intravenous (IV) and intramuscular (IM) routes can be used but intravenous route is preferred. IM route is preferred when cerebral edema is present.

IV infusion: Administer as a diluted solution over 8–12 hours or continuously over 24 hours.

For IM injection: Divide the daily dose into 2–3 equal doses and administer by deep IM injection 8–12 hours apart. Procaine hydrochloride or lidocaine may be added to minimize pain at injection site. When dimercaprol is also used inject into a separate site.

Dose reduction in renal disease. No dose modification in hepatic disease.

Pregnancy/breastfeeding: It is a pregnancy category B drug. No well-controlled studies in pregnant women.

Chelation therapy should be initiated with blood lead levels more than or equal to 45 µg/dL. If blood levels are more than 70 µg/dL or clinical features suggest lead encephalopathy, chelation therapy should be initiated irrespective of trimester.

Nursing mothers with blood lead levels more than or equal to 40 µg/dL should avoid breastfeeding. Calcium supplementation may reduce the amount of lead in breast milk.

Cadmium poisoning (off-label): May be beneficial in some cases. Chelation is effective only up to 24–48 hours postexposure.

Therapy is for 5 days with a dose of about 75 mg/kg/day divided into 3–6 doses. Total dose for 5 days should not exceed 500 mg/kg. A repeat course may be considered based on blood cadmium levels after 2 days.

DANTROLENE

It is a skeletal muscle relaxant used for the treatment of malignant hyperthermia and neuroleptic malignant syndrome (off label). It prevents the release of calcium from the sarcoplasmic reticulum in the skeletal muscle and thus decreases myoplasmic calcium concentrations.

Malignant Hyperthermia[15]

The Malignant Hyperthermia Association of the United States (MHAUS) recommendation is followed.

Dantrolene is administered at a dose of 2.5 mg/kg by intravenous route.

Dose may be repeated every 5–15 minutes till symptoms abate or a cumulative dose of 10 mg/kg is reached.

Post-crisis Management

As per MHAUS protocol, administer 1 mg/kg every 4–6 hours (route not specified) or a continuous IV infusion of 0.25 mg/kg/hour for at least 24 hours.

Administration

Doses are administered as rapid IV push during crisis. Follow-up doses are administered over at least 1 minute.

Adverse Effects

- Dantrolene is hepatotoxic and is reported at variable drug doses.

Risk of hepatotoxicity is higher in women (>35 years) and elderly patients.
- Begin treatment with the lowest possible effective dose.
- Monitor liver function tests routinely.

Pregnancy/Breastfeeding

It is a pregnancy category C drug. Dantrolene crosses placenta and small amounts are also present in breast milk.

DEFEROXAMINE

It is a chelating agent that forms complexes with ferric ions to form ferrioxamine, which is excreted by the kidneys. 100 mg of deferoxamine binds to 8.5 mg of free circulating elemental iron (85 mg per 1,000 mg dose). It does not bind to iron from transferrin or hemoglobin. It reduces the cytoplasmic free iron levels and thus free iron-induced disruption of mitochondrial cell membranes and enzyme systems. Ferrioxamine produces a pink- to red- or orange-colored urine. It is the drug of choice for iron poisoning.

Iron Poisoning[16]

- Severe intoxication with serum iron more than or equal to 500 µg/dL irrespective of symptoms.
- Severe symptomatic toxicity characterized by coma, metabolic acidosis, shock, gastrointestinal bleeding and cardiovascular collapse.
- Initial dose is 5 mg/kg/hour, which is gradually titrated up to 15 mg/kg/hour if well tolerated.
- Repeat dose of 500 mg every 4 hours can be administered for a maximum of two doses.
- Subsequent doses are administered at 4–12 hour intervals to a maximum of 6 g in 24 hours.
- Optimal duration of therapy is unknown. Therapeutic endpoints include serum iron level less than 350 µg/dL and resolution of signs of toxicity.
- Intravenous route is preferred. Rarely, intramuscular route may be used but is not recommended.

Dose Modification

No dose modification in hepatic disease. Contraindicated in severe renal disease or anuric patients[17] (Table 4).

Pregnancy and Breastfeeding

It is a pregnancy category C drug. Deferoxamine is not known to cross the placenta or excreted in breast milk. Use with caution.

DIMERCAPROL

It is also called British anti-Lewisite (BAL). It is used for the treatment of arsenic, gold and mercury poisoning. It provides sulfhydryl groups which combine with heavy metals to form nontoxic soluble chelates which are excreted in urine. The dosing regimens of dimercaprol is mentioned in Box 4.

Premedication with a H_1 histamine antagonist such as diphenhydramine is recommended.

Dose Modification

No renal dose modification. It is contraindicated in hepatic dysfunction except in hepatocellular injury secondary to arsenic.

Table 4: Dose modification of deferoxamine in renal dysfunction.

Creatinine clearance	>50 mL/min	10–50 mL/min or CRRT	<10 mL/min hemodialysis Peritoneal dialysis
Dose modification	No adjustment	Give 25–50% of dose	Contraindicated

Box 4: Dosing regimens of British anti-Lewisite (BAL) in arsenic, gold and mercury poisoning.

Arsenic or gold poisoning (Mild): 2.5 mg/kg every 6 hours for 2 days, then every 12 hours for 1 day, followed by once daily for 10 days

Arsenic or gold poisoning (Severe): 3 mg/kg every 4 hours for 2 days, then every 6 hours for 1 day, followed every 12 hours for 10 days

Inorganic mercury poisoning: 5 mg/kg initially, followed by 2.5 mg/kg 1–2 times/day for 10 days

Lead poisoning[13] *(No guideline or recommendation at present):* 3–5 mg/kg IM followed by 3–4 mg/kg along with $CaNa_2EDTA$ every 4–6 hours for 3–5 days. Lower doses (2–3 mg/kg) may be used in the absence of encephalopathy

Note: Urine alkalization stabilizes the dimercaprol-metal complex, and is recommended during chelation therapy to prevent kidney damage.
All injections are administered deep intramuscular.

Adverse Effects

- British anti-Lewisite is nephrotoxic. Maintain alkaline urine pH.
- Use with caution in G6PD patients as it can lead to hemolysis.

Pregnancy and Breastfeeding

Pregnancy category C drug. Not known if secreted in breast milk. Use with caution and only if benefits outweigh risks.

DIGOXIN-SPECIFIC ANTIBODY FRAGMENTS

They are purified preparations of the Fab portion of the IgG anti-digoxin antibodies which are derived from immunized sheep. They bind to free digoxin to form immune complexes which are freely excreted in urine. As the free digoxin levels decrease in blood, digoxin dissociates from the sodium-potassium ATPase channel (Na-K-ATPase) along the concentration gradient thereby alleviating toxic symptoms. Hemodialysis is an ineffective treatment modality as the digoxin-immune fragment complexes are of large molecular size.

DigiFab is one of the commercial preparations and each vial contains 40 mg of Fab fragments which binds 0.5 mg of digoxin. It lacks the Fc portion of the antibody and hence allergic reactions are uncommon. However, individuals with allergies to sheep or papaya extracts (papain), which are used to cleave the antibody, are at risk.

Fab is used for the treatment of digitalis poisoning associated with life-threatening arrhythmias (Tachyarrhythmias—VT/VF, bradyarrhythmias—heart block, symptomatic bradycardia), hemodynamic instability and hyperkalemia.

It is also used for other cardiac glycoside toxicities such as oleander, quill and toad venom.

For acute toxicity the dose is calculated by various methods depending upon the clinical scenario (Table 5).[18,19]

Chronic Digoxin Ingestion

Lower dose of digoxin-Fab is used as the total body digoxin load is lower. Usually half the normal dose is given. One way is to administer 1 vial of Fab and observe for clinical response. If no response is seen in 1 hour a second ampule is given.

Nonpharmacological Cardiac Glycoside Poisoning

The serum concentrations do not correlate well and cannot be used to calculate the dose of Fab. Dose is 10 vials of Fab initially which is repeated if clinical response is inadequate.

Administration

- Administer slowly over 30 minutes in all cases
- Administer by slow IV push in cases of cardiac arrest or in whom arrest is imminent.

FLUMAZENIL[20]

It is an antidote used for the treatment of benzodiazepine poisoning and reversal of benzodiazepine induced sedation. It is an imidazobenzodiazepine derivative and is a competitive benzodiazepine receptor antagonist. It inhibits the activity at the benzodiazepine receptor site on the GABA/benzodiazepine receptor complex. Flumazenil does not antagonize the effect of drugs

Table 5: FAB dose for acute digitalis toxicity.		
Digoxin level, *or* Amount ingested unknown	Amount of Digoxin ingested known but Digoxin concentration unknown	Digoxin concentration known
Empirical treatment 10 vials of DigiFab Repeat if no clinical response	Calculate total body load (TBL) TBL for digoxin = Dose in mg x 0.8 (0.8 – refers to bioavailability of digoxin and is a constant) No. of vials = TBL/0.5 (round off to nearest whole no.)	Number of vials = (Digoxin conc. ng/mL) (Wt kg) 100 or Digitoxin (ng/mL) × Wt (kg) 1,000

(FAB: antibody fragments; conc: concentration; Wt: weight))

affecting GABA-ergic neurons and does not reverse the effects of opioids.

Benzodiazepine Poisoning

Initial dose is 0.2 mg over 30 seconds

↓ Response (regain of consciousness) is inadequate after 30 seconds

Repeat 0.3 mg over 30 seconds after 1 minute

↓ Response inadequate

Repeat 0.5 mg over 30 seconds at 1-minute intervals

↓

Maximum cumulative dose: 3 mg (usual total dose: 1 to 3 mg)

For patients with partial response at total dose of 3 mg, additional doses up to a total dose of 5 mg may be required. If no response after a total of 5 mg consider alternative diagnosis or effect of coingestants.

Monitor for at least 2 hours for sedation, respiratory depression, benzodiazepine withdrawal, and residual effects of benzodiazepines.

Although not FDA approved, IV infusion of 0.1–1 mg/hour may be used in certain cases of re-sedation.

Always administer into a large vein with a freely running intravenous fluid.

Dose modification is not needed for the initial doses in patients with hepatic impairment. However, subsequent doses may need to be reduced or frequency decreased. No renal dose modification required.

Adverse Effect

A notable adverse effect is seizures. They are mostly seen in patients on long-term benzodiazepine for sedation or in cases with signs of tricyclic antidepressant overdose. Keep a benzodiazepine at bedside in case of seizure.

Pregnancy and Breastfeeding

Pregnancy category C drug. Avoid used during labor and delivery. Not known if secreted in breast milk. Use with caution.

FOMEPIZOLE (4-METHYLPYRAZOLE)

Fomepizole is a competitive inhibitor of the enzyme alcohol dehydrogenase which catalyzes the metabolism of ethanol, ethylene glycol, and methanol. Methanol is metabolized to formaldehyde by alcohol dehydrogenase and by a series of subsequent reactions to formic acid. Formic acid leads to metabolic acidosis and visual impairment in methanol poisoning. Similarly, ethylene glycol is metabolized to glycoaldehyde and finally oxidized to form glycolate and oxalate. These compounds lead to metabolic acidosis and kidney damage. Hence, fomepizole is used for the treatment of ethylene glycol and ethanol poisoning.

Ethylene Glycol and Methanol Poisoning[21,22]

Begin treatment immediately.

Dose

Loading dose of 15 mg/kg, followed by 10 mg/kg 12 hourly for 2 days, followed by 15 mg/kg every 12 hours, until

- Ethylene glycol or methanol concentrations are less than 20 mg/dL *or*
- Patient is asymptomatic
- Acidosis is resolved.

Dose modification in hemodialysis[23] *(Table 6)*

Dose modification in liver disease: Fomepizole is metabolized in the liver. However, no dose modification has been described in hepatic impairment.

Table 6: Dosing schedule of fomepizole in patients on hemodialysis (HD).	
Before	Determine when the last dose was given If given <6 hours: No additional dose required If ≥6 hours: Administer the next dose prior to HD
During	Administer fomepizole every 4 hours *or* Loading dose of 10–20 mg/kg followed by infusion at 1–1.5 mg/kg/hour
After	Determine when the last dose was given Last dose < 1 hour prior to completion—No additional dose Last dose 1–3 hour prior to completion—Administer half the scheduled dose Last dose > 3 hour prior to completion—Administer full scheduled dose after completion Maintenance dose when dialysis is stopped is 10–15 mg/kg every 12 hours.

General Management of Poisoning or Overdose

Role of hemodialysis in toxic alcohol poisoning:
- In severe cases hemodialysis may be required along with antidote. Hemodialysis should be considered as an adjunct to fomepizole.
- Indications of hemodialysis are renal failure, refractory metabolic acidosis and high alcohol concentrations more than 50 mg/dL.

Administration

All IV doses should be administered by slow infusion over 30 minutes. Do not administer as a bolus injection or in undiluted form.

Adverse Effects

- Hypersensitivity to fomepizole or components is contraindication to its use.
- Nausea and headache are common adverse effects.

Pregnancy/Breastfeeding

Pregnancy category C drug. Not known whether it is secreted in breast milk.

FOLIC ACID (VITAMIN B$_9$)

Folic acid is used as a cofactor for various metabolic reactions in the body. It is essential for purine and pyrimidine synthesis, nucleoprotein synthesis, maturation of RBCs and production of WBCs and platelets.

It has an off-label use for methanol poisoning[22] as it increases the metabolism of formic acid to nontoxic metabolites. It is used as an adjunct and should not be used as the sole agent for treatment.

Dose

It can be administered by both IV and oral route.[24]
- *Intravenous:* 50–70 mg every 4 hours
- *Oral:* 50 mg every 3–4 hours
  Continue treatment till both methanol and formic acid are undetectable.
  For dialysis patients administer the dose after completion of dialysis irrespective of timing of last dose.

Administration

- Administered by oral, IV, IM, and SC routes. Oral route preferred.

- Dose less than or equal to 5 mg administered undiluted over more than or equal to 1 minute or dilute in 50 mL of NS or D$_5$W and infuse over 30 minutes.

Pregnancy/Breastfeeding

Folic acid crosses placenta and is present in breast milk. Requirements of folic acid increase during pregnancy and supplementation is necessary.

GLUCAGON

Glucagon is a hormone which increases cyclic AMP production by stimulating adenylate cyclase. This increases glycogenolysis and gluconeogenesis in the liver leading to an increase in blood sugar. It also induces relaxation of smooth muscles especially in the stomach and gut. Glucagon also has a positive chronotropic and inotropic effect in the heart which is mediated by glucagon receptors. This mechanism makes it a treatment option for β-blocker or CCB poisoning induced myocardial depression.[25] It is used as an adjunct in cases not responding to standard therapy.

Dose

A bolus dose of 0.05–0.15 mg/kg (5–10 mg) is given over 1 minute followed by an infusion of 3–5 mg/hour (or 0.05–0.1 mg/kg/hour). Titrate infusion to clinical response and a target mean arterial pressure (MAP) of 65 mm Hg.[12] No hepatic/renal dose adjustments.

It is contraindicated in patients with pheochromocytoma, insulinoma, and glucagonoma. No adverse effect has been reported in pregnancy and breastfeeding.

Pregnancy/Breastfeeding

No reported adverse events. Use with caution.

HIGH-DOSE INSULIN THERAPY

High-dose insulin therapy (HDIT) is used for the treatment of β-blocker and CCB toxicity refractory to standard therapy.[26]

The exact mechanism of action is unknown. Both β-blockers and CCBs interfere with fatty acid metabolism in myocytes. This leads to insulin resistance and glucose dependence for functioning in the myocardial cells. In addition, secretion of insulin from beta cells of pancreas

Box 5: Protocol for high-dose insulin therapy.
High-dose insulin therapy
Bolus dose: 1 unit/kg of regular, short-acting insulin by IV route followed by *Continuous infusion*: 0.5 units/kg/hour IV
Titrate infusion till hypotension is rectified or to a maximum dose of 10 units/kg/hour is reached. Hemodynamic response may be delayed for 30–60 minutes
Maintain euglycemia by a continuous IV infusion of 5–10% dextrose (0.5–1 g of dextrose/kg/hour)
Monitor glucose levels every 15–30 minutes initially and then every 1 hour until several hours after completion of therapy
Monitor potassium levels every 30 minutes initially and then 1–2 hourly. Maintain potassium in low normal range.
Magnesium supplementation may be needed in some cases.

is inhibited. Hence, high-dose insulin is of help in such cases. Since, the dose of insulin administered is very large the risk of hypoglycemia is very high (Box 5).

Pregnancy/Breastfeeding

Insulin is present in breast milk and is detected in cord blood. It is recommended for treatment in pregnant and nursing mothers. Watch for hypoglycemia.

HYDROXOCOBALAMIN

It is a water soluble vitamin used for the treatment of cyanide poisoning. It is a precursor to cyanocobalamin (vitamin B_{12}). Cyanocobalamin acts as a coenzyme for carbohydrate and fat metabolism and protein synthesis. In the presence of cyanide each molecule of hydroxocobalamin binds with one cyanide ion forming cyanocobalamin, which is excreted in urine.[27,28]

Dose

- Single dose 70 mg/kg (maximum 5 g) as an infusion over 15 minutes.
- May repeat an additional dose of 5 g.
- Maximum cumulative dose is 10 g.
- No hepatic/renal dose modifications.
- No contraindications have been reported.

Adverse Effects

Can cause urine and skin discoloration which can persist for up to 5 weeks. Headache and hypertension are commonly reported.

Pregnancy and Breastfeeding

Pregnancy category C. Unknown if secreted in breast milk. Advised to avoid nursing in lieu of unknown adverse effects in infant.

HYPERBARIC OXYGEN

The benefits of hyperbaric oxygen therapy (HBOT) are based on the relationship between volume, pressure and concentration of gas. HBOT helps to increase oxygen content and delivery, reduces the size of gas bubbles, improves wound healing and antagonizes the effects of carbon monoxide poisoning.[29]

Patients are exposed to 100% oxygen under supra-atmospheric conditions. This reduces the half-life of carboxyhemoglobin (COHb), from approximately 90 minutes to approximately 30 minutes and also increases the amount of dissolved oxygen from approximately 0.3–6.0 mL/dL. Thus, oxygen delivery to tissues is increased.

Carbon Monoxide Poisoning[30,31]

No clear-cut recommendation for use of HBOT as evidence is mixed.

The greatest benefit is achieved if administered within 6 hours. Suggested in cases where:
- Carbon monoxide level > 25% or >20% in a pregnant patient
- Metabolic acidosis (pH < 7.1)
- Unconscious or comatose state
- Evidence of end-organ damage.

Dose

The optimal number of treatment sessions, duration and treatment pressure are not clearly defined.

Normally each treatment session consists of administering oxygen at a pressure of 2.5–3 ATM for 60–100 minutes.

Depending on response, further treatment sessions are recommended. The contraindications to the use of HBOT are mentioned in Table 7.

Complications

- Middle ear barotrauma—most common adverse effect
- Sinus squeeze/sinus barotrauma—second most common effect
- Reversible myopia

General Management of Poisoning or Overdose

Table 7: Contraindication to hyperbaric oxygen therapy (HBOT).

Contraindications	
Absolute	*Relative*
Untreated pneumothorax	Obstructive airway diseases
	Asymptomatic pulmonary blebs or bullae on Chest X-ray
	Upper respiratory or sinus infections
	Recent ear surgery
	Recent thoracic surgery
	Uncontrolled fever
	Claustrophobia

- Pulmonary barotrauma—rare
- Oxygen toxicity
- Seizures.

METHYLENE BLUE

It is a phenothiazine derivative used for its vasoplegic and antidotal properties.

Uses[32]

- Methemoglobinemia (drug-induced/acquired)
- Cyanide toxicity
- Ifosfamide-induced encephalopathy
- Vasoplegia syndrome.

Dose

Methemoglobinemia

- 1–2 mg/kg over 5–30 minutes
- Repeat dose after 1 hour, if levels more than 30%
- Glucose-6-phosphate dehydrogenase (G6PD) is essential for methylene blue to function.
- If no response after two doses of methylene blue, do not give more.

  At low concentrations, it accelerates the conversion of methemoglobin to hemoglobin; however, at high concentrations, it has opposite effects.

Ifosfamide-induced Encephalopathy

- Encephalopathy may improve spontaneously and treatment is not always required.
- 50 mg PO every 4–8 hours until symptoms improve.

Vasoplegia

- No validated dosing regimens
- Single dose of 1.5–2 mg/kg over 20–60 minutes, *or*

- Bolus dose of 1 mg/kg followed by an infusion of 0.5–1 mg/kg/hour.
- Methylene blue inhibits nitric oxide synthase and guanylate cyclase enzyme thus increasing vascular tone.

Renal/Hepatic Dose Modifications

No dose modifications.

Administration

Routes: Oral, intravenous (IV):
- IV—administer slowly as undiluted injection over 5–30 minutes. Use only 5% dextrose for dilution. For infusions, always use central line.
- Oral: Administer with juice to mask the taste.
  Topical: Used as a diagnostic aid and is sprayed or applied directly to the affected mucosa.

  Do not administer subcutaneously or intrathecally.

Adverse Effects

- Discoloration of body fluids (urine—blue green)
- Dizziness, chest pain, nausea, and vomiting.

Special Populations

- *G6PD deficiency*: Use with caution or avoid as it can precipitate hemolysis.
- *Concomitant drugs*: Avoid in patients on selective serotonin reuptake inhibitor (SSRI), serotonin and norepinephrine reuptake inhibitors (SNRI), monoamine oxidase inhibitors (MAO) inhibitors as fatal serotonin syndrome may be precipitated.

Pregnancy/Breastfeeding

- Pregnancy category X
- Not known, if secreted in breast milk. Preferable to avoid feeding for up to 8 days after completion of therapy.

NALOXONE

- It is pure opioid antagonist. It is a competitive antagonist of μ, κ, and σ opiate receptors in the central nervous system. It has maximum affinity for μ receptor.
- Used for the treatment of opioid overdose/poisoning.

Antidotes

Dose[33]

- 0.4–2 mg by IV, intramuscular (IM), and subcutaneous (SC) route.
- May repeat dose every 2–3 minutes.
- Use a lower initial dose (0.1–0.2 mg) in patients with opioid dependence to avoid acute withdrawal.
- After reversal, may readminister dose at later intervals (20–60 minutes) depending on the type of opioid.
- If no response is achieved after a total of 10 mg, consider other causes of respiratory depression.
- Endotracheal route (off-label) may be used in some cases. Dose is 2–2.5 times the initial IV dose (i.e. 0.8–5 mg).

Continuous Infusion (Off-label Dosing)[34]

Uses

- Long-acting opioids (e.g. methadone)
- Sustained release product, and
- Symptomatic body packers after initial naloxone response
- Dose is usually two-thirds of the initial effective naloxone dose
- Administer ½ the initial dose to maintain serum levels of naloxone followed by infusion
- Titrate infusion rate to ensure adequate ventilation as well as prevent withdrawal.

Other Routes of Administration

Nebulization

Dilute 3 mg of naloxone with 3 mg of normal saline for nebulization. The usual nebulization masks are used.

Intranasal Spray

- Place the patient in the supine position
- Tilt the head back
- Alternate nostrils with each dose
- Turn patient sideways after administration
- Each container contains a single intranasal spray, do not reuse
- Use a new container with each administration.

Renal/Hepatic Dose Modification

No renal or hepatic dose modifications.

Pregnancy/Breastfeeding

- Pregnancy category C. Naloxone is not recommended in pregnant women except is life-threatening emergency as it crosses the placenta and may precipitate opioid withdrawal in the fetus.
- Unknown, if naloxone is secreted in breast milk. However, opioids may be present in breast milk and may be transferred to the nursing infant.

PENICILLAMINE

It is a chelating agent, which forms soluble complexes with lead, copper, mercury, and other heavy metals. These complexes are excreted in urine. Penicillamine is not US-FDA approved for lead chelation therapy. It is no longer recommended for arsenic or mercury toxicity.[35]

It is recommended for chelation in the treatment of lead poisoning as third-line agent.

Lead Poisoning

Dose

- Chelation therapy indicated, if blood lead level is more than 45 µg/dL in children and more than 70 µg/dL in adults.
- *Oral*: 900–1,500 mg/day in three divided doses for 1–2 weeks, then 750 mg/day.
- Start with a small dose and increase it gradually.
- Continue treatment till blood lead concentrations are less than 60 µg/dL or urinary lead excretion less than 500 µg/L for 2 consecutive months.

Renal/Hepatic Dose Modification

- Dose adjustment required in renal impairment. Avoid if creatinine clearance (CrCl < 50 mL/min). Penicillamine is dialyzable. In chronic kidney disease, dose reduction to 250 mg three times per week is advisable.
- No hepatic dose modification.

Administration

- Oral doses less than or equal to 500 mg may be administered as a single dose
- Doses more than 500 mg should be given in divided doses

General Management of Poisoning or Overdose

- Administer on an empty stomach (1 hour before or 2 hours after meals) and do not administer with other drugs, milk, antacids, and zinc-containing products or at least 2 hours apart from iron-containing products.

Adverse Effects

- High rate of adverse reactions of 33%.
- Reactions include nausea, vomiting, leukopenia, thrombocytopenia, aplastic anemia, nephrotic syndrome, proteinuria, incontinence, teratogenicity.

Pregnancy/Breastfeeding

Pregnancy category D. Birth defects (congenital cutis laxa) have been reported. Unknown if secreted in breast milk. Contraindicated during feeding.

PHYSOSTIGMINE

It is an inhibitor of the enzyme acetylcholinesterase thereby potentiating the effects of acetylcholine. It is used for reversing the effects of anticholinergic toxidrome.[36]

Dose

Dose is 0.5–2 mg. Administer as a slow IV push no faster than 1 mg/min. May repeat every 10–30 minutes to achieve adequate response. It may be given by intramuscular route.

Rapid administration can lead to bradycardia, respiratory distress, or seizures.

Renal/Hepatic Dose Modification

No dose modification.

Contraindications

- Gastrointestinal or genitourinary obstruction
- Asthma
- Gangrene
- Cardiovascular disease
- Coadministration of choline esters and depolarizing neuromuscular-blocking agents (e.g. succinylcholine).

Adverse Effects

It may cause cholinergic side effects—salivation, lacrimation, urination, diaphoresis, emesis, bronchorrhea.

Pregnancy/Breastfeeding

May be used in pregnant, if benefits outweigh risks. Unknown, if secreted in breast milk.

PHYTONADIONE (VITAMIN K₁)

It is a fat-soluble vitamin, which promotes the synthesis of clotting factors (II, VII, IX, and X) in the liver.

Indications

- Warfarin toxicity leading to coagulopathy
- Intracranial hemorrhage in association with vitamin K antagonists
- Hypoprothrombinemia.

Warfarin Toxicity

Dose:
Usual doses are 2.5–10 mg given by oral or intravenous route as a single dose. Dose may be repeated in 12–48 hours based on INR values. Anticoagulation reversal begins within 4–6 hours after intravenous administration and about 24 hours after oral administration. Dosing regimens may be based on the levels of INR and the presence or absence of bleeding (Table 8).

Intracranial Hemorrhage in Association with Vitamin K Antagonists (Off-label Use)

- Intravenous vitamin K 10 mg and four factor PCC, if INR more than 1.4
- Monitor INR levels. If values more than or equal to 1.4 within 24–48 hours a repeat dose of Vitamin K (10 mg) is given.[39]

Hypoprothrombinemia Secondary to Drugs (Other than Coumarin Derivatives) or Factors-limiting Absorption or Synthesis

- *Oral*: 2.5–25 mg (rarely up to 50 mg)
- *Intravenous*: Initial: 2.5–25 mg (rarely up to 50 mg). Measure INR after 6–8 hours and repeat dose, if needed.
- *Coagulopathy secondary to acute liver failure*: IV vitamin K 5–10 mg (at least one dose).[40]

Anticoagulant Rodenticide Poisoning[41]

- High doses of vitamin K are administered.
- In adults, 25–50 mg is administered PO two to four times per day. In children, 0.4 mg/kg per dose is administered two to four times per day.

Table 8: Dosing regimens for vitamin K based on international normalized ratio (INR) levels and evidence of bleeding.

INR and bleeding	Dose
<4.5 No bleeding	Hold next dose of warfarin Frequently monitor INR Restart warfarin at a low dose when INR is near normal range[37]
4.5–10 No bleeding	Hold warfarin Against routine use of vitamin K as per ACCP guidelines (2012)[38] Monitor INR frequently Some recommend a low dose of vitamin K (oral 1–2.5 mg), if risk factors for bleeding are present
INR > 10 No bleeding	Hold warfarin Administer oral vitamin K (dose not specific but 2.5–10 mg may be given) as per the 2012 ACCP guidelines Monitor INR and give additional vitamin K as necessary (Hirsh, 2008)
If minor bleeding at any INR elevation	Hold warfarin Administer vitamin K 2.5–5 mg PO Monitor INR Repeat doses may be necessary, if INR correction is incomplete
If major bleeding at any INR elevation	Administer IV vitamin K 5–10 mg and four factor Prothrombin complex concentrate (PCC) as per 2012 ACCP guidelines Hold warfarin

(ACCP: American College of Chest Physicians)

- INR levels are monitored 6–8 hourly and repeat doses are administered based on values.
- Alternatively, IV 10 mg two to four times per day is administered in those unable to take oral medication.

Note: High doses of vitamin K (>10 mg) lead to warfarin resistance for more than 1 week. During this time period, heparin (UFH or LMWH) may be needed till the INR responds.[42]

Administration

Oral route is preferred. If parenteral routes are used, intravenous route is preferred. Subcutaneous and intramuscular routes are not commonly used.

Intravenous administration should be slow with infusion not exceeding 1 mg/min. If dilution is required, it should be done in 50 mL normal saline and given via infusion pump over at least 20 minutes. No renal or hepatic dose modifications. Use with caution in patients on mechanical heart valves.

Adverse Effects

Chest pain, flushing, tachycardia, hypotension, dizziness, and anaphylactoid reaction.

Specific Concerns

- *Aluminum toxicity*: Certain parenteral forms contain aluminum, which may accumulate in patients with renal dysfunction or those receiving high doses of vitamin K. Premature neonates are at high risk. High-aluminum exposures of more than 4–5 µg/kg/day leads to neurological and bone toxicity.
- *Benzyl alcohol and derivatives*: Certain preparations contain benzyl alcohol, which in large amounts (≥99 mg/kg/day) have been associated with a fatal "gasping syndrome" especially in neonates. The "gasping syndrome" consists of abnormal respirations (gasping), metabolic acidosis, neurological dysfunction (convulsions, intracranial hemorrhage), hypotension, and cardiovascular collapse.[43]
- *Polyoxyethylated castor oil*: Can lead to hypersensitivity reactions.
- *Polysorbate 80 (Tweens)*: Can cause delayed hypersensitivity reactions in certain individuals.

Thrombocytopenia, pulmonary dysfunction, and kidney and hepatic failure have been reported in premature neonates.

Pregnancy/Breastfeeding

Vitamin K crosses placenta and is present in breast milk. The dietary requirements are same for pregnant and nonpregnant and breastfeeding and nonbreastfeeding women. It is advisable to use preservative-free preparations in breastfeeding women.

PRALIDOXIME (2-PAM)

It is used for the treatment of organophosphate poisoning. It reactivates the enzyme cholinesterase that had been rendered inactivated by organophosphate compound. It removes the phosphoryl group from the active site of the enzyme thus reactivating cholinesterase activity.

Organophosphate Poisoning

Always administered in conjunction with atropine. Response to atropine needs to be established before

General Management of Poisoning or Overdose

Table 9: Dosing regimen for organophosphate (OP) poisoning.	
Intravenous route:[44-46] Loading dose: 30 mg/kg (maximum: 2,000 mg) or 2,000 mg to be administered over 15–30 minutes followed by: Maintenance dose of 8–10 mg/kg/hour (maximum: 650 mg/hour or 500 mg/hour) Rate not to exceed 200 mg/min	Intramuscular route: Depending on the symptoms, 600 mg is administered by IM route Doses are repeated every 15 minutes to a maximum of 1,800 mg

administering PAM. Dosing regimen is discussed in Table 9.

Adverse Effects

- Tachycardia, hypertension, cardiac arrest, dizziness, drowsiness, and apnea.
- No absolute contraindications to its use.

Special Situations

- *Carbamate poisoning*: PAM is *not* indicated for carbamate poisoning as acetylcholinesterase is weakly affected by carbamates.
- *Nonanticholinesterase poisoning*: PAM is *not* indicated for the treatment of poisoning with substances (phosphorus, inorganic phosphates, or organophosphates) without anticholinesterase activity.
- *Myasthenia gravis*: Use with caution as it may precipitate a myasthenic crisis.
- *Renal dysfunction*: Use with caution in patients with renal impairment; dosage modification is required.

Pregnancy/Breastfeeding

Pregnancy category C. Unknown, if secreted in breast milk. Use with caution.

PROTAMINE SULFATE

Protamine is a positively charged alkaline molecule while heparin is a negatively charged strongly acidic molecule. Protamine forms a stable complex with heparin with no anticoagulant activity. However, it only partially reverses the antifactor Xa activity in the presence of LMWH. It is important to emphasize that at high doses, protamine itself has a weak anticoagulant activity.[47]

Uses

- Heparin/LMWH overdose
- Neutralization of heparin
- Intracranial hemorrhage associated with heparin/LMWH.

Heparin Overdose

One mg of protamine neutralizes 100 units of unfractionated heparin. Amount of protamine to be administered depends upon the time elapsed since heparin administration. Table 10 describes the dose of protamine needed for heparin overdose with respect to time of administration.

Low-molecular-weight Heparin Overdose

Protamine does not completely neutralize factor Xa activity (maximum 60–75%). The doses of protamine to neutralize various formulations of LMWH are described in Box 6.

Table 10: Neutralization dose of protamine for intravenous (IV) heparin overdosage.[48]	
Time since administration	Dose of protamine (mg) to neutralize 100 units of heparin
Immediate	1–1.5
30–60 minutes	0.5–0.75
>2 hours	0.25–0.375

Box 6: Neutralization dose of protamine for low-molecular-weight heparins.

Enoxaparin:
- Less than or equal to 8 hours—1 mg protamine for 1 mg enoxaparin
- More than 8 hours or if aPTT is prolonged after 2–4 hours of the first dose—0.5 mg of protamine for every 1 mg of enoxaparin administered

Dalteparin/tinzaparin:
- 1 mg protamine for each 100 anti-Xa units of dalteparin or tinzaparin
- If PTT prolonged after 2–4 hours of the first dose or in cases with persistent bleeding: Repeat dose of 0.5 mg for each 100 anti-Xa units of dalteparin or tinzaparin

(aPTT: activated partial thromboplastin time; PTT: partial thromboplastin time)

Intracranial Hemorrhage Associated with Heparin/LMWH

Recommendations from the Neurocritical Care Society/Society of Critical Care Medicine (NCS/SCCM):[39]

Unfractionated heparin-mediated:

- One mg protamine for every 100 units of heparin administered in the previous 2–3 hours; maximum single dose is 50 mg.
- A repeat dose of 0.5 mg protamine for every 100 units of heparin, if aPTT is prolonged after 2–4 hours
- Also reverse prophylactic SC heparin when aPTT is prolonged.

LMWH-mediated (full therapeutic dose):

- LMWH for prophylaxis (i.e. not a full therapeutic dose), the NCS/SCCM guidelines suggest against reversal.
- Dose is same as mentioned in Box 6.

Unknown amount of heparin:

Neutralization is based on the activated coagulation time (ACT) (Table 11).

Administration

Only for IV use. Administer by slow IV infusion (50 mg over 10 minutes). Rapid infusion can cause hypotension. No renal or hepatic dose modifications.

Adverse Effects

- *Hypersensitivity reactions*: Hypotension, cardiovascular collapse, noncardiogenic pulmonary edema, pulmonary vasoconstriction, and pulmonary hypertension. Patients with diabetes on neutral protamine Hagedorn (NPH) insulin are at high risk. Other risk factors include high doses of protamine, fish allergy, and severe left ventricular dysfunction.

Table 11: Neutralization dose of protamine based on activated coagulation time (ACT) for unknown quantity of heparin administered.

ACT	Dose
≤150 seconds	No protamine
300–500 seconds	Dose of 1.2 mg/kg protamine IV (maximum 50 mg) over 15 minutes
ACT is not available, and time of administration is unknown	Administer 25–50 mg protamine IV as an initial dose (maximum 50 mg) Monitor aPTT levels frequently

(aPTT: activated partial thromboplastin time)

- Heparin rebound associated with bleeding has been reported. Typically seen after 8–9 hours of protamine administration.
- *Infusion-related reactions*: Rapid administration can cause hypotension and anaphylactoid reactions.

Pregnancy/Breastfeeding

- Pregnancy category C. Unknown, if secreted in breast milk. Use with caution.

PYRIDOXINE (VITAMIN B₆)

It is a water soluble vitamin. It is essential for protein, fat, and carbohydrate metabolism, synthesis of GABA in CNS and release of glycogen from storage sites.[49]

Indications

- Isoniazid-induced seizures
- Ethylene glycol poisoning
- False morel toxicity.

Isoniazid-induced Seizures[50]

Dose of pyridoxine is equal to the amount of isoniazid ingested. Maximum dose of pyridoxine is 5 g. The calculated dose is administered at the rate of 0.5-1 g/min till seizures stop or maximum dose is reached. If seizures stop before the total dose is administered then the remaining dose can be administered over 4–6 hours. A repeat dose may be administered after 5–10 minutes, if seizures persist. If amount of isoniazid ingested is unknown then 5 g is administered at 0.5–1 g/min.

Ethylene Glycol Toxicity

Pyridoxine is used as an adjunct and is not the sole therapy. The mechanism of benefit is unclear but pyridoxine is said to increase the formation of glycine, which is a nontoxic metabolite. Dose is 100 mg/day till clinical features of toxicity abate.

False Morel Toxicity[51]

They are gyromitrin-containing mushrooms, which can lead to seizures. Pyridoxine is administered at 25 mg/kg over 15–30 minutes. Repeat doses may be needed, if seizures persist.

Administration

Administered by oral and parenteral routes (IV and IM). Parenteral routes are preferred in acute toxicity. No renal or hepatic dose modification.

Adverse Effects

- *Peripheral neuropathy*: Long-term administration with doses more than 2 g/day.
- Hypersensitivity reactions
- Ataxia, paresthesias
- *Aluminum toxicity*: Parenteral preparations contain aluminum, which can lead to aluminum toxicity.

Pregnancy/Breastfeeding

Pregnancy category A and is present in breast milk. Maternal requirements increase during pregnancy and breastfeeding.

SODIUM NITRITE

- Used for the treatment of cyanide poisoning.[28,52]
- Sodium nitrite promotes the formation of methemoglobin, which combines with the cyanide ion to form cyanomethemoglobin. Thus, cytochrome oxidase if free for aerobic metabolism to continue.

Dose

- Sodium nitrite is given in conjunction with sodium thiosulfate.
- Always administer sodium nitrite first.
- Usual dose is 0.2 mL/kg (usually 300 mg; 10 mL of a 3% solution).

Since administration of sodium nitrite causes methemoglobinemia, some authorities suggest dosing based on hemoglobin levels, especially in patients with pre-existing comorbidities, wherein oxygen delivery is hampered. Such cases include and are not restricted to ischemic heart disease, cardiomyopathies, chronic lung diseases, etc.

Table 12 is used for dose calculation based on hemoglobin levels.[53]

If symptoms of cyanide toxicity recur, half the original dose of sodium nitrite and sodium thiosulfate can be administered.

Monitor for methemoglobin levels. If levels exceed 30% withhold sodium nitrite.

Table 12: Dose on sodium nitrite solution based on hemoglobin levels.

Hemoglobin level (g/dL)	Dose (3% sodium nitrite solution)
7	0.19
8	0.22
9	0.25
10	0.27
11	0.3
12	0.33
13	0.36
14	0.39

Administration

Administered as a slow IV injection (2.5–5 mL/min) followed by immediate administration of sodium thiosulfate. Slow the infusion rate if hypotension occurs.

Special Cases

- *Anemia*: Anemic patients tend to form more methemoglobin. Dose reduction is required. Refer to Table 12 for appropriate doses.
- *Glucose-6-phosphate dehydrogenase deficiency*: Sodium nitrite can lead to hemolysis in G6PD patients. Alternative treatment options may need to be explored. Monitor for an acute drop in hemoglobin and hematocrit. Exchange transfusion may be required.
- *Renal impairment*: Sodium nitrite is excreted renally. Risk for adverse events may be increased.
- *Elderly*: Use cautiously as they usually have decreased renal function.
- *Fire victims*: Fire victims may present with both cyanide and carbon monoxide poisoning. Administration of sodium nitrite in such cases may worsen tissue hypoxia by promoting methemoglobinemia, which decreases the O_2-carrying capacity of hemoglobin. Hydroxocobalamin is the agent of choice in such cases for cyanide toxicity. Sodium nitrite (and methemoglobinemia induction) is contraindicated till carbon monoxide levels decline to normal levels. Sodium thiosulfate may be used alone for cyanide toxicity but hydroxocobalamin is preferred.

Adverse Effects

- Hypotension can occur during administration. Maintain euvolemia.
- Methemoglobinemia.

Pregnancy/Breastfeeding

- Pregnancy category C. Teratogenic effects have been observed. Fetal methemoglobin reductase levels are lower than that in adults and hence they are at increased risk of nitrite-induced prenatal hypoxia.
- Unknown, if sodium nitrite is excreted in breast milk. Use with caution.

Note: Sodium nitrite is also used for hydrogen sulfide poisoning as an off-label medication. The dose remains the same as previously mentioned for cyanide poisoning.

SODIUM THIOSULFATE

Sodium thiosulfate is used in conjunction with sodium nitrite for cyanide poisoning. It serves as a sulfur donor for the formation of thiocyanate. Thiocyanate is less toxic than cyanide.[28,52]

Dose

- Administered immediately after sodium nitrite
- Dose is 12.5 g (25% solution). Half the dose may be repeated, if symptoms recur
- The total dose is administered by slow IV infusion over 10–30 minutes. Infusion rate may need to be decreased, if hypotension occurs.
- No hepatic or renal dose modifications. Use with caution in patients with renal dysfunction as risk of adverse events is increased.

Adverse Effects

Hypotension can occur with rapid administration. Nausea, vomiting, altered sensorium, and prolonged bleeding time have been reported. No absolute contraindications to its use. Hypersensitivity to sulfite should not preclude its use.

Pregnancy/Breastfeeding

Pregnancy category C. No teratogenic effect has been reported in animal studies. Unknown, if excreted in breast milk. Use with caution.

SUCCIMER [DIMERCAPTOSUCCINIC ACID (DMSA)]

Succimer is an analog of dimercaprol. Succimer binds to heavy metals to form water-soluble chelates, which are easily excreted renally.

It is used for lead poisoning in adults, mercury, and arsenic poisoning.[13,54] (*Note*: All indications are off label). Off-label treatment decisions should be made after consultation with a toxicologist and on a case-by-case basis.

Dose

- Lead poisoning (adults)
- Treat, if lead levels more than 50 µg/dL with symptoms, or
- Levels more than or equal to 100 µg/dL with/without symptoms
- Available only as oral capsule
- Dose for adults is not clearly defined
- 10 mg/kg/dose (maximum 500 mg) may be used. Administer 500 mg TDS for 5 days followed by 500 mg BD for 14 days
- Lead may be released from storage sites leading to a rebound increase in the blood levels and subsequent toxicity
- Succimer may be repeated, but at a 2-week interval.

There are no recommended dosing regimens for arsenic and mercury poisoning. The same treatment course for lead poisoning may be used.

No dose modifications in renal impairment. However, succimer is dialyzable but the chelates are not. No hepatic dose modification required. In patients with history of or pre-existing liver disease, liver function test may need to be monitored frequently due to risk of transaminitis.

Dose modification is required in cases of succimer toxicity leading to neutropenia. If absolute neutrophil count is less than 1,200 mm^3, succimer should not be administered. Succimer may be re-initiated cautiously once ANC is more than 1,500 mm^3.

Administration

It is available only in capsule form. If patient is unable to swallow the capsule, the contents can be sprinkled on food or mixed with a fruit drink.

Adverse Effects

- Raised hepatic transaminases
- Arrhythmias
- Neutropenia.

Pregnancy/Breastfeeding

Adverse events were observed in animal reproduction studies. Unknown, if excreted in breast milk. Use with caution.

SILYMARIN

Silymarin and silibinin are flavonoids. Their exact mechanism of action is unknown.[55] They have antioxidant properties and regulate the intracellular levels of glutathione. They have membrane stabilizing properties, which prevent hepatotoxic substances from entering hepatocytes. They also stimulate rRNA synthesis-induced liver regeneration and inhibit transformation of stellate cells into myofibroblasts and subsequent fibrosis and cirrhosis. Free radical scavenging is said to be the key player among the above mechanisms.

Uses

Hepatotoxicity secondary to:
- Mushroom poisoning (Amanita phalloides)
- Ethanol
- Paracetamol
- Carbon tetrachloride.

Amanita Phalloides (Mushroom Poisoning)

Silymarin prevents amanitin (toxic principle) from entering the hepatocytes and thus has hepatoprotective effects. It also inhibits the effects of tumor necrosis factor and lipid peroxidation.

Dose

Doses range from 280 mg/day to 800 mg/day. Exact doses have not been studied. Suggested dose is 140 mg three times/day.

Adverse Effects

- Allergic reactions, anaphylaxis, abdominal pain, bloating, rash, and pruritis.

- Use with caution or avoid in patients with hypersensitivity to chrysanthemums, daisies, marigolds, etc.

Pregnancy/Breastfeeding

Pregnancy category is unknown. Not known whether secreted in breast milk.

SODIUM BICARBONATE

Sodium bicarbonate diffuses to sodium and bicarbonate ion. The bicarbonate ion neutralizes hydrogen ion raising blood and urinary pH.

Uses

- Tricyclic antidepressants (TCA) poisoning/toxicity
- Salicylate poisoning/toxicity
- Methotrexate toxicity
- Toxic alcohol poisoning.

TCA Poisoning/Toxicity[56]

Indicated with:
- Hypotension
- Widened QRS complex more than 100 ms
- Ventricular arrhythmia.

Probable benefit is secondary to increase in blood pH levels and extracellular sodium concentrations. Alkalosis prevents drug (TCA) dissociation and thus prevents binding to sodium channels. Also, increase in extracellular sodium increases the electrochemical gradient across cardiac cell membranes and thus attenuates TCA-induced blockade of sodium channels.

Dose:
- Sodium bicarbonate 1–2 mEq/kg
- Given by rapid IV administration.

One approach used is administration of 150 mL of 8.4% sodium bicarbonate as a bolus. Depending on the response, the dose may be repeated after 5 minutes.

Continuous ECG monitoring is mandatory during therapy to look for narrowing of QRS complex, reduced amplitude of R wave in lead aVR and resolution of arrhythmia. Once QRS complex narrows, a continuous infusion is started. 150 mEq of $NaHCO_3$ is mixed with 1 L of 5% dextrose and started at 250 mL/hour. Sodium bicarbonate therapy is tapered when ECG changes resolve, which may take days to weeks. It is suggested

Antidotes 53

Chapter 4

to taper infusion rate by 25% every hour for 4 hours and monitor for widening of QRS complex. In case QRS widens administer a bolus dose followed by original infusion rate.

Monitor arterial blood pH levels (goal 7.5–7.55). Watch for hypernatremia, fluid overload, metabolic alkalosis, and hypokalemia.

Salicylate Poisoning[57]

Alkalinization therapy (both serum and urine) is the mainstay of treatment of salicylate poisoning.

Salicylic acid is a weak acid, which dissociates at equilibrium to form hydrogen ion and salicylate ion:

$$H^+ + Sal^- \leftrightarrow HSal$$

Alkalosis shifts the equation to the left thus reducing salicylic acid levels. As plasma salicylic acid levels reduce, the salicylic acid in the brain diffuses down the concentration gradient into the extracellular fluid. As CNS levels reduce, the equation shifts to the right further forming salicylic acid. This further diffuses down the concentration gradient attenuating the toxic effects of salicylic acid. Urine alkalinization also increases tubular excretion.

Dose:
- Bolus dose 1–2 mEq/kg followed by infusion
- For infusion, dilute 150 mEq of sodium bicarbonate in 1 L of 5% dextrose and initiate at around 150–250 mL/hour. Titrate infusion rate to target a urine pH of 7.5–8 and a serum pH of 7.50–7.55.

Note: Respiratory alkalosis is not a contraindication to alkalinization therapy.

Alkalinization is discontinued when:
- Serum salicylate levels less than 40 mg/dL
- Metabolic acidosis is resolved
- Symptoms resolved with normal respiratory rate and effort
- Monitor ABG and serum salicylate levels every 1–2 hours and urine pH every 1 hour after discontinuation of alkalinization.

Methotrexate Toxicity

Methotrexate precipitates in acidic urine. Alkalinization increases solubility and prevents precipitation in renal tubules.

Sodium bicarbonate (150 mEq in 1 L of 5% dextrose) is started at an infusion of 125–150 mL/hour. Target urine pH more than 7. Sodium bicarbonate may be administered by IV bolus at 1 mEq/kg every 4–6 hours or as oral tablets (650 mg) 2–5 tablets every 2–4 hours.

Toxic Alcohol (Methanol and Ethylene Glycol) Poisoning:[21,22] Sodium bicarbonate may be used to treat refractory life-threatening metabolic acidosis. It may help to improve hemodynamic parameters but is used only as an adjunct and as a short term rescue therapy. Dose is 1 mEq/kg IV bolus. Dose is repeated depending on blood pH levels.

LEUCOVORIN (FOLINIC ACID)

Leucovorin calcium is the reduced form of folic acid. It restores folate stores by competing with methotrexate for transport sites and intracellular binding sites.

Indications

- Methotrexate toxicity
- Methanol poisoning.

Methotrexate Toxicity[58]

- Dose is equal to or more than the dose of methotrexate.
- Usual dose is 10–25 mg/m² 6 hourly
- Higher doses (100 mg/m² 3–6 hourly) are used in the following cases:
  ○ Serum creatinine increase more than 50% at 24 hours post-MTX administration
  ○ 24 hour MTX level more than 5 micromolar
  ○ 48 hour MTX level more than 0.9 micromolar.

Goal is to increase serum concentration of leucovorin higher than MTX and reduce MTX level less than 0.01 micromolar.

Methanol Toxicity[21]

Formic acid is the toxic metabolite in methanol poisoning. 10-tetrahydrofolate dehydrogenase metabolizes formic acid to carbon dioxide and water. Leucovorin serves as a source of tetrahydrofolate thus helping in eliminating formic acid.

Dose is 1 mg/kg IV (maximum 50 mg) every 4–6 hours. It is administered over ½ to 1 hour.

Administration

- Administered by IM and IV routes. Oral preparations are also available. Never to be administered intrathecally. Never to be administered concurrently

General Management of Poisoning or Overdose

with MTX. It is usually started 24 hours after MTX administration. Due to calcium content never to infuse at a rate faster than 160 mg/min.
- No hepatic or renal dose modification.
- Contraindicated in pernicious anemia and vitamin B$_{12}$ deficiency states.

Pregnancy/Breastfeeding

Pregnancy category C. Leucovorin is the active form of folate and is routinely recommended in pregnancy and breastfeeding.

LEVOCARNITINE

Levocarnitine is a dietary supplement, which works as a carrier molecule for long-chain fatty acids (LCFA) in the mitochondria. It is principally used for the treatment of carnitine deficiency. One off-label use is acute valproic acid toxicity.[59] The exact mechanism of action in valproic acid toxicity is unknown but it is said to increase beta-oxidation of valproic acid whereby toxic metabolite and ammonia production decrease.

Dose[60,61]

- *Bolus dose*: 100 mg/kg IV followed by
- *Infusion*: 50 mg/kg to be infused over 30 minutes every 8 hours
- Continue therapy till ammonia levels decrease or patient shows clinical improvement.
- In some studies, lower maintenance doses of 15 mg/kg every 4–6 hours have been used.

Administration

- Available as oral solution and IV preparation.
- *Oral solution*: Only for oral use. Consume slowly after dissolution in a drink. Administer doses every 3–4 hours. This route is not usually used for acute valproic acid toxicity.
- *Parenteral preparation*: IV preparation to be administered either as a bolus or slowly over 15–30 minutes.
- For hemodialysis patients administer after each dialysis session in the venous return line.
- No renal or hepatic dose modification for oral/ IV carnitine. Use with caution.

Adverse Effects

- Hypersensitivity reactions to both oral and IV formulations, especially in dialysis patients.
- Use with caution in patients with seizures as it can precipitate seizures.

Pregnancy/Breastfeeding

No teratogenic effects observed in animal studies. Use with caution.

OCTREOTIDE

It is a somatostatin analog, which mimics endogenous somatostatin. It inhibits the secretion of serotonin, gastrin, VIP, insulin, secretin, motilin and pancreatic polypeptide.

Uses

- Acromegaly
- Carcinoid
- VIPomas
- Diarrhea (chemotherapy induced)
- *Decompensated chronic liver disease*: Esophageal varices, hepatorenal syndrome
- Sulfonylurea-induced hypoglycemia.

Sulfonylurea-induced Hypoglycemia

The exact indications and the dosage are not clearly defined. However, it is used in patients when hypoglycemia is not responding to standard therapy with dextrose.[62,63]

Dose:
- *SC*: Administer 50 µg every 6 hours. Repeat doses on the basis of blood glucose concentrations.
- *IV*: A bolus dose of 50 µg is given, infusions up to 125 µg/hour have been used
- Levels of octreotide peak in about 1 hour. Always administer glucose with octreotide
- Monitor blood sugar levels and for symptoms of hypoglycemia after stopping octreotide for at least 24 hours
- No role in hypoglycemia secondary to biguanides (metformin) and insulin.

Administration

- It is administered by subcutaneous (SC), intravenous push (over 3 minutes), and intravenous infusion (over

15–30 minutes) routes. Only in emergency situations, it is administered as IV bolus. For SC administration, use the smallest quantity and rotate the injection site.
- Administer injection only after bringing to room temperature.
- No renal dose adjustments. However, in patients on dialysis, the clearance of octreotide is reduced by 50% and dose modification may be needed. No hepatic dose adjustments but the half-life (t1/2) and clearance are reduced in cirrhotics.

Adverse Effects

- Hypersensitivity reactions
- Hypothyroidism—suppresses thyroid-stimulating hormone (TSH) secretion.
- Pancreatitis—alters absorption of fats
- Sinus bradycardia, palpitations, and chest pain
- Abdominal pain, dyspepsia, and bloating
- Abnormal Schilling's test—with long-term use.

Pregnancy/Breastfeeding

Pregnancy category B. Octreotide crosses placenta and is present in breast milk. No teratogenic effects reported from use in case reports. The Endocrine Society suggests using short-acting octreotide prior to planned pregnancy. Avoid long-acting and depot formulations.

THIAMINE (VITAMIN B$_1$)

It is a water-soluble vitamin, which is essential for carbohydrate metabolism.

Indications[64,65]

- Wernicke's encephalopathy
- Thiamine deficiency (Beriberi)
- Ethylene glycol toxicity.

Wernicke's Encephalopathy

- High-dose IV thiamine (200–500 thrice daily) for 7 days followed by
- 250 mg IV/IM once per day for 3–5 days followed by
- Oral thiamine 30 mg twice per day or 100 mg/day for 7–14 days followed by
- 100 mg orally once daily.
- Always administer thiamine prior to parenteral glucose.

Ethylene Glycol Toxicity

- IV thiamine 100 mg once a day till signs and symptoms of toxicity resolve
- It is used as an adjunct and is not the sole form of therapy
- In ethylene glycol toxicity, thiamine is said to increase the formation of glycine, which is a nontoxic metabolite.

Administration

It is available in oral and parenteral forms. Parenteral forms are administered by IV or IM routes. For doses up to 100 mg, administer over 5 minutes while for doses exceeding 100 mg extended infusion times are preferred. Preferable to administer in large proximal veins to prevent local injection reactions. No renal or hepatic dose modifications.

Adverse Effects

- Hypersensitivity reactions, anaphylaxis, angioedema.
- Flushing, restlessness.
  Note: Thiamine should always be administered before dextrose or symptoms of acute thiamine deficiency may be precipitated.

Pregnancy/Breastfeeding

Pregnancy category A. Being water soluble, it crosses placenta and is also present in breast milk.

POTASSIUM IODIDE

It is used an antidote during nuclear radiation emergencies for thyroid block. It blocks the uptake of radioactive iodine by the thyroid gland and thereby reduces the risk of thyroid cancer.

Dose[66]

- Oral potassium iodide 130 mg per day for 10–14 days or as directed by public officials.
- It may have to be continued till the risk of exposure has reduced or other safety measures have been instituted.
- It is also to be administered to pregnant and lactating women. However, use the lowest possible dose due to risk of hypothyroidism in the neonate.

General Management of Poisoning or Overdose

> **Box 7:** Dosing regimen for potassium iodide.
>
> *Dose based on age and weight:*
>
> - *Children > 12 years and adolescents weighing ≥ 68 kg*: 130 mg once daily
> - *Children > 12 years and adolescents weighing < 68 kg*: 65 mg once daily
> - *Children > 3 to ≤ 12 years*: 65 mg once daily
> - *Infants > 1 month to children ≤ 3 years*: 32.5 mg once daily
> - *Infants ≤ 1 month*: 16.25 mg once daily

- Most efficacious when administered with 3–4 hours of exposure. Efficacy decreases by 50% after 6 hours of exposure.
- Monitor thyroid function tests, especially in pregnant, nursing mothers, neonate, and infants, if more than one dose is administered (Box 7).

Administration

Available as oral tablet or solution. Dilute with water, juice, or milk. Maximum one dose in 24 hours. No renal or hepatic dose modification.

Adverse Effects

- Hypersensitivity reactions to iodide
- Acne, dermatitis
- Hypothyroidism (with prolonged use).

Contraindications

- Iodine allergy
- Vasculitis with hypocomplementemia
- Dermatitis herpetiformis
- Nodular thyroid disease.

Pregnancy/Breastfeeding

Pregnancy category D. It is secreted in breast milk. Use with caution only in consultation with a medical toxicologist or as directed by public officials.

ANTI-SNAKE VENOM (ASV)

Antivenom is the mainstay of therapy in patients with life-threatening envenomation. It neutralizes the circulating venom in the body. Antivenin consists of immunoglobulins developed against whole venom. They are of two types, i.e. monovalent and polyvalent. Monovalent antivenoms act against a single species while polyvalent antivenins act against various species, which are usually confined to a geographical area. In India, only polyvalent ASV is available, which is used against cobra, Indian common krait, Russell's viper, and Saw-scaled viper. Each mL neutralizes 0.6 mg of dried Indian cobra venom, 0.45 mg of dried common krait venom, 0.6 mg of dried Russell's, and 0.45 mg dried Saw-scaled viper.

Indications (Box 8)

Confirmed or suspected snake bite with signs and symptoms of envenomation.

Dose

- Dose is dependent on the species.
- No difference in dose between adults and children.
- If the species can be identified and the respective ASV is available then it is preferable to administer the monovalent ASV.
- Due to lack of clinical trials, the exact dose is not determined. WHO has recommended the initial dose should be 10 vials (of Indian polyvalent ASV)

> **Box 8:** Indications of anti-snake venom (ASV) in life-threatening envenomation.
>
> | **Systemic envenomation** |
> | --- |
> | *Hematological:*
• Spontaneous systemic bleeding
• Coagulopathy
[Deranged 20 minute whole blood clotting time (WBCT) or prothrombin time], or
Thrombocytopenia (<100,000/mm^3) |
> | *Neurological:* Ptosis, external ophthalmoplegia, and paralysis |
> | *Cardiovascular:*
• Hypotension, shock, arrhythmias
• Renal
• Acute kidney injury presenting as oliguria/anuria, azotemia, uremia
• Hemoglobinuria
• Myoglobinuria
• Rhabdomyolysis |
> | **Local envenomation** |
> | • Local swelling involving more than half of the limb (in the absence of a tourniquet) within 48 hours of the bite
• Swelling after bites on the digits
• Rapid extension of swelling within a few hours of bite on the hands or feet
• Enlarged tender lymph node draining the bitten limb |

- For vasculotoxic snake bites, doses may need to be repeated depending on the whole blood clotting time. For neuroparalytic snake bites, a single infusion of 20 vials is administered.

Administration

- It is usually administered by intravenous route (IV). Intramuscular route may also be used but absorption is erratic. In severe life-threatening situations with difficult IV access, intraosseous route may also be used.
- ASV is either diluted (normal saline) or administered after reconstitution without dilution. To be administered slowly over 30–60 minutes.
- Local administration of ASV at the site of bite is not recommended. During treatment with ASV, a number of parameters are monitored (Box 9).

Adverse Effects

A significant number of individuals (>10%) develop adverse reactions to ASV. The adverse effects are divided into early (within hours) anaphylactic reactions, pyrogenic reactions, and late (5 days or more) reactions. Box 10 describes the type of adverse reactions and their treatment.

Contraindications

- No absolute contraindications to ASV
- Use with caution in patients with history of atopy, asthma, and previous reaction to horse/sheep serum-containing products.

CONCLUSION

Antidotes are available for a multitude of drugs, poisons, and toxins. In depth knowledge and understanding of the specific poison will help to utilize the antidote in the most effective way. When in doubt, always consult a medical toxicologist or a poison control center.

Box 10: Adverse reactions to anti-snake venom (ASV).

Early anaphylactic reactions
- Develops within 2–3 hours. Not true allergic reactions (i.e. not IgE mediated) and are complement mediated
- Present with itching, dry cough, urticaria, nausea, vomiting, and abdominal pain
- Life-threatening anaphylactic shock is seen only in a minority of patients.

Treatment
- Stop ASV infusion
- Injection adrenaline 0.5 mg (1:1,000 dilution) IM for adult and 0.01 mg/kg for children
- Injection chlorpheniramine maleate 10 mg IV
- Injection hydrocortisone 100 mg IV
- Injection ranitidine—50 mg IV

Pyrogenic reactions
- Develop within 1–2 hours
- Present with fever, chills, and rigors. Febrile convulsions may be precipitated in children
- These reactions are caused by contamination with pyrogens during manufacturing

Treatment
- Oral paracetamol SOS
- External cooling
- IV fluids

Late (serum sickness) reactions
- Develops within 1–12 days with an average of 7 days
- Present with fever, nausea, vomiting, itching, urticaria, myalgias, arthralgias, lymphadenopathy, mononeuritis multiplex, proteinuria with immune complex nephritis and, encephalopathy.

Treatment
- Oral antihistamine
- Steroid (prednisolone 5 mg every 6 hours may be required in unresponsive cases)

KEY POINTS

- Antidotes act by various mechanisms
- Patient-tailored approach is necessary
- Whenever an antidote is available for a specific poison, it should be administered.

REFERENCES

1. Green JL, Heard KJ, Reynolds KM, et al. Oral and intravenous acetylcysteine for treatment of acetaminophen toxicity: A systematic review and meta-analysis. West J Emerg Med. 2013;14(3):218-26.

Box 9: Monitoring parameters for response to anti-snake venom (ASV).

Response to ASV
- General improvement in patient well-being
- Stoppage of systemic bleeding (usually takes in 15–30 minutes)
- Resolution of coagulopathy (measured by 20 WBCT)—usually takes 3–9 hours
- Resolution of hypotension, bradycardia, and arrhythmias
- Improvement in neurological symptoms

(WBCT: whole blood clotting time)

2. Wong A, Graudins A. Simplification of the standard three-bag intravenous acetylcysteine regimen for paracetamol poisoning results in a lower incidence of adverse drug reactions. Clin Toxicol (Phila). 2016;54(2):115-9.

3. Michael E, Nick AB, Peter E, et al. Management of acute organophosphorus pesticide poisoning. The Lancet. 2008;371(9612):597-607.

4. Abedin MJ, Sayeed AA, Basher A, et al. Open-label randomized clinical trial of atropine bolus injection versus incremental boluses plus infusion for organophosphate poisoning in Bangladesh. J Med Toxicol. 2012;8(2):108-17.

5. Hill SE, Iqbal R, Cadiz CL, et al. Foodborne botulism treated with heptavalent botulism antitoxin. Ann Pharmacother. 2013;47(2):e12.

6. Food and Drug Administration. BabyBIG (BIG-IV) (botulism immune globulin) [prescribing information]. Westlake Village, CA: Baxter Healthcare Corporation; 2015.

7. Strawn JR, Keck PE Jr, Caroff SN. Neuroleptic malignant syndrome. Am J Psychiatry. 2007;164(6):870-6.

8. Gude AB, Hoegberg LC, Angelo HR, et al. Dose-dependent adsorptive capacity of activated charcoal for gastrointestinal decontamination of a simulated paracetamol overdose in human volunteers. Basic Clin Pharmacol Toxicol. 2010;106(5):406-10.

9. Chyka PA, Seger D, Krenzelok EP, et al. American Academy of Clinical Toxicology; European Association of Poisons Centres and Clinical Toxicologists. Position Paper: Single-Dose Activated Charcoal, Clin Toxicol (Phila). 2005;43(2):61-87.

10. Krenzelok EP, Lush RM. Container residue after the administration of aqueous activated charcoal products. Am J Emerg Med. 1991;9(2):144-6.

11. Bailey B. Are there teratogenic risks associated with antidotes used in the acute management of poisoned pregnant women? Birth Defects Res A Clin Mol Teratol. 2003;67(2):133-40.

12. Vanden Hoek TL, Morrison LJ, Shuster M, et al. Part 12: cardiac arrest in special situations: 2010 American Heart Association Guidelines for Cardiopulmonary Resuscitation and Emergency Cardiovascular Care. Circulation. 2010;122(18 Suppl 3):S829-61.

13. Kosnett MJ, Wedeen RP, Rothenberg SJ, et al. Recommendations for medical management of adult lead exposure. Environ Health Perspect. 2007;115(3):463-71.

14. Howland M. Antidotes in depth: edetate calcium disodium (CaNa2EDTA). In: Hoffman RS, Howland MA, Lewin NA (Eds). *Goldfrank's Toxicologic Emergencies*, 10th edition. New York, NY: McGraw-Hill Companies, Inc; 2015.

15. Malignant Hyperthermia Association of the United States (MHAUS). (2011). Annual Report. [online] Available from https://www.mhaus.org/about/financial-reports/2011-2012-annual-report/. [Accessed December, 2018].

16. Sheth S. Iron chelation: an update. Curr Opin Hematol. 2014;21(3):179-85.

17. Aronoff GR, Bennett WM, Berns JS, et al. Drug Prescribing in Renal Failure: Dosing Guidelines for Adults and Children, 5th edition. Philadelphia, PA: American College of Physicians; 2007. p. 116.

18. Chan BS, Buckley NA. Digoxin-specific antibody fragments in the treatment of digoxin toxicity. Clin Toxicol (Phila). 2014;52(8):824-36.

19. Bayer MJ. Recognition and management of digitalis intoxication: implications for emergency medicine. Am J Emerg Med. 1991;9(2 Suppl 1):29-32; discussion 33-4.

20. An H, Godwin J. Flumazenil in benzodiazepine overdose. CMAJ. 2016;188(17-18):E537.

21. Barceloux DG, Bond GR, Krenzelok EP, et al. American Academy of Clinical Toxicology practice guidelines on the treatment of methanol poisoning. J Toxicol Clin Toxicol. 2002;40(4):415-46.

22. Barceloux DG, Krenzelok EP, Olson K, et al. American Academy of Clinical Toxicology Practice Guidelines on the Treatment of Ethylene Glycol Poisoning. Ad Hoc Committee. J Toxicol Clin Toxicol. 1999;37(5):537-60.

23. Jobard E, Harry P, Turcant A, et al. 4-Methylpyrazole and hemodialysis in ethylene glycol poisoning. J Toxicol Clin Toxicol. 1996;34(4):373-7.

24. Zakharov S, Pelclova D, Navratil T, et al. Fomepizole versus ethanol in the treatment of acute methanol poisoning: Comparison of clinical effectiveness in a mass poisoning outbreak. Clin Toxicol (Phila). 2015;53(8):797-806.

25. Bailey B. Glucagon in beta-blocker and calcium channel blocker overdoses: a systematic review. J Toxicol Clin Toxicol. 2003;41(5):595-602.

26. Olson KR. What is the best treatment for acute calcium channel blocker overdose? Ann Emerg Med. 2013;62(3):259-61.

27. Anseeuw K, Delvau N, Burillo-Putze G, et al. Cyanide poisoning by fire smoke inhalation: a European expert consensus. Eur J Emerg Med. 2013;20(1):2-9.

28. Reade MC, Davies SR, Morley PT, et al. Review article: management of cyanide poisoning. Emerg Med Australas. 2012;24(3):225-38.

29 Gill AL, Bell CN. Hyperbaric oxygen: its uses, mechanisms of action and outcomes. QJM. 2004;97(7):385-95.

30. Ernst A, Zibrak JD. Carbon monoxide poisoning. N Engl J Med. 1998;339(22):1603-8.

31. Rose JJ, Wang L, Xu Q, et al. Carbon Monoxide Poisoning: Pathogenesis, Management, and Future Directions of Therapy. Am J Respir Crit Care Med. 2017;195(5):596-606.

32. Clifton J 2nd, Leikin JB. Methylene blue. Am J Ther. 2003;10(4):289-91.

33. Kampman K, Jarvis M. American Society of Addiction Medicine (ASAM) National Practice Guideline for the Use of Medications in the Treatment of Addiction Involving Opioid Use. J Addict Med. 2015;9(5):358-67.

34. Goldfrank L, Weisman RS, Errick JK, et al. A dosing nomogram for continuous infusion intravenous naloxone. Ann Emerg Med. 1986;15(5):566-70.

35. Aronoff GR, Bennett WM, Berns JS, et al. Drug Prescribing in Renal Failure: Dosing Guidelines for Adults and

Children, 5th edition. Philadelphia, PA: American College of Physicians; 2007. p. 104.

36. Howland M. Antidotes in depth: physostigmine salicylate. In: Hoffman RS, Howland MA, Lewin NA (Eds). Goldfrank's Toxicologic Emergencies, 10th edition. New York, NY: McGraw-Hill; 2015.

37. Patriquin C, Crowther M. Treatment of warfarin-associated coagulopathy with vitamin K. Expert Rev Hematol. 2011;4(6):657-65; quiz 666-7.

38. Guyatt GH, Akl EA, Crowther M, et al. Executive summary: Antithrombotic Therapy and Prevention of Thrombosis, 9th edition. American College of Chest Physicians Evidence-Based Clinical Practice Guidelines. Chest. 2012;141(2 Suppl):7S-47S.

39. Frontera JA, Lewin JJ, Rabinstein AA, et al. Guideline for Reversal of Antithrombotics in Intracranial Hemorrhage: A Statement for Healthcare Professionals from the Neurocritical Care Society and Society of Critical Care Medicine. Neurocrit Care. 2016;24(1):6-46.

40. Lee WM, Stravitz T, Larson AM. (2011). AASLD Position Paper: The management of acute liver failure: update 2011. [online] Available from http://aasld.org/sites/default/files/guideline_documents/AcuteLiverFailureUpdate201journalformat1.pdf. [Accessed December, 2018].

41. Watt BE, Proudfoot AT, Bradberry SM, et al. Anticoagulant rodenticides. Toxicol Rev. 2005;24(4):259-69.

42. Ansell J, Hirsh J, Hylek E, et al. Pharmacology and management of the vitamin K antagonists: American College of Chest Physicians Evidence-Based Clinical Practice Guidelines (8th Edition). Chest. 2008;133 (6 Suppl):160S-198S.

43. Centers for Disease Control (CDC). Neonatal deaths associated with use of benzyl alcohol—United States. MMWR Morb Mortal Wkly Rep. 1982;31(22):290-1.

44. Howland MA. Antidotes in Depth-Pralidoxime. In: Hoffman RS, Howland MA, Lewin NA, Nelson LS, Goldfrank LR (Eds). Goldfrank's Toxicologic Emergencies, 10th edition. New York, NY: McGraw Hill; 2015. pp. 1419-34.

45. Roberts DM, Aaron CK. Management of acute organophosphorus pesticide poisoning. BMJ. 2007;334 (7594):629-34.

46. World Health Organization (WHO); United Nations Environment Programme (UNEP). (2006). Sound management of pesticides and diagnosis and treatment of pesticide poisoning: a resource tool. [online] Available from http://www.who.int/whopes/recommendations/IPCSPesticide_ok.pdf?ua=1. [Accessed December, 2018].

47. Pai M, Crowther MA. Neutralization of heparin activity. Handb Exp Pharmacol. 2012;(207):265-77.

48. Caravati EM. Protamine sulfate. In: Dart RC (Ed). Medical Toxicology, 3rd edition. Philadelphia, PA: Lippincott Williams and Wilkins; 2004. pp. 243-4.

49. Howland MA. Antidotes in Depth: Pyridoxine. In: Flomenbaum NE, Goldfrank LR, Hoffman RS (Eds). Goldfrank's Toxicologic Emergencies, 10th edition. New York, NY: McGraw-Hill Companies Inc.; 2015. pp. 872-5.

50. Morrow LE, Wear RE, Schuller D, et al. Acute isoniazid toxicity and the need for adequate pyridoxine supplies. Pharmacotherapy. 2006;26(10):1529-32.

51. Lheureux P, Penaloza A, Gris M. Pyridoxine in clinical toxicology: a review. Eur J Emerg Med. 2005;12(2):78-85.

52. Gracia R, Shepherd G. Cyanide poisoning and its treatment. Pharmacotherapy. 2004;24(10):1358-65.

53. Berlin CM Jr. The treatment of cyanide poisoning in children. Pediatrics. 1970;46(5):793-6.

54. Kosnett MJ. The role of chelation in the treatment of arsenic and mercury poisoning. J Med Toxicol. 2013;9(4):347-54.

55. Valenzuela A, Garrido A. Biochemical bases of the pharmacological action of the flavonoid silymarin and of its structural isomer silibinin. Biol Res. 1994;27(2):105-12.

56. Hoffman JR, Votey SR, Bayer M, et al. Effect of hypertonic sodium bicarbonate in the treatment of moderate-to-severe cyclic antidepressant overdose. Am J Emerg Med. 1993;11(4):336-41.

57. Proudfoot AT, Krenzelok EP, Vale JA. Position Paper on urine alkalinization. J Toxicol Clin Toxicol. 2004; 42(1):1-26.

58. Widemann BC, Adamson PC. Understanding and managing methotrexate nephrotoxicity. Oncologist. 2006;11(6):694-703.

59. Perrott J, Murphy NG, Zed PJ. L-carnitine for acute valproic acid overdose: a systematic review of published cases. Ann Pharmacother. 2010;44(7-8):1287-93.

60. Russell S. Carnitine as an antidote for acute valproate toxicity in children. Curr Opin Pediatr. 2007;19(2): 206-10.

61. Howland MA. Antidotes in depth: L-carnitine. In: Nelson L, Lewin N, Howland MA, Hoffman R, Goldfrank L, Flomenbaum N (Eds). Goldfrank's Toxicologic Emergencies, 9th edition. New York, NY: McGraw-Hill Companies, Inc.; 2011. p. 711.

62. Barkin JA, Block HM, Mendez PE. Octreotide: a novel therapy for refractory sulfonylurea-induced hypoglycemia. Pancreas. 2013;42(4):722-3.

63. Dougherty PP, Klein-Schwartz W. Octreotide's role in the management of sulfonylurea-induced hypoglycemia. J Med Toxicol. 2010;6(2):199-206.

64. Latt N, Dore G. Thiamine in the treatment of Wernicke encephalopathy in patients with alcohol use disorders. Intern Med J. 2014;44(9):911-5.

65. Hoffman RS. Antidotes in depth: thiamine. In: Flomenbaum NE, Goldfrank LR, Hoffman RS, (Eds). Goldfrank's Toxicologic Emergencies, 10th edition. New York, NY: McGraw-Hill Companies, Inc.; 2015.

66. American Academy of Pediatrics Committee on Environmental Health. Radiation disasters and children. Pediatrics. 2003;111(6 Pt 1):1455-66.

5
CHAPTER

Lipid Emulsion Therapy

Omender Singh, Deven Juneja

INTRODUCTION

There are several indications for use of intravenous lipids in critically ill patients. In these patients, they are mostly prescribed as nutritional supplement to provide for the essential fatty acids and calories. Presently, their clinical indications have expanded and they are regularly being used as an antidote in patients with lipophilic drug overdose.[1] Other indications for lipids include as a carrier vehicle for drug delivery and for attenuation of reperfusion injury.[1]

The Association of Anesthetists of Great Britain and Ireland (AAGBI), in their 2007 guidelines for the management of local anesthetic systemic toxicity (LAST) have recommended the use of lipid emulsion therapy (LET). They even recommended that lipid emulsions should be easily available at all places in the hospital where potentially toxic doses of local anesthetics (LAs) may get administered.[2]

Several studies have suggested the utility of LET in the management of severe LAST and it has become an accepted therapy. It is now increasingly been used in patients with less severe form of LAST also.[3-6] Moreover, its role as an antidote, in the management of other drug overdoses has now been recognized and it has been used successfully in the overdoses of several antiepileptic, cardiovascular (CV), and psychotropic medications.[7-11] As per the recent estimates, there are reports of LET being tried in 65 unique substances, with varying results.[12] However, in these patients, its utility is largely restricted to patients with cardiac arrest or life-threatening arrhythmias who are not responding to the standard medical therapies.[13,14]

As is true for several other therapies used in the management of poisoning and overdose, there is a dearth of large randomized control trials (RCTs) assessing the efficacy of LET in these patients. Hence, all the recommendations presently are based on case reports. Patient registries and larger trials are needed before this therapy can be applied more regularly.

MECHANISM OF ACTION

Several mechanisms of action for LET have been suggested as the exact mechanism is unknown. These proposed theories include the following:

The Lipid Sink Theory

This is the most widely accepted mechanism of action in the management of acute poisonings. As per this theory, when large volumes of lipids are infused intravenously, they act as a "lipid sink", where lipophilic drugs are accumulated and absorbed.[5] This removes large quantities of these potentially harmful drugs from their target sites and hence reduce their harmful effects

Fatty Acid Metabolism Theory

The myocardium utilizes fatty acids for production of energy in the normal aerobic conditions. These fatty acids generate 80–90% of the cardiac adenosine triphosphate (ATP).[15] LAs inhibit the metabolism of fatty acids by the myocardium and hence interferes with energy production. Large volumes of lipids provide the myocardium with an alternate source of energy, thereby, reducing the harmful effects of the LA and restoring the normal function of the myocardium.[16]

Ion Channel Modulation Theory

High-dose lipid emulsion causes increase in the serum fatty acid levels which affect the functioning of the sodium and calcium ion channels present in the myocardium.[17,18] This theory also suggests that LET may also have a direct cardiotonic effect as it affects the carnitine transport which improves fatty acid utilization by the myocardium causing a positive inotropic effect and improved cardiac function.[19,20] This effect may especially explain the utility of LET in resuscitation of patients in cardiac arrest situation.[21]

Nitric Oxide Synthase Inhibition

This theory proposes that the release of nitric oxide may contribute to the hypotension associated with LAST. By inhibiting endothelial nitric oxide synthase, LET may reduce the nitric oxide induced vasodilation and hence may improve hypotension.[22]

LIPID PREPARATIONS

Numerous lipid preparations have been used clinically for different indications. These preparations have different lipid concentrations and the lipid source. Preparations of 10%, 20%, and 30% lipid solutions are available commercially in different unit doses ranging from 100–1,000 mL. The most commonly prescribed and studied lipid formulation is the 20%, which contains 20% soybean oil, 1.2% egg yolk phospholipids and 2.25% glycerine.[23] It can be given easily through a peripheral line as its osmolality is approximately 350 mOsm/kg water.[23] Generally, lipid emulsions incorporating fish and olive oils, which are commonly prescribed as parenteral nutrition, are used less frequently as antidotes.

These different emulsions are prescribed for different indications when used for providing parenteral nutrition. But for its use as an antidote in the management of LAST, there are no guidelines which suggest use of one formulation over the other. There are reports which suggest that long-chained triglycerides based lipid emulsions may be 2.5 times more efficient when used as an antidote in the management of LAST.[24] But other reports have failed to show similar efficacy.[25] As most of the literature pertains to use of 20% lipid formulation, this preparation is mostly recommended for use in patients with LAST.[26]

DOSE AND DELIVERY

Initial Management

As with any other patient requiring acute care, the initial management of any patient with LAST includes airway, breathing and circulation (ABC) of resuscitation.

Treatment of Seizures

Seizures are a common complication or presentation of LAST. Benzodiazepines are the drugs of choice for management of these seizures.

Initiation of Lipid Emulsion Therapy

A bolus dose is recommended, 1.5 mL/kg of 20% lipid emulsion intravenously over 1 minute, which should be followed by a maintenance dose. The bolus dose of LET may be repeated up to two times, with 5-minute intervals, if adequate circulation is not restored.[26]

Maintenance Therapy

Infusion of 20% lipid emulsion should be initiated at a rate of 0.25 mL/kg/min. The infusion rate can be doubled (up to 0.50 mL/kg/min), if there is no hemodynamic improvement after 5 minutes of initiation of therapy. The end points of infusion therapy are less clear. The American College of Medical Toxicology (ACMT) recommends that the infusion should be continued for at least 60 minutes.[27] However, longer regimens of up to 6.5 hours have also been tried, without any significant side effects.[28] It is generally accepted to continue the

General Management of Poisoning or Overdose

infusion for at least 10 minutes till after achieving the hemodynamic stability.

It should be kept in mind that the total dose of lipids should not exceed 10 mL/kg over 30 minutes for 20% lipid emulsion, as the rate of complications may increase beyond this dose.[26]

As per the AAGBI guidelines recommendations, the maximum total dose should not exceed 12 mL/kg, in the management of LAST.[2]

ADVERSE EFFECTS

Lipid therapy, be it for parenteral nutrition or as an antidote, may be associated with a few adverse effects.[29] As the dose used as an antidote is much higher, higher complications rates may be expected. However, most of the reports have suggested that LET may be used effectively and safely in most of the patients.[30] But still, awareness of potential side effects associated with this therapy should be there. The associated complications may be divided into immediate and delayed complications.[31]

Immediate Adverse Effects

These include pyrogenic reactions and fat overload. The commonly associated side effects of LET may be related to administration site contamination and irritation of the veins secondary to other fluids coinfused with lipid emulsion. Nausea, vomiting, headache, dizziness, somnolence, dyspnea, hyperthermia, diaphoresis, allergic reactions and pain at injection site are other side effects which may occur in the immediate initiation period.[23] Hence, it becomes imperative that the patients be monitored closely for development of any allergic reactions especially during the initial infusion.

Delayed Adverse Effects

These adverse effects may be dose related and include:

Interference with Laboratory Studies

The use of high-dose lipids in the form of LET obviously leads to lipemia which may make the blood sample analysis difficult. Several commonly used tests like complete blood cell counts, serum glucose, electrolytes, creatinine, albumin, total protein, alanine aminotransferase, bilirubin, creatine kinase, amylase and lipase may get affected. Lipemia may also affect the analysis of arterial blood gases. Hence, the possibility of this interference should always be kept in mind when the patient is on LET and interpretation of the laboratory tests results should be done with caution. Moreover, it should also be kept in mind that this interference may persist even up to 24 hours after stopping the LET.[32-35]

Acute Pancreatitis

It is a rare but dreaded side effect associated with use of LET.[32] This side effect seems to be dose related and the risk is highest in those patients who receive several doses or a prolonged lipid infusion.

The exact mechanism for the development of acute pancreatitis secondary to hypertriglyceridemia is not known. However, it is suggested that when triglycerides are hydrolyzed by pancreas to form free fatty acid, it results in free radical formation which may further lead to inflammation causing pancreatitis.[36,37] It is believed that serum triglyceride levels of >1,000 mg/dL are necessary to cause acute pancreatitis.[38] It is, therefore, recommended to regularly monitor serum triglyceride levels in patients on high dose of lipids. It is recommended that if the patient develops hypertriglyceridemia (triglyceride levels >400 mg/dL), then the dose of LET should be reduced, but if the serum triglyceride levels exceed 1,000 mg/dL, then LET should be completely stopped.[39]

Acute Lung Injury

Cases of acute lung injury have been reported after the initiation of LET which may lead to acute hypoxia. However, other causes of hypoxia, in these patients, must also be kept in mind. These causes include acute bronchospasm after a rapid lipid infusion and fat or pulmonary embolism.[35]

Fat Accumulation

This may occur especially when large doses or prolonged lipid infusion is administered. This may clinically manifest as hemolytic anemia, fat embolism or hyperlipidemia.[31,35,37] Fat accumulation may also cause steatosis, cholestasis and gallbladder sludge.

Recurring Toxic Effects

Several reports of delayed or recurring toxicity have been reported following LET. These effects may appear even after 24 hours of stopping lipid infusion and may exhibit as worsening of sensorium, development of seizures,

Lipid Emulsion Therapy

arrhythmias, or even cardiac arrest. Hence, every patient should be monitored for development of such complications even after stopping LET.[36]

Miscellaneous

Other rare side effects which have been reported to be associated with use of LET include deep vein thrombosis, acute renal failure, and digital amputation. LET use may also cause derangement in liver function tests, coagulopathy, thrombocytopenia, leukopenia, and spleen and liver enlargement. These effects are generally mild and reversible on stopping the therapy. Nevertheless, caution must be exercised when LET is used in patients with pregnancy, underlying severe liver or pulmonary disease, coagulation disorders, or anemia.[23]

INDICATIONS OF USE

Local Anesthetic Systemic Toxicity

We use LAs regularly in our day-to-day clinical practice. Even though the side effects are rare, there is always a potential for severe toxicity if these agents are inadvertently given systemically, rather than locally. Systemic administration may lead to LAST, which has a reported incidence of 7.5–20 cases per 10,000 peripheral blockades performed.[40] The reported incidence of LAST is slightly lower, 4 out of 10,000, when LAs are used for epidural anesthesia.[40]

The initial symptoms of LAST are secondary to central nervous system (CNS) involvement as LAs first suppress the inhibiting pathways in the brain. Initial clinical symptoms may include metallic taste, slurred speech, visual changes, light headedness, altered sensorium and seizures. These symptoms may worsen with increasing serum levels of the LA involved. Later in the course, the excitatory pathways get affected leading to inhibition of respiration, apnea and coma.

Cardiovascular toxicity may exhibit clinically as development of arrhythmias and myocardial depression, secondary to inhibition of sinoatrial and atrioventricular node conduction. This may manifest on an electrocardiogram (ECG) as prolonged PR, widening of QRS complex and atrioventricular blocks of varying degrees. Patient may develop bradycardias and re-entrant tachyarrhythmias along with life-threatening ventricular tachycardia or fibrillation. These CV manifestations might be refractory to general supportive treatment. Presence of CV symptoms at the time of presentation indicates severe toxicity and poor outcomes.[41]

Several factors may determine the clinical severity of LAST. These include:[42]

- Speed of administration of LA
- Site of LA administration
- Total dose of LA given
- Protein binding of the involved LA
- Route of administration of LA (intravenous or intra-arterial)
- Coadministration of epinephrine.

The systemic absorption of LA depends on the vascularity of the site of injection. If the LA involved is highly protein bound, it reduces the serum concentration of the free drug and hence systemic toxicity.[42] Moreover, epinephrine is sometimes coadministered to reduce bleeding, which causes local vasoconstriction and therefore inhibit the absorption and hence, systemic levels of LA.[41]

If a patient with LAST develops cardiac arrest, it may be refractory to standard resuscitative measures, more so if the involved agent is a long-acting LA like bupivacaine.[41,43] In such a clinical scenario, before the use of LET, the only available therapeutic option was cardiopulmonary bypass.

Lipid emulsion therapy has been in clinical use for more than a decade now with the first reported human case in LAST being published in 2006.[44] This report described a case of 58-year-old male who had developed seizures followed by asystolic cardiac arrest after being administered with 20 mL of 1.5% mepivacaine and 20 mL of 0.5% bupivacaine. He was administered 20% lipid emulsion at a rate of 0.5 mL/kg/min for 2 hours, when he failed to respond to standard resuscitative measures. He showed remarkable recovery without development of any side effects.[44]

The American Society of Regional Anesthesia (ASRA) has recommended the use of LET in the management of patients with severe LAST as an adjunct to airway management and good cardiopulmonary resuscitation (CPR).[45] They have further stated that LET may be helpful in reducing the toxicity of LA by providing a "lipid sink" and hence reducing the LA concentration in the cardiac tissue and improve cardiac contractility, conduction and also the coronary perfusion.[45]

It is argued that early initiation of LET may be more beneficial and may be associated with better patient outcomes. As CNS symptoms appear before CV symptoms, the current evidence suggests initiating LET before the patient develops severe CV symptoms or

General Management of Poisoning or Overdose

cardiac asystole. It is also important to understand that in the presence of hypoxia, the deleterious effects of LET may be more pronounced.[46] In addition, underlying acidosis may also affect the binding of lipids with LA, thereby reducing its clinical efficacy.[47]

As per the current evidence, it seems prudent to keep stocks of 20% lipid emulsions in all the areas, within the hospital, where LAs are routinely used. These should include at least the operation theaters, emergency rooms and intensive care units (ICUs). As 20% lipid can be kept at room temperature (<25°C), it can easily become a standard component of resuscitation trolleys or crash carts. As per the ASRA recommendations, lipid emulsions should be stored as 500 mL bags, because these are more likely to be sufficient for resuscitation of an adult patient.[26]

Toxicities Other than Local Anesthetics

It was postulated that LET may be beneficial in patients with other lipophilic drug toxicities as it may be useful in removing the offending agent from its site of activity by providing a "lipid sink". Hence, the antidotal role of LET was expanded and it has been tried in various other drug overdoses too including β-blockers, calcium channel blockers (CCBs), herbicides, parasiticides, tricyclic antidepressants (TCAs) and several other psychotropic drugs (Box 1), with varying efficacy.[12]

Certain group of drugs like β-blockers, CCBs and TCAs share many properties including lipophilic nature, with LA.[48] Hence, it was postulated that the principles of "lipid sink" should apply to these drugs too and LET may be beneficial in these drug overdoses.

Lipid emulsion therapy has been tried in other drug toxicities for a long time with the first successful case

being published in 2008.[49] The authors reported a case of a 17-year-old female who suffered from cardiac arrest after administration of a large dose of bupropion and lamotrigine. Twenty percent lipid emulsion was initiated after a prolonged unsuccessful resuscitative effort lasting for 70 minutes. She showed a dramatic response within 1 minute of LET administration and achieved return of spontaneous circulation and showed remarkable clinical recovery with no observed side effects.[49]

In view of the expanding clinical applications regarding LET, it is generally accepted that conduction of RCTs might not be possible for evaluating its efficacy. Therefore, the Lipid Injection for the Purpose of Antidotal Effect in lipophilic Medicine IntoxiCation (LIPAEMIC) study group was formed in 2009 with the objective of initiating a prospective registry enrolling all the patients in whom LET is being used. The results from this "LIPID REGISTRY" were published in 2014 in which they reported use of LET in 48 patients from 61 centers across the world.[30] The results showed that the LET was being primarily used in patients with non-LA toxicities and presence of neurological symptoms were the primary indication for starting LET. Use of LET led to improvement of 2 points in Glasgow Coma Score (GCS) in patients with neurological dysfunction and a significant improvement in blood pressure, in patients with hemodynamic instability, within 30 minutes of initiation. The reported side effects were few with only one patient developing serious adverse event and two patients developing minor side effects. The authors concluded that LET can be used safely and effectively as an antidote in patients with LA and non-LA drug toxicities.[30]

The last decade witnessed growing interest in the use of LET as an antidotal therapy with publication of many systematic reviews. In addition, several clinical associations

---

Box 1: Drugs which may benefit by use of lipid emulsion therapy.[12]

Probable benefit
- *All local anesthetics:* Bupivacaine, mepivacaine, ropivacaine, levobupivacaine, prilocaine, lignocaine, lidocaine

Possible benefit
- *Antiepileptics:* Carbamazepine, lamotrigine
- *Antipsychotics:* Chlorpromazine, haloperidol, olanzapine, quetiapine
- *Antihistamine:* Diphenhydramine
- *Barbiturates:* Pentobarbital, phenobarbital, thiopental
- *Beta-blockers:* Atenolol, carvedilol, metoprolol, nebivolol, propranolol
- *Calcium channel blockers:* Amlodipine, diltiazem, felodipine, nifedipine, verapamil
- *Disease-modifying antirheumatic drug:* Hydroxychloroquine
- *Tricyclic antidepressants:* Amitriptyline, clomipramine, dosulepin, dothiepin, doxepin, imipramine
- *Other antidepressants:* Bupropion, venlafaxine
- *Others:* Baclofen, cocaine, endosulfan, flecainide, propanone

Lipid Emulsion Therapy

have also released their guidelines and recommendations on use of LET.[20,50-53] The largest systematic analysis on the use of LET has been recently published by a workgroup established by the American Academy of Clinical Toxicology. Their primary aim was to analyze the available clinical evidence on the efficacy of LET in patients with non-LA drug poisoning.[12] Their analysis included 203 articles (141 human studies and 62 animal studies). Even though, most of these articles were case reports, they also included three human RCTs and one observational study. However, because of the low quality of evidence, they reported that the efficacy of LET in the management of various non-LA poisonings remains heterogenous.[12]

As per the current evidence, the LET has been accepted as a standard of care in the management of severe toxicity associated with LA. However, more clinical evidence is required, before it can be recommended regularly in the management of non-LA toxicities. But in patients who develop severe hemodynamic compromise, with a background of non-LA toxicity, LET must be considered especially when standard resuscitation measures have not been effective. Even in cases where drug overdose is suspected, but the offending agent is unknown and the standard measures have been unsuccessful, LET must be considered strongly to improve patient outcomes. There is dearth of data, as far as the dosing regimens are concerned, in patients with non-LA toxicities. However, it is safe to presume that the regimens recommended for LAST should be effective in these patients also.

CONCLUSION

Lipid emulsion therapy is being increasingly used in management of drug overdoses. Presently, it is recommended for management of severe toxicities related to LA overdose. However, its role is expanding, and it should be considered in the management of patients with severe hemodynamic compromise secondary to overdose of lipophilic cardiotoxic drugs, especially when other standard therapies have proven to be ineffective. Because of potentially life-threatening nature of LAST, lipid emulsions should be readily available in hospital areas where LAs are routinely used.

KEY POINTS

- Lipid emulsion therapy is an effective and safe therapeutic option which can be used in the management of LAST

- Lipid emulsion therapy should also be considered in cases of suspected or proven drug overdoses if the patient is having CV collapse or refractory shock, not responding to standard resuscitative measures
- The therapeutic role of LET is unclear in patients with less severe drug toxicities.

REFERENCES

1. Buys M, Scheepers PA, Levin AI. Lipid emulsion therapy: non-nutritive uses of lipid emulsions in anaesthesia and intensive care. SAJAA. 2015;21(5):124-30.
2. The Association of Anaesthetists of Great Britain and Ireland. Guidelines for the management of severe local anaesthetic toxicity. August 2007. [online] Available from https://www.aagbi.org/sites/default/files/la_toxicity_2010_0.pdf [Assessed July, 2018].
3. Neal JM, Mulroy MF, Weinberg GL. American Society of Regional Anesthesia and Pain Medicine checklist for managing local anesthetic systemic toxicity: 2012 version. Reg Anesth Pain Med. 2012;37(1):16-8.
4. Vanden Hoek TL, Morrison LJ, Shuster M, et al. Part 12: Cardiac arrest in special situations: 2010 American Heart Association guidelines for cardiopulmonary resuscitation and emergency cardiovascular care. Circulation. 2010;122(18 Suppl 3):S829-S861.
5. Weinberg GL. Lipid emulsion infusion: resuscitation for local anesthetic and other drug overdose. Anesthesiology. 2012;117(1):180-7.
6. Picard J, Ward SC, Zumpe R, et al. Guidelines and the adoption of 'lipid rescue' therapy for local anaesthetic toxicity. Anaesthesia. 2009;64:122-5.
7. Brent J. Poisoned patients are different-sometimes fat is a good thing. Crit Care Med. 2009;37:1157-8.
8. Picard J, Harrop-Griffiths W. Lipid emulsion to treat drug overdose: past, present and future. Anaesthesia. 2009;64:119-21.
9. Jamaty C, Bailey B, Larocque A, et al. Lipid emulsions in the treatment of acute poisoning: a systematic review of human and animal studies. Clin Toxicol (Phila). 2010;48:1-27.
10. Cave G, Harvey M. Intravenous lipid emulsion as antidote beyond local anesthetic toxicity: a systematic review. Acad Emerg Med. 2009;16:815-24.
11. Cave G, Harvey M, Willers J, et al. LIPAEMIC Report: Results of clinical use of intravenous lipid emulsion in drug toxicity reported to an online lipid registry. J Med Toxicol. 2014;10:133-42.
12. Levine M, Hoffman RS, Lavergne V, et al. Systematic review of the effect of intravenous lipid emulsion therapy for non-local anesthetics toxicity. Clin Toxicol (Phila). 2016;54:194-221.
13. Jamaty C, Bailey B, Larocque A, et al. Lipid emulsions in the treatment of acute poisoning: a systematic review

14. Rothschild L, Bern S, Oswald S, et al. Intravenous lipid emulsion in clinical toxicology. Scand J Trauma Resusc Emerg Med. 2010;18:51.

15. Collins-Nakai RL, Noseworthy D, Lopaschuk GD. Epinephrine increases ATP production in hearts by preferentially increasing glucose metabolism. Am J Physiol. 1994;267:H1862-71.

16. Partownavid P, Umar S, Li J, et al. Fatty acid oxidation and calcium homeostasis are involved in the rescue of bupivacaine-induced cardiotoxicity by lipid emulsion in rats. Crit Care Med. 2012;40(8):2431-7.

17. Stehr SN, Ziegler JC, Pexa A, et al. The effects of lipid infusion on myocardial function and bioenergetics in l-bupivacaine toxicity in the isolated rat heart. Anesth Analg. 2007;104(1):186-92.

18. Mottram AR, Valdivia CR, Makielski JC. Fatty acids antagonize bupivacaine induced I(Na) blockade. Clin Toxicol (Phila). 2011;49(8):729-33.

19. Weinberg GL, Palmer JW, VadeBoncouer TR, et al. Bupivacaine inhibits acylcarnitine exchange in cardiac mitochondria. Anesthesiology. 2000;92(2):523-8.

20. Waring WS. Intravenous lipid administration for drug-induced toxicity: a critical review of the existing data. Expert Rev Clin Pharmacol. 2012;5(4):437-44.

21. Cave G, Harvey MG. Should we consider the infusion of lipid emulsion in the resuscitation of poisoned patients? Crit Care. 2014;18:457.

22. Ok SH, Sohn JT, Baik JS, et al. Lipid emulsion reverses levobupivacaine-induced responses in isolated rat aortic vessels. Anesthesiology. 2011;114:293-301.

23. Intralipid® 20% (a 20% I.V. fat emulsion in Excel® container) [package insert]. Deerfield, IL: Baxter Healthcare Corporation; 2006.

24. Mazoit JX, Le Guen R, Beloeil H, et al. Binding of long-lasting local anesthetics to lipid emulsions. Anesthesiology. 2009;110:380-6.

25. Candela D, Louart G, Bousquet PJ, et al. Reversal of bupivacaine-induced cardiac electrophysiologic changes by two lipid emulsions in anesthetizes and mechanically ventilated piglets. Anesth Analg. 2010;10:1473-9.

26. Neal JM, Bernards CM, Butterworth JF 4th, et al. ASRA practice advisory on local anesthetic systemic toxicity. Reg Anesth Pain Med. 2010;35:152-61.

27. American College of Medical Toxicology. ACMT position statement: interim guidance for the use of lipid resuscitation therapy. J Med Toxicol. 2011;7:81-2.

28. Fettiplace MR, Akpa BS, Rubinstein I, et al. Confusion about infusion: rational volume limits for intravenous lipid emulsion during treatment of oral overdoses. Ann Emerg Med. 2015;66:185-8.

29. Levine M, Skolnik AB, Ruha AM, et al. Complications following antidotal use of intravenous lipid emulsion therapy. J Med Toxicol. 2014;10:10-4.

30. Cave G, Harvey M, Willers J, et al. LIPAEMIC Report: Results of clinical use of intravenous lipid emulsion in drug toxicity reported to an online lipid registry. J Med Toxicol. 2014;10:133-42.

31. Turner-Lawrence DE, Kearns W II. Intravenous fat emulsion; a potential novel antidote. J Med Toxicol. 2008;4:109-14.

32. Bucklin MH, Gorodetsky RM, Wiegand TJ. Prolonged lipemia and pancreatitis due to extended infusion of lipid emulsion in bupropion overdose. Clin Toxicol (Phila). 2013;51(9):896-8.

33. Smith NA. Possible side effects of lipid rescue therapy. Anaesthesia. 2010;65(2):210-1.

34. Grunbaum AM, Gilfix BM, Gosselin S, et al. Analytical interferences resulting from intravenous lipid emulsion. Clin Toxicol (Phila). 2012;50(9):812-7.

35. Geib AJ, Liebelt E, Manini AF; Toxicology Investigators' Consortium (ToxIC). Clinical experience with intravenous lipid emulsion for drug-induced cardiovascular collapse. J Med Toxicol. 2012;8(1):10-4.

36. Levine M, Brooks DE, Franken A, et al. Delayed-onset seizure and cardiac arrest after amitriptyline overdose, treated with intravenous lipid emulsion therapy. Pediatrics. 2012;130:e432-e438.

37. Lekka ME, Liokatis S, Nathanali C, et al. The impact of intravenous fat emulsion administration in acute lung injury. Am J Respir Crit Care Med. 2004;169:638-44.

38. Tsuang W, Navaneethan U, Ruis L, et al. Hypertriglyceridemic pancreatitis: presentation and management. Am J Gastroenterol. 2009;104:984-91.

39. Adolph M, Heller AR, Koch T, et al. Lipid emulsions. Guidelines on parenteral nutrition. Ger Med Sci. 2009;18:7-23.

40. Manavi MV. Lipid infusion as a treatment for local anesthetic toxicity: a literature review. AANA J. 2010;78:69-78.

41. Cox B, Durieux ME, Marcus MA. Toxicity of local anaesthetics. Best Pract Res Clin Anaesthesiol. 2003;17(1):111-36.

42. Faccenda KA, Finucane BT. Complications of regional anaesthesia: incidence and prevention. Drug Safety. 2001;24(6):413-42.

43. Weinberg GL, Massad MG. Metabolic modulation for cardiac protection. Expert Rev Cardiovasc Ther. 2007;5(2):135-8.

44. Rosenblatt MA, Abel M, Fischer GW, et al. Successful use of a 20% lipid emulsion to resuscitate a patient after a presumed bupivacaine-related cardiac arrest. Anesthesiology. 2006;105:217-8.

45. Weinberg GL. Treatment of local anesthetic systemic toxicity (LAST). Reg Anesth Pain Med. 2010;35:188-93.

46. Harvey M, Cave G, Kazemi A. Intralipid infusion diminishes return of spontaneous circulation following hypoxic cardiac arrest in rabbits. Anesth Analg. 2009;108:1163-8.

47. Mazoit JX, Le Guen R, Beloeil H, et al. Binding of long-lasting local anesthetics to lipid emulsions. Anesthesiology. 2009;110:380-6.

48. Leskiw U, Weinberg GL. Lipid resuscitation for local anesthetic toxicity: is it really lifesaving? Curr Opin Anaesthesiol. 2009;22:667-71.

49. Sirianni AJ, Osterhoudt KC, Calello DP, et al. Use of lipid emulsion in the resuscitation of a patient with prolonged cardiovascular collapse after overdose of bupropion and lamotrigine. Ann Emerg Med. 2008;51:412-5.

50. Harvey M, Cave G. Intravenous lipid emulsion as antidote beyond local anesthetic toxicity: a systematic review. Acad Emerg Med. 2009;16:815-24.

51. Leelach R, Bern S, Oswald S, et al. Intravenous lipid emulsion in clinical toxicology. Scand J Trauma Resusc Emerg Med. 2010;18:51-9.

52. Jamaty C, Bailey B, Larocque A, et al. Lipid emulsions in the treatment of acute poisoning: a systematic review of human and animal studies. Clin Toxicol. 2010;48:1-27.

53. Cave G, Harvey M, Graudins A. Intravenous lipid emulsion as antidote: a summary of published human experience. Emerg Med Australas. 2011;23:123-41.

6 CHAPTER

Forensic Toxicology for the Critical Care Specialist

Sudhir K Gupta, Neha Sharma

INTRODUCTION

As per World Health Organization (WHO), poisoning occurs when people drink, eat, breathe, inject or touch enough of a hazardous substance (poison) to cause illness or death. Some poisons can cause illness or injury in very small amounts. When a poisoned patient is brought to hospital, the primary duty of the doctor is to save the life of patient by decontamination of the ingested/injected/inhaled poison by antidote, gastric lavage and supportive management. But the doctor also has a legal responsibility toward his patient, by marking the case as a medicolegal case (MLC) and by providing information to police.

DEFINITIONS

Toxicology: The science that deals with the source, the physical and chemical properties, the physiological action, the detection, the estimation and the treatment of ill effects resulting from the consumption or administration of poisonous substances. It can be divided into two divisions:
1. *Forensic toxicology*: The science dealing with medicolegal aspects of the harmful effects of the chemicals on the human body
2. *Clinical toxicology*: Deals with the clinical diagnosis of poisoning and management of sign and symptoms.

Poison: A poison may be defined as any substance which, if introduced into or brought into contact with a living body, produces ill health, disease or death. If such a substance, even if it is nontoxic, is administered with the intention of killing or causing injury to a person, the person who administered it is punishable under law.

Drugs: Natural or synthetic substances, which are used to treat human diseases and have physiological or psychological effect on the consumer.

Overdose: Accidental or intentional ingestion of a drug or other substance which leads to harmful effects over the body.

Lethal dose (fatal dose): Lethal dose (LD) for a poison is the dose which can cause death of an individual. It is generally considered as minimum LD, i.e. the dose fatal to 50% of animals (LD 50).

LAWS RELATING TO POISONS

Many therapeutic substances are poisonous to human body. Statutory restrictions on the import, export, manufacture, possession and sale of drugs are necessary to prevent dangers arising from abuse. Various laws have been made and amended from time to time.

Drugs and Cosmetics Act (1940, Amended in 1964)

The most important provision of the Drugs Act of 1940 is that no person shall import or exhibit for sale, or distribute patent or proprietary medicines, unless there is displayed on its label or container either the true formula or the list of ingredients in it in a manner readily intelligible to members of the medical profession. The Act further empowers the Central Government to prescribe conditions of packing of bottles, packages and other containers of imported drugs and to prescribe maximum proportion of any poisonous substances contained in any imported drug.

Drugs and Cosmetics Rules (1945)

The rules were framed to implement under the Drugs and Cosmetics Act 1940 by the Central Government to regulate import of drugs into India, the functions and procedures of the Central Drugs Laboratory, and the manufacture, distribution, and sale of drugs in India.

These rules have classified all therapeutic drugs into various schedules as follows:
- *Schedule C*: Biological products
- *Schedule E*: Poisons
- *Schedule F*: Vaccines and sera
- *Schedule G*: Hormonal preparations
- *Schedule H*: Drugs to be sold only on prescriptions
- *Schedule J*: List of diseases, drugs for which should not be advertised
- *Schedule L*: Antibiotics (like schedule H drugs to be sold only on prescription)
- *Schedule O*: Standards to be followed with regard to disinfectant fluid
- *Schedule S*: Standards to be followed with regard to cosmetics and allied products
- *Schedule X*: Barbiturates and other sedatives.

Narcotic Drugs and Psychotropic Substances Act (1985, Amended in 1988, 2001 and 2004)

The Act was made to consolidate and amend the law relating to narcotic drugs, to make stringent provisions for the control and regulation of operations relating to narcotic drugs and psychotropic substances. As per this Act, a narcotic drug could be an opiate, cannabis or cocaine. The term psychotropic substance is with reference to mind altering drugs such as lysergic acid diethylamide (LSD), phencyclidine, amphetamines, barbiturates, methaqualone, benzodiazepines, mescaline, psilocybin and designer drugs. The Act imposes complete prohibition on the cultivation, manufacture, sale, purchase use, or transport of any of the mentioned drugs except for

medical or scientific purpose. The punishment term may range from minimum 6 months to a maximum imprisonment of 20 years and fine as decided by the court of law. There is also scope for enhanced punishment for repeat offences which includes even death penalty.[1,2]

LEGAL PROVISIONS PERTAINING TO POISONING

The treating doctor should be aware of these legal provisions, to be able to act accordingly:
- *Section 175 Indian Penal Code (IPC)*: Medical practitioner is legally bound to give information about MLCs including poisoning cases to an authorized public servant or investigating officer whenever the latter summons him.
- *Section 176 IPC*: Omission to give notice or information to public servant by person legally bound to give it. Punishment is simple imprisonment for a term which may extend to 6 months
- *Section 201 IPC*: Causing disappearance of evidence of offence, or giving false information to screen offender. Punishment is imprisonment for a term which may extend to 7 years
- *Section 202 IPC*: Intentional omission to give information of offence by person bound to inform. Punishment is imprisonment for a term which may extend to 6 months
- *Section 284 IPC*: Negligent conduct with respect to poisonous substance in his possession as is sufficient to guard against any probable danger to human life from such poisonous substance, shall be punished with imprisonment of either description for a term which may extend to 6 months, or with fine
- *Section 299 IPC*: Culpable homicide including that caused through administration of some poisonous substance
- *Section 300 IPC*: Murder including that caused through administration of poisonous substance with the intention of causing death
- *Section 328 IPC*: Causing hurt by means of poison, etc. with intent to commit an offence. Whoever administers to or causes to be taken by any person any poison or any stupefying, intoxicating or unwholesome drug, or other thing with intent to cause hurt to such person, or with intent to commit or to facilitate the commission of an offence or knowing it to be likely that he will thereby cause hurt, shall be punished with imprisonment of either description

for a term which may extend to 10 years, and shall also be liable to fine.[3]

Administration of drug causing poisoning is a criminal offence on the basis of intent:

- To kill
- To cause injury
- Stupefying for commission of a crime
- Causing abortion.

CIRCUMSTANCES OF POISONING

Poisoning can be homicidal, accidental or suicidal.

Suicidal Poisoning

This is the most common manner among poisoning cases due to easy availability of certain household and agricultural poisons. In recent times, many instances of doctors committing suicides injecting some medicinal drugs and anesthetic agents, like thiopental have come to light.

Homicidal Poisoning

A medical practitioner must keep in mind the homicidal manner of poisoning and should keep an eye on the visitors and relatives of the patient in case of suspicion. Homicidal poisoning can be acute or chronic, i.e. chronically given in small doses leading to chronic disease and death. Some poison mimic signs and symptoms of a natural disease and cause confusion among the doctor regarding its diagnosis.

Accidental Poisoning

Though the manner of poisoning is rare but there is sharp rise in the number of cases due to accidental poisoning especially inhalation poisons, e.g. carbon dioxide, hydrogen sulfide, etc. Bhopal gas tragedy is a well-known example of accidental poisoning. Few other examples are workers dying in abandoned wells or gutters due to the inhalation of poisonous gases, insecticides spraying leading to death of farmers/workers, suffering from bite of a poisonous snake, etc. It is also a common manner among children who carelessly take some easily available household poison or some organic plant poison. The accidental poisoning usually takes place as a result of the carelessness/negligence leading to death or damage to body.

DUTIES OF A MEDICAL PRACTITIONER IN A PATIENT OF SUSPECTED POISONING

Medical Duties

The first and the foremost duty of a doctor is to save the life of a patient. He should find out the nature of poisoning by looking for symptoms and signs carefully so that he can apply appropriate treatment immediately.

Legal Duties

When a doctor is called to attend a suspected case of poisoning, he must exercise certain precautions.

- Preliminaries of the patient like name, sex, age, address, name of attendant, time of admission and address should be noted properly
- A registered medical practitioner is bound to inform all such cases to police and under Section 39 of Criminal Procedure Code, if a private practitioner is convinced regarding the homicidal manner of poisoning, then he must inform police. However, it is advisable to inform all the cases of poisoning to the police as a doctor may not always be right to differentiate manner of the case. This is also in the interest of the practitioner and the investigating agencies, as it will avoid unnecessary complications
- He should avoid giving any opinion whether verbal or in writing on a mere suspicion. If proved wrong, action for damages can be brought against him
- Doctor must notify the health authority in case he comes across cases of food poisoning involving several people at same time from same source of a public eating places like hotel, cafeteria, hostel canteen, restaurant, etc. or at a mass eating place such as at a wedding party dinner or any such other group/festival occasions eating in common place
- Doctor must make every attempt to collect, preserve and dispatch all the suspected materials (vomited material, urine, feces and suspected food or medicine) to the Chemical Examiner. In the event of noncompliance to this, the doctor is held responsible for the loss or disappearance of evidence and punishable (Section 201 IPC)
- To arrange for recording dying declaration, if the patient is about to die. However, if there is any delay in arrival of magistrate, and death is imminent, doctor himself can record the dying declaration [Section 32, Clause 1 of Indian Evidence Act (IEA)]

- If the victim dies, withhold issuing of the death certificate and arrange for the medicolegal autopsy examination at the earliest
- Doctor must always maintain a detailed written record of every case of poisoning treated by him and kept under safe custody labeling MLC

Special attention must be given to the following:
- The character of symptoms and time of their occurrence
- If related to taking food, drink or medicines
- If the signs and symptoms ceased or increased in severity with time
- If the patient was apparently healthy before suspected poisoning incidence
- If symptoms appeared after taking food, if yes whether he had taken similar food previously and with what effects
- Any suspicion on kith and kin for poisoning.[4,5]

EVIDENCE COLLECTION AND PRESERVATION OF SAMPLES IN A PATIENT OF SUSPECTED POISONING

Proper sampling and evidence collection is of utmost importance in reference to forensic toxicology. It is essential for the screening, confirmation, interpretation by chemical analysis and also in negligible cases of reanalysis. So, the sample collection and its preservations need to be fool proof, as it not only provides a definitive diagnosis for treatment but also holds a crucial position for medicolegal provision. In a live patient, the collection and preservation comes under the duty of the treating doctor, which refers to whosoever treats the patient either in emergency department or in intensive care and is engaged in removal of unabsorbed and absorbed poison along with supportive and resuscitative care. So, along with treatment they must preserve samples. There is limitation to the samples to be collected from living than from nonliving as from dead we can collect variety of samples for analytical detection. It is a challenge for the doctor to collect sample in order to detect unknown substance. The doctors are recommended to collect and preserve the following sample properly and immediately while treating the patient.

Gastric Lavage

Irrigation of stomach is indicated both medically and legally when the patient who has ingested poison by whatever manner (suicidal/homicidal/accidental) in large quantity comes to the casualty. However, it is not indicated in certain poisonings like corrosives (except carbolic acid), unconscious patients, and strychnine poisoning. The first wash samples with plain lukewarm water or isotonic salt solutions should be preserved and send for chemical analysis as a whole in a container which should be duly sealed, labeled and handed over to the police officer for further analysis. The containers recommended are preferably disposable hard plastic and labeling requires complete preliminaries of the patient for easy tracking.[6]

Urine

It is probably the best sample to be collected for comprehensive screening of drugs, poisons and their metabolites, as these get accumulated in urine in high concentrations. A minimum 20 mL of sample is sufficient for the chemical analysis. It should be collected in a glass vial and fluoride as preservative may be added but not necessarily.

Blood

It is the sample most preferred for quantification and interpretation of concentration of drug/poison and their metabolites. In addition to above, blood samples are also useful in detection of gaseous poisons, e.g. carbon monoxide, hydrogen sulfide, etc. which should be covered on the top with paraffin wax to avoid exposure to atmosphere. A minimum of 10–20 mL of blood is sufficient to collect for sampling and it should be collected in a glass tube preferably made of amber glass to avoid photodegeneration and preserved with sodium fluoride at a concentration of 2% weight by volume or 20 mL of blood in 10 mg/mL of sodium fluoride. An additional 5 mL of blood should be preserved in potassium ethylenediaminetetraacetic acid (EDTA) vials in case of suspected fluoride poisoning. The vial should be sealed and labeled and kept at the temperature on 4°C or a frozen fraction may be maintained for a better analysis and stability.

Hair

Sample of hair is one of the most important sample and evidence in cases of delayed poisoning or chronic poisoning cases. Hair (100–200 mg) should be collected from the posterior region of head by cutting near to the scalp or plucking. These should be tied together, covered in an aluminum foil, wrapped in an envelope and stored in room temperature till analysis.

Nails

Just like hair sample, nail samples are helpful in detection of poisoning which is chronic in nature, as in heavy metals. Nails should be trimmed in living and the nail clippings should be collected in an aluminum foil or parchment paper, properly wrapped in an envelope, sealed, labeled and stored in room temperature till analysis.[7-9]

IMPORTANT POINTS FOR DISPATCH OF SAMPLE FOR CHEMICAL ANALYSIS

- All the containers and vials should be sealed correctly, pasted with a label containing reference number of the case, date, name of the patient, nature of material, the nature of the preservative and signature of the Medical Officer
- It is advisable to take three copies of the label using carbon paper. The original of the label is cut out and pasted on the bottles. One copy is sent to the Chemical Examiner along with the materials. The second copy is kept in the office for future reference
- The labels are affixed on the containers and tightly closed with the screw cap, which are then wrapped with paper
- The Medical Officer should have a metal seal showing the identity. Sealing wax is applied at all junctions
- If sealing is not done, it will not be accepted by the Chemical Examiner. The entire procedure must be done in such a manner that the container cannot be opened without breaking the seals
- Medical Officer should send the sample along with the requisite form which should be made in three copies (chemical analysis, police and office reference) along with a report containing brief history and relevant particulars of the case including details of symptoms, differential diagnosis and detail of any high-risk case [hepatitis B, human immunodeficiency virus (HIV)]
- The material objects are forwarded to the Chemical Examiner through police. The Medical Officer should maintain a register showing the details of materials forwarded to the Chemical Examiner.[9]

ALGORITHM OF MANAGEMENT OF A PATIENT WITH SUSPECTED POISONING

The management of a patient with suspected poisoning is shown in Flowchart 1.

TOXIDROME APPROACH

The word "toxidrome" is a combination of the words "toxic" and "syndrome". Toxidromes are a specific group of signs and symptoms that are caused by overdose of certain medications or chemicals. Proper recognition, identification and assessment lead to diagnosis and treatment. Common toxidromes experienced in day-to-day life are according to Table 1.[4]

LIST OF COMMON POISONS AND THEIR ANTIDOTES

Antidotes (Table 2) are substances which counteract the effects of poisons and are divided into three groups—physical (mechanical), chemical and physiological.[10]

REASON FOR NEGATIVE CHEMICAL ANALYSIS REPORT IN A PATIENT WITH POSITIVE HISTORY OF POISONING

There may be instances where in spite of positive history of consumption of a specific poison by the patient and

Flowchart 1: Management of a patient with suspected poisoning.

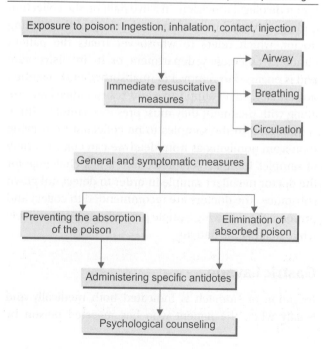

Forensic Toxicology for the Critical Care Specialist

Table 1: Common toxidromes experienced in day-to-day life.

Toxidrome	Drugs/medicines	Mental status	Pupils	Signs	Antidote
Anticholinergic	Atropine, dhatura	Hypervigilant, agitated, delirium, hallucination, coma	Mydriasis	Raised temperature, blood pressure, heart rate, respiratory rate, dryness, flushed dry mucous, urinary retention	Physostigmine
Sympathomimetic	Cocaine, amphetamines, caffeine	Hypervigilant, agitated, hallucinations, paranoid	Mydriasis	Raised temperature, blood pressure, heart rate, respiratory rate, tremors, seizures, hyper-reflexia	β-blockers
Opioid	Heroin, morphine, methadone	CNS depression, coma	Miosis	Decreased temperature, blood pressure, heart rate, respiratory rate, pulmonary edema, hyporeflexia	Naloxone
Cholinergic	Organophosphorus, insecticide, pilocarpine	Confusion, coma	Miosis	Raised heart rate, blood pressure, decreased heart rate, respiratory rate. Muscarinic: Diarrhea, diaphoresis, urination, bronchial secretions, emesis, lacrimation, lethargic, salivation. Nicotinic: Weakness tremors, fasciculation, seizures	Atropine, oximes (oximes are contraindicated in carbamates)
Hallucinogenic	Phencyclidine, lysergic acid diethylamide, amphetamines, designer drugs	Hallucinations, depersonalization, agitation	Mydriasis	Raised temperature, blood pressure, heart rate, respiratory rate, nystagmus	Supportive
Sedative hypnotic/alcoholic	Barbiturates, ethyl alcohol	Sedation, hyporeflexia, coma, confusion, stupor	Miosis	Decreased temperature, blood pressure, heart rate, respiratory rate, diplopia, paresthesia, slurred speech	Supportive

(CNS: central nervous system)

presence of typical signs and symptoms, the chemical analysis report may be negative for the poison. There can be several reasons like:[11-13]

- Improper collection
- Inadequate collection
- Improper preservation of the sample
- Elimination of the poison
- Chemical disintegration of the poison in the sample, e.g. morphine, anesthetic agents
- Presence of metabolites and residues in analysis
- Poisons not detected in routine examination, e.g. sulfmethemoglobin, solvents, radioactive compounds, calcium channel blockers, etc.
- Lack of suitable chemical test
- Negligible amount of poison in samples
- Difficult extraction

- Tampering of the samples
- Specific poison which are difficult to detect by chemical analysis, e.g. thallium, polonium, insulin, heroine, snake venom, photolabile poisons, etc.

CONCLUSION

Critical care specialist needs to be updated about the management of patient with alleged poisoning not only medically but also medicolegally. The foremost duty of the doctor is to save the life of patient but we must be aware of the forensic aspects of medicine and toxicology. Suitable samples to be collected preserved and handed over to investigating authorities. In case the patient dies, no death certificate should be issued and the police informed regarding the death to follow further proceedings.

General Management of Poisoning or Overdose

Table 2: Poisons and their antidotes.

Poisons	Antidotes
Organophosphorus compounds	Pralidoxime, atropine
Digitalis	Digoxin-specific Fab antibody
Heavy metals	Chelating agents
Methyl alcohol, ethylene glycol	Ethyl alcohol, fomepizole
Benzodiazepines	Flumazenil
Local anesthetics	Intravenous lipid emulsion
Acetaminophen	N-acetyl cysteine
Opioid	Naloxone
Nitrites, sulfonamides	Methylene blue
Carbon monoxide	Hyperbaric oxygen
Cyanide	Sodium nitrite, sodium thiosulfate
Sodium channel blocker	Sodium bicarbonate
Anticoagulant rodenticides	Vitamin K1
Insulin, oral hypoglycemics	Dextrose
Snake venom	Antisnake venom
Tricyclic antidepressants	Sodium bicarbonate

KEY POINTS

- Any unconscious patient presenting to emergency department could be suspected to have consumed poison
- Doctor's role is to try to save the patient's life and also to perform medicolegal documentation
- Toxidrome approach should be applied while managing a patient with poisoning
- Antidote, if available, should be promptly administered
- Police must be informed about all patients with suspected poisoning
- Death certificate should not be issued in any suspected poisoning cases.

REFERENCES

1. Matiharan K, Patnaik AK. Modi's Medical Jurisprudence and Toxicology, 2nd section, 23rd edition, 5th reprint. Nagpur: Lexis Nexis; 2010. pp. 22-43.
2. Vij K. Textbook of Forensic Medicine and Toxicology: Principles and Practice, 5th edition. New Delhi: Elsevier; 2011. pp. 446-7.
3. Justice Thomas KT, Rashid MA. The Indian Penal Code- as amended by the Criminal Law (Amendment) Act, 2013, 34th edition. Lexis Nexis; 2014. pp. 336-81.
4. Aggarwal A. Textbook of Forensic Medicine and Toxicology, 1st edition. New Delhi: Avichal Publishing Company; 2014. pp. 543-80.
5. Bhullar DS. Role of toxicologist in the management of poisoning cases in the casualty department. J Karnataka Medicolegal Soc. 2002;2:23-4.
6. Pathak AK, Rathod B, Mahajan A. Significance of gastric lavage in viscera of death due to poisoning. JIAFM. 2013;35(1):7-9.
7. Levine B. Principles of Forensic Toxicology. Washington, DC: American Association for Clinical Chemistry; 2006.
8. Society of Forensic Toxicologists/American Academy of Forensic Sciences. Forensic Toxicology Laboratory Guidelines (2006). [online] Available from www.soft-tox.org [Accessed October, 2018].
9. Jaiswal AK, Millo T. Handbook of Forensic Analytical Toxicology. New Delhi: Jaypee Brothers; 2014. pp. 450-62.
10. Pillay VV. Textbook of Forensic Medicine and Toxicology, 17th edition. Paras Medical Publication; 2016. pp. 470-96.
11. Giroud C, Mangin P. Drug assay and interpretation of results. In: Payne-James, Busuttil A, Smock W (Eds). Forensic Medicine: Clinical and Pathological Aspects. London: Greenwich Medical Media Ltd; 2003. pp. 609-22.
12. Yadav A, Gupta SK, Prasad KB, et al. Death is due to poisoning: Negative viscera report intricacies thereof. Indian Police Journal. 2015;216-27.
13. Malik Y, Chaliha RR, Malik P, et al. Toxicology unit in Department of Forensic Medicine emphasis from a study from North East India. JIAFM. 2012;34(4):23-7.

SECTION 2

Drugs of Abuse

7. **Central Nervous System Depressants: Overdose and Management**
   Mradul Kumar Daga, Lalit Kumar, Jitendra Shukla

8. **Sympathomimetic Drugs**
   Anish Gupta, Omender Singh

9. **Cocaine Intoxication**
   Omender Singh, Anish Gupta

10. **Newer Drugs of Abuse**
    Omender Singh, Rajesh Chawla, Deven Juneja

7
CHAPTER

Central Nervous System Depressants: Overdose and Management

Mradul Kumar Daga, Lalit Kumar, Jitendra Shukla

INTRODUCTION

Central nervous system (CNS) depressants are a class of drug that produce global decline in functions of the nervous system to produce sedation and in larger doses coma. These include the barbiturates, benzodiazepine (BZD), i.e. sedative and hypnotics, opioids and a wide variety of agents like gamma-hydroxybutyric acid (GHB). Cannabinoids on the other hand, have both CNS excitatory as well as inhibitory properties. A sedative is prescribed to calm down the subject and alleviate anxiety while hypnotic induces sleep.[1] Opioids are used mainly for pain relief and anesthesia while cannabinoids are active compounds present in the hemp plant *Cannabis indica* used for recreational purposes. These drugs are easily available to the general population especially in settings where their sale and prescription is not regulated and hence have abuse potential.

A population-based retrospective study done in United Kingdom estimated that for every million prescriptions of BZD 3–7.9 deaths occur as a result of overdose.[2] In 2013, BZD prescription overdose was found in 31% of the estimated 22,767 deaths in a study conducted in United States.[3] Their toxicity is rarely fatal, if adequate timely measures are taken during management.[4] In 2015, globally 122,000 people died because of opioid toxicity. In United States, the number of deaths due to opioids

prescribed for medical illness was 20,100 while number of deaths due to heroin overdose was 13,000. Another astonishing thing was the fact that opioids caused more than 60% of drug overdose deaths.[5,6] According to Drug Use Epidemiology in 2017, marijuana overdose although commonly due to widespread use, did not cause any mortality in United States.

In this review, we will discuss the commonly used CNS depressants, their mechanism of action, uses and how a patient with toxicity presents in the emergency along with its management. Finally, a brief discussion on party drugs will be done.

COMMON CENTRAL NERVOUS SYSTEM DEPRESSANTS: MECHANISM OF ACTION AND USES

Barbiturates

- Barbiturates are derived from barbituric acid and include phenobarbitone, thiopentone and methohexitone. They act on gamma-aminobutyric acid (GABA) BZD receptor chloride channel complex to potentiate the GABAergic inhibition by increasing the duration of chloride channel opening. They are lipid soluble and well absorbed from the gastrointestinal tract

Drugs of Abuse

- Phenobarbitone is used in the management of status epilepticus while thiopentone is useful as anesthetic agent.

Benzodiazepines

- Benzodiazepines include diazepam, midazolam, alprazolam, flurazepam, lorazepam, oxazepam and chlordiazepoxide
- Benzodiazepines increase the pre- and postsynaptic inhibition by acting on a specific BZD receptor, which is an integral part of the $GABA_A$ receptor chloride channel complex in the ascending reticular formation and limbic system
- They have overshadowed the barbiturates due to their high therapeutic index, lower incidence of side effects like respiratory and cardiovascular depression, low potential for abuse with less drug seeking behavior and the availability of the antidote, flumazenil in case of overdose
- Commonly used BZDs include diazepam which is used as anxiolytic, hypnotic, muscle relaxant, anesthetic and antiepileptic in status epilepticus. Alprazolam and flurazepam are commonly employed as anxiolytic and hypnotic.

Nonbenzodiazepine Hypnotics

- These include zolpidem, zopiclone and zaleplon
- These compounds differ in structure from BZD but still they act like agonist on alpha-1 unit containing BZD receptors to produce hypnotic and amnesic action but only weak antianxiety, muscle relaxant and anticonvulsant effects
- These are used for short-term treatment of insomnia or as a replacement strategy in chronic insomniacs with BZD seeking behavior.

Opioid

- The commonly used opioids include morphine, oxycodone, hydrocodone, fentanyl, naloxone and naltrexone
- Opioids act on the opioid receptors in the CNS and other tissues of the body. There are three types of opioid receptors: the mu (1, 2 and 3), kappa, delta and opioid-like receptor-1 to produce a variety of effects. All these receptors are G protein coupled receptors which act at GABAergic transmission. Some opioids may act as agonist at one receptor while antagonist at other receptors
- Opioids are mainly used for pain relief predominantly chronic pain in malignancies. Other uses include as cough suppressants and also for diarrhea and dyspnea in advanced cases of chronic obstructive pulmonary disease (COPD) and cancer.[7-9]

Cannabinoids

- The cannabis plant contains more than 400 active substances but the most important ones include tetrahydrocannabinol, cannabidiol and cannabivarin
- Cannabinoids act on the CB receptor which is of two types (type 1 and type 2). CB1 receptor is found predominantly in the brain and is responsible for the psychological effects of tetrahydrocannabinol while CB2 receptor is found on the cells that make up the immune system
- Cannabinoids are mainly used for recreational purposes.

Gamma-hydroxybutyric Acid

- It is a psychoactive drug which acts on the GHB receptor and also a weak agonist at the $GABA_B$ receptor
- Due to its quick onset of action of 5–15 minutes, it has been used as a general anesthetic, along with for treatment of cataplexy, narcolepsy, fibromyalgia and alcoholism
- Gamma-hydroxybutyric acid uses include abuse by athletes to enhance their performance and may be detected in urine samples
- Due to its colorless and odorless nature with the ability to dissolve easily in drinks, it is used as date rape drug. Its street names are G, liquid G and liquid X.

CENTRAL NERVOUS SYSTEM DEPRESSANT OVERDOSE AND ITS MANAGEMENT

Sedative Hypnotics

- Since barbiturates are less commonly used, the main chunk of overdose cases is due to BZD. Patient presents within hours of ingestion
- Central nervous system symptoms predominate the clinical picture with the patient looking intoxicated,

sleepy, slurring of speech, loss of recent memory, i.e. amnesia, loss of balance and impaired motor function leading to ataxia and hypotonia. Patients attendant may also give history of frequent vomiting episodes.[10,11] Some patients may present with hyperexcitability features as anxiety, delirium, hallucinations and aggression. This paradoxical stimulation is especially seen in flurazepam overdose

- With increased dose, respiratory depression may occur and patient lands up in coma which is life threatening. Patient may aspirate and features of cardiovascular collapse may manifest leading to cardiac arrest and death. These symptoms typically last for 12–36 hours post-overdose[11]
- Pure BZD overdose is rarely fatal and features of severe toxicity is seen when these drugs are combined with other CNS depressants like alcohol and opioids to make a cocktail for recreational purpose, suicidal intent or accidental overdose. Combination of heroin and sedatives is particularly dangerous
- Many studies done in the past have established that different BZD have different levels of toxicity. In 1993, a British study analyzed the deaths of patients who died because of drug overdose and concluded that flurazepam followed by temazepam had higher mortality rates per million prescriptions of the drug when they were compared with the then other available BZD.[12] An Australian study done in 1995 conclude that oxazepam had less toxicity and sedative potential than temazepam.[13] Another Australian study done in 2004 which analyzed overdose admissions during 1987–2002 found out that alprazolam was more toxic than diazepam.[14] Zopiclone was found out to be having a comparable toxicity profile with other BZD in a study done in New Zealand in 2003[15]
- Blood levels of any particular BZD is not helpful in predicting the clinical course or outcome.[15] To diagnose a case of BZD overdose, a careful clinical history focusing on the amount of drug ingested, time at which drug was taken along with history of intake of other concomitant drugs is enough. This should be followed by a detailed neurological examination[16]
- A possibility of suspected case of suicidal intent should be noted and patient should always be examined for other evidences of any type of body harm. However, the ABC (airway, breathing and circulation) care to the patient should not be delayed due to any cause.

MANAGEMENT OF SEDATIVE HYPNOTIC OVERDOSE AND ROLE OF FLUMAZENIL

- A case of sedative hypnotic overdose is managed by frequent observation of the patients vital signs to look for any early deterioration, use of Glasgow coma scale scoring, intravenous (IV) fluid administration and maintenance of airway including artificial ventilation if the need arises like in cases of respiratory depression or pulmonary aspiration.[17] Hypotension is managed by aggressive fluid therapy, although occasionally patient may require ionotropic support. Bradycardia is managed by atropine
- A thorough gastric decontamination with activated charcoal should be performed in a patient with suspected sedative hypnotic overdose, especially if the patient has undertaken a cocktail of CNS depressants and that too if they present within first 4 hours of ingestion. Both gastric lavage and bowel irrigation are not recommended at present[18]
- For barbiturate overdose, urinary alkalinization with sodium bicarbonate may be beneficial. The optimum urinary pH which needs to be achieved is >7.5 and urine output should be more than 2 mL/kg/min. Forced diuresis is unlikely to have any benefit in a case of BZD overdose due to high-lipid solubility along with high volume of distribution.[19] Similarly, there is no role of hemodialysis
- Supportive measures are always given priority than specific antidotes like flumazenil which may only be beneficial in pure BZD overdose or in patients who are not on chronic BZD intake which constitute less than 10% of overdose cases[19]
- Flumazenil is contraindicated in patients who are on BZD for long term, patients with toxicity due to drugs which may lower the seizure threshold and patients which have a wide complex tachycardia in electrocardiogram (ECG), or patients showing anticholinergic symptoms.[20-22] It is given in a dose of 0.1–0.2 mg IV over 30–60 seconds, and repeated every 1–2 minutes to a total of 1–2 mg. The half-life of flumazenil is less than 1 hour, so multiple doses may be needed in patients or in such a scenario it may be given as a continuous infusion at a rate of 0.3–1 mg/hour for a duration of 3–6 hours.[23,24]

OPIOID OVERDOSE AND ITS MANAGEMENT

- Opioid toxicity is the leading cause of death due to drug overdoses. The onset of symptoms depends on the route, with IV route showing early toxicity
- Opioid overdose manifests as nausea, vomiting, sedation, drowsiness, respiratory depression and urinary retention. Patients are usually unconscious and pupils are pin point
- Those who survive the period of early toxicity may develop late complications of drug overdose like pulmonary edema, rhabdomyolysis, compartment syndrome and permanent neurological sequelae
- Opioids dependence, injectable drug user, patients with chronic illness and mood disorders are more likely to consume more dose of drug and hence are especially at risk. Use with other CNS depressants is particularly dangerous
- Like BZD, patient with toxicity are managed aggressively with focus on basic life support care otherwise death will ensue. Adequate hydration therapy must be given
- Naloxone is given to all patients of opioids overdose as an antidote.[25,26] Naloxone is a competitive antagonist at all the opioids receptor site. It is given as 0.4–0.8 mg IV every 2–3 minutes to a maximum of 10 mg dose
- It should be realized that most of the deaths are due to overprescription of these agents and there should be national level programs that monitor the drug prescription rates as well as may also decrease doctor shopping which is done by addicted patients.

CANNABINOIDS TOXICITY

- Mortality due to cannabis overdose is very rare as the lethal dose of cannabis is much higher than the usuaul dose taken
- The psychological effects of cannabinoids that one gets on smoking or ingesting the drug include feeling of high, euphoria, anxiety, increased creativity, increased libido and ataxia. Auditory, visual hallucinations, depersonalization and derealization may occur with very high doses
- The physiological effects include tachycardia, dry mouth, constipation, reddening of eyes, decreased intraocular pressure and feeling of relaxation of muscle and joints

- The basic life supportive measures should be provided to the patients till they are symptomatic
- Special care needs to be taken with regards to predisposition to arrhythmia and ECG monitoring should be done along with serial measurements of creatinine kinase.

GAMMA-HYDROXYBUTYRIC ACID OVERDOSE

- Gamma-hydroxybutyric acid overdose is a difficult condition to treat due to its multiple effects on the body
- Gamma-hydroxybutyric acid acts like a CNS depressant at higher doses and as a stimulant at lower doses. Thus euphoria, disinhibition, enhanced libido and empathogenic state is seen at lower dose, while nausea, dizziness, drowsiness, visual disturbance, breathing difficult, amnesia, unconsciousness and death are seen at higher doses
- A dose of 3,500 mg produces unconsciousness while a dose of 7,000 mg causes respiratory depression, bradycardia, and cardiac arrest. Its toxicity is increased when taken with other CNS depressants especially alcohol which may have a lethal combination. Zvosec et al. investigated 226 deaths due to GHB of which 213 deaths were due to cardiorespiratory arrest and 13 were due to accident-related cause[27]
- The management of GHB overdose is supportive only
- Regular ECG monitoring to look for bradycardia and life-threatening bradycardia should be managed by atropine
- Convulsions are managed by BZDs like diazepam. BZDs act on $GABA_A$ which is not the site of action of GHB and hence dual depression of CNS is rare
- A new drug called SCH-50911 is being used as antidotes in experimental animals.

The common CNS depressants and their fatal doses are summarized in Table 1.

PARTY DRUGS

- Party drugs also known as rave drug, club drug are commonly used these days mainly in discotheques, night-clubs, house parties and rave parties
- These include MDMA (3,4-methylenedioxy-methamphetamine), 2C-B (2,5-dimethoxy-4-

Central Nervous System Depressants: Overdose and Management

Table 1: Common central nervous system depressants and their fatal dose.

Drug	Therapeutic dose used for specific indication	Available strength in market	Usual lethal dose
Phenobarbitone	15–18 mg/kg IV for status epilepticus 1–3 mg/kg/day oral for seizures 100–200 mg PO for insomnia	15 mg, 30 mg, 60 mg in tablet 30–130 mg/mL in IV form	5,000–10,000 mg
Thiopentone	50–75 mg for induction of anesthesia	Available as a powder, to be dissolved in the reconstitution fluid	1,500 mg
Alprazolam	0.25–0.5 mg TDS for anxiety 0.5 mg TDS for panic disorder	0.25 mg, 0.5 mg, 1 mg, 2 mg as tablet 1 mg/mL as oral syrup	7,500 mg
Diazepam	1 mg/mL and 5 mg/mL as IV, 5 mg/ml as IM	2 mg, 5 mg, 10 mg as oral tablet	3,000–4,000 mg
Midazolam	70–80 µg/kg 30–60 minutes before surgery for sedation 300–350 µg/kg IV for anesthetic purpose	2 mg/mL as syrup 1 mg/mL and 5 mg/mL for IV/IM injection	3,000–4,000 mg
Flurazepam	15–30 mg PO for insomnia	15 mg, 30 mg oral tablet	3,300 mg
Morphine	10–20 mg PO q4hr, 5–10 mg q4hr, 2.5–5 mg q 3–4hr for pain relief	15 mg, 30 mg, 60 mg, 100 mg, 200 mg as oral tablet/capsules 0.5 mg/mL, 1 mg/mL, 2 mg/mL, 4 mg/mL, 10 mg/mL as IV or IM injection	250 mg
Hydrocodone	10–90 mg capsule used in chronic pain*	10 mg, 15 mg, 30 mg, 45 mg, 60 mg, 90 mg as oral tablet	90 mg
Oxycodone	10–30 mg divided 6 hourly for pain relief†	5 mg, 10 mg, 15 mg, 20 mg, 30 mg as oral tablet	80 mg
Fentanyl	50–100 µg slow IV/IM 30–60 minutes prior to surgery Increase dose to up to 2–20 µg/kg/dose followed by 1–2 µg/kg/h infusion for major surgery	0.05 mg/mL as IV injection	80 mg

*not available in medicine
†not used in India
(IM: intramuscular; IV: intravenous; PO: per oral; q6hr: every 6 hours; TDS: three times a day)

bromophenethylamine) and inhalants (nitrous oxide and poppers), stimulants (amphetamine and cocaine), depressants/sedatives (GHB, Rohypnol), and psychedelic and hallucinogenic drugs [LSD and dimethyltryptamine (DMT)]

- The MDMA, also commonly known as ecstasy and molly, is synthetic compound which affects CNS and has stimulant and hallucinogenic action leading to sense of increased energy, pleasure and emotional warmth. The effect lasts for 3–6 hours and in higher doses leads to nausea, vomiting, blurring of vision, sweating and depression. Treatment is supportive only. The blood levels of 0.1–0.25 mg/L are seen in patients who take drug for recreational purpose, while most fatal cases have blood levels of 0.5–10 mg/L.

- The use of these drugs is illegal in many countries, but is commonly used in night parties
- Party drugs are commonly used in mixed form as additive to other drugs and alcohol leading to difficulty in identifying the exact offending drug, thus difficult to treat and are often fatal
- The treatment is supportive in form of correction of hydration level, vital monitoring and observation, in absence of antidote.

CONCLUSION

Central nervous system depressants are prescribed to a large number of patients for their medicinal indications. Overdosage is mostly due suicidal intent or recreational purpose. Children, elderly and frail persons are susceptible to severe toxicity. A combination of drugs is most dangerous. The management of overdose is generally supportive with a focus on airway breathing and circulation. A thorough gastric decontamination is advised, if patients present early. Respiratory compromise should be suspected early and patient should be put on mechanical ventilation to salvage the life.

Flumazenil use should be restricted to patients who may actually benefit from it like in case of pure BZD overdose or patients who are not on its chronic use. Patients with opioid toxicity may benefit from naloxone and it should be given to all patients with suspected opioid overdose.

Whatever the antidote available, life saving measures especially protection of airway, breathing and circulation strategy are the cornerstone of management.

KEY POINTS

- Central nervous system depressants overdose is a medical emergency and timely intervention may save a life
- Airway, breathing and circulation stabilization is the most important cornerstone of management
- Detailed history about the possible drugs involved along with a complete neurological examination is the most important diagnostic test
- Do a thorough gastric decontamination, but avoid gastric lavage and whole bowel irrigation
- Respiratory depression in a case of sedative hypnotic overdose is dangerous and mechanical ventilation must be initiated in its presence
- Overenthusiastic use of flumazenil may actually do more harm than benefiting the patient; give it only in cases of pure BZDs overdose or those who are BZD naïve
- Naloxone should be given in all suspected cases of opioid overdose.

REFERENCES

1. Taylor S, McCracken CF, Wilson KC, et al. Extent and appropriateness of benzodiazepine use. Results from an elderly urban community. Br J Psychiatry. 1998;173(5): 433-8.
2. Buckley NA, McManus PR. Changes in fatalities due to overdose of anxiolytic and sedative drugs in the UK (1983–1999). Drug Saf. 2004;27:135-41.
3. Bachhuber MA, Hennessy S, Cunningham CO, et al. Increasing benzodiazepine prescriptions and overdose mortality in the United States, 1996-2013. Am J Public Health. 2016;106(4):686-8.
4. Ngo AS, Anthony CR, Samuel M, et al. Should a benzodiazepine antagonist be used in unconscious patients presenting to the emergency department? Resuscitation. 2007;74(1):27-37.
5. GBD 2015 Mortality and Causes of Death, Collaborators. (8 October 2016). Global, regional, and national life expectancy, all-cause mortality, and cause-specific mortality for 249 causes of death, 1980-2015: a systematic analysis for the Global Burden of Disease Study 2015. Lancet. 2016;388(10053):1459-544.
6. American Society of Addiction Medicine. Opioid Addiction 2016 Facts & Figures. Rockville: ASAM; 2016.
7. Gallagher R. The use of opioids for dyspnea in advanced disease. CMAJ. 2011;183(10):1170.
8. Wiseman R, Rowett D, Allcroft P, et al. Chronic refractory dyspnoea--evidence based management. Aust Fam Physician. 2013;42(3):137-40.
9. Rocker G, Horton R, Currow D, et al. Palliation of dyspnoea in advanced COPD: revisiting a role for opioids. Thorax. 2009;64:910-5.
10. Wiley CC, Wiley JF. Pediatric benzodiazepine ingestion resulting in hospitalization. J Toxicol Clin Toxicol. 1998;36(3):227-31.
11. Gaudreault P, Guay J, Thivierge RL, et al. Benzodiazepine poisoning. Clinical and pharmacological considerations and treatment. Drug Saf. 1993;6(4):247-65.
12. Serfaty M, Masterton G. Fatal poisonings attributed to benzodiazepines in Britain during the 1980s. Br J Psychiatry. 1993;163(3):386-93.
13. Buckley NA, Dawson AH, Whyte IM, et al. Relative toxicity of benzodiazepines in overdose. BMJ. 1995;310(6974):219-21.
14. Isbister GK, O'Regan L, Sibbritt D, et al. Alprazolam is relatively more toxic than other benzodiazepines in overdose. Br J Clin Pharmacol. 2004;58(1):88-95.
15. Reith DM, Fountain J, McDowell R, et al. Comparison of the fatal toxicity index of zopiclone with benzodiazepines. J Toxicol Clin Toxicol. 2003;41(7):975-80.
16. Perry HE, Shannon MW. Diagnosis and management of opioid- and benzodiazepine-induced comatose overdose in children. Current Opinion in Pediatrics. 1996;8(3):243-7.
17. Rumpl E, Prugger M, Battista HJ, et al. Short latency somatosensory evoked potentials and brain-stem auditory evoked potentials in coma due to CNS depressant drug poisoning. Preliminary observations. Electroencephalogr Clin Neurophysiol. 1988;70(6):482-9.
18. el-Khordagui LK, Saleh AM, Khalil SA. Adsorption of benzodiazepines on charcoal and its correlation with in vitro and in vivo data. Pharmaceutica Acta Helvetiae. 1987;62(1):28-32.
19. Whyte IM. Benzodiazepines. Medical Toxicology. Philadelphia: Williams & Wilkins; 2004. pp. 811-22.

20. Nelson LH, Flomenbaum N, Goldfrank LR, et al. Antidotes in depth: Flumazenil. Goldfrank's Toxicologic Emergencies, 8th edition. New York: McGraw-Hill; 2006. pp. 1112-7.

21. Spivey WH. Flumazenil and seizures: analysis of 43 cases. Clin Ther. 1992;14(2):292-305.

22. Marchant B, Wray R, Leach A, et al. Flumazenil causing convulsions and ventricular tachycardia. BMJ. 1989;299(6703):860.

23. Weinbroum AA, Flaishon R, Sorkine P, et al. A risk-benefit assessment of flumazenil in the management of benzodiazepine overdose. Drug Saf. 1997;17(3):181-96.

24. Penninga EI, Graudal N, Ladekarl MB, et al. Adverse events associated with flumazenil treatment for the management of suspected benzodiazepine intoxication: a systematic review with meta-analyses of randomised trials. Basic Clin Pharmacol Toxicol. 2016;118:37-44.

25. Etherington J, Christenson J, Innes G, et al. Is early discharge safe after naloxone reversal of presumed opioid overdose. CJEM. 2000;2(3):156-62.

26. Leo B, Scott CB, Alex HK. Closing death's door: Action steps to facilitate emergency opioid drug overdose reversal in the United States. SSRN Electronic Journal. 2009.

27. Zvosec DL, Smith SW, Porrata T, et al. Case series of 226 gamma hydroxybutyrate associated deaths: lethal toxicity and trauma. Am J Emerg Med. 2011;29(3):319-32.

8 CHAPTER

Sympathomimetic Drugs

Anish Gupta, Omender Singh

INTRODUCTION

Substance or drug abuse is an emerging problem worldwide sparing no age group, including children and the elderly. The exact reasons are not known but changes in cultural values, social and peer pressure, monetary issues and multiple stressors have led to this emerging epidemic. As per the World Health Organization (WHO), substance abuse is defined as the harmful use of psychoactive substances.[1] It refers to patterned use of these substances in quantities not recommended and leads to self-harm. Such substances are varied in nature and include alcohol, cocaine, opiates, amphetamines, hallucinogens, recreational drugs and designer drugs.

All psychoactive substances can lead to dependence syndromes, toxicity due to excessive doses and withdrawal syndromes. The critical care specialist and emergency physician should be aware of the physiological and pathological effects of these compounds as their early diagnosis and appropriate management may play a crucial role in the outcome.

The drugs of abuse can be classified into the following categories as mentioned in Table 1.

Table 1: Classification of drugs of abuse.[2]	
Class	*Drugs/Toxins*
Stimulants	Amphetamines, methamphetamine, cocaine, 3,4-methylenedioxymethamphetamine (MDMA) (ecstasy), nicotine, caffeine
Depressants	Barbiturates, benzodiazepines (BZDs), gamma-hydroxybutyrate, antihistaminics
Hallucinogens	Lysergic acid diethylamide (LSD), mescaline, psilocybin (mushrooms), dextromethorphan (DXM)
Dissociative anesthetics	Ketamine, phencyclidine (PCP) and analogs (angel dust)
Cannabinoids	Ganja, hashish, marijuana (pot, grass, weed, Mary Jane)
Opiates	Opium, heroin, morphine, fentanyl, codeine, oxycodone, tramadol
Inhalants (converted to vapor at room temperature)	Acetone, aerosol sprays, paint thinner , gases (nitrous oxide), glue, amyl nitrite, gasoline, Iodex, pen ink, marker, room deodorizers
Others	Alcohol, anabolic steroids

CENTRAL NERVOUS SYSTEM STIMULANTS

Amphetamines (Ma-huang, Khat, Propylhexedrine, Meow)

Amphetamine is a central nervous system (CNS) stimulant belonging to the phenethylamine group. Historically, it was used as a nasal decongestant and weight loss drug. Then, it was a common agent used by military personnel to increase alertness and reduce fatigue, but eventually came into vogue for its euphoric effects.

Being lipophilic amphetamines have large volumes of distribution and can readily cross the blood-brain barrier.[3] The $t_{1/2}$ varies from 2 hours to 24 hours and depends on the compound consumed. They are metabolized in the liver and are excreted in urine. Urinary excretion is primarily pH dependent as amphetamines are alkaline in nature. Acidic urine enhances excretion.[4]

The chemical structure of amphetamines resembles epinephrine, norepinephrine and to a certain extent dopamine. Hence, the clinical features of amphetamine intoxication are secondary to sympathomimetic effects and action on dopaminergic pathways. The constellation of signs and symptoms of amphetamine intoxication form a part of the sympathomimetic toxidrome.[4] However, a number of coingestants may aggravate or blunt the classic clinical features of amphetamine intoxication. The commonly abused substances with amphetamines are alcohol, cocaine, cannabis and 3,4-methylenedioxymethamphetamine (MDMA).[5]

The clinical effects are secondary to stimulation of α- and β-adrenergic receptors. Studies have also shown a role of amphetamine in competitively inhibiting the enzyme monoamine oxidase (MAO) which oxidatively metabolizes epinephrine and norepinephrine. As a result, the effects of these adrenergic neurotransmitters are prolonged with their resultant systemic effects.

The toxic dose of amphetamine varies on the type of user as well as the dose consumed. Naïve users may develop toxicity at doses of 1 mg/kg while in chronic abusers the toxic doses may be higher.

Clinical Features

The cardiovascular and nervous systems are commonly involved.

Cardiovascular: Stimulation of the cardiac β-receptors leads to adrenergic effects with increase in heart rate, palpitations and blood pressure. There is associated bronchodilatation, anxiety and tremulousness. Patients present with chest pain, diaphoresis and arrhythmias. Myocardial ischemia, dysfunction and cases of myocarditis have been reported with acute intoxication.[6]

Central nervous system: Since amphetamines easily cross the blood-brain barrier, neurological symptoms are common. A neuropsychiatric syndrome is described wherein cases present with anxiety, agitation, violent and aggressive behavior, confusion, hallucinations, tremors, myoclonus and seizures.[7] Hyponatremia with altered mental status and cerebral edema has been reported in some cases.[8]

Other systems: Amphetamines can cause mydriasis and weight loss. Skin tracks with thrombophlebitis, local abscess and cellulitis, can occur after intravenous use.[9] Dyselectrolytemias (hypokalemia/hyperkalemia, hypermagnesemia and hyponatremia) and high anion gap metabolic acidosis can occur in severe cases. Renal ischemia leading to acute kidney injury and acute tubular necrosis have also been reported.[10]

Tolerance can develop in chronic abusers with physical or psychological dependence. Abusers may present with mental impairment, increased sleep, emotional instability and loss of weight and appetite.

Diagnosis

Amphetamine is routinely detected in urine toxicology screen. However, urine assays should be analyzed with caution as false-positive results are seen with selegiline, pseudoephedrine and bupropion.[11] At present, there is no specific test to diagnose amphetamine toxicity. Serum drug levels can be measured but are cumbersome and time consuming thus mitigating their role in acute intoxication.

The diagnosis is made on the basis of history of particular drug abuse and clinical features suggestive of sympathomimetic toxidrome.

The management of amphetamine toxicity is similar to methamphetamine intoxication and is discussed in the following section.

Methamphetamine (Sisa, Speed, Crank, Crystal, Chalk, Tina, Gak, Poor Man's Coke, Redneck)

Methamphetamine (similar to amphetamine) is a sympathomimetic amine belonging to phenethylamine group.

It differs slightly from amphetamine in chemical structure with a second methyl group in the carbon chain. It exists as two isomers dextro- and levo-isomer. These features increase the lipophilicity of methamphetamine as compared to amphetamine.

The mechanism of toxicity is similar to amphetamine. However, unlike amphetamine, methamphetamine does not have direct adrenergic effects. Methamphetamine enters the presynaptic nerve terminals and displaces epinephrine, norepinephrine, dopamine and serotonin from their vesicles into the cytosol. As the cytosolic concentration of these amines increases they diffuse out of the neuron into the synaptic spaces and bind to their respective postsynaptic receptors. Methamphetamine also inhibits the reuptake of these amines by inactivating transporter systems. This leads to surge in sympathetic stimulation.[4]

Methamphetamine is absorbed by oral, intravenous, intramuscular, rectal and vaginal routes. Peak plasma concentrations vary depending on the route of administration and ranges from 5 minutes for intranasal to 2–3 hours for oral route. The $t_{1/2}$ is 12–36 hours.[12]

Toxic Features

Methamphetamine intoxication has features similar to sympathomimetic toxidrome. The commonly involved systems are cardiovascular, respiratory, neurological and gastrointestinal.

Cardiovascular: Methamphetamine causes dose-dependent increase in heart rate and blood pressure. Acute coronary syndrome occurs rarely. Valvular dysfunction can occur and is secondary to serotonergic effects. Sudden cardiovascular collapse has been reported with severe intoxications.[13]

Central nervous system: Choreiform movements are typical and secondary to abnormal dopaminergic transmission.[14] Focal neurological deficits, seizures and hyperactive delirium are commonly seen in acute intoxication. A variety of psychiatric symptoms, i.e. anxiety, hallucinations, paranoia, psychosis and suicidal ideation have been reported but mainly in chronic abusers.[15]

Respiratory: Tachypnea and breathlessness are often seen at presentation. Acute pulmonary edema and pulmonary hypertension may be the presenting features. Pneumonia, pneumothorax, pneumomediastinum, pulmonary hemorrhage and acute respiratory distress syndrome, have all been reported with acute methamphetamine intoxication.[16,17]

Meth mouth: A typical finding in chronic methamphetamine abusers. It is extensive tooth decay and distortion secondary to poor dental hygiene, repeated grinding of teeth and decreased salivation.

Others: Vomiting, diarrhea and abdominal pain are seen in some cases. Methamphetamine can cause bowel ischemia especially in cases of body packing.[18] Abuse during pregnancy can lead to placental insufficiency and abruptio placenta.[19] "Track marks" may be present in chronic intravenous abusers.

Diagnosis

Diagnosis is similar to that mentioned in amphetamine intoxication. A patient presenting with a sympathomimetic toxidrome and a positive assay for the drug in urine is diagnosed as a case of methamphetamine intoxication. A number of drugs may present with clinical features similar to methamphetamine toxicity and include cocaine, phencyclidine derivatives, MAO inhibitors, salicylates, lithium, tricyclic antidepressants and synthetic cathinones, etc. Some nontoxicologic conditions like cerebral hemorrhage, thyrotoxicosis, pheochromocytoma and hyperthermic disorders (heat stroke) can mimic methamphetamine intoxication.

Baseline investigations include complete hemogram, kidney and liver function tests and blood glucose levels. An electrocardiogram (ECG) should be done in all cases to rule out conduction abnormalities. A pregnancy screening test should be done in all women of childbearing age.

A urine toxicology screen can detect methamphetamine. The test is not specific and has false-positive and false-negative results.[11] Bupropion, benzphetamine, selegiline and nasal inhalers (containing L-desoxyephedrine) may yield false-positive results.[20,21]

Management

One specific feature to methamphetamine intoxication is that patients may become severely agitated and violent without any provocation. The principal strategy for management of patients includes prevention and control of agitation and hyperthermia.

Airway management: The indications for endotracheal intubation are severely intoxicated patients with hyperthermia, severe agitation not responding to benzodiazepines and antipsychotics, muscle rigidity and worsening acidosis. Nondepolarizing neuromuscular blocking agents (rocuronium, vecuronium) are preferred for paralysis. Succinylcholine is contraindicated as it can precipitate life-threatening hyperkalemia in hyperthermic and severely agitated patients. Some authors recommend giving soda bicarbonate prior to endotracheal intubation to target a pH > 7.1. This recommendation is not based on any randomized controlled trials.

Sedation: Severely agitated patients can pose a threat to themselves and others. Control of violent behavior is of utmost importance. Benzodiazepines are the drugs of choice. Midazolam 3–5 mg or lorazepam 2–6 mg can be given IV. The doses can be repeated every 5–10 minutes until patient is sedated or agitation is controlled. In some cases, a second benzodiazepine may need to be added if poor control is achieved with the first one. Antipsychotic medications are administered as an adjunct when high doses of benzodiazepines are unable to achieve control of psychotic symptoms. Butyrophenones (haloperidol) are the preferable agents but can prolong QT interval and precipitate fatal arrhythmias.[22,23]

Avoid sole physical restraints: Agitated patients solely with physical restraints are at risk of sudden cardiac death. This is explained by the fact that struggle against restraints by these patients leads to isometric muscle contractions which can lead to hyperthermia and lactic acidosis which may be life-threatening. Always use chemical sedation in combination with physical restraints and discontinue them as soon as possible.

Control of tachycardia and hypertension: Tachycardia is usually well tolerated. However, in patients with coronary artery disease, it can precipitate acute coronary syndrome. Benzodiazepines reduce the heart rate by decreasing central catecholamine release. The doses are the same as mentioned above. Calcium channel blockers (diltiazem 15–30 mg TDS) can be used for rate control in addition to benzodiazepines. Avoid pure β-blockers and combined α- and β-blockers as they increase the risk of vasoconstriction.[24]

Hypertension is a common finding in intoxicated patients and usually responds to sedation with benzodiazepines. However, in some cases, intravenous antihypertensives may be needed. Preferable agents include nitroprusside, nitroglycerin and phentolamine.

Avoid β-blockers during the acute phase as they can lead to unopposed alpha agonistic actions.

Hyperthermia: Temperature should be controlled aggressively with external and in some extreme cases internal cooling methods. Benzodiazepines are often used to reduce temperature but in some cases neuromuscular paralysis may be warranted. Antipyretics have no role in the management of methamphetamine-induced hyperthermia.

Gastric decontamination: Activated charcoal has no routine role as methamphetamine is not commonly consumed orally but is smoked, inhaled or injected. Activated charcoal helps in cases of body packing or stuffing.

Urine acidification: No role at present. It was used in the past to increase elimination.

HALLUCINOGENS

A hallucinogen is a substance which alters mood, thought process and sensory perception. Hallucinogens occur naturally or are artificially synthesized. The first synthetic hallucinogen is lysergic acid diethylamide (LSD). It was synthesized by Albert Hofmann in 1938 and is considered the prototype hallucinogen.[25] Hallucinogens are abused for their psychedelic effects. Two common terms are used to describe the hallucinogenic effects in individuals namely "Trip" and "Flashback". A Trip refers to acute toxic effects of hallucinogens and can be a good or a bad trip. Flashback refers to the recurrence of toxic symptoms after the acute phase has worn off.

Pharmacology

The exact mechanisms of effects are unknown but a common feature to all is their ability to bind to 5-hydroxytryptamine (5-HT) 2A receptors.[26,27] Various neurotransmitters have been implicated in the hallucinogenic process namely serotonin, dopamine and glutamate. A unique hallucinogen is Salvinorin A, which has κ-opioid agonistic activity.[28] Most hallucinogens are administered by oral route and have different pharmacokinetics depending upon the substance consumed.

Features of Intoxication

The most common presenting features are neuropsychiatric. The clinical manifestations are euphoria, altered

Drugs of Abuse

mental status (impaired perception of time), distorted perception of sensory stimuli and heightened experience of mystical and spiritual feelings. A peculiar feature is blending of senses called synesthesia. Individuals may hear objects or see sounds. Tachycardia, hypertension and hyperthermia are commonly observed. Negative symptoms include fear, anxiety attacks, panic episodes and sense of impending doom. Although uncommon some may present with frank psychosis.

A typical manifestation of hallucinogens (LSD, MDMA) is Serotonin Syndrome which is characterized by a triad of altered mentation, myoclonus and autonomic hyperactivity.

Lysergic Acid Diethylamide (Lysergide)

It is an indole alkylamine and a potent hallucinogen. Generally, it is consumed orally as a pill, capsule or liquid. Commonly available as small blotting paper strips impregnated with liquid LSD, where each strip is equivalent to one dose. The usual recreational doses are 20–80 µg. It produces psychedelic effects for 8–12 hours.[29] Individuals have impaired perception of time, visual illusions or hallucinations, blurred vision, euphoria, synesthesia and depersonalization. Life-threatening toxicity leading to cardiovascular collapse is uncommon and is reported with ingestions >400 µg.[30] Most cases of death are due to impaired judgment leading to accidents and not due to LSD toxicity. It is metabolized in the liver and excreted mainly in bile. It can be detected in urine for 1–2 days post-ingestion.

Dextromethorphan

Dextromethorphan (DXM) is a common component of over-the-counter (OTC) cough and cold remedies. DXM abuse is most commonly observed in adolescents and young adults. Although it is commonly abused for recreational purposes, suicidal attempts have also been reported. In children and infants, toxicity is usually accidental (e.g. miscalculation of dose for viral illness). DXM is frequently coingested with ethanol and history of all possible coingestants should be elicited. DXM poisoning is usually secondary to a single large ingestion but chronic use can also lead to toxicity.

Dextromethorphan is a D-isomer of codeine analog, levorphanol and is chemically D-3-methoxy-N-methylmorphine. The addictive and sedative properties of DXM are considered to be negligible. However,

cases of drug dependence have been reported. The therapeutic dose is 15–30 mg given three to four times per day (maximum 120 mg/day). At therapeutic doses, DXM causes tachycardia, dry mouth and decreases concentration (anticholinergic syndrome). At high doses, it produces a dissociative state called "robo-tripping", "robo-copping", "robo-ing" or "going pharming".[31] The dissociative effects and adrenergic effects are secondary to antagonism of N-methyl-D-aspartate (NMDA) receptors. DXM also has some action on serotonergic receptors (5-HT2) and hence can precipitate serotonin syndrome in abusers.[32,33] The ease of access has made it a commonly used recreational drug and is referred by adolescents as a "legal high".

Dextromethorphan toxicity occurs in a dose-dependent manner. Toxic symptoms become manifest at doses greater than 1.5 mg/kg. There are different stages of toxicity which are called as "plateaus" amongst abusers (Table 2).[34]

Mechanism of toxicity of DXM has been shown in Flowchart 1.

Toxic Manifestations

In acute overdose, DXM produces tachycardia, mydriasis, euphoria, hallucinations, agitation, dissociative symptoms and in extreme cases coma. Tachycardia is a consistent finding. The absence of tachycardia rules out the possibility of DXM poisoning except in cases where patients are on atrioventricular node blocking agents (β-blockers, calcium channel blockers). Agitation can be severe leading to rhabdomyolysis and metabolic acidosis.[31,35]

Serotonin syndrome can be precipitated in large ingestions or concomitant ingestion of serotonergic drugs (MAO-inhibitors, tramadol, linezolid).[36]

Respiratory depression, coma and dystonic reactions have been reported in infants and children.[35]

The OTC medications do not always contain DXM as the sole agent. There are additional drugs in

Table 2: Various stages (plateaus) of toxicity of dextromethorphan poisoning.

1st Plateau	100–200 mg	Tachycardia, hypertension, diaphoresis, mydriasis
2nd Plateau	200–300 mg	Hallucinations, euphoria
3rd Plateau	300–600 mg	Dissociative symptoms
4th Plateau	600 mg	Coma, unresponsiveness

Flowchart 1: Mechanism of toxicity of dextromethorphan.

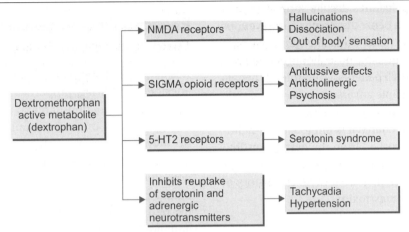

combination namely antihistaminics, decongestants (pseudoephedrine, phenylephrine) and acetaminophen. Overdose may lead to toxic features of these co-ingestants in addition to those of DXM.

Antihistaminics block H1 receptors and toxicity is manifested as anticholinergic poisoning with tachycardia, hypertension, mydriasis, hyperthermia, warm flushed skin, urinary retention and delirium.[31] Excess of decongestants (α-1 adrenergic agonist) can lead to headache, hypertension with reflex bradycardia or tachycardia. Acetaminophen can lead to acute or delayed liver cell failure. Acetaminophen poisoning is discussed in detail in a separate chapter.

Bromism: The salt of DXM found in OTC medications is DXM hydrobromide. In chronic abusers, bromide toxicity may occur and manifest as fatigue, headache, memory loss and ataxia. An elevated chloride concentration and a negative anion gap metabolic acidosis should raise the concern for bromism.[37]

Diagnosis

Dextromethorphan toxicity/poisoning is diagnosed on the basis of history and clinical features. Typical cases are young adults with sudden change in behavior with gait disturbances, visual hallucinations, tachycardia and hypertension.

Routinely available urine drug assay tests do not detect DXM as they use immunoassay technology.[38] However, tests which use the liquid chromatography technique may detect DXM but may give false-positive results for phencyclidine and derivatives.[39] Quantitative and qualitative assays use gas chromatography or mass spectroscopy and are for reference laboratories. DXM levels in blood are usually performed for forensic purposes.

Psilocybin

It is an hallucinogen belonging to the tryptamine group.[40] They are also known as "magic mushrooms" or "shrooms". Recreational doses vary from 10 mg to 50 mg. Other similar tryptamines include α-methyltryptamine, N,N-dimethyltryptamine and 5-methoxy-dimethyltryptamine (foxy methoxy). The neuropsychiatric effects of all tryptamines are similar to LSD. In addition, gastrointestinal symptoms (nausea, vomiting, diarrhea) are frequently present. Serotonin syndrome is a common presentation as tryptamines have structural similarity to serotonin.

Management of Hallucinogenic Intoxication

Most patients who present with acute intoxication with hallucinogens have self-limited toxic features and only need supportive care. The main goal of care is to limit the sensory input as intoxicated patients distort and augment the sensory input.[41,42] Patients should be nursed in a calm and quiet environment with frequent monitoring of vital parameters.[42]

Patients occasionally may present with serious symptoms. Assessment and stabilization of airway, breathing and circulation is first done in such patients.

Benzodiazepines (midazolam, diazepam, lorazepam) are the first-line agents for psychomotor agitation. Benzodiazepines should be administered preferably by

Drugs of Abuse

the intravenous route. Neuroleptic medications are added for those with psychotic features despite supportive care and optimal therapy with benzodiazepines.[43] Intravenous haloperidol 2–5 mg is used to abate the psychotic symptoms. The minimal possible dose should be used. It is imperative to monitor such patients as neuroleptic agents by itself can lead to multiple adverse effects (neuroleptic malignant syndrome, broad QRS complex).

The role of activated charcoal is limited, since hallucinogens are rapidly absorbed from the gastrointestinal tract. Activated charcoal is given only in cases which present within 1 hour of presentation or there is a history of coingestion with other drugs/toxins.

Control of Hyperthermia

Cooling methods should be instituted promptly. Evaporative cooling is the best modality as it is noninvasive and effective. Some experts are of the opinion that patients with severe hyperthermia (>40°C) should be intubated and paralyzed as it reduces muscle activity. No routine role of antipyretics (paracetamol) as there is no change in the temperature set point in the hypothalamus.

Role of Urinary Acidification

Acidification of urine has been used in the past to increase the excretion of certain hallucinogens, in particular LSD which is a weak base. However, the effect was minimal with a propensity to cause harm. At present, urinary acidification is not recommended to treat intoxication with hallucinogens.

Antidotal Therapy

At present, there is no specific antidote for any of the hallucinogens and treatment is symptomatic and supportive.

Naloxone

Naloxone is an opioid receptor antagonist. Hence, it helps reverse respiratory depression and coma in patients with DXM poisoning.[44] It is administered at a dose of 0.1 mg/kg to a maximum dose of 2 mg. All patients on naloxone will need hospital admission and invasive monitoring. Patients may not respond to the initial doses and repeat doses may be needed. Total doses may approach 10 mg.

DISSOCIATIVE ANESTHETICS

Phencyclidine (Angel Dust, Embalming Fluid, Killer Weed, Peace Pill)

It is a synthetic arycycloalkylamine and is a dissociative anesthetic.[45,46] It has properties similar to ketamine. At low doses, it has non-narcotic anesthetic effects while at higher doses it causes cataplexy. Phencyclidine acts by noncompetitively inhibiting NMDA receptors,[47] inhibiting the uptake of biogenic amines (epinephrine, norepinephrine and dopamine)[48] and binding to sigma opioid receptors.[49] The recreational doses vary from 1 mg to 6 mg and is available as powder, tablets, crystals and liquid. Toxicity depends on the dose and route of administration. Symptoms commence at a dose of 0.05 mg/kg. Distortion of body image occurs at 0.1 mg/kg and there are reports of catatonic stupor at 10 mg.[46] Neurological symptoms are the most common. Symptoms may wax or wane and include agitation, bizarre behavior or in some rare cases coma. In one case series, the neurological features are named as "acute brain syndrome" with defining features as disorientation, confusion, amnesia and lack of judgement.[50] Hallucinations (visual, auditory and tactile) have been reported. Psychosis is seen in a significant number of patients. Nystagmus (horizontal, vertical or rotatory) is a common toxic manifestation.[51] Urine and serum phencyclidine levels can be measured. Usually qualitative tests are performed as quantitative levels do not correlate with toxic features.[51] Gas chromatography is used for confirmation but is not routinely used. False-positive tests are seen with ketamine, DXM, venlafaxine and tramadol. Management includes initial assessment and stabilization of airway, breathing and circulation. The mainstay of management is control of psychomotor agitation and benzodiazepines are used for the same. Butyrophenones are added as adjuncts in uncontrolled cases.[52] Gastrointestinal decontamination with activated charcoal has a limited role. Urine acidification and charcoal hemoperfusion have no role.

Ketamine (Street Names K, Special K, Kit Kat, Vitamin K, Ket and Super K)

Ketamine, like phencyclidine, is an arylcycloalkylamine used as an induction and maintenance agent in general anesthesia. It is a dissociative anesthetic agent with hallucinogenic properties. It is an NMDA receptor antagonist with sympathomimetic properties. It also has some opioid receptor activity. Its main site of action is the thalamocortical projection system. The therapeutic dose is based on patients' age and type of procedure. Usual doses are up to 5 mg/kg.[53] Recreational doses vary from 75 mg to 300 mg and depend on the route of administration. Some analogs of ketamine (methoxetamine, methoxyketamine and tiletamine) called Designer drugs have gained popularity due to ease of availability.[54] In small doses, it has hallucinogenic effects and decreases alertness, alters sensory perception and causes ataxia and nystagmus.[55] In overdose, it can cause severe psychomotor agitation and fear. At therapeutic doses, it causes increase in heart rate and blood pressure while in large doses cardiac effects are unpredictable. Ketamine can precipitate acute coronary syndrome as it increases myocardial oxygen consumption.[56] It is important to emphasize that ketamine is commonly abused with other illicit drugs like cocaine, amphetamines and MDMA.[57] There is no definitive laboratory test for ketamine and diagnosis is based on history and clinical features. There is no specific antidote for ketamine intoxication and management is mainly supportive.

CONCLUSION

Sympathomimetic drugs are compounds which mimic the endogenous agonists of the sympathetic nervous system, directly or indirectly. Most of these are CNS stimulants, with possible abuse potential, and the ability to induce tolerance and/or physical dependence. Overdose resembles a sympathomimetic toxidrome, with features like hyperactivity, anxiety, hyper-reflexia, hyperthermia, altered mentation, hypertension, etc. Commonly abused ones include amphetamine, cocaine, and MDMA. Management of overdose is mostly supportive and symptomatic.

KEY POINTS

- The clinical features of amphetamine and methamphetamine overdose resemble a sympathomimetic toxidrome
- The cornerstone of management of CNS stimulant intoxication is prevention and control of agitation and hyperthermia. Benzodiazepines are the mainstay of therapy
- Hallucinogens produce a trip or flashback
- Dextromethorphan produces dose-related toxicity with different stages called as "plateaus"
- Bromide toxicity can be seen with DXM overdose

- Naloxone can be used for management of respiratory depression in DXM toxicity
- "Acute brain syndrome" is seen with phencyclidine toxicity.

REFERENCES

1. World Health Organization. (2018). Substance abuse. [online] Available from http://www.who.int/topics/substance_abuse/en/ [Accessed October, 2018].
2. Nahas GG. A pharmacological classification of drugs of abuse. Bull Narc. 1981;33(2):1-19.
3. Baselt RC. Disposition of Toxic Drugs and Chemicals in Man, 7th edition, Foster City: Biomedical Publications; 2004.
4. Chiang WK. Amphetamines. In: Goldfrank LR (Ed). Goldfrank's Toxicologic Emergencies, 9th edition, New York: McGraw-Hill; 2011. p. 1078.
5. Winstock AR, Mitcheson LR, Deluca P, et al. Mephedrone, new kid for the chop? Addiction. 2011;106(1):154-61.
6. Nicholson PJ, Quinn MJ, Dodd JD. Headshop heartache: acute mephedrone 'meow' myocarditis. Heart. 2010;96(24):2051-2.
7. Durham M. Ivory wave: the next mephedrone? Emerg Med J. 2011;28(12):1059-60.
8. Wood DM, Davies S, Puchnarewicz M, et al. Recreational use of mephedrone (4-methylmethcathinone, 4-MMC) with associated sympathomimetic toxicity. J Med Toxicol. 2010;6(3):327-30.
9. Dorairaj JJ, Healy C, McMenamin M, et al. The untold truth about "bath salt" highs: a case series demonstrating local tissue injury. J Plast Reconstr Aesthet Surg. 2012;65(2):e37-41.
10. Adebamiro A, Perazella MA. Recurrent acute kidney injury following bath salts intoxication. Am J Kidney Dis. 2012;59(2):273-5.
11. elSohly MA, Jones AB. Drug testing in the workplace: could a positive test for one of the mandated drugs be for reasons other than illicit use of the drug? J Anal Toxicol. 1995;19:450.
12. Meredith CW, Jaffe C, Ang-Lee K, et al. Implications of chronic methamphetamine use: a literature review. Harv Rev Psychiatry. 2005;13(3):141-54.
13. Hawley LA, Auten JD, Matteucci MJ, et al. Cardiac complications of adult methamphetamine exposures. J Emerg Med. 2013;45(6):821-7.
14. Sperling LS, Horowitz JL. Methamphetamine-induced choreoathetosis and rhabdomyolysis. Ann Intern Med. 1994;121(12):986.
15. Zweben JE, Cohen JB, Christian D, et al. Psychiatric symptoms in methamphetamine users. Am J Addict. 2004;13(2):181-90.
16. Wells SM, Buford MC, Braseth SN, et al. Acute inhalation exposure to vaporized methamphetamine causes lung injury in mice. Inhal Toxicol. 2008;20(9):829-38.
17. Schaiberger PH, Kennedy TC, Miller FC, et al. Pulmonary hypertension associated with long-term inhalation of "crank" methamphetamine. Chest. 1993;104:614.

18. Johnson TD, Berenson MM. Methamphetamine-induced ischemic colitis. J Clin Gastroenterol. 1991;13(6):687-9.

19. Oro AS, Dixon SD. Perinatal cocaine and methamphetamine exposure: maternal and neonatal correlates. J Pediatr. 1987;111(4):571-8.

20. Nixon AL, Long WH, Puopolo PR, et al. Bupropion metabolites produce false-positive urine amphetamine results. Clin Chem. 1995;41(6 Pt 1):955-6.

21. Cody JT, Valtier S. Detection of amphetamine and methamphetamine following administration of benzphetamine. J Anal Toxicol. 1998;22(4):299-309.

22. Richards JR, Derlet RW, Duncan DR. Methamphetamine toxicity: treatment with a benzodiazepine versus a butyrophenone. Eur J Emerg Med. 1997;4(3):130-5.

23. Delbridge TR, Yealy DM. Wide complex tachycardia. Emerg Med Clin North Am. 1995;13:903.

24. Paratz ED, Cunningham NJ, MacIsaac AI. The cardiac complications of methamphetamines. Heart Lung Circ. 2016;25(4):325-32.

25. Hoffman A. LSD: My Problem Child. Ott J (Trans), Saline, MI: McNaughton and Gunn; 2005.

26. Nichols DE. Hallucinogens. Pharmacol Ther. 2004;101(2):131-81.

27. Fantegrossi WE, Murnane KS, Reissig CJ. The behavioral pharmacology of hallucinogens. Biochem Pharmacol. 2008;75(1):17-33.

28. Roth BL, Baner K, Westkaemper R, et al. Salvinorin A: a potent naturally occurring nonnitrogenous kappa-opioid selective agonist. Proc Natl Acad Sci USA. 2002;99(18):11934-9.

29. Dolder PC, Schmid Y, Steuer AE, et al. Pharmacokinetics and pharmacodynamics of lysergic acid diethylamide in healthy subjects. Clin Pharmacokinet. 2017;56(10):1219-30.

30. Klock JC, Boerner U, Becker CE. Coma, hyperthermia and bleeding associated with massive LSD overdose. West J Med. 1974;120(3):183-8.

31. Kirages TJ, Sule HP, Mycyk MB. Severe manifestations of Coricidin intoxication. Am J Emerg Med. 2003;21:473-5.

32. Carr BC. Efficacy, abuse, and toxicity of over-the-counter cough and cold medicines in the pediatric population. Curr Opin Pediatr. 2006;18(2):184-8.

33. Weinbroum AA, Rudick V, Paret G, et al. The role of dextromethorphan in pain control. Can J Anaesth. 2000;47(6):585-96.

34. Logan BK, Yeakel JK, Goldfogel G, et al. Dextromethorphan abuse leading to assault, suicide, or homicide. J Forensic Sci. 2012;57(5):1388-94.

35. Paul IM, Reynolds KM, Kauffman RE, et al. Adverse events associated with pediatric exposures to dextromethorphan. Clin Toxicol (Phila). 2017;55(1):25-32.

36. Ganetsky M, Babu KM, Boyer EW. Serotonin syndrome in dextromethorphan ingestion responsive to propofol therapy. Pediatr Emerg Care. 2007;23(11):829-31.

37. Ng YY, Lin WL, Chen TW, et al. Spurious hyperchloremia and decreased anion gap in a patient with dextromethorphan bromide. Am J Nephrol. 1992;12(4):268-70.

38. Boyer EW. Dextromethorphan abuse. Pediatr Emerg Care. 2004;20(12):858-63.

39. Schier J. Avoid unfavorable consequences: dextromethorphan can bring about a false-positive phencyclidine urine drug screen. J Emerg Med. 2000;18(3):379-81.

40. Halpern JH. Hallucinogens and dissociative agents naturally growing in the United States. Pharmacol Ther. 2004;102(2):131-8.

41. Solursh LP, Clement WR. Use of diazepam in hallucinogenic drug crises. JAMA. 1968;205(9):644-5.

42. Taylor RL, Maurer JI, Tinklenberg JR. Management of "bad trips" in an evolving drug scene. JAMA. 1970;213(3):422-5.

43. Spain D, Crilly J, Whyte I, et al. Safety and effectiveness of high-dose midazolam for severe behavioural disturbance in an emergency department with suspected psychostimulant-affected patients. Emerg Med Australas. 2008;20(2):112-20.

44. Schneider SM, Michelson EA, Boucek CD, et al. Dextromethorphan poisoning reversed by naloxone. Am J Emerg Med. 1991;9(3):237-8.

45. Pali MJ, Tharratt RS, Albertson TE. Phencyclidine and its congeners. In: Brent J, Wallace KL, Burkhart KK, et al. (Eds). Critical Care Toxicology, 1st edition, Philadelphia: Mosby; 2005.

46. Aniline O, Pitts FN Jr. Phencyclidine (PCP): a review and perspectives. Crit Rev Toxicol. 1982;10(2):145-77.

47. Javitt DC, Zukin SR. Recent advances in the phencyclidine model of schizophrenia. Am J Psychiatry. 1991;148(10):1301-8.

48. Akunne HC, Reid AA, Thurkauf A, et al. [3H]1-[2-(2-thienyl)cyclohexyl]piperidine labels two high-affinity binding sites in human cortex: further evidence for phencyclidine binding sites associated with the biogenic amine reuptake complex. Synapse. 1991;8(4):289-300.

49. Wolfe SA Jr, De Souza EB. Sigma and phencyclidine receptors in the brain-endocrine-immune axis. NIDA Res Monogr. 1993;133:95-123.

50. McCarron MM, Schulze BW, Thompson GA, et al. Acute phencyclidine intoxication: clinical patterns, complications, and treatment. Ann Emerg Med. 1981;10(6):290-7.

51. Barton CH, Sterling ML, Vaziri ND. Phencyclidine intoxication: clinical experience in 27 cases confirmed by urine assay. Ann Emerg Med. 1981;10(5):243-6.

52. Giannini AJ, Nageotte C, Loiselle RH, et al. Comparison of chlorpromazine, haloperidol and pimozide in the treatment of phencyclidine psychosis: DA-2 receptor specificity. J Toxicol Clin Toxicol. 1984-1985;22(6):573-9.

53. Miller RD. Miller's Anesthesia, 6th edition, New York: Elsevier Churchill Livingstone; 2005.

54. Ward J, Rhyee S, Plansky J, et al. Methoxetamine: a novel ketamine analog and growing health-care concern. Clin Toxicol (Phila). 2011;49(9):874-5.

55. Green SM, Li J. Ketamine in adults: what emergency physicians need to know about patient selection and emergence reactions. Acad Emerg Med. 2000;7(3):278-81.

56. Weiner AL, Vieira L, McKay CA, et al. Ketamine abusers presenting to the emergency department: a case series. J Emerg Med. 2000;18(4):447-51.

57. Wood DM, Nicolaou M, Dargan PI. Epidemiology of recreational drug toxicity in a nightclub environment. Subst Use Misuse. 2009;44(11):1495-502.

9
CHAPTER

Cocaine Intoxication

Omender Singh, Anish Gupta

INTRODUCTION

Coca is the oldest known stimulant with history dating back to 3000 BC when ancient Incas used to chew coca leaves for spiritual and religious purposes. It is one of the most common illegal drugs used for recreational purposes in the world. Cocaine is derived from the leaves of coca plant *(Erythroxylum coca)* and was first isolated by Albert Niemann (German chemist) in 1859.[1] Cocaine is the principal alkaloid in cocoa leaves and exists in the chemical form called benzoylmethylecgonine.[2]

Cocaine abuse is commonly seen in adolescents and young adults (age 15–35 years).[3] Unemployed men are the predominant abusers. It is used to increase vitality, alertness, social disinhibition, euphoria and to decrease fatigue.[4-6] A term called "total body orgasm" is used for this intensely pleasurable experience.[4]

Cocaine is consumed by various ways including oral, intravenous (IV), insufflation, inhalational, rectal and vaginal routes. The most common route is nasal insufflation by snorting, sniffing or blowing. It is coingested with a variety of substances such as opiates, alcohol, benzodiazepines (BZDs) and cannabinoids.

It rapidly passes through the nasal mucosa and enters the blood stream. The half-life $(t_{1/2})$ of cocaine in blood is 1–2 hours. It is metabolized to various compounds namely benzoylecgonine (BE), ecgonine methyl ester, norcocaine, meta-hydroxy BE (mOH-BE) and para-hydroxy BE (p-OH-BE).[7-9] These metabolites have longer $t_{1/2}$ and can be spotted in urine for many days after administration. Cocaine ingested along with alcohol produces a metabolite, cocaethylene, which has longer $t_{1/2}$ and similar toxic effects as cocaine.[10,11]

PATHOPHYSIOLOGY

The effects of cocaine are due to sodium channel blockade, increased concentration of excitatory amino acids and inhibition of reuptake of biogenic amines.[12,13] Cocaine inhibits the recovery of neuronal and cardiac sodium channels and slows sodium current. It increases the levels of excitatory neurotransmitters such as glutamate and aspartate in the brain.[13] It also blocks the reuptake of biogenic amines like serotonin, epinephrine, norepinephrine and dopamine. Increased levels of these catecholamines lead to stimulation of alpha- and beta-receptors with their consequent physiological effects.

CLINICAL FEATURES

Cocaine abuse produces dose-dependent toxicity leading to multisystem involvement, predominantly affecting the cardiovascular and central nervous system (CNS).

Cardiovascular

Cocaine has a positive chronotropic and inotropic effect on the heart causing an increase in heart rate and blood pressure, leading to increased myocardial oxygen demand.

Cardiotoxicity occurs secondary to coronary vasoconstriction and accelerated atherosclerosis.[14,15] Vasospasm is primarily alpha receptor mediated. Cocaine also stimulates platelet aggregation and production of plasminogen activator inhibitor 1, thus increasing thrombus formation.[16] These effects can lead to myocardial ischemia and in severe cases acute coronary syndrome. It is estimated that about 5% of cases presenting to the triage have ischemia. Acute intoxication can also cause tachyarrhythmias (both supraventricular and ventricular) or conduction blocks which occur secondary to myocardial ischemia or direct myocardial toxicity. The most common arrhythmias are supraventricular (paroxysmal atrial tachycardia, atrial fibrillation, sinus tachycardia). Rarely, aortic dissection and rupture have been reported with cocaine abuse.

Central Nervous System

Cocaine is a stimulant which increases arousal, alertness, vigilance and provides a sense of euphoria or exultation. Intoxication can lead to headache, psychomotor agitation, hallucinations, seizures, coma, intracranial (IC) bleeds and focal neurological deficits.[13] Increased levels of excitatory amines and neurotransmitters and vasoconstriction are implicated in the pathogenesis of CNS effects. Seizures occur in 3–4% cases.[17] Focal neurological effects occur secondary to intracerebral hemorrhage or ischemia. It is important to note that IC bleeds are more common than ischemic strokes.

Hyperthermia

Hyperthermia is commonly seen and is associated with a high mortality to a tune of 30%.[18] It occurs secondary to agitation and concurrent peripheral vasoconstriction. As a result, there is increased heat production with inadequate heat loss. Severe cases may present with rhabdomyolysis with elevated creatine kinase (CK), myoglobin levels, hyperkalemia, hypocalcemia, metabolic and lactic acidosis and acute kidney injury.

Respiratory

The respiratory effects are secondary to the mode of cocaine administration and direct effects on the respiratory airways and parenchyma. Sniffing, snorting or inhalational cocaine can lead to pneumothorax and pneumomediastinum.[19,20] It can precipitate bronchospasm or exacerbate pre-existing airway disease. Some forms of cocaine (crack) need high temperatures to be smoked. The heated fumes can lead to pharyngeal and laryngeal burns. Though uncommon pulmonary infarction can occur secondary to vasospasm and accelerated atherosclerosis. Crack lung is a serious complication of inhalational cocaine use. Patients present with dyspnea, tachypnea, chest pain, hemoptysis and acute respiratory distress syndrome.[21,22]

Gastrointestinal

Cocaine increases gastric acid formation leading to peptic ulcer disease and gastrointestinal perforations.[23] It can lead to local ischemia in gut causing intestinal infarction and ischemic colitis.

Body Packer Syndrome

Body packers are individuals who swallow large quantities of prepackaged drugs for the purpose of smuggling. They are referred to by several names like couriers, mules or internal carriers.[24] In contrast body stuffers swallow smaller quantities of drugs.

Ocular

Cocaine causes pupillary dilatation secondary to sympathetic stimulation. Pupillary reaction to light is preserved. It can lead to loss of vision and can precipitate acute angle closure glaucoma.[25]

Effects of Adulterants

Levamisole and Clenbuterol are common adulterants found in cocaine. Levamisole causes agranulocytosis, leukoencephalopathy, cutaneous vasculitis and necrosis.[26,27] Clenbuterol has beta-agonistic activity and can cause tachycardia, palpitations, arrhythmias, hyperglycemia and hypokalemia.[28]

Pregnancy

Cocaine readily crosses the placenta and is secreted in breast milk. It can lead to fetal malformations, mental retardation, delayed milestones and development with possibility of drug dependence in neonates.[29] It can lead to abruptio placenta and subsequent antepartum hemorrhage.

DIAGNOSIS

Cocaine and its metabolites can be detected in various body fluids and tissues. They include urine (most common), blood, saliva and hair.[30] Benzoylecgonine is the major metabolite of cocaine. The time frame for detection of cocaine is shorter than for benzoylecgonine. Rapid point-of-care tests are available which can detect cocaine metabolites in urine for up to 10 days depending on the quantity consumed.[31] Normally the metabolites are detectable for up to 72 hours after cocaine consumption. However, it is important to understand that detection of benzoylecgonine confirms cocaine abuse but does not establish acute toxicity. Concordance between clinical features and laboratory assays is important to establish a firm diagnosis.

Specialized techniques such as gas chromatography-mass spectrometry (GC-MS) are used for detection of these metabolites.

Blood levels of cocaine and its metabolites are not routinely measured. Cocaine can be detected in blood for 12 hours while benzoylecgonine can be detected for 48 hours after acute intoxication. The blood levels do not correlate well with severity of symptoms and have a limited role.[32] Testing of sweat and hair for cocaine has no role in acute intoxication as they have long detection periods. Hair samples have the longest detection period and can test positive for years after cocaine consumption while sweat samples may test positive for weeks.[33]

Cardiovascular Findings

- *Electrocardiography (ECG):* Obtain an ECG in all patients with chest pain following cocaine abuse. Rule out ST-elevation myocardial infarction (STEMI), supraventricular tachycardias, ventricular tachycardias and ventricular fibrillation. QT prolongation and broad QRS complex type may be seen secondary to sodium channel blockade. Brugada like ECG pattern (ST elevation in V1–V4) and early repolarization changes may be seen in some patients
- *Cardiac troponins:* Troponin T and I to be measured in all cases with cardiovascular symptoms. Troponin I is more specific than CK-MB for diagnosis of cocaine induced ACS
- *Two-dimensional echocardiography (2D ECHO):* Transthoracic echo should be performed in patients with chest pain to rule out findings suggestive of acute coronary syndrome. A detailed assessment is done to rule out regional wall motion abnormality, valvular regurgitation, vegetations on valves (injection drug abusers), septal defects and to calculate ejection fraction.

Radiology

A chest X-ray (CXR) should be performed in all patients presenting with acute intoxication. A widened mediastinum with chest pain may be suggestive of aortic dissection which may warrant further investigation and emergent treatment. Bilateral infiltrates on CXR with hypoxia may suggest acute respiratory distress syndrome (crack lung). An X-ray of the abdomen should be done in cases with suspicion of body packing/stuffing which may show multiple radiopaque packets.

Routine investigation such as complete hemogram, renal function test, liver function test and blood sugar levels should be done in all cases. Blood/serum ethanol, acetaminophen and salicylate levels should be measured as these are common coingestants.

Any patient who presents to emergency room (ER) with unexplained tachycardia, hypertension and hyperthermia and history of sympathomimetic toxidrome, cocaine intoxication should be rule out.

MANAGEMENT

General Management

The general approach to and the management of a patient with poisoning is discussed elsewhere. Supplemental oxygen is administered as per target oxygen saturation. Protect airway, optimize ventilation and maintain adequate circulation. During endotracheal intubation it is best to avoid succinylcholine for neuromuscular paralysis. Succinylcholine and cocaine are both metabolized by plasma cholinesterase, hence, coadministration may either increase cocaine related toxicity or prolong the effects of succinylcholine. It is preferable to use nondepolarizing neuromuscular blocking agent. The preferred induction agents are BZDs, etomidate and propofol.

Specific Management

Cardiovascular Toxicity

Cardiovascular symptoms account for the majority of hospital emergency department visits with chest pain accounting for about 40% cases.[34]

Benzodiazepines are the first-line agents to alleviate cardiovascular symptoms. It is given to anxious and agitated patients. BZDs reduce sympathetic flow and hence decrease tachycardia and hypertension. IV lorazepam can be given in 1 mg aliquots until sedation is achieved.

Chest pain

Oxygen is administered to all hypoxic patients to maintain oxygen saturation (SpO_2) more than 94%. Chest pain and hypertension can be managed with nitroglycerine (NTG). NTG is given sublingually at a dose of 0.4 mg. It can be repeated at 5 minutes intervals for a maximum of three doses. For persistent chest pain an IV infusion of NTG can be started and titrated to effect (relief of pain).

Calcium channel blockers (IV diltiazem, IV verapamil, IV nicardipine) are administered as adjunctive therapy in patients with refractory symptoms despite optimal dose of NTG.

Phentolamine is an alpha-antagonist. It helps reduce coronary artery vasospasm. It is given in bolus doses of 1–2 mg every 5–15 minutes. It is administered in patients with chest pain and hypertension refractory to BZDs.[35]

Acute Coronary Syndrome

Aspirin is administered to all patients with cocaine induced acute coronary syndrome except in cases of suspected aortic dissection. The initial dose of aspirin is similar to that recommended by AHA for ACS, i.e. 162–325 mg.

Role of Beta-blockers

The major difference in management of cocaine induced myocardial ischemia/infarction is the contraindication to the use of beta-blockers, especially in cases when cocaine abuse is within less than 24 hours.[36] Beta-blockers can lead to unopposed alpha-adrenergic stimulation, which can cause hypertension and coronary arterial vasoconstriction, further exacerbating myocardial ischemia and infarction.[37] The use of combined alpha/beta-blockers (e.g. labetalol) is controversial with inconclusive evidence with regard to their safety and efficacy. Some authors believe that labetalol with mixed alpha and beta-blocking properties (beta:alpha = 3:1 for oral and 7:1 for IV preparation) may be useful.

In case beta-blockers need to be given, they should be given along with an alpha antagonist or a vasodilator.

Patients should be monitored under close observation with frequent hemodynamic monitoring and ECGs.

The management of patients with non-NSTEMI or STEMI is similar to AHA guidelines for management of ACS. Primary percutaneous coronary intervention (PCI) is preferred over fibrinolytic therapy in cocaine induced acute MI as rate of ICH is higher in patients who received fibrinolytic therapy for cocaine induced MI. Also, young individuals have early repolarization changes (J point elevation) on ECG which may mimic STEMI and lead to inadvertent administration of fibrinolytic therapy.[38] For primary PCI bare metal stents are considered superior to drug eluting stents as patients are at a greater risk of stent thrombosis[39] and long-term compliance with antiplatelet therapy is a matter of concern.

Management of Arrhythmias[40]

The etiology of arrhythmias in acute intoxication is multifactorial. Blockade of sodium and potassium channels, catecholamine excess and acute coronary syndrome have been implicated in the etiology of arrhythmias.

Sodium channel blockade is manifested as prolonged QRS duration while potassium channel blockade prolongs QT interval. Hypertonic sodium bicarbonate is administered if the QRS complex is substantially prolonged or patient has tachyarrhythmias (ventricular arrhythmias). The optimal dose is not clear but usually a bolus of 1–2 mEq/kg is given followed by intermittent boluses or as an infusion. There is no fixed duration of therapy. Sodium bicarbonate is continued till hemodynamic parameters are optimized and QRS duration is decreased or normalized. Infusions can be discontinued if the pH rises above 7.5. If bicarbonate therapy fails to correct arrhythmias, lidocaine 1–1.5 mg/kg is administered as a bolus followed by continuous infusion at the rate 1–3 mg/min. Lidocaine is a class 1B antiarrhythmic agent. All class 1A and 1C antiarrhythmic are contraindicated for treating arrhythmias. The role of amiodarone is unclear and unsupported at present. Electrolyte disturbances such as hypokalemia and hypomagnesemia should be corrected.

Hypertension

Raised blood pressure is commonly seen with cocaine intoxication. There are no cocaine specific blood pressure goals. In case of hypertensive emergencies, the blood pressure should be lowered rapidly but not exceeding an initial fall of 25% in mean arterial pressure. BZDs are first-line medications. Phentolamine, NTG, and sodium nitroprusside can be added to BZDs in case target goals are not achieved. Nonselective beta-blockers may be used with caution.

Crack Lung

Management includes symptomatic and supportive care. Maintain adequate oxygenation. Patient may need ventilatory support (noninvasive or invasive) for hypoxemia and to reduce work of breathing.

Body Packers and Body Stuffers

Symptomatic patients are treated with gastrointestinal decontamination with activated charcoal or whole bowel irrigation.[41] Activated charcoal is given at a dose of 1 g/kg (maximum 50 g) every 4 hours. Whole bowel irrigation can be done using polyethylene glycol until the gut is clear of all packets. Avoid oil-based laxatives as they can lead to rupture of the packets.[42] Endoscopic management may be needed to remove the packets. Surgery with emergent removal of packets is recommended for symptomatic patients or those with intestinal obstruction. The management of cocaine induced toxicity is same as mentioned earlier.

Neuropsychiatric Symptoms

Benzodiazepines are the drugs of choice for cocaine induced psychomotor agitation. BZDs can lead to respiratory depression and hypotension and patients need to be monitored closely. Midazolam (1–2 mg), diazepam (5–10 mg IV every 3–5 min) or lorazepam (1 mg every 3–5 min) can be administered.

Hyperthermia

Aggressive cooling is recommended. Target temperatures should be achieved within 30 minutes. The target core body temperature is less than 102°F. External cooling with cooling blankets, ice packs, immersion in ice water or evaporative cooling can be used. Internal cooling with cold IV fluids, cold gastric lavage or cold inspired oxygen can be used for severe cases. If there is evidence of rhabdomyolysis then regular CPK monitoring and fluid resuscitation with urinary alkalinization (if CPK >5,000) is recommended.

PROGNOSIS

The overall prognosis is good. However, patients with myocardial infarction (MI) secondary to cocaine are prone for more complications as compared to patients with MI without cocaine. Timely and prompt management may help alleviate adverse events.

CONCLUSION

Cocaine is one of the most common causes of drug related emergency department visits. Over the years, a number of adulterants have been mixed with cocaine, which, if in excess, can lead to significant deleterious effects. Knowledge of these adulterants is imperative to improve patient care. Also, every visit to the ED should be used as an opportunity to counsel patients to seek treatment and help for drug abuse. In addition, laws should be enforced strongly to prevent smuggling and illicit use of cocaine.

KEY POINTS

- The toxic effects of cocaine are due to blockade of sodium channels, increased concentration of excitatory amino acids and inhibition of reuptake of biogenic amines
- Levamisole and clenbuterol are two common adulterants found in cocaine which can produce toxic effects
- Benzoylecgonine is the main metabolite of cocaine and is easily detected in urine
- Benzodiazepines are the first-line agents to alleviate cardiovascular symptoms
- Beta-blockers are contraindicated in the management of cocaine induced MI. The role of mixed alpha- and beta-blockers (labetalol) is not clearly established.

REFERENCES

1. Grzybowski A. The history of cocaine in medicine and its importance to the discovery of the different forms of anaesthesia. Klin Oczna. 2007;109(1-3):101-5.
2. Damodaran S. Cocaine and beta-blockers: the paradigm. Eur J Intern Med. 2010;21(2):84-6.
3. Center for Behavioral Health Statistics and Quality. 2015 National Survey on Drug Use and Health: Detailed Tables. Rockville: Substance Abuse and Mental Health Services Administration; 2016.
4. Angrist, B. Clinical effects of central nervous system stimulants: a selective update. In: Engel J, Oreland L, Ingvar DH (Eds). Brain Reward Systems and Abuse. New York: Raven Press; 1987. pp. 109-27.

5. Baselt RC. Drug Effects on Psychomotor Performance. Foster City: Biomedical Publications; 2001.

6. Fischman MW, Foltin RW. Cocaine self-administration research: implications for rational pharmacotherapy. In: Higgins ST, Katz JL (Eds). Behavior, Pharmacology, and Clinical Applications. San Diego: Cocaine Abuse Academic Press; 1998. pp. 181-207.

7. Warner A, Norman AB. Mechanisms of cocaine hydrolysis and metabolism in vitro and in vivo: a clarification. Ther Drug Monit. 2000;22(3):266-70.

8. Cone EJ. Pharmacokinetics and pharmacodynamics of cocaine. J Anal Toxicol. 1995;19(6):459-78.

9. Gorelick DA. Pharmacokinetic strategies for treatment of drug overdose and addiction. Future Med Chem. 2012;4(2):227-43.

10. Pennings EJ, Leccese AP, Wolff FA. Effects of concurrent use of alcohol and cocaine. Addiction. 2002;97(7):773-83.

11. Baker J, Jatlow P, Pade P, Ramakrishnan V. Acute cocaine responses following cocaethylene infusion. Am J Drug Alcohol Abuse. 2007;33(4):619-25.

12. Tella SR, Schindler CW, Goldberg SR. Cocaine: cardiovascular effects in relation to inhibition of peripheral neuronal monoamine uptake and central stimulation of the sympathoadrenal system. J Pharmacol Exp Ther. 1993;267(1):153-62.

13. Smith JA, Mo Q, Guo H, et al. Cocaine increases extraneuronal levels of aspartate and glutamate in the nucleus accumbens. Brain Res. 1995;683(2):264-9.

14. Afonso L, Mohammad T, Thatai D. Crack whips the heart: a review of the cardiovascular toxicity of cocaine. Am J Cardiol. 2007;100:1040-3.

15. Lange RA, Cigarroa RG, Yancy CW Jr, et al. Cocaine-induced coronary-artery vasoconstriction. N Engl J Med. 1989;321(23):1557-62.

16. Moliterno DJ, Lange RA, Gerard RD, et al. Influence of intranasal cocaine on plasma constituents associated with endogenous thrombosis and thrombolysis. Am J Med. 1994;96:492-6.

17. Koppel BS, Samkoff L, Daras M. Relation of cocaine use to seizures and epilepsy. Epilepsia. 1996;37(9):875-8.

18. Marzuk PM, Tardiff K, Leon AC, et al. Ambient temperature and mortality from unintentional cocaine overdose. JAMA. 1998;279(22):1795-800.

19. Maeder M, Ullmer E. Pneumomediastinum and bilateral pneumothorax as a complication of cocaine smoking. Respiration. 2003;70(4):407.

20. Kloss BT, Broton CE, Rodriguez E. Pneumomediastinum from nasal insufflation of cocaine. Int J Emerg Med. 2010;3(4):435-7.

21. Forrester JM, Steele AW, Waldron JA, et al. Crack lung: an acute pulmonary syndrome with a spectrum of clinical and histopathologic findings. Am Rev Respir Dis. 1990;142(2):462-7.

22. Ettinger NA, Albin RJ. A review of the respiratory effects of smoking cocaine. Am J Med. 1989;87(6):664-8.

23. Chander B, Aslanian HR. Gastric Perforations Associated With the Use of Crack Cocaine. Gastroenterol Hepatol (NY). 2010;6(11):733-5.

24. Traub SJ, Hoffman RS, Nelson LS. Body packing—the internal concealment of illicit drugs. N Engl J Med. 2003;349:2519.

25. Hoffman RS, Reimer BI. "Crack" cocaine-induced bilateral amblyopia. Am J Emerg Med. 1993;11(1):35-7.

26. Gross RL, Brucker J, Bahce-Altuntas A, et al. A novel cutaneous vasculitis syndrome induced by levamisole-contaminated cocaine. Clin Rheumatol. 2011;30(10):1385-92.

27. Chang A, Osterloh J, Thomas J. Levamisole: a dangerous new cocaine adulterant. Clin Pharmacol Ther. 2010;88(3):408-11.

28. Centers for Disease Control and Prevention (CDC). Atypical reactions associated with heroin use—five states, January-April 2005. MMWR Morb Mortal Wkly Rep. 2005;54:793.

29. Addis A, Moretti ME, Ahmed Syed F, et al. Fetal effects of cocaine: an updated meta-analysis. Reprod Toxicol. 2001;15(4):341-69.

30. Verstraete AG. Detection times of drugs of abuse in blood, urine, and oral fluid. Ther Drug Monit. 2004;26(2):200-5.

31. Preston KL, Epstein DH, Cone EJ, et al. Urinary elimination of cocaine metabolites in chronic cocaine users during cessation. J Anal Toxicol. 2002;26(7):393-400.

32. Blaho K, Logan B, Winbery S, et al. Blood cocaine and metabolite concentrations, clinical findings, and outcome of patients presenting to an ED. Am J Emerg Med. 2000;18(5):593-8.

33. Gambelunghe C, Rossi R, Ferranti C, et al. Hair analysis by GC/MS/MS to verify abuse of drugs. J Appl Toxicol. 2005;25(3):205-11.

34. Brody SL, Slovis CM, Wrenn KD. Cocaine-related medical problems: consecutive series of 233 patients. Am J Med. 1990;88(4):325-31.

35. Lange RA, Hillis LD. Cardiovascular complications of cocaine use. N Engl J Med. 2001;345(5):351-8.

36. Hoffman RS. Cocaine and beta-blockers: should the controversy continue? Ann Emerg Med. 2008;51(2):127-9.

37. Richards JR, Hollander JE, Ramoska EA, et al. β-Blockers, Cocaine, and the Unopposed α-Stimulation Phenomenon. J Cardiovasc Pharmacol Ther. 2017;22(3):239-49.

38. Hollander JE, Wilson LD, Leo PJ, et al. Complications from the use of thrombolytic agents in patients with cocaine associated chest pain. J Emerg Med. 1996;14(6):731-6.

39. McKee SA, Applegate RJ, Hoyle JR, et al. Cocaine use is associated with an increased risk of stent thrombosis after percutaneous coronary intervention. Am Heart J. 2007;154(1):159-64.

40. Hoffman RS. Treatment of patients with cocaine-induced arrhythmias: bringing the bench to the bedside. Br J Clin Pharmacol. 2010;69(5):448-57.

41. Tomaszewski C, McKinney P, Phillips S, et al. Prevention of toxicity from oral cocaine by activated charcoal in mice. Ann Emerg Med. 1993;22(12):1804-6.

42. Traub SJ, Hoffman RS, Nelson LS. Body packing--the internal concealment of illicit drugs. N Engl J Med. 2003;349(26):2519-26.

10
CHAPTER

Newer Drugs of Abuse

Omender Singh, Rajesh Chawla, Deven Juneja

INTRODUCTION

Drugs which are abused are the drugs which are easily accessible and popular with peer groups. Hence, the drugs which are commonly abused differ according to the geographic location and the social demographics. These drugs also differ depending on the age of the users. Historically, the drugs most commonly abused included marijuana, cocaine and amphetamine. However, increasing legislative measures made these drugs less easily available. Hence, "street pharmacists" had to come up with novel drugs, by slightly altering the chemical structure of these drugs, and producing drugs which are not illegal. These "designer drugs" or "legal highs" have become very popular, especially among the young population because of their ease of availability and lack of any legislative restrictions. These drugs are readily available at retail shops, street dealers and even on the Internet. They are sold under various street or generic names which make their identification difficult.

SUBSTITUTED CATHINONES OR "BATH SALTS"

Synthetic analogs of cathinone are termed as substituted cathinones. Cathinone is a monoamine alkaloid which is naturally present in the "khat" plant.[1] These drugs are derived from phenethylamines and have a beta-keto group on the side chain. Certain cathinones, like pyrovalerone and diethylpropion, have been used medically and bupropion is even recommended for smoking cessation.

They were introduced as recreational drugs in the mid-2000s and have become very popular, especially among the youths. These were initially marketed as "legal highs" and are still legal in several countries. However, more and more legislative changes are being made to change their legal status and get these drugs under government's control. Subtle changes in their chemical structure are also common, as there is no standardization of their manufacturing process. They are commercially sold under different street names each having subtle differences in their basic chemical structure (Table 1).[2,3]

Modes of Administration

These drugs are commercially available as powders, and can be administered orally, by snorting or intravenously. The typical dose consumed varies according to the type of cathinone derivative and the route of administration. The typical dose of mephedrone or methylone ranges between 50 mg and 100 mg for first time users but it may go up to 150–250 mg in experienced users.[4] Drug doses are generally smaller when used as insufflation, with the typical dose ranging between 15 mg and 25 mg going up to 75–125 mg.[4]

Drugs of Abuse

Table 1: Common street/brand names for substances containing synthetic cathinones and cannabinoids.[2,3]

Synthetic cathinones	Synthetic cannabinoids
Bath salts	Aroma
Bubbles	Aztec fire
Cloud 9	Aztec thunder
Energy-1	Banana cream nuke
Explosion	Black mamba
Hurricane Charlie	Blaze
Impact	Bliss
Ivory wave	Blueberry posh
Khat	Bombay blue
MCAT	Bonzai
Meow meow	Buddha-blue
NRG-1	C-Liquid
Red dove	Chaos mint/original/cherry
Scarface	Chill out
Vanilla sky	Clover spring
White dove	Eclipse
White lightning	Egypt
White rush	Exclusive original/cherry/mint
	Fake weed
	Genie
	Happy tiger incense
	Herbal e-liquid
	K2
	Krypton
	Moon rocks
	Mr Smiley
	Red merkury
	Sensation vanilla/orange/blackberry
	Smoke
	Spice
	Spice arctic synergy
	Spice diamond
	Spice gold
	Spice silver
	Spicy XXX
	Tai fun blackberry/orange/vanilla
	Yucatan fire
	Zohai
	Zen
	Zen ultra

Recreational Effects

These agents act by releasing the catecholamines and preventing their reuptake in the central nervous system (CNS) and the peripheral nervous system (PNS). These drugs have a CNS stimulatory and entactogenic effects leading to desirable effects like empathy, increased libido, reduced inhibition, euphoria, enhancement of sensory senses, increased sociability, and energy levels.[1] After recreational use, serum levels of cathinone derivatives generally remain below 0.1 mg/L. However, in patients with acute toxicity, these levels may dramatically increase but these levels may not correlate with clinical picture or prognosis.

Adverse/Toxic Effects

The adverse effects associated with these drugs involve the CNS and cardiovascular system and patients may present with agitation, hallucinations, paranoia, seizures, tachycardia, and hypertension.[1] "Bath salts" abuse may even lead to multiorgan failure.[5] Patients with severe toxicity may present with signs and symptoms of excessive serotonin activity, like metabolic acidosis, hyperthermia, and rhabdomyolysis. These drugs have been shown to induce a strong craving and have an addictive potential in most users.[6]

Laboratory Analysis

Apart from the basic laboratory investigations, cardiac markers, creatinine kinase and urinary myoglobin levels must be done to rule out rhabdomyolysis.[7] The commonly available urine toxicology screens fail to detect most of the cathinones derivatives. However, urine toxicology screening should be done to rule out coingestions.

Recently, several analytical methods have been developed to analyze the constituents of these drugs. Immunoassay screening methods which are employed to detect methamphetamines, are generally not effective in detecting cathinone derivatives.[8] Gas-liquid chromatography-mass spectrometry (GC-MS) remains the method of choice which can be used to rapidly identify cathinones derivatives in powders.[9,10] Liquid chromatography-mass spectrometry (LC-MS) has also been used to identify cathinones in urine, oral fluids, blood, postmortem tissues, and even dried blood spots useful in forensic toxicology.[11,12] Presently, it is the only approved technique to identify and quantify cathinones derivatives in biological fluids.

Other newer techniques which may be employed include direct analysis in real time mass spectrometry (DART-MS) or portable mass-spectrometer equipped with desorption electrospray ionization-mass spectrometry (DESI-MS).[13]

Clinical Management

There is no specific antidote available for these agents and clinical experience with their overdose is also limited. Hence, most of the literature related to management of acute toxicity has been extrapolated from data related to cocaine or amphetamine overdose.

Early identification and management of complications like seizures, hyponatremia, hyperthermia and dysrhythmias is vital in improving patient outcomes. Benzodiazepines may be used to control agitation and seizures. Generally, use of dopamine blocking antipsychotic drugs should be avoided as they may exacerbate thermoregulatory disturbances.[1]

SYNTHETIC CANNABINOIDS

Another newer classes of psychoactive drugs which have become increasingly popular over the last decade are synthetic cannabinoids (SCs). SCs were developed in the 1970s and SCs like nabilone or dronabinol have also been used therapeutically as antiemetic, in the treatment of chemotherapy-induced nausea and vomiting and as orexigenics for the management of anorexia. Their analgesic property has also been utilized in the management of neuropathic pain associated with multiple sclerosis.

Pharmacologically, SCs bind to CB1 and/or CB2 receptors. CB1 receptor agonism is responsible for the recreational effects of the SCs. Some SCs bind to these receptors more strongly than others and even natural cannabinoids, which may result in more potent, unpredictable and sometimes even dangerous effects.

They are also promoted as "legal highs" as they mimic the euphoric effects of cannabis and are not illegal to use in many countries. American studies have reported use of SCs in 1.4–10% of population studies[14,15] with increasing incidence among the adolescents, especially males living in urban areas.[16]

Modalities of Administration

They are commonly sprayed on natural herbs and marketed as "herbal incense" or "herbal smoking blends".[17] These are typically sold in metal foil sachets mixed with dried vegetable matter. These are available easily at convenience stores or internet and marked as "not for human consumption" and sold under different street names like "K2", "spice" and "black mamba" (Table 1).[2,3]

Newer formulations of SCs are also available in the solution form to be used in e-cigarettes. Ingestion of SCs is rarely reported and other modes of administration like nasal insufflation and intravenous injection are even more rare.[18-20]

Recreational Effects

The psychoactive effects of SCs are similar to cannabis. Users may feel a sense of euphoria, calmness, relaxation, lowering of inhibitions, disorientation, and a sense of altered perception. These effects generally appear within a few minutes after inhalation and last for 2–6 hours.[17]

Adverse/Toxic Effects

Use of SCs is associated with several adverse effects, which are predominantly neurological (61.9%) or cardiovascular (43.5%).[21] In a large case series, the most commonly reported adverse effect was tachycardia (41.6%), followed by drowsiness/lethargy (24.3%), nausea/vomiting (21.6%), agitation/irritability (18.5%), and hallucinations/delusions (10.8%). Even though the adverse effects were not life threatening in majority of patients, a large proportion of these patients (61%) had adverse effects serious enough to require medical intervention.[22,23] Seizures are also commonly reported among these patients and serious effects like stroke and acute myocardial infarction have also been reported after "K2" abuse.[24,25] SCs have also shown to have addictive potential and patients may develop symptoms of agitation, tachycardia, irritability, anxiety, and mood swings after acute withdrawal.[26]

Diagnostic Tests

Routine laboratory tests include random blood sugar (RBS), complete blood counts (CBCs), liver function test (LFT), kidney function test (KFT), coagulation studies, and cardiac markers. Electrocardiogram (ECG) and electromyogram (EMG) may also be required in some patients, depending upon their clinical presentation. Urine toxicology screen does not detect SCs but may be useful in detecting other possible coingestions.

Immunochemistry

The immunoassay screening methods generally employed to detect cannabis are unable to detect SCs. Hence, specialized enzyme-linked immunosorbent assays (ELISAs) or homogeneous enzyme immunoassays have been recently developed for detection of SCs in urinary samples.[27-29]

Other laboratory tests like gas-liquid chromatography (LC) along with electron impact mass spectrometry (GC-MS) may also be utilized to rapidly identify and quantify

Drugs of Abuse

SCs in herbal and powder materials.[30] These are the only methods which can be utilized to rapidly identify and quantify SCs in biological specimens like urine, serum, blood, oral fluid, or hair.[31]

Clinical Management

There is no typical toxidrome associated with SC toxicity. Clinical picture may further be complicated by different mixes of SC compounds which are available on the market. As there is limited data related to management of patients with SCs toxicity, treatment is generally guided based on the data extrapolated from the experiences with management of cannabis. There is no specific antidote for management of SC toxicity and hence, general management includes early aggressive care with intravenous fluids along with management and prevention of complications. Patients presenting with withdrawal symptoms, may require treatment with benzodiazepines like diazepam and antipsychotics drugs like quetiapine.[32]

SUBSTITUTED PHENETHYLAMINES (2C DRUGS)

Recent years have witnessed appearance of several new synthetic derivatives of amphetamine. These substituted phenethylamines also share their basic structure with catecholamines, synthetic cathinones, and many other drugs and are called 2C class of drugs.[33,34] Examples of these drugs include 3,4-methylenedioxy-N-hydroxyamphetamine (MDOH) and 4,5-methylenedioxy-3-methoxy-phenethylamine (MMDPEA).[35]

Their use is common in dance clubs and rave parties with a reported use of 17.6% for 2C-B and 11.2% for 2C-I drugs.[36] These are generally available in tablet or powder forms.[37] Party revelers seeking ecstasy are frequently exposed to 2C drugs as contaminants or substitutes. Most of the users tend to be young males and most of them have a history of polydrug use.[38]

Clinical Effects

Phenethylamines exhibit both stimulatory and hallucinogenic properties. Users may develop nausea, vomiting, diarrhea, headaches, dizziness, hallucinations, body aches, depression, and confusion.[33,34,38] Seizures and serotonin syndrome with hyperthermia have also been reported after ingestion of 2C drugs.[39]

Clinical Management

There is no specific test which is recommended for phenethylamine ingestion as these drugs cannot be detected using standard laboratory tests or urine toxicology screening. However, GC/MS or LC-MS/MS or thin-layer chromatography (TLC) may be useful in confirming the exposure.[40,41] Treatment consists of symptom-based goal-directed care as there is no specific antidote for 2C drug toxicity.[34]

PIPERAZINES

These are fully synthetic recreational drugs which were initially developed as antihelminthic drugs and were also used clinically as antidepressants.[40] There are two main types of piperazines which are used for recreational purposes; these are benzylpiperazines (BZPs) and phenylpiperazines.[33]

They are commonly sold as mixtures of multiple piperazine derivatives or in combinations with other drugs of abuse especially ecstasy or amphetamines and form an active ingredient of "party pills". These are frequently marketed as "legal" alternatives to amphetamine and ecstasy [3,4-methylenedioxy methamphetamine (MDMA)] and sold with street names like "Legal E" and "Herbal ecstasy". These are commonly abused by younger males and can be purchased on the Internet. Rather, piperazines form the most common active ingredient found in recreational drugs purchased on the Internet.[42]

It is sold in pills or powder form.[43] Dosage, time to onset and duration of effects differ among different piperazines. The typical dosage for 1-BZP, the most commonly used piperazine range from 50 mg to 250 mg, and its effects may last for 6–8 hours.[40]

Piperazines are generally consumed orally, but may also be consumed by sniffing. Their effects are unpredictable and may be dangerous, even after consumption of small doses.[44]

Clinical Effects

The effects produced by piperazines are similar to that produced by amphetamine, albeit with lower intensity. Apart from the desirable recreational euphoriant and stimulant effects, patients with toxicity may present with nausea, vomiting, tremors, insomnia, anxiety, headaches, dizziness, palpitations, breathlessness, confusion, hallucinations and paranoia. Prolonged QT interval, seizures, hyperthermia, rhabdomyolysis, renal failure, disseminated intravascular coagulation and hyponatremia are potentially serious adverse effects of piperazine toxicity. Because of the serotonergic effects of piperazines, patients may be at risk of developing serotonin syndrome, especially if there is coingestion of other serotonergic agents.[40]

Clinical Management

No commercially available immunoassay is useful in detecting piperazines. However, use of piperazines may cause these tests to be falsely positive for amphetamines. Routinely employed urine toxicology screens are also negative. Tests like GC-MS, LC-MS, TLC may be employed to confirm the exposure to piperazines but they are not useful in clinical situations as they are neither easily available nor economically viable.[41,45]

TRYPTAMINES

Tryptamines are a heterogeneous group of compounds which are derivatives of the amino acid tryptophan. All of these have hallucinogenic properties but some even have stimulant properties.[46] Lysergic acid diethylamide (LSD), which also belongs to this group, is the most hallucinogenic compound known.[46] These compounds are known to cause euphoria, increase creativity, enhance libido, and increase sensory perceptions.[47]

Tryptamines occurring naturally include serotonin, melatonin, bufotenine, and psilocin/psilocybin.[48] Naturally occurring tryptamines can only be eaten or drunk, whereas, synthetic tryptamines can be smoked, sniffed or injected also.

Patients may present with tachycardia, hypertension, agitation, psychosis, excited delirium and mydriasis. These compounds may also lead to rhabdomyolysis and acute renal failure.

KRATOM

It is a naturally occurring compound, extracted from a Southeast Asian tree [*Mitragyna speciosa* (Korth)]. Its stimulant, euphoric and analgesic properties were recognized even in late 1800s, when it was used by manual laborers of these regions.[49] Several other beneficial properties have now been recognized including anti-inflammatory, antidiarrheal, antipyretic, antihypertensive, hypoglycemic, and procirculatory

properties.[2] Moreover, kratom also has been used for opium withdrawal and to enhance sexual prowess.[2,49] Because of these properties, it has gained popularity among the young population and is increasingly sold over the Internet.[50]

Its main recreational use is because of its hallucinogenic properties. Lower doses may produce cocaine like simulant effects. Kratom is generally smoked or ingested after brewing in tea. The time of onset of effects is generally 5 minutes and their duration is around 1 hour, but these properties are dose dependent.

Due to its multiple effects, patients may present with signs and symptoms suggestive of sympathomimetic or opioid effects or even opioid withdrawal. Long-term users may become addicted to kratom and may develop symptoms of kratom withdrawal, which is clinically similar to opioid withdrawal. Rarely patients may develop life-threatening complications like generalized tonic-clonic seizures.[51] There are no specific tests for the diagnosis and the management is generally supportive as there is no specific antidote.

SALVIA

Salvia is a member of the mint family and is native to Mexico. There are hundreds of species but *Salvia divinorum* is clinically most relevant species. Historically, salvia has been used in religious ceremonies and has been known to have hallucinogenic properties.[52] It can be smoked, or ingested after brewing in tea. Plant leaves can also be chewed to give the desired effects and is commonly sold in convenient stores or on the Internet as prepackaged crushed leaves. It is also sold under the street names of "mystic sage", "magic mint", and "Sally D".

Salvia causes serotonin receptor agonism, which is responsible for its hallucinogenic effects.

It can be smoked, ingested or chewed. Traditionally, salvia is smoked like marijuana, with deep inhalation with valsalva.[53] Buccal absorption may stimulate kappa-opioid receptors which may clinically manifest as pseudohallucinations, perceptual distortions, and an altered sense of self and environment.

There is rapid onset of effects, ranging from 30 seconds to 10 minutes, depending on the route of exposure and these effects last for only 30 minutes.[52,53] The effects are brief but intense, and may be further exaggerated in younger users. Some of them have even reported having out of body experiences, visual distortions of body image, and hearing colors.[52]

As the effects are short lived, most of the users do not seek treatment and hence, experience with medical management is very limited.[54] However, the most commonly reported adverse symptoms include tachycardia, hypertension, giddiness, confusion, disorientation, hallucinations, and a flushed sensation. The only medical management required in most of the cases is benzodiazepine administration, for symptom control.[54]

HAWAIIAN BABY WOODROSE

Lysergamide (LSA) is a naturally occurring ergot alkaloid and is the chief psychoactive component of the seeds of the morning glory (*Ipomoea violacea*) and Hawaiian baby woodrose (*Argyreia nervosa*). Its chemical structure is similar to that of synthetic lysergamide or LSD and has an abuse potential because of its hallucinogenic properties.

Convenience stores and online websites account for the majority of sale of these seeds across the United States and Europe.[55] The seeds from the woodrose may be eaten directly or in extract form after being soaked in water. Generally, five to ten seeds are ingested to have the desired effects, which roughly correspond to a dose of 2–5 mg of LSA. The resultant hallucinogenic effects may last for 4–6 hours.[56]

The desired recreational effects are similar to that of other hallucinogenic agents, with users experiencing euphoria, happiness, altered perceptions of colors and textures, and enhanced mood. However, users may also experience untoward clinical effects like tachycardia, hypertension, nausea, vomiting, anxiety, vertigo, mydriasis, sedation, and a sense of derealization.[56-58] After prolonged use, users may also have depression, feelings of loneliness, depression, and suicidal tendency.[58]

DESOMORPHINE

Desomorphine is a newer opioid analog which is pharmacologically similar to heroin. It is commonly known as "krokodil/crocodile" because of the characteristic skin lesions it causes in the users. It was introduced in the United States in 1932, and promoted as an alternative to morphine.[59] However, it is increasingly being abused for recreational purposes now.[60]

It is a μ-receptor agonist and has analgesic effects which are ten times stronger than morphine. The onset of action is rapid, within 1–2 minutes, and duration of action is also shorter (1–2 hours) than morphine. These properties increase its abuse potential and also chance for addiction and withdrawal.[61,62]

Desomorphine is easy to synthesize and hence, it is produced widely at in-home laboratories at low cost with easy to procure chemicals, further increasing its abuse potential.[59] This also increases the variability in chemical composition and may cause unpredictable clinical effects.

Its adverse effects profile is similar to other opioids. Intravenous injections may cause damage to injection site and may also lead to more systemic effects like bacteremia, osteomyelitis, meningitis and other organ dysfunction. Due to potentially serious side effects, the reported survival from its first use is 2 years.[62]

There is limited data regarding the specific management. The basic management principles are similar to that of other opioid toxicities. Naloxone administration may be attempted but caution must be exerted to prevent symptoms of opioid withdrawal.

CONCLUSION

Recent years have witnessed a renewed interest in chemically synthesizing several recreational drugs as "legal" alternatives to commonly abused stimulants like cocaine and amphetamine/methamphetamine. These drugs are increasingly being marketed as "designer drugs" or "legal highs" and are being targeted to young population. Additionally, their increasing popularity and lack of legislative controls have further fuelled process of introducing subtle chemical modifications leading to increase in diversity of these agents. Physicians dealing with toxicology patients are very likely to encounter patients who have consumed these drugs. However, because of lack of any specific toxidrome or laboratory tests, diagnosis may be difficult. As the basic management principles remain the same (Box 1), general understanding of broad clinical classification of these drugs becomes important to understand the clinical implications of their abuse.

KEY POINTS

- Drugs of abuse post a serious challenge for the treating physicians as they keep evolving by manipulation of basic chemical structures of various compounds.
- Understanding of individual names and their underlying chemical formulations may not be possible. Hence, a general understanding of broad clinical classification of these drugs becomes important to understand the clinical implications of their abuse.
- Abuse of majority of these newer synthetic drugs cause psychoactive and sympathomimetic effects.

Box 1: Common features of newer drugs of abuse.

- Legal to use in many countries and hence are marketed as "legal highs"
- Newer drugs are frequently introduced by making subtle changes in the basic structure to avoid legislative measures
- Most of the users are young males, with a history of polydrug use
- Available under different street names at convenience stores, rave parties, dance clubs and over the Internet
- No toxidrome, and coingestions may further complicate clinical picture
- Difficult to diagnose, routine urine toxicology screens do not detect these compounds
- There is no specific antidote and hence, treatment is mainly symptomatic

- The side effects may sometimes be serious and are often unpredictable.
- The general management consists of aggressive resuscitation and symptom-based goal-directed supportive care.

REFERENCES

1. Prosser JM, Nelson LS. The toxicology of bath salts: a review of synthetic cathinones. J Med Toxicol. 2012;8:33-42.
2. Rosenbaum CD, Carreiro SP, Babu KM. Here today, gone tomorrow and back again? A review of herbal marijuana alternatives (K2, Spice), synthetic cathinones (bath salts), kratom, Salvia divinorum, methoxetamine, and piperazines. J Med Toxicol. 2012;8(1):15-32.
3. Nelson ME, Bryant SM, Aks SE. Emerging drugs of abuse. Emerg Med Clin North Am. 2014;32(1):1-28.
4. Forrester MB. Synthetic cathinone exposures reported to Texas poison centers. Am J Drug Alcohol Abuse. 2012;38(6):609-15.
5. Borek HA, Holstege CP. Hyperthermia and multiorgan failure after abuse of "bath salts" containing 3,4-methylenedioxypyrovalerone. Ann Emerg Med. 2012;60(1):103-5.
6. Brunt TM, Poortman A, Niesink RJ, et al. Instability of the ecstasy market and a new kid on the block: mephedrone. J Psychopharmacol. 2011;25(11):1543-7.
7. Mas-Morey P, Visser MH, Winkelmolen L, et al. Clinical toxicology and management of intoxications with synthetic cathinones ("bath salts"). J Pharm Pract. 2013;26(4):353-7.
8. Ojanperä LA, Heikman PK, Rasanen IJ. Urine analysis of 3,4-methylenedioxypyrovalerone in opioid-dependant patients by gas chromatography-mass spectrometry. Ther Drug Monitoring. 2011;33:257-63.
9. Brandt SD, Freeman S, Sumnall HR, et al. Analysis of NRG 'legal highs' in the UK: identification and formation of novel cathinones. Drug Test Anal. 2011;3(9):569-75.

10. McDermott SD, Power JD, Kavanagh P, et al. The analysis of substituted cathinones. Part 2: an investigation into the phenylacetone-based isomers of 4-methylmethcathinone and N-ethylcathinone. Forensic Sci Int. 2011;212(1-3):13-21.
11. Wyman JF, Lavins ES, Engelhart D, et al. Postmortem tissue distribution of MDPV following lethal intoxication by "bath salts". J Anal Toxicol. 2013;37(3):182-5.
12. O'Byrne PM, Kavanagh PV, McNamara SM, et al. Screening of stimulants including designer drugs in urine using a liquid chromatography tandem mass spectrometry system. J Anal Toxicol. 2013;37(2):64-73.
13. Lesiak AD, Musah RA, Cody RB, et al. Direct analysis in real time mass spectrometry (DART-MS) of "bath salt" cathinone drug mixtures. Analyst. 2013;138(12):3424-32.
14. Wohlfarth A, Scheidweiler KB, Castaneto M, et al. Urinary prevalence, metabolite detection rates, temporal patterns and evaluation of suitable LC-MS/MS targets to document synthetic cannabinoid intake in US military urine specimens. Clin Chem Lab Med. 2015;53(3):423-34.
15. Palamar JJ, Acosta P. Synthetic cannabinoid use in a nationally representative sample of US high school seniors. Drug Alcohol Depend. 2015;149:194-202.
16. Martz G, Tankersley W, Mekala HM, et al. Rates of synthetic cannabinoid use in adolescents admitted to a treatment facility. Prim Care Companion CNS Disord. 2018;20(5).17m02265.
17. Auwärter V, Dresen S, Weinmann W, et al. 'Spice' and other herbal blends: harmless incense or cannabinoid designer drugs? J Mass Spectrum. 2009;44(5):832-7.
18. Lapoint J, James LP, Moran CL, et al. Severe toxicity following synthetic cannabinoid ingestion. Clin Toxicol (Phila). 2011;49(8):760-4.
19. Lonati D, Buscaglia E, Papa P, et al. MAM-2201 (analytically confirmed) intoxication after "Synthacaine" consumption. Ann Emerg Med. 2014;64(6):629-32.
20. Debruyne D, Le Boisselier R. Emerging drugs of abuse: current perspectives on synthetic cannabinoids. Subst Abuse Rehabil. 2015;6:113-29.
21. Forrester MB, Kleinschmidt K, Schwarz E, et al. Synthetic cannabinoid exposures reported to Texas poison centers. J Addict Dis. 2011;30(4):351-8.
22. Forrester MB. Adolescent synthetic cannabinoid exposures reported to Texas poison centers. Pediatr Emerg Care. 2012;28(10):985-9.
23. Hoyte CO, Jacob J, Monte AA, et al. A characterization of synthetic cannabinoid exposures reported to the National Poison Data System in 2010. Ann Emerg Med. 2012;60(4):435-8.
24. Freeman MJ, Rose DZ, Myers MA, et al. Ischemic stroke after use of the synthetic marijuana "spice". Neurology. 2013;81(24):2090-3.
25. McKeever RG, Vearrier D, Jacobs D, et al. K2—not the spice of life; synthetic cannabinoids and ST elevation myocardial infarction: a case report. J Med Toxicol. 2015;11(1):129-31.
26. Palmer S. Synthetic cannabinoid JWH-018 and psychosis: an explorative study. Drug Alcohol Depend. 2011;117 (2-3):152-7.
27. Arnston A, Ofsa B, Lancaster D, et al. Validation of a novel immunoassay for the detection of synthetic cannabinoids

and metabolites in urine specimens. J Anal Toxicol. 2013;37(5):284-90.

28. Mohr A, Ofsa B, Keil A, et al. Enzyme-linked immuno-sorbent assay (ELISA) for the detection of use of the synthetic cannabinoid agonists UR-144 and XLR-11 in human urine. J Anal Toxicol. 2014;38(7):427-31.

29. Barnes AJ, Young S, Spinelli E, et al. Evaluation of a homogenous enzyme immunoassay for the detection of synthetic cannabinoids in urine. Forensic Sci Int. 2014;241:27-34.

30. Simolka K, Lindigkeit R, Schiebel HM, et al. Analysis of synthetic cannabinoids in "spice-like" herbal highs: snapshot of the German market in summer 2011. Anal Bioanal Chem. 2012;404(1):157-71.

31. Kneisel S, Speck M, Moosmann B, et al. LC/ESI-MS/MS method for quantification of 28 synthetic cannabinoids in neat oral fluid and its application to preliminary studies on their detection windows. Anal Bioanal Chem. 2013;405(14):4691-706.

32. MacFarlane V, Christie G. Synthetic cannabinoid withdrawal: a new demand on detoxification services. Drug Alcohol Rev. 2015;34(2):147-53.

33. Hill SL, Thomas SH. Clinical toxicology of newer recreational drugs. Clin Toxicol. 2011;49:705-19.

34. Dean BV, Stellpflug SL, Burnett AM, et al. 2C or not 2C: phenethylamine designer drug review. J Med Toxicol. 2013;9:172-8.

35. Freeman S, Alder JF. Arylethylamine psychotropic recreational drugs: a chemical perspective. Eur J Med Chem. 2002;37(7):527-39.

36. Winstock AR, Mitcheson LR, Deluca P, et al. Mephedrone, new kid for the chop? Addiction. 2010;106:154-61.

37. Caudevilla-Galligo F, Riba J, Ventura M, et al. 4-Bromo-2,5-dimethoxyphenethylamine (2C-B): presence in the recreational drug market in Spain, pattern of use and subjective effects. J Psychopharmacol. 2012;26:1026-35.

38. Sanders B, Lankenau SE, Bloom JJ, et al. "Research chemicals": tryptamine and phenethylamine use among high-risk youth. Subst Use Misuse. 2008;43:389-402.

39. Bosak A, LoVecchio F, Levine M. Recurrent seizures and serotonin syndrome following "2C-I" ingestion. J Med Toxicol. 2013;9:196-8.

40. Schep LJ, Slaughter RJ, Vale JA, et al. The clinical toxicology of the designer "party pills" benzylpiperazine and trifluoromethylphenylpipeazine. Clin Toxicol. 2011;49:131-41.

41. Arbo MD, Bastos ML, Carmo HF. Piperazine compounds as drugs of abuse. Drug Alcohol Depend. 2012;122:174-85.

42. Davies S, Wood DM, Smith G, et al. Purchasing 'legal highs' on the Internet—is there consistency in what you get? QJM. 2010;103:489-93.

43. Wikström M, Holmgren P, Ahlner J. A2 (N-benzylpiperazine) a new drug of abuse in Sweden. J Anal Toxicol. 2004;28(1):67-70.

44. Gee P, Gilbert M, Richardson S, et al. Toxicity from the recreational use of 1-benzylpiperazine. Clin Toxicol (Phila). 2008;46:802-7.

45. Gee P, Jerram T, Bowie D. Multiorgan failure from 1-benyzlpiperazine ingestion—legal high or lethal high? Clin Toxicol (Phila). 2010;48:230-3.

46. Baumann MH, Partilla JS, Lehner KR, et al. Powerful cocaine-like actions of 3,4-methylenedioxypyrovalerone (MDPV), a principal constituent of psychoactive "bath salts" products. Neuropsychopharmacology. 2013;38:552-62.

47. Dargan P, Wood D. Novel Psychoactive Substances: Classification, Pharmacology and Toxicology. Cambridge, MA: Academic Press; 2013.

48. Hohmann N, Mikus G, Czock D. Effects and risks associated with novel psychoactive substances: mislabeling and sale as bath salts, spice, and research chemicals. Dtsch Arztebl Int. 2014;111:139-47.

49. Shellard EJ. Ethnopharmacology of Kratom and the Mitragyna alkaloids. J Ethnopharmacol. 1989;25:123-4.

50. Boyer EW, Babu KM, Macalino GE, et al. Self-treatment of opioid withdrawal with a dietary supplement, Kratom. Am J Addict. 2007;16:352-6.

51. Nelson JL, Lapoint J, Hodgman MJ, et al. Seizures and coma following Kratom (*Mitragyna speciosa* Korth) exposure. J Med Toxicol. 2010;6:424-6.

52. Kelly BC. Legally tripping: a qualitative profile of Salvia divinorum use among young adults. J Psychoactive Drugs. 2011;43:46-54.

53. Baggott MJ, Erowid E, Erowid F, et al. Use patterns and self-reported effects of Salvia divinorum: an internet-based survey. Drug Alcohol Depend. 2010;111:250-6.

54. Rais V, Seefeld A, Cantrell L, et al. Salvia divinorum: exposures reported to a statewide poison control system over 10 years. J Emerg Med. 2011;40:643-50.

55. Schmidt MM, Sharma A, Schifano F, et al. "Legal highs" on the net: evaluation of UK-based websites, products and product information. Forensic Sci Int. 2011;206:92-7.

56. Klinke HB, Muller IB, Steffenrud S, et al. Two cases of lysergamide intoxication by ingestion of seeds from Hawaiian baby woodrose. Forensic Sci Int. 2010;197:e1-5.

57. Kremer C, Paulke A, Wunder C, et al. Variable adverse effects in subjects after ingestion of equal doses of Argyreia nervosa seeds. Forensic Sci Int. 2012;214: e6-8.

58. Juszczak GR, Swiergiel AH. Recreational use of D-lysergamide from the seeds of Argyreia nervosa, Ipomoea tricolor, Ipomoea violacea, and Ipomoea purpurea in Poland. J Psychoactive Drugs. 2013;45:79-93.

59. Grund J-PC, Latypov A, Harris M. Breaking worse: the emergence of krokodil and excessive injuries among people who inject drugs in Eurasia. Int J Drug Policy. 2013;24:265-74.

60. DESOMORPHINE (Dihydrodesoxymorphine; dihydrodesoxymorphine-D; Street Name: Krokodil, Crocodil). Available from: http://www.deadiversion.usdoj.gov/drug_chem_info/desomorphine.pdf. Accessed November 21, 2018.

61. Thekkemuriyi DV, John SG, Pillai U. "Krokodil"—a designer drug from across the Atlantic, with serious consequences. Am J Med. 2014;127:e1-2.

62. Gahr M, Freudenmann RW, Hiemke C, et al. Desomorphine goes "crocodile." J Addict Dis. 2012;31:407-12.

SECTION 3

CNS Toxins

11. **Toxin-induced Seizures**
Dinesh Chaudhari, Anjali Chaudhari, Omender Singh

12. **Toxic Alcohols**
Michael E Nelson, Farah Dadabhoy, Timothy B Erickson

13. **Botulism**
Anjali Chaudhari, Deven Juneja

14. **Anticonvulsant Overdose**
Rohit Yadav, Deven Juneja

SECTION 3

CNS Toxins

11
CHAPTER

Toxin-induced Seizures

Dinesh Chaudhari, Anjali Chaudhari, Omender Singh

INTRODUCTION

Conceptual definition of an "epileptic seizure" is abnormal and excessive neuronal activity in the brain leading to transient signs and/or neuronal symptoms.[1] The International League Against Epilepsy (ILAE) has defined refractory seizures as drug-resistant seizures which occur when a patient fails to remain seizure free with two class of antiepileptic medications (appropriately chosen for the patient's seizure type and tolerated well by the patient).[2] The new definition of status epilepticus (SE) proposed by ILAE is: failure of seizure termination mechanisms or initiation of mechanisms leading to abnormally, prolonged seizures (after time point t_1). The long-term consequences, such as neuronal injury and neuronal death occur later (after time point t_2). It is a conceptual definition of two operational dimensions: first is the seizure length (t_1), beyond which it is considered to be continuous seizure activity.[3] The time of ongoing seizure activity leading to long-term consequences is the second dimension (t_2). For a convulsive SE, both time points (t_1 at 5 min and t_2 at 30 min) are based on clinical research and animal experiments. Refractory SE is defined as SE which is refractory to two intravenous antiepileptic drugs (AEDs), one of which is a benzodiazepine.[4] Super-refractory status epilepticus (SRSE) is SE that goes on for 24 hours or more, even after the use of intravenous anesthetic drugs, including SE cases which recur on weaning of anesthesia.[5] Various toxins and drugs can potentially lead to such refractory seizures.

TOXIN-INDUCED SEIZURES

Amongst the important causes of seizures is toxic chemicals exposure. These toxins cause abnormal hyperactivity in the brain. A lot of household chemicals can precipitate seizures when exposed at higher doses, but the major culprit still remains waste from industries, pesticide use in agriculture and occupational hazards.[6]

Epidemiology

Incidence of toxin related seizures still remains unknown. In the studies done so far on patients with first convulsive seizure, suggest that 8.5% patients with age above 25 years and around 11% patients with age above 60 years have a toxin-related etiology. For patients with age of 40–65 years, 24% of them have toxic, metabolic or vascular etiology for seizure.[7]

Pathophysiology

Toxin-induced seizures occur due to disturbances in excitation-inhibition coupling mechanisms. The balance is maintained by excitatory neurotransmitters [e.g. glutamate, N-methyl-D-aspartate (NMDA)] and inhibitory neurotransmitters [e.g. gamma-aminobutyric acid (GABA)]. Reduction in the levels of inhibitory neurotransmitters or their receptor function, or increase in excitatory activity, can cause seizures. Certain drugs that reduce levels of GABA [e.g. isoniazid (INH)] can precipitate seizures. A sudden withdrawal of drugs like ethanol having inhibitory functions can precipitate withdrawal seizures.[8]

Electrolyte abnormalities causing seizures include hyponatremia, hypernatremia, hypomagnesemia, hypocalcemia, hypoglycemia, and hyperglycemia.[9] There are certain toxins such as cyanide and carbon monoxide (acting as hypoglycemic agents) that may result in increased excitatory amino acids (EAA) levels and precipitate seizure. Oral hypoglycemic agents such as sulfonylureas can also precipitate seizures via hypoglycemia, compounds such as 3,4-Methylenedioxymethamphetamine (MDMA) via hyponatremia and salicylates by causing cerebral edema.[10]

Various Molecular Mechanisms Associated with Toxin-induced Seizures

GABA and NMDA Receptors

When stimulated, GABA receptors modulate chloride ion flux, inhibiting membrane depolarization.[11] On the contrary GABA antagonism or deficiency increases membrane depolarization and reduces seizure thresholds. Certain withdrawal seizures attributed to ethanol, sedative hypnotics, and baclofen also happen due to loss of GABA mediated inhibition.[12] Hydrazines like INH or *Gyromitra* species of mushrooms block the enzyme pyridoxal 5-phosphate, which is a cofactor in the synthesis of GABA hence resulting in its deficiency. Under this circumstance use of benzodiazepines and barbiturates would not be useful due to insufficient levels of GABA to exert their effects. Pyridoxine (vitamin B_6) is therefore the treatment of choice in seizures of hydrazine toxicity, and is proposed to be useful in theophylline toxicity as well.[7]

The excitatory amino acid (glutamate) after binding to the glutamate receptors can cause influx of sodium, resulting in depolarization and excessive neuronal excitation that may result in seizures.[10]

Disturbances of Ion Flux

Depolarization is caused by the opening of Na^+ channels and voltage-gated K^+ channels are essential in the repolarization and hyperpolarization. Seizures result due to a disequilibrium, and shifting from a given state of homeostasis. Deviation from this homeostasis in any direction can cause seizure. It could be due to increased sodium channel opening or blockade, or simply because of the changes in the cholinergic tone. Local anesthetics (LA) is one such example which can be possibly used for the treatment of SE due to its virtue of Na^+ channel blockade and precipitate seizures in the overdose. Similarly carbamazepine, which is used as an anticonvulsant in therapeutic doses but may precipitate seizures in overdoses.[12] Various toxins that induce seizures via ion flux mechanism are mentioned in Table 1.[7]

Adenosine Antagonism

Adenosine receptors are located in central nervous system (CNS). Presynaptic adenosine receptors reduce the release of glutamate and postsynaptic receptors directly inhibit excitatory pathways. Therefore drugs such as theophylline and caffeine which are adenosine antagonists can reduce seizure threshold.[8] Seizures occurring due to theophylline or caffeine poisoning which are not responding to benzodiazepines are also not likely to respond to phenytoin as well, but may respond to barbiturates.[7]

Other Biogenic Amines

Other neurotransmitters known to be playing a role in seizure induction include serotonin, acetylcholine (ACh), norepinephrine, dopamine, and histamine. Ethanol withdrawal causes increased norepinephrine release and can precipitate seizures due to autonomic overstimulation.[12] Cholinergic overstimulation caused by carbamates, organophosphates and nerve gas may also result in seizures.[13]

Table 1: Examples of toxins that induce seizure via ion flux mechanism.

1	Sodium channel openers	Pyrethroids, ciguatoxin
2	Sodium-channel blockers	Phenytoin, lidocaine, quinidine
3	Potassium-channel openers	Barium, apamin (bee venom)
4	Potassium channel blockers	Aminopyridine
5	Beta-blockers	Propranolol

The organophosphates and carbamates are acetylcholinesterase inhibitors (the hydrolyzing enzyme for the neurotransmitter ACh that degrades it into choline and acetic acid) causing overstimulation of cholinergic receptors. The mainstay of treatment is atropine and pralidoxime.

Clinical Presentation and Differential Diagnosis

To differentiate between drug and toxin-induced seizures from other causes is difficult unless there is a pertaining history of overdose. A thorough history of the medications patient has access to should be assessed. In case of focal seizures, seizure is unlikely to be drug related if there is no history of altered sensorium or postictal period.[10] Certain clinical scenarios may help in narrowing down the differential diagnosis. Patients with psychiatric disorders may have overdosed on their own medications. Patients with a history of exposure to wild plants or mushrooms may have unknowingly ingested water hemlock or Gyromitra.[12] Sympathomimetic toxidrome preceding the seizure is suggestive of substance abuse with cocaine or amphetamines. Seizures with wide QRS interval on electrocardiogram (ECG) may be secondary to tricyclic antidepressants, venlafaxine, propoxyphene, diphenhydramine, etc. If a patient presents with seizure and has recent history of Mantoux test or antitubercular treatment, INH is likely to be the cause for seizure.[12] Presentation of seizure as myoclonic activity with or without altered mental status may be caused by strychnine[14] and serotonin syndrome.[15]

Drugs Causing Seizures

Drugs causing seizures are broadly classified as psychotropic and nonpsychotropic agents. Psychotropic drugs include antipsychotics, antidepressants, and antiepileptics. Few examples of nonpsychotropic drugs are narcotics, anticholinergics, methylxanthines, and other miscellaneous drugs (Table 2).[16]

Toxins Causing Seizures

List of seizurogenic chemicals includes toxic industrial chemicals, pesticides, and natural toxins (Table 3).[6]

Seizure Causing Chemicals which Modulate Ion Channels

Organochlorines [e.g. dichlorodiphenyltrichloroethane (DDT), pyrethroids] interrupt the functions of sodium channels, leading to repetitive firing of the nerve impulse causing tremors and seizures.[17] No specific antidotes are available for organochlorine pesticides. So benzodiazepines are their first-line therapy and rest is supportive management.[18]

Natural Agents

Certain natural agents are notorious for causing seizures. *Water hemlock* (*Cicuta douglasii*) is a highly toxic plant containing cicutoxin, a neurotoxin that causes intractable seizures and has no specific antidote (Table 4).[19] The cytotoxic mushroom *Gyromitra esculenta* contains gyromitrins, a family of hydrazines, structurally similar to INH. Ingestion may cause

Table 2: Common drugs causing seizures.	
Class of drugs	*Examples*
Analgesics	Tramadol, mefenamic acid, meperidine, propoxyphene, salicylates
Antiepileptics	Carbamazepine, phenytoin, vigabatrin, lamotrigine
Drug abuse	Amphetamines, cocaine, MDMA
Antidepressants and antipsychotics	SSRI, venalafaxine, TCA, lithium, citalopram, clonazepine, olanzepine, haloperidol, quetiapine
Withdrawal	Ethanol, baclofen, sedative-hypnotics
Natural substances	Mushrooms (*Gyromitra esculenta*), ephedra, *datura*, water hemlock
Cellular asphyxiants	Cyanide, carbon monoxide, hydrogen sulfide
Miscellaneous agents	Methylxanthines, isoniazid, camphor, chloroquines, quinines, iron, and asphyxiants

(MDMA: 3,4-methylenedioxymethamphetamine; SSRI: selective serotonin re-uptake inhibitors; TCA: tricyclic antidepressants)

CNS Toxins

Table 3: Chemical agents causing seizures.

Mode of action	Chemical class	Examples
Over stimulation of cholinergic receptors	Organophosphates and carbamates	Parathion, carbaryl, aldicarb, chlorpyrifos
	Warfare and nerve gas agents	Sarin, soman
Action on voltage-gated sodium channels	Pyrethroid pesticides and organochlorine	DDT, permethrin
	Biotoxins	Scorpion toxin
Glutamate receptor activation	Industrial chemicals	Cyanides, azides
Glycine receptor inhibition	Pesticides	Strychinine
GABA receptor inhibition	Pesticides	Tetramethylenedisulfotetramine, Lindane

(DDT: dichloro-diphenyl-trichloroethane; GABA: gamma amino butyric acid)

Table 4: Examples of some specific antidotes.

Agents	Specific antidotes
Arsenic, lead	BAL/EDTA
INH, theophylline, hydrazines, gyrometria mushroom	Pyridoxine
OP insecticides, nerve gas agents	Atropine/pralidoxime
Thallium	Prussian blue
Carbon monoxide	Hyperbaric oxygen
Insulin, OHA agents	Dextrose
Sulfonylureas	Octreotide
Salicylates, lithium, theophylline	Hemodialysis

(BAL: British anti-Lewisite; EDTA: ethylenediaminetetraacetic acid; INH: isoniazid; OHA: oral hypoglycemic agents; OP: organophosphate)

seizures, delayed gastrointestinal symptoms and renal or hepatic failure.[20] Picrotoxin (a toxic plant compound) a noncompetitive antagonist of the GABA receptor has been used in models to study seizures.[21] Strychnine is a proconvulsant because of its antagonistic activity at glycine receptors, mostly in the spinal cord, causing hyperactivity of both sensory and motor functions. Strychnine poisoning usually requires an aggressive airway protection, anticonvulsant treatment, and sometimes even neuromuscular blockade.[22]

Heavy Metals

Exposure to heavy metals like arsenic, thallium and lead, leads to multiple toxic effects. Presentation may include severe neurologic and gastrointestinal symptoms, including confusion, encephalopathy, delirium or seizures.[23]

Investigations

As a part of routine work up, blood sugar levels, complete metabolic panel, serum electrolytes and a 12 lead ECG should be done. Other important investigations which should be done are:

- *Urinary toxicology panel* is done to look for common drugs of abuse like cocaine, amphetamines, opioids, cannabinoids (marijuana), etc.
- *Computed tomography (CT)* of head should be selectively done if any focal neurological deficit is present along with seizures.
- *Electroencephalograph (EEG)* may help to know if there is any underlying structural brain lesion. It is also indicated when there is doubt about presence of seizure activity.[7]

Treatment of Drug- and Toxin-associated Seizures

The first and foremost attention is paid to the supportive management that includes airway protection and mechanical ventilation, hemodynamic stabilization with the blood pressure and heart rate monitoring. Bedside blood glucose and arterial blood gas (ABG) measurement with the core body temperature monitoring as mentioned in Flowchart 1. Majority of drug and toxin-induced seizures present as generalized tonic-clonic motor seizures and are often self-limited. But a prolonged convulsive activity can lead to complications such as, hyperthermia, hypoxia, hypercarbia, rhabdomyolysis, lactic acidosis, and aspiration of gastric contents. A permanent neurological sequelae is also likely due to uncontrolled seizure activity.[8]

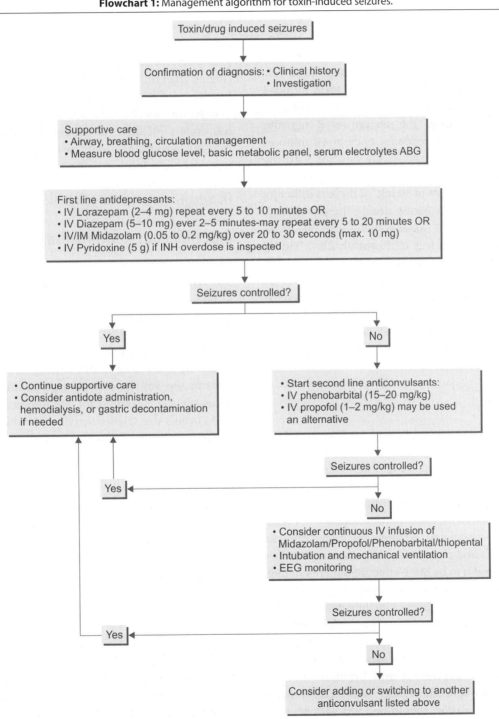

Flowchart 1: Management algorithm for toxin-induced seizures.

Hyperthermia is a dreaded complication of SE and needs urgent intervention to prevent death and serious end-organ damage. If the muscle contractions persist despite initial anticonvulsant therapy and the temperature exceeds above 40°C, then neuromuscular relaxants may be used with external cooling measures.[12] EEG monitoring is recommended to monitor response to anticonvulsants.

Benzodiazepines

Benzodiazepines are the first-line drugs used for anticonvulsant therapy in drug and toxin-induced seizures.[8] Intravenous lorazepam is the preferred benzodiazepine, used in the dosage of 2 mg/min up to 4 mg and can be repeated once at 10 minutes if needed. Diazepam is used in the dose of 5–10 mg intravenous in adults repeated every 10 minutes if needed up to a maximum of 30 mg.[7] If there is difficulty securing an intravenous access during the emergency, then midazolam (more water-soluble) can be given intramuscularly (IM) as it is more readily absorbed by this route.[24] According to a Cochrane review and a large randomized controlled trials (RCTs) for SE, intravenous lorazepam was found to be better than intravenous phenytoin or intravenous diazepam for cessation of SE.[25,26] As a life-saving measure, high doses of midazolam have also been used to terminate seizures refractory to other agents.

Barbiturates

Barbiturates are the second-line of anticonvulsants if patient does not respond to benzodiazepines. Amongst barbiturates, phenobarbital is the drug of choice, given in the doses of 15–20 mg/kg intravenous (bolus), rate not exceeding 1 mg/kg/min. A repeat dose of 5–10 mg/kg can be given after 10 minutes. Barbiturates are effective in fluvoxamine-associated seizures not responding to benzodiazepines and phenytoin.[27] Experimental studies have also reported it to be more effective than phenytoin in prevention and treatment of theophylline-induced seizures.[28] The other barbiturates include pentobarbital, thiopental, and secobarbital. They have higher potency, better lipid solubility, and more rapid onset as compared to phenobarbital. However they also carry a greater risk of respiratory depression and hypotension. The combination of benzodiazepines and barbiturates together or in succession should be used with caution due to the risk of respiratory depression. These two drugs work synergistically, where benzodiazepines increase the frequency and barbiturates increase the duration of GABA chloride channel opening.[29]

Propofol

Propofol is an alternative second-line anticonvulsant for drug-induced seizures. It is an intravenous anesthetic agent with synergistic effects with benzodiazepines and barbiturates.[28] The dose for ceasing SE is 2–5 mg/kg (higher than the dose used for sedation) and the patient may require endotracheal intubation with mechanical ventilation. The harmful effects of high-dose propofol infusions include hypertriglyceridemia, propofol infusion syndrome, and neuroexcitation. Prolonged propofol infusion can result in propofol infusion syndrome manifesting as hypotension, bradycardia, rhabdomyolysis, and metabolic acidosis.[8]

Miscellaneous Anticonvulsant Agents

Pyridoxine is the ideal drug for seizures induced by INH toxicity. Empirically dose of 5 g intravenously (70 mg/kg in pediatric) is given if the ingested dose of INH is not known. But, if the amount of drug ingested is known, then it is gram for gram replacement with pyridoxine. It has also been used in poisonings by theophylline where it acts by increasing GABA concentrations. Phenytoin acts on the voltage-dependent sodium channels and increases the threshold for membrane depolarization that curtails the seizure activity.[7] However, it has been shown to be ineffective in terminating withdrawal seizures in a number of cases,[30] and may even be harmful in cases of theophylline, lidocaine or tricyclic antidepressants toxicity.[31] As a last resort there may be a role of inhalational anesthetic agents such as isoflurane in case of refractory SE.[7] An upcoming drug whose definite role has still not been proved is valproic acid. Drugs like ketamine are also under evaluation for treatment of refractory SE. Its efficacy has been proved in cases of tetramine poisoning and where benzodiazepines and thiopental failed to control the seizures.[32]

Other Treatment Modalities

Patients undergoing gastrointestinal decontamination procedures should have a protected airway. Activated charcoal (dose of 1 g/kg) may be considered for agents that are known to adsorb to it such as methylxanthines or carbamazepine. The airway should be protected for the risk of aspiration. Bowel irrigation may be done in cases of heavy metal toxicity, sustained release drugs, body stuffers and packers. Not recommended in cases of hemodynamic instability, active seizures or ileus. Hemodialysis can enhance the elimination of drugs such as salicylates, lithium, and methylxanthines.[12]

STATUS EPILEPTICUS

Drugs that may precipitate SE either by lowering the threshold or by increasing the clearance of antiepileptic drugs are enumerated in Table 5.

Complications of Status Epilepticus

Prolonged seizure activity can lead to several complications. Respiratory complications include apnea, respiratory failure, and hypoxia with risk for ventilator-associated pneumonia, adult respiratory distress syndrome (ARDS), atelectasis, and neurogenic pulmonary edema. Metabolically patient has a risk

Table 5: Category of drugs with examples.

Category of drugs	Examples
Antiepileptics	Tiagabine, levetiracetam, valproate, lamotrigine, carbamazepine, pregablin, and phenytoin
Antipsychotics	Clozapine, lithium, chlorpromazine
Tricyclic antidepressants	Clomipramine, imipramine
Tetracyclic antidepressants	Maprotiline, amoxapine
Monocyclic antidepressant	Bupropion
Selective serotonin reuptake inhibitor (SSRI)	Sertraline, paroxetine, fluoxetine
Recreational drugs	Alcohol withdrawal, amphetamines, cocaine, MDMA (ectasy)
Antibiotics	Carbapenems—imipenem Cephalosporins—ceftazidime, cefepime Quinolones—ciprofloxacin, oflaoxacin, alatrofloxacin Macrolides—clarithromycin Isoniazid Metronidazole

(MDMA: 3,4-methylenedioxymethamphetamine)

for hyperkalemia, hyperglycemia then hypoglycemia, volume depletion.

Other complications include cerebral edema with raised intracranial pressure, hypertension, arrhythmias, myocardial dysfunction, stress ulcers with gastrointestinal bleed, renal failure with rhabdomyolysis, disseminated intravascular coagulation, venous stasis, and possible thrombosis. It is important to detect these potentially life-threatening early and institute prompt treatment.[33]

Refractory Status Epilepticus (RSE)

About 30% of the patients with SE may show resistant to the standard treatment with the first-line anticonvulsant agents of benzodiazepines and phenytoin. The patients of refractory status epilepticus (RSE), not responding to first line of AEDs are unlikely to respond to an alternate drug from the same category. If seizures fail to terminate after administration of lorazepam and fosphenytoin in appropriate dosages, a provisional diagnosis of RSE can be made. These patients usually need intensive care unit (ICU) care for monitoring and more rigorous treatment with assisted mechanical ventilation. Recently a randomized trial concluded the efficacy of valproate in terminating generalized convulsive SE (GCSE) refractory to phenytoin in 15 out of 19 (79%) of patients.[34] It has a desirable safety profile as a nonsedating drug and can be used (in the doses of 30 mg/kg) in patients with cardiorespiratory impairment with do not ventilate status. Other relatively newer AEDs include IV levetiracetam and oral topiramate. These two drugs are gaining popularity for their nonsedating properties and hence can be tried without ventilator assistance. Intravenous preparation of levetiracetam has been used safely up to a max dosage of 3,000 mg given over 15 mins. Oral topiramate in the doses of 300–1,600 mg/day when administered via nasogastric tube have also been found to be effective in terminating RSE.[33]

Pharmacological treatment algorithm after failure of first and second-line anticonvulsants is as described in Flowchart 2. In GCSE, intravenous anesthetics are usually recommended (treatment pathway 1). But a third nonanesthetic agent such as phenobarbital or valproic acid can also be used before using the intravenous anesthetics (treatment pathway 2). In nonconvulsive status epilepticus (NCSE), pathway 2 is recommended and anesthetics are preferably avoided.[35]

Flowchart 2: Treatment algorithm for refractory status epilepticus.[35]

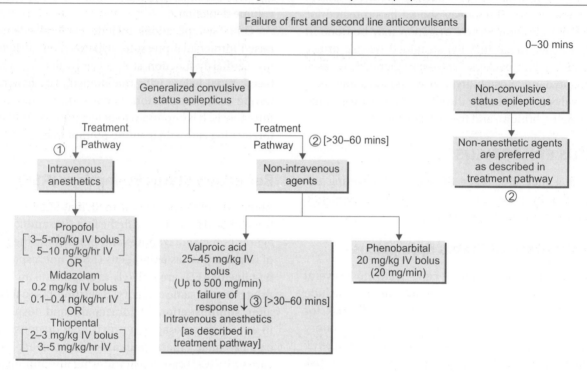

CONCLUSION

Certain chemicals are highly toxic and have deleterious effects on nervous system. A wide variety of such agents lead to seizures. A thorough clinical history regarding exposure to such agents and physical examination is probably more useful than diagnostic testing.

KEY POINTS

- In this modern era of medicine, all critical care physicians must have an awareness and basic knowledge about the drugs and toxins with seizurogenic potential.
- Majority of toxin-induced seizures respond to anticonvulsants.
- Serum blood glucose levels, ABG, and serum electrolytes should be checked on presentation.
- Use of pyridoxine needs to be considered when INH-related seizure is suspected.
- In cases of NCSE nonanesthetic agents such as valproic acid may be preferred over anesthetic agents for termination of seizures.
- Certain newer agents such as topiramate and levetiracetam are still under study for treatment of drug-induced RSE.

REFERENCES

1. Fisher RS, Acevedo C, Arzimanoglou A, et al. ILAE official report: a practical clinical definition of epilepsy. Epilepsia. 2014;55(4):475-82.
2. Kwan P, Arzimanoglou A, Berg AT, et al. Definition of drug resistant epilepsy: Consensus proposal by the ad hoc Task Force of the ILAE Commission on Therapeutic Strategies. Epilepsia. 2010;51(6):1069-77.
3. Trinka E, Cock H, Hesdorffer D, et al. A definition and classification of status epilepticus—Report of the ILAE task force on classification of status epilepticus. Epilepsia. 2015;56(10):1515-23.
4. Rossetti AO, Lowenstein DH. Management of refractory status epilepticus in adults: Still more questions than answers. Lancet Neurol. 2011;10(10):922-30.
5. Dubey D, Kalita J, Misra UK. Status epilepticus: Refractory and super-refractory. Neurol India. 2017;65:S12-7.
6. Jett DA. Chemical toxins that cause seizures. Neurotoxicology. 2012;33(6):1473-5.
7. Sharma AN, Hoffman RJ. Toxin-related seizures. Emerg Med Clin North Am. 2011;29(1):125-39.

8. Chen HY, Albertson TE, Olson KR. Treatment of drug-induced seizures. Br J Clin Pharmacol. 2016;81(3):412-9.

9. Delanty N, Vaughan CJ, French JA. Medical causes of seizures. Lancet. 1998;352(9125):383-90.

10. Pooja HV, Anup UP. Drugs implicated in seizures and its management. J Pharmacol Clin Res. 2017;3(2):555-607.

11. Fountain NB, Lothman EW. Pathophysiology of status epilepticus. J Clin Neurophysiol. 1995;12(4):326-42.

12. Wills B, Erickson T. Drug- and toxin-associated seizures. Med Clin N Am. 2005;89(6):1297-321.

13. Yokoyama H, Sato M, Iinuma K, et al. Centrally acting histamine H1 antagonists promote the development of amygdala kindling in rats. Neurosci Lett. 1996;217 (2-3):194-6.

14. Shadnia S, Moiensadat M, Abdollahi M. A case of acute strychnine poisoning. Vet Hum Toxicol. 2004;46(2):76-9.

15. Walker IA, Slovis CM. Lidocaine in the treatment of status epilepticus. Acad Emerg Med. 1997;4(9):918-22.

16. Franson KL, Hay DP, Neppe V, et al. Drug-induced seizures in the elderly. Causative agents and optimal management. Drugs Aging. 1995;7(1):38-48.

17. Chang LW, Dyer RS. Handbook of Neurotoxicology. New York: Marcel Dekker; 1995.

18. Bradberry SM, Cage SA, Proudfoot AT, et al. Poisoning due to pyrethroids. Toxicol Rev. 2005;24(2):93-106.

19. From the Centers for Disease Control and Prevention. Water hemlock poisoning—Maine, 1992. JAMA. 1994;271(19):1475.

20. Michelot D, Toth B. Poisoning by Gyromitra esculenta—a review. J Appl Toxicol. 1991;11(4):235-43.

21. Baden DG, Bourdelais AJ, Jacocks H, et al. Natural and derivative brevetoxins: historical background, multiplicity, and effects. Environ Health Perspect. 2005;113(5): 621-5.

22. Philippe G, Angenot L, Tits M, et al. About the toxicity of some Strychnos species and their alkaloids. Toxicon. 2004;44(4):405-16.

23. Toxicologic profiles ATSDR. [online] Available from http://www.atsdr.cdc.gov/toxprofiles. [Accessed Nov., 2004].

24. Silbergleit R, Durkalski V, Lowenstein D, et al. Intramuscular versus intravenous therapy for prehospital status epilepticus. N Engl J Med. 2012;366(7):591-600.

25. Prasad M, Krishnan PR, Sequeira R, et al. Anticonvulsant therapy for status epilepticus. Cochrane Database Syst Rev. 2014;9:CD003723.

26. Treiman DM, Meyers PD, Walton NY, et al. A comparison of four treatments for generalized convulsive status epilepticus. Veteran Affairs Status Epilepticus Cooperative Study Group. N Engl J Med. 1998;339(12):792-8.

27. Wood DM, Rajalingam Y, Greene SL, et al. Status epilepticus following intentional overdose of fluvoxamine: a case report with serum fluvoxamine concentration. Clin Toxicol. 2007;45(7):791.

28. Blake KV, Massey KL, Hendeles L, et al. Relative efficacy of phenytoin and phenobarbital for the prevention of theophylline-induced seizures in mice. Ann Emerg Med. 1988;17(10):1024-8.

29. Tunnicliff G. Basis of the antiseizure action of phenytoin. Gen Pharmacol. 1996;27(7):1091-7.

30. Rathlev NK, D'Onofrio G, Fish SS, et al. The lack of efficacy of phenytoin in the prevention of recurrent alcohol-related seizures. Ann Emerg Med. 1994;23(5):513-8.

31. Callaham M, Schumaker H, Pentel P. Phenytoin prophylaxis of cardiotoxicity in experimental amitriptyline poisoning. J Pharmacol Exp Ther. 1988;245(1):216-20.

32. Chau CM, Leung AKH, Tan IKS. Tetramine poisoning. Hong Kong Med J. 2005;11(6):511-4.

33. Cherian A, Thomas SV. Status epilepticus. Ann Indian Acad Neurol. 2009;12(3):140-53.

34. Misra UK, Kalita J, Patel R. Sodium valproate vs phenytoin in status epilepticus: a pilot study. Neurology. 2006;67(2):340-2.

35. Holtkamp M. The anaesthetic and invasive care of status epilepticus. Curr Opin Neurol. 2007;20:188-93.

12 CHAPTER

Toxic Alcohols

Michael E Nelson, Farah Dadabhoy, Timothy B Erickson

ETHANOL

Ethanol is the most commonly used recreational substance worldwide and consumption per capita is increasing. In the United States, ethanol is the third leading cause of preventable death and alcoholism permeates all levels of society. The widespread incidence and deleterious effects of alcoholism are well-known to the critical care clinician. Almost all societies that consume alcohol show related health and social problems.[1] The effects of acute and chronic alcoholism not only affect the individual drinker but also have far-reaching implications for the family, community, and workplace. Ethanol consumption is responsible for nearly 4% of global mortality, 5% of disability-adjusted life-years (DALY) lost due to premature death, and is projected to take on increasing importance over time.[2,3] Alcohol contributes to 88,000 deaths and $249 billion in societal costs annually in the United States.[4] Additionally in the United States, at least 24–31% of emergency department (ED) patients meet National institute alcohol abuse and Alcoholism (NIAAA) criteria for "at-risk" drinking.[3] At-risk drinking is defined as an average of 15 or more standard drinks per week or 5 or more on an occasion for men and 8 or more drinks weekly or 4 or more on an occasion for women as well as people older than 65 years of age.[5] The lifetime prevalence of alcohol use disorder (AUD) in the general population is 18%, and of dependence is 12%.[6] AUD consists of loss of control of alcohol intake with compulsive alcohol use and a negative emotional state, if not using alcohol. AUD also has varying degrees of severity from mild to severe based on criteria as outlined in the diagnostic and statistical manual of mental disorders (DSM). AUD is common in all developed countries and is more prevalent in men than in women, with lower but still substantial rates in developing countries. The prevalence of AUD is higher in specialized populations, affecting about 40% of patients presenting to the emergency department and 60% of trauma patients.[7]

In the United States, alcohol is the recreational substance most commonly used by youth. "Binge drinking" tendencies (five or more consecutive drinks on one occasion) have been reported in 7.3–21% of 9th through 12th graders, respectively, and up to 32% of college students.[5,6] Intermittent ethanol exposure in adolescence is associated with lasting changes in the adult brain that can increase the risk for alcohol use disorder and dependence as well as all the complications of alcoholism.[7]

In China, high school pooled male drinking rate in a recent meta-analysis was 36.5%, while middle school male drinking rate was 23.6% over 30 days.[8] In East Africa, the prevalence of alcohol use in secondary school students was 33%, with problem drinking ranging from 3% to 15%.[9] According to a 2-year prospective study in Norway, 46% of poisonings in 8- to 15-year-old children involved ethanol.[10] In parts of India, adolescent drinking has dramatically increased over the last two decades, with estimates being as high as 74% for those born between 1981 and 1985.[11]

Pharmacokinetics and Pathophysiology

Ethanol undergoes hepatic metabolism via two metabolic pathways: alcohol dehydrogenase and the microsomal ethanol oxidizing system (MEOS). Alcohol dehydrogenase (ADH) is the major metabolic pathway and the rate-limiting step in converting ethanol to acetaldehyde. Acetaldehyde is then metabolized by aldehyde dehydrogenase (ALDH) into acetic acid, which is then converted to water and carbon dioxide. With consumption of large quantities of ethanol, the cytochrome P450 2E1 enzyme contributes to ethanol metabolism. In general, nontolerant individuals metabolize ethanol at 10–25 mg/dL/hour, and those with tolerance can metabolize it up to a rate of 30 mg/dL/hour.[12] Children may ingest large amounts of ethanol in relation to their body weight, resulting in rapid development of high blood concentrations. In children, the ability to metabolize ethanol is diminished because of immature hepatic ADH activity.

Clinical Presentation

Ethanol is a selective central nervous system (CNS) depressant at low concentrations and a general depressant at high concentrations. Initially, ethanol produces euphoria and loss of inhibition, which progresses to lack of coordination, ataxia, slurred speech, gait disturbances, drowsiness, and ultimately stupor and coma. The intoxicated patient may demonstrate a flushed face, dilated pupils, excessive sweating, gastrointestinal (GI) distress, hypoventilation, hypothermia, and hypotension. Death from respiratory depression may occur at serum ethanol concentrations more than 500 mg/dL. Convulsions and death have been reported in children with acute ethanol intoxication owing to alcohol-induced hypoglycemia.

Hypoglycemia results from inhibition of hepatic gluconeogenesis and is most common in chronic malnourished alcoholics and children younger than 5 years. It does not appear to be directly related to the quantity of ethanol ingested and it is not uniformly present in all cases of pediatric ethanol ingestion.[13]

Laboratory Studies

In symptomatic patients who have suspected ethanol intoxication, the most critical laboratory tests are the serum ethanol and glucose concentrations.[14] Although blood ethanol concentrations roughly correlate with clinical signs, the physician must treat patients based on their clinical status, not the absolute level as tolerant individuals will require higher concentrations to achieve CNS depression.[15] If the ethanol level does not correlate with the clinical picture (such as a comatose patient with a low serum ethanol concentration), the intensivist should consider coingestants or other causes of altered mental status. If patients have experienced fluid losses, measure serum electrolytes and assess their acid-base status.

Management

The mainstay of treatment for most patients with acute ingestions of ethanol is supportive care and allowing the patient to metabolize the ethanol until of no longer clinically intoxicated. Attention is directed toward management of the patient's airway, circulation, and blood sugar status. If hypoglycemia is present, administer 2–4 mL/kg of D25W in children less than 50 kg, and 1 amp of D50W to those adults more than 50 kg. Serial glucose levels are followed to detect recurrent hypoglycemia. In obtunded patients, naloxone 0.01 mg/kg intravenous (IV) push can be given for suspected opiate co-intoxication. Gastric decontamination is not indicated in ethanol-poisoned patients because ethanol is absorbed rapidly from the stomach. Hemodialysis does increase ethanol clearance by three to four times and may be considered in massive ethanol ingestions with significant metabolic disturbances and in patients who do not respond to conventional therapy although this is rarely needed.

Disposition

Patients with significantly altered mental status following acute ethanol ingestion should be admitted or observed for monitoring of respiratory and blood sugar status and for management of fluids and electrolytes. Asymptomatic patients may be discharged home with reliable caretakers. Patients should be referred for counseling in an alcohol

CNS Toxins

addiction program if a recurrent pattern of problematic ethanol use is suspected.

METHANOL

Methanol is present in a variety of substances found around the home and workplace, including paint solvents, gasoline additives, air or brake line antifreeze, canned-heat products, windshield washer fluid, and embalming fluid, and is manufactured as an intermediate in many chemical reactions. It is also known as wood alcohol, as it was distilled from wood in the 1920s to 1930s prohibition era.[15] Despite vast knowledge about the deleterious effects of methanol, it is still implicated in many recent mass poisonings, including Norway (2002–2004), Estonia 2007, Libya (2013), Iran (2013), and Kenya (2014).[16-18] According to Dawn news, the largest English newspaper, there were 317 deaths in Pakistan over the last 13 years due to suspected methanol contamination.[19] The largest outbreak was documented in Toba Tek Singh in 2016 with 42 deaths.[20] In India, over the last three decades, methanol has been implicated in over 2000 fatalities. As recently as 2015, it is estimated that 80–100 people died after consuming toxic methanol in Mumbai alone.

Pharmacokinetics and Pathophysiology

Methanol is rapidly absorbed following ingestion, with an average absorption half-life of 5 minutes. Peak serum concentration can be reached as early as 30–60 minutes after ingestion. As with ethanol, methanol is primarily metabolized by hepatic ADH. Its immediate metabolite is formaldehyde, which is rapidly metabolized (half-life of 1–2 minutes) to formic acid. The half-life of methanol at toxic concentrations may be as long as 24 hours, but in the presence of ADH inhibition (such as with fomepizole or coingested ethanol), it extends upward of 50 hours.[21-23] Elimination of methanol is mainly via zero-order kinetics, but at low concentrations can have first-order metabolism.[21,24,25] Methanol is harmless; however, its metabolite, formic acid, is extremely toxic. Formic acid inhibits mitochondrial cytochrome oxidase thus impairing oxidative metabolism and promotes lactic acidosis.

It affects the optic disc of the retina due to low levels of mitochondria and cytochrome oxidase.[26] Formic acid combines with tetrahydrofolate (THF) and is metabolized into water and carbon dioxide. Fatalities

have been reported after ingestion of as little as 15 mL of a 40% methanol solution, although 30 mL is generally considered a minimal lethal dose. Ingestion of only 10 mL can lead to blindness. Adults have survived ingestions of 500 mL.

Clinical Presentation

The onset of symptoms following methanol ingestion varies from 1 hour to 72 hours. Initial symptoms are similar to ethanol intoxication and include mental status depression, inebriation, ataxia, slurred speech, and potential gastric irritation. The classic triad of methanol poisoning consists of visual complaints, abdominal pain, and metabolic acidosis. The accumulation of formic acid leads to the delayed development of ophthalmologic signs and symptoms. Reported visual disturbances and findings include blurred vision ("snowstorm" appearance), photophobia, constricted visual fields, blindness, hyperemia of the optic disk, retinal edema, and reduced pupillary light response. The outcomes of patients who develop blindness cannot be predicted, as partial visual recovery can occur.[27,28]

Patients typically complain of nausea and vomiting and can experience GI bleeding and acute pancreatitis. Unlike other alcohols, these patients often lack the odor of ethanol on their breath and can have a clear sensorium. Methanol toxicity should be suspected in patients with altered mental status and metabolic acidosis of unclear etiology, especially if they have complaints involving vision.[29] Prognosis correlates with degree of acidosis, time from ingestion to presentation, and timing to initiation of treatment.[16,30] Necrosis of the putamen and subcortical white matter can lead to permanent neurologic complications such as a Parkinson-like extrapyramidal syndrome, polyneuropathy, and cognitive deficits.[31,32]

Laboratory Studies

Definitive diagnosis requires direct measurement of the serum methanol concentration. Additional recommended studies include a complete blood cell count, serum electrolytes and blood glucose, serum ethanol, lipase, blood urea nitrogen (BUN), and serum creatinine, a urinalysis, and a blood gas. If the type of toxic alcohol ingested is unclear, a serum ethylene glycol is also recommended along with the methanol concentration. Classically, methanol-intoxicated patients develop an elevated anion gap (AG) metabolic acidosis, although this may not be present, if the patient presents before a significant quantity of formic acid has been generated.[33] The AG is calculated using the equation:

$$AG = (Na^+) - (Cl^- + HCO_3^-) \ (N = 8\pm4 \ mEq/L).$$

The presence of an elevated-osmolar gap can suggest methanol ingestion but is not specific for methanol (or ethylene glycol, discussed later). The osmolar gap is the difference between the measured and calculated serum osmolarities. An elevated osmolar gap indicates the presence of an unmeasured osmotically active substance in the serum. The formula for calculating the serum osmolarity is:

$$Calculated \ Osm \ (mOsm/kg) = 2(Na^+) + glucose/18 + BUN/2.8$$

Normally, the difference between the measured and calculated serum osmolarities is less than 10 mOsm. Additional causes of an elevated-osmolar gap include ethanol, ethylene glycol, and isopropanol. Nontoxicological causes of an elevated-osmolar gap include diabetic ketoacidosis, alcoholic ketoacidosis, renal failure, critical illness, and multiple organ failure. A normal osmolar gap does not rule-out toxic alcohol poisoning[32,33] because the toxic alcohol may have been metabolized prior to patient presentation. Additionally, patients may have different baseline osmolarities resulting in a wide range of osmolar gap in the population from –15 mOsm to +10 mOsm. Thus, if a person begins with a negative osmolar gap, they could have a "normal" calculated osmolar gap with significant toxic alcohol ingestion. Generally, peak methanol concentrations of less than 20 mg/dL do not produce toxicity but peak levels of more than 50 mg/dL indicate significant risk.[15] Ocular effects occur at levels of more than 100 mg/dL, and fatalities have been reported in untreated victims with levels of more than 150 mg/dL.[32] Regardless of measured methanol concentration, comatose presentation and pH less than 7.0 are strong predictors of morbidity and mortality.[30]

Management

Due to the rapid absorption of alcohols from the GI tract, gastric decontamination is not indicated. Initial management consists of standard supportive care and fluid resuscitation. The main priorities in methanol or ethylene glycol poisonings are correction of acidosis, inhibition of toxic acid generation, and elimination of the parent alcohol and toxic metabolites. If a significant ingestion of methanol (or ethylene glycol) is likely, begin empiric treatment with the IV ADH inhibitor fomepizole prior to confirmatory laboratory tests, thus inhibiting the generation of toxic metabolites.[34,35] The initial loading dose of fomepizole is 15 mg/kg followed by 10 mg/kg every 12 hours. After 48 hours of treatment with fomepizole, increase dosing to 15 mg/kg every 12 hours, as repeated administration of fomepizole induces its own metabolism via the cytochrome P4502E1 enzyme.[36,37] Specific indications for fomepizole therapy include serum methanol (or ethylene glycol) concentrations of more than or equal to 20 mg/dL, history of ingestion with osmolar gap greater than 10 mOsm/L, or suspected ingestion with acidemia (pH <7.30).[38] Fomepizole therapy should be continued until the methanol or ethylene glycol concentration is less than 20 mg/dL.

If fomepizole is unavailable (which is generally the case in low-middle income countries), then ethanol, a preferential substrate of ADH, may be administered.[39] Fomepizole is preferable due to its safety profile and ease of administration compared to ethanol.[40] To prevent toxic metabolite formation, ethanol levels are maintained between 100 mg/dL and 150 mg/dL. An IV solution of 10% ethanol in 5% dextrose in water (D5W) is optimal, with a loading dose of 0.6 g/kg. A simplified approximation of the loading dose is 1 mL/kg of 10% diluted absolute ethanol. Close monitoring of the ethanol level every 1–2 hours is necessary in order to titrate the infusion to maintain the serum ethanol within the desired range. If IV ethanol preparations are unavailable, oral ethanol therapy can be instituted. Hypoglycemia is a potential complication of ethanol therapy in young children, thus serum glucose concentrations must be closely monitored. Additional adverse effects of ethanol include CNS and respiratory depression, hypotension, phlebitis, nausea, and vomiting.[40] Unlike ethanol, fomepizole does not cause CNS depression and hypoglycemia.

Additional therapies include IV sodium bicarbonate for pH less than 7.3. Correction of acidosis may improve ophthalmologic symptoms.[13,36] Bicarbonate may be given as bolus 1–2 mEq/kg or infusion at 150 mEq/L in 5% dextrose at 1.5–2 times maintenance fluid rate until no longer acidemic. Folate, the active form of folic acid, is a coenzyme in the metabolic step converting the toxic metabolite formic acid to CO_2 and H_2O and can be administered to the methanol-poisoned patient.

Give 1 mg/kg up to 50 mg of folate intravenously every 4–6 hours until the acidosis is corrected and methanol concentrations fall below 20 mg/dL.[15,16]

Hemodialysis removes methanol and formic acid. Indications for dialysis include visual impairment, metabolic acidosis (pH <7.3), renal failure, electrolyte imbalance, and methanol concentration of more than 50 mg/dL (with or without clinical signs or symptoms). Hemodialysis can be discontinued once acid-base disturbances are corrected and methanol concentrations are less than 20 mg/dL. Since, fomepizole and ethanol are readily dialyzed, dose adjustments are required. For fomepizole, the recommendation is to increase the frequency of dosing to every 4 hours during hemodialysis.[15]

Disposition

Any patient who is comatose and has abnormal vital signs, visual complaints, metabolic acidosis, or high methanol concentrations requires admission to an intensive care unit. Asymptomatic patients without evidence of acidosis and with a methanol level of less than 10 mg/dL may be discharged after observation in the emergency department.

ETHYLENE GLYCOL

Ethylene glycol is an odorless, sweet-tasting compound that is found in antifreeze products, coolants, preservatives, industrial solvents, hydraulic brake fluids, paints, glycerin substitutes, and certain paints and cosmetics.

Pharmacokinetics and Pathophysiology

Ethylene glycol undergoes rapid absorption from the GI tract, and initial signs of intoxication may occur as early as 30 minutes after ingestion. It undergoes hepatic metabolism via ADH to form glycolaldehyde. Glycolaldehyde is metabolized by ALDH into glycolic acid, which is then metabolized to glyoxylate and oxalic acid. Pyridoxime and thiamine act as cofactors in the metabolism of glyoxylate. Half-life of ethylene glycol ranges from 3 hours to 8.6 hours but can increase up to 20 hours with ADH inhibition.[41-43] Oxalic acid can combine with calcium to form calcium oxalate crystals that precipitate in the proximal renal tubules and lead to acute tubular necrosis and renal failure.[44,45] Additionally, hypocalcemia can occur due to this reaction.[46]

Clinical Presentation

The clinical effects of ethylene glycol poisoning classically are divided into three stages: Stage I (acute neurologic stage) occurs within the first 12 hours of ingestion with CNS symptoms similar to that experienced with ethanol and methanol, including slurred speech, nystagmus, ataxia, vomiting, lethargy, and coma. Unique to ethylene glycol, convulsions, myoclonic jerks, and tetanic contractions may occur because of hypocalcemia. As in methanol poisoning, patients can have an anion gap acidosis with an elevated-osmolar gap. In approximately one-third of cases, calcium oxalate crystals will be found in the urine (Fig. 1).

Stage II (cardiopulmonary stage) occurs within 12–24 hours after ingestion and is characterized by rapidly progressive tachypnea, cyanosis, metabolic acidosis, pulmonary edema, adult respiratory distress syndrome, and cardiomegaly. Death is most common during this stage. Stage III (renal stage) occurs 2 to 3 days after ingestion and is heralded by flank pain, oliguria, proteinuria, anuria, and renal failure.

Like methanol, delayed neurologic sequelae can occur with bulbar palsy, diplopia, nystagmus, facial droop, dysphagia, hearing loss, and autonomic nerve dysfunction.[47,48] Poor prognostic factors include severe acidosis, renal failure, seizures, comatose state, hyperkalemia, and a delay to treatment.[47,48] Also, like methanol, the degree of acidosis does predict mortality outcomes as well as morbidity, particularly the development of renal insufficiency.[33,41,49] Ethylene glycol

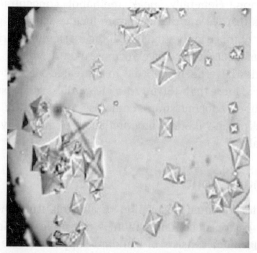

Fig. 1: Calcium oxalate crystals found with ethylene glycol poisoning.

poisoning is possible in any inebriated patient lacking an odor of ethanol who has severe acidosis, oxalate crystalluria, hematuria, or renal failure. This diagnosis should be considered in a patient with a metabolic acidosis of an unclear etiology.[50]

Laboratory Studies

Definitive diagnosis requires direct measurement of serum ethylene glycol concentrations. Additional recommended studies include complete blood cell count, serum electrolytes, blood glucose, serum ethanol, calcium, creatine kinase, an arterial or venous blood gas, BUN, serum creatinine, serum osmolarity, and urinalysis for crystals, protein, and blood. If the specific type of toxic alcohol ingested is unclear, a serum methanol level should also be measured in addition to the ethylene glycol concentration. Calculate both anion and osmolar gaps (as for methanol ingestion). Compared to other alcohols, ethylene glycol's contribution to the osmolar gap is relatively small, and toxic serum ethylene glycol concentrations will only cause an 8- to 10- mOsm elevation.[39] Therefore, an elevated-osmolar gap can suggest ethylene glycol exposure, but a normal gap does not exclude it. Because of the potential for severe cardiopulmonary toxicity, a chest radiograph and an electrocardiogram are recommended. Peak serum ethylene glycol concentrations less than 20 mg/dL do not cause significant toxicity.[41,47]

Management

Many of the management principles of ethylene glycol are similar to methanol. Gastric decontamination is not indicated because ethylene glycol is rapidly absorbed from the GI tract. Implement standard supportive care and treat seizures with benzodiazepines and barbiturates as needed.

Correct acidosis (pH <7.3) with sodium bicarbonate boluses or continuous infusion, as it may increase urinary excretion of ethylene glycol and delay calcium oxalate-induced renal failure.[33] Start ADH blockade as soon as possible with fomepizole 15 mg/kg loading dose followed by 10 mg/kg every 12 hours for a total of 48 hours. After 48 hours, increase the dose to 15 mg/kg every 12 hours due to fomepizole inducing its own metabolism.[37,38] If fomepizole is not available, administer ethanol as for methanol (see previous discussion). Since, ethylene glycol has a shorter half-life than methanol, certain cases

can be managed with fomepizole alone,[41,47,51,52] as long as there is no renal compromise or acidosis.

Hemodialysis effectively removes ethylene glycol and its metabolites. Indications for dialysis include metabolic acidosis (pH <7.3), renal failure, electrolyte imbalance, and ethylene glycol concentrations of more than 50 mg/dL. Hemodialysis can be discontinued once acid-base disturbances are corrected and ethylene glycol concentrations are less than 20 mg/dL. Since, fomepizole and ethanol are readily dialyzed, dose adjustments are required.

Monitor serum calcium levels, and if the patient develops clinical signs of hypocalcemia, treat with 10% calcium gluconate. Calcium replacement is not indicated for hypocalcemia alone, since this will encourage the formation of calcium oxalate crystals. In addition, thiamine and pyridoxine (vitamin B6) act as cofactors in ethylene glycol metabolism and can be administered but have not been proven to be effective in changing clinical outcomes.[36] Give thiamine 0.25–0.5 mg/kg to maximum 100 mg and pyridoxine 1–2 mg/kg to maximum 50 mg every 6 hours.

Disposition

Any patient with altered mental status, metabolic acidosis, high ethylene glycol serum concentration, or evidence of renal dysfunction should be admitted to a pediatric intensive care unit. Asymptomatic patients without acidosis and an ethylene glycol serum concentration of less than 10 mg/mL can be discharged with close out patient follow-up.

ISOPROPYL ALCOHOL

Isopropyl alcohol (isopropanol, IPA) is a common solvent and disinfectant with CNS-depressant properties similar to ethanol. The majority of exposures (up to 90%) occur in children younger than 6 years. Exposure to IPA occurs more frequently in children than methanol or ethylene glycol ingestions. Toxicity results from both accidental and intentional ingestions, as well as inhalation and dermal exposures in patients given "rubbing alcohol" sponge baths for fever.

Pharmacokinetics and Pathophysiology

Isopropanol is rapidly absorbed across the gastric mucosa, with acute intoxication occurring within

CNS Toxins

30 minutes of ingestion. IPA can be absorbed transdermally, rectally, or via inhalation. The folk remedy of dermal application of IPA for fever reduction places children at risk for systemic symptoms.[53,54] IPA is metabolized by ADH, but unlike methanol and ethylene glycol, it is metabolized into acetone and not an aldehyde or significant acid byproducts. Acetone, the chief metabolite, also acts as a CNS depressant but to a lesser extent than IPA. Respiratory elimination of acetone causes a fruity odor on the patient's breath similarly observed in diabetic ketoacidosis. Since, IPA is a potent inebriant that is about twice as intoxicating as ethanol, a level of 50 mg/dL is comparable to an ethanol level of 100 mg/dL.[55] Elimination of IPA is primarily renal via first-order kinetics with a half-life of 2.5–8 hours. Acetone elimination is slower, with a half-life of 7.7–27 hours.[56]

Clinical Presentation

Isopropanol acts as a CNS depressant and a peripheral vasodilator. Significant IPA ingestions cause varying degrees of inebriation ranging from lethargy and stupor to comatose state. Due to peripheral vasodilation and cardiac depression, hypotension and a reflex tachycardia can occur. Hypotension represents severe ingestion and confers increased risk of mortality. Due to IPA GI irritant effects, nausea, vomiting, abdominal pain, and a hemorrhagic gastritis can occur.[54] Aspiration can cause a hemorrhagic tracheobronchitis.[55] Other effects include hypotonia, hyporeflexia, respiratory depression, and hypothermia. Acetone production can cause a fruity odor on the breath. Deep coma develops at levels of more than 150 mg/dL, and death has been associated with concentration of more than 200 mg/dL.[56] Serum concentrations, however, do not correlate well with clinical outcomes.

Laboratory Studies

Like ethanol, methanol, and ethylene glycol, IPA produces an elevated-osmolar gap. Due to IPA metabolism to acetone, however, an acidosis does not ensue[31] (Table 1). Test blood and urine for acetone or ketones. Unlike diabetic ketoacidosis, the acetone is typically found in the absence of glycosuria, hyperglycemia, or acidemia. Indicated laboratory studies include a complete blood cell count, serum electrolytes, an arterial or venous blood gas, blood

Table 1: Comparisons of toxic alcohols parameter.

	Methanol	Ethylene Glycol	Isopropanol
Anion gap	+	+	–
Acidosis	+	+	–
Osmolar gap	+	+	+
CNS depression	+	+	+
Eye findings	+	–	–
Renal failure	–	+	–
Ketones	–	–	+
Oxalate crystals	–	+	–

(CNS: central nervous system)

glucose, serum ethanol level, serum osmolarity, BUN, and creatinine. Acetone can cause a "pseudo" elevation in creatinine due to interference with the laboratory assay.[57,58] Definitive diagnosis relies on direct measurement of IPA concentrations.

Management

Supportive care is the primary management intervention in IPA ingestions.[56] Close monitoring for respiratory depression, airway protection, and cardiovascular symptoms is paramount. Hypotension typically responds to IV crystalloid fluid but can be supplemented with vasopressors or inotropes, if necessary. Since, IPA is so rapidly absorbed from the GI tract, gastric decontamination is not indicated. Treat hemorrhagic gastritis with a proton pump inhibitor or H2 antagonist. Hemodialysis removes IPA and should be considered for prolonged coma, hypotension, and IPA levels more than 400 mg/dL. The decision for hemodialysis should not be based solely on an IPA concentration but on the clinical status of the patient.[56]

Disposition

Isopropanol-intoxicated patients who are lethargic should be admitted to an intensive care unit setting. Asymptomatic children may be safely discharged from the emergency department after 6 hours of observation.

CONCLUSION

Alcohol is the most consumed recreational substance worldwide, permeates all levels of society, and is a leading cause of preventable morbidity and mortality. In children, ethanol overdose may result in coma and hypoglycemia. Methanol and ethylene glycol can result in severe cellular dysfunction resulting in significant complications and mortality, if unrecognized and untreated. Methanol is commonly found in gasoline additives, air or brake line antifreeze, canned-heat products, and windshield washer fluid. Methanol poisoning is manifested by metabolic acidosis, visual disturbance, and potential multiorgan system failure. Ethylene glycol is a compound that is found in antifreeze products, coolants, preservatives, industrial solvents and hydraulic brake fluids. Ethylene glycol poisoning is manifested by metabolic acidosis, renal failure, and potential multiorgan system failure. Isopropyl alcohol is a common solvent and disinfectant with CNS-depressant properties similar to ethanol. Isopropyl alcohol will result in medical complications but has lower mortality outcomes than methanol or ethylene glycol. Isopropanol may also cause GI bleeding and hypotension but generally does not cause metabolic acidosis. All alcohols can produce an osmolar gap but the absence of an osmolar gap does not exclude toxic alcohol ingestion.

Definitive diagnosis relies on direct measurement of specific concentrations, however inhibition of alcohol dehydrogenase should be initiated promptly, if there is strong clinical suspicion for ingestion of methanol or ethylene glycol. Fomepizole is the only Food and Drug Administration (FDA) approved antidote for ethylene glycol and methanol poisoning however in the absence of access to fomepizole, ADH inhibition can be achieved with ethanol. Hemodialysis effectively removes the parent alcohol and its metabolites. It is indicated for toxic alcohol poisoning not responsive to supportive and antidote therapy or in patients with evidence of end-organ damage or severe acidosis. Despite widespread understanding of these substances and their management, significant complications and outbreaks still continue to occur, thus the clinician should consider these poisons in the appropriate clinical setting.

KEY POINTS

- Methanol poisoning classically presents with metabolic acidosis, visual disturbance, and multi-organ system failure.
- Ethylene glycol poisoning classically presents with metabolic acidosis, renal failure, and multiorgan system failure.
- Isopropanol may cause CNS depression and hypotension but does not cause metabolic acidosis.
- All alcohols can produce an osmolar gap, but the absence of an osmolar gap does not exclude toxic alcohol ingestion.
- Fomepizole is the antidote for ethylene glycol and methanol poisoning, and it should be administered if there is strong clinical concern for toxicity.
- Hemodialysis is indicated for toxic alcohol poisonings not responsive to supportive measures and antidote therapy or in patients with severe metabolic acidosis and/or end organ damage.

REFERENCES

1. Rehm J, Mathers C, Popova S, et al. Global burden of disease and injury and economic cost attributable to alcohol use and alcohol use disorders. Lancet. 2009;373(9682):2223-33.
2. Zhang M, Wu R, Jiang J, et al. The presence of hepatitis B core antibody is associated with more advanced liver disease in alcoholic patients with cirrhosis. Alcohol. 2013;47(7):553-8.
3. Trillo AD, Merchant RC, Baird JR, et al. Sex differences in alcohol misuse and estimated blood alcohol concentrations among emergency department patients: implications for brief interventions. Acad Emerg Med. 2012;19(8):924-33.
4. Centers for Disease Control and Prevention (2018). Fact Sheets – Alcohol Use and Your Health [online] Available from: https://www.cdc.gov/alcohol/fact-sheets/alcohol-use.htm. [Accessed November 2018].
5. Friedmann PD. Clinical practice. Alcohol use in adults. N Engl J Med. 2013;368(4):365-73.
6. Kann L, McManus T, Harris WA, et al. Youth Risk Behavior Surveillance—United States, 2017. MMWR Surveill Summ. 2018;67(SS-8):1-114.
7. Maldonado JR, Sher Y, Ashouri JF, et al. The "Prediction of alcohol withdrawal severity scale" (PAWSS): systematic literature review and pilot study of a new scale for the prediction of complicated alcohol withdrawal syndrome. Alcohol. 2014;48(4):375-90.
8. Feng Y, Newman IM. Estimate of adolescent alcohol use in China: a meta-analysis. Arch Public Health. 2016;74(45):1-14.
9. Francis JM, Grosskurth H, Changalucha J, et al. Systematic review and meta-analysis: prevalence of alcohol use among young people in eastern Africa. Trop Med Int Health. 2014;19(4):476-88.
10. Rajka T, Heyerdahl F, Hovda K, et al. Acute child poisonings in Oslo: A 2 year prospective study. Acta Pediatr. 2007;96(9):1355-9.
11. Pilai A, Nayak MB, Greenfield TK, et al. Adolescent drinking onset and it adult consequences among men:

12. Jones AW. Evidence-based survey of the elimination rates of ethanol from blood with applications in forensic casework. Forensic Sci Int. 2010;200(1-3):1-20.
13. Minera G, Robinson E. Accidental acute alcohol intoxication in infants: review and case report. J Emerg Med. 2014;47(5):524-6.
14. Erickson T, Brent J. Toxic Alcohols. In: Erickson T, Ahren W, Aks S, Baum C, Ling L (Eds). Pediatric Toxicology Diagnosis and Management of the Poisoned Child, 1st edition. New York, NY: McGraw-Hill; 2005. pp. 326-32.
15. Barceloux DG, Bond RG, Krenzelok EP, et al. American Academy of Clinical Toxicology Ad Hoc Committee: AACT practice guidelines on the treatment of methanol poisoning. J Toxicol Clin Toxicol. 2002;40(4):415-46.
16. Zakharov S, Pelclova D, Urban P, et al. Czech mass methanol outbreak 2012: epidemiology, challenges, and clinical features. Clin Toxicol. 2014;52:1013-24.
17. Rostrup M, Edwards JK, Abukalish M, et al. The methanol poisoning outbreaks in Libya 2013 and Kenya 2014. PLoS One. 2016;11(3):1-10.
18. Hassanian-Moghaddam H, Nikfarjam A, Mirafzal A, et al. Methanol mass poisoning in Iran: role of case finding in outbreak management. J Public Health (Oxf). 2015;37(2):354-9.
19. Palatnick W, Redman LW, Sitar DS, et al. Methanol half-life during ethanol administration: Implications for management of methanol poisoning. Ann Emerg Med. 1995;26:202-7.
20. Hovda KE, Andersson KS. Methanol and formate kinetics during treatment with fomepizole. Clin Toxicol. 2005;43:221-7.
21. Brent J, McMartin K, Phillips S, et al. Methylpyrazole for Toxic Alcohols Study Group: Fomepizole for the treatment of methanol poisoning. N Engl J Med. 2001;344:424-9.
22. Haffner HT, Besserer K, Graw M, et al. Methanol elimination in non-alcoholics: inter- and intraindividual variation. Forensic Sci Int. 1997;86:69-76.
23. Wu AB, Kelly T, McKay C, et al. Definitive identification of an exceptionally high methanol concentration in an intoxication of a surviving infant: methanol metabolism by first order elimination kinetics. J Forensic Sci. 1995;40:315-20.
24. Sharpe JA, Hostovsky M, Bilbao JM, et al. Methanol optic neuropathy: a histopathological study. Neurol. 1982;32:1093-100.
25. Erickson T. Toxic alcohol poisoning: when to suspect and keys to diagnosis. Consultant. 2000;40:1845-56.
26. Sanaei-Zadeh H, Zamani N, Shadnia S. Outcomes of visual disturbances following methanol poisoning. Clin Toxicol. 2011;49:102-7.
27. Brent J, Lucas M, Kulig K, et al. Methanol poisoning in a 6 week old infant. J Pediatr. 1991;118:644-6.
28. Paasma R, Hovda KE, Hassanian-Moghaddam H, et al. Risk factors related to poor outcome after methanol poisoning and the relation between outcome and antidotes – a multicenter study. Clin Toxicol. 2012;50(9):823-31.
29. Reddy NJ, Sudini M, Lewis LD. Delayed neurological sequelae from ethylene glycol, diethylene glycol and methanol poisonings. Clin Toxicol. 2010;48:967-73.
30. Paasma R, Hovda KE, Jacobsen D. Methanol poisoning and long term sequelae—a six years follow-up after a large methanol outbreak. BMC Clin Pharmacol. 2009;9:5.
31. Kraut J, Kraut I. Toxic alcohol ingestions: clinical features, diagnosis and management. Clin J Am Soc Nephrol. 2008;3(1):208-25.
32. Hoffman RS, Smilkstein MJ, Howland MA, et al. Osmol gaps revisited: normal values and limitations. Clin Tox. 1993;31(1):81-93.
33. Glaser DS. Utility of the serum osmol gap in the diagnosis of methanol or ethylene gylcol ingestion. Ann Emerg Med. 1996;27(3):343-6.
34. Liu JJ, Daya MR, Carrasquill O, et al. Prognostic factors in patients with methanol poisoning. J Toxicol Clin Toxicol. 1998;36:175.
35. Brent J, McMartin K, Phillips S, et al. Fomepizole for the treatment of methanol poisoning. N Engl J Med. 2001;344:424-9.
36. Mégarbane B, Borron SW, Baud FJ. Current recommendations for treatment of severe toxic alcohol poisonings. Intensive Care Med. 2005;31:189-95.
37. Brent J. Fomepizole for ethylene glycol and methanol poisoning. N Engl J Med. 2009;360(21):2216-23.
38. Jacobsen D, McMartin KE. Antidotes for methanol and ethylene glycol poisoning. J Toxicol Clin Toxicol. 1997;35:127.
39. Lepik KJ, Levy AR, Sobolev BG, et al. Adverse drug events associated with antidotes for methanol and ethylene gylcol poisoning: a comparison of ethanol and fomepizole. Ann Emerg Med. 2009;53(4):439-50.
40. Barceloux DG, Krenzelor E, Olson K, et al. American Academy of Clinical Toxicology Ad Hoc Committee: Guidelines on the treatment of ethylene glycol poisoning. J Toxicol Clin Toxicol. 1999;37:537-60.
41. Sivilotti MLA, Burns MJ, McMartin KE, et al. Toxicokinetics of ethylene glycol during fomepizole therapy: implications for management. Ann Emerg Med. 2000; 36(2):114-25.
42. Levine M, Curry SC, Ruha AM, et al. Ethylene glycol elimination kinetics and outcomes in patients managed without hemodialysis. Ann Emerg Med. 2012;59(6): 527-31.
43. McMartin K. Are calcium oxalate crystals involved in the mechanism of acute renal failure in ethylene glycol poisoning? Clin Toxicol. 2009;47:859-69.
44. Guo C, Cenac TA, Li Y, et al. Calcium oxalate, and not other metabolites, is responsible for the renal toxicity of ethylene glycol. Toxicol Lett. 2007;173:8-16.
45. Kraut JA, Mullins ME. Toxic alcohols. NEJM. 2018;378(3):270-80.
46. Kruse JA. Methanol and ethylene glycol intoxication. Crit Care Clin. 2012;28:661-711.

47. Rahman SS, Kadakia S, Balsam L, et al. Autonomic dysfunction as a delayed sequelae of acute ethylene glycol ingestion. J Med Toxicol. 2012;8:124-9.

48. Hylander B, Kjellstrand CM. Prognostic factors and treatment of severe ethylene glycol intoxication. Intensive Care Med. 1996;22(6):546-52.

49. Lung DD, Kearney TE, Brasiel JA, et al. Predictors of death and prolonged renal insufficiency in ethylene glycol poisoning. J Intensive Care Med. 2015;30(5): 270-7.

50. Coulter CV, Farquhar SE, McSherry CM, et al. Methanol and ethylene glycol acute poisonings – predictors of mortality. Clin Toxicol. 2011;49:900-6.

51. Woolf AD, Wynshaw-Boris A, Rinaldo P, et al. Intentional infantile ethylene glycol poisoning presenting as an inherited metabolic disorder. J Pediatr. 1992;120: 421-4.

52. Brent J. Fomepizole for the treatment of pediatric ethylene and diethylene glycol, butoxyethanol, and methanol poisonings. Clin Toxicol. 2010;48(5):401-6.

53. Boyer EW, Mejia M, Woolf A, et al. Severe ethylene glycol ingestion treated without hemodialysis. Pediatrics. 2001;107(1):172-4.

54. Dyer S, Mycyk MB, Ahrens WR, et al. Hemorrhagic gastritis from topical isopropanol exposure. Ann Pharmacother. 2002;36(11):1733-5.

55. McFadden SW, Haddow JE. Coma produced by topical application of isopropanol. Pediatrics. 1969;43(4):622-3.

56. Trummel J, Ford M, Austin P. Ingestion of unknown alcohol. Ann Emerg Med. 1996;27:368-74.

57. Slaughter RJ, Mason RW, Beasley DMG, et al. Isopropanol poisoning. Clin Toxicol. 2014;52:470-8.

58. Hawley PC, Falko JM. "Pseudo" renal failure after isopropyl alcohol intoxication. South Med J. 1982;75(5):630-1.

13 CHAPTER

Botulism

Anjali Chaudhari, Deven Juneja

INTRODUCTION

Botulism is a naturally occurring potentially lethal paralytic illness causing descending flaccid paralysis. It results from the action of a potent neurotoxin produced by *Clostridium botulinum* which is an anerobic, spore forming, Gram-positive rod. These spores are found in dust, soil, and aquatic sediments. Botulinum toxin has been investigated as a biologic agent since the time of World War II. It is known to be the most lethal substance, with a lethal dose (LD50) of 1 ng/kg body weight.[1] There are eight known serotypes of botulism, A to G, and Cα and Cβ subgroups. All most all human botulism cases are attributed to toxin types A, B, and E. Types C and D cause outbreaks in birds and animals. No human disease has been documented so far by type Cb or type G.[2]

EPIDEMIOLOGY

Occurrence of food botulism dates back to late 1700s in the countries of Europe. Back in those days it was mainly associated with the sausage production and consumption. Presently the highest incidence is found in Republic of Georgia and Asia, attributed to improper food handling. US has a low incidence rate with maximum percentage of 70–75% of infant botulism followed by foodborne botulism 20–25%.[3] A total of 139 cases of food botulism were reported between 2001 and 2007 in US, with neurotoxin type A being the culprit in

more than half of the cases. Incidence of infant botulism throughout the world has been mostly implicated to honey consumption. Incidences of wound botulism have been on a rise, especially after intravenous injection use of black tar heroin. Confirmed cases have been largely under reported in India due to lack of diagnostic enzyme-linked immunosorbent assay (ELISA) kits. Hence, mostly mouse neutralization test and molecular tests such as polymerase chain reaction (PCR) are done.[4]

CLASSIFICATION

Classically three forms of disease have been described:
1. *Foodborne botulism*, caused by ingestion of preformed toxin, usually occurs after consumption of inadequately cooked food, home canned food or fermented meat. More than half of the cases are attributed to type A toxin.[5] Normally adults can consume the spores (e.g. raw vegetables) without any effects. If the food is contaminated, the spores have the capacity of germinating under anaerobic conditions producing the toxin. Standard cooking does not kill *C. botulinum* spores (which requires heating at a specific temperature and pressure), but the toxins are heat labile and temperature sensitive.[6]
2. *Wound botulism*, caused by wound contamination with *Clostridium* spores, which germinate and multiply under anaerobic conditions producing toxin.

Approximately 80% cases of this class are attributed to toxin type A and 20% to toxin type B.[5] Seen in intravenous drug abusers and postsurgical cases.

3. *Intestinal colonization botulism*, usually seen in infants (rarely in adults as intestinal toxemia) is a result of colonization of the infant's colon. Multiple proved factors have been associated with the development of this form of botulism including age (2–4 months) and ingestion of honey.[2]

Adult-type Infant Botulism (Classification Undetermined)

A subtype identified by Centers for Disease Control and Prevention (CDC). Includes cases in noninfantile age group for which no vehicle is identified.[7]

Inadvertent Botulism

This type although rare can occur in patients receiving treatment with injections of botulinum toxin for dystonia and similar disorders. In December 1989 Food and Drug Administration (FDA) approved crystalline botulinum toxin type A for treatment of spasmodic muscle disorders.[6] Both the types of toxins, i.e. botox (type A toxin) and myobloc (type B toxin) have been used to treat spastic myopathies.

PATHOGENESIS

Botulinum toxin majorly acts on the cholinergic nerve terminal. It acts by binding to the presynaptic acetylcholine containing vesicles, inhibiting its release. The toxin has a large molecular mass (150,000 d), rendering its entry into the blood-brain barrier difficult, therefore its manifestations and symptoms are mostly restricted to peripheral nervous system only. It can also inhibit cholinergic transmission at sympathetic and parasympathetic ganglia, and at parasympathetic postganglionic sites.[8]

The botulinum toxin is made up of a light and heavy chain linked by a disulfide bond which is taken up into the presynaptic nerve ending by the process of endocytosis. The light chain after separating free from the heavy chain attacks on the SNARE (soluble N-ethylmaleimide sensitive fusion protein attachment receptor) protein inside the neuron. This SNARE protein is involved in the release of acetylcholine into the synaptic cleft. Hence, the disruption of SNARE protein complex inhibits the muscle contraction by inhibiting acetylcholine release causing flaccid paralysis.[9]

CLINICAL PRESENTATION

Usually the disease in case of foodborne botulism begins with the prodromal symptoms such as nausea and vomiting (diarrhea usually not seen) that appear within 18–36 hours of ingestion of contaminated food.[10] This is followed by the constellation of neurological symptoms that begin with the involvement of ocular muscles resulting in diplopia, ptosis followed by facial muscle paralysis, muscles of mastication and swallowing and then the larger groups of muscles of limbs. It is a classical descending type of symmetrical flaccid paralysis and many patients present with signs of bulbar palsies to emergency room. If the illness goes undiagnosed and untreated it may involve intercostal muscles with other muscles of respiration including the diaphragm resulting in respiratory failure and need for mechanical ventilation. The bulbar palsy presents with motor involvement of cranial nerves with signs and symptoms of blurring of vision, diplopia, nystagmus, dilated pupils, sore throat, dysphagia, dysphonia, diminished gag reflexes (Table 1).

The gastrointestinal symptoms are absent in case of wound botulism and incubation period is longer (4–14 days).[2] In both the types, patient is notably afebrile and features of inflammation and markers of systemic infection such as leukocytosis is usually absent (unless a superimposed secondary infection).[9,11] There is usually

Table 1: Signs and symptoms of botulism.[6]	
Gastrointestinal	Nausea, vomiting, pain abdomen, constipation
Cranial nerves	Ptosis, diplopia, blurring of vision, difficulty lifting head, dysarthria, dysphagia, dysphonia, facial weakness
Peripheral nerve system	Respiratory muscle weakness, weakess of limb muscles, loss of deep tendon reflexes, ataxia
Autonomic nervous system	Postural hypotension, paralytic ileus, dry mouth, urinary incontinence/retention, and respiratory failure.

CNS Toxins

no sensory or central neurological involvement seen. Patients generally have an intact consciousness status unless there is hypoxic injury secondary to respiratory failure. However patients may show features of autonomic dysfunction such as dry mouth or fixed dilated pupils.[6]

Infant botulism occurs 95% times in babies younger than 6 months of age.[12] Presentation includes poor sucking and swallowing, lethargic, weak cry, hypotonic floppy appearance with inability to hold the head upright. Constipation is also a remarkable feature.[13]

DIFFERENTIAL DIAGNOSIS

Common causes of motor and bulbar neuropathies that may mimic botulism include myasthenia gravis, Miller Fisher variant of Guillain-Barré syndrome, paralytic shell fish poisoning, tick paralysis, Lambert-Eaton syndrome and poliomyelitis (Table 2).

DIAGNOSIS

The first basic assessment to aid in clinical diagnosis includes motor and cranial nerve examination where features of cranial neuropathy with loss of deep tendon reflexes may be identified. Classical botulism usually

spares the cognitive and sensory system. Initial panel of investigations includes complete blood count (absence of leukocytosis), renal function test, and electrolytes (normal electrolytes levels). A suspicion of impending respiratory failure mandates arterial blood gas (ABG) analysis and repeated assessment of vital capacity.[14]

For toxin assays adequate sample such as serum, stools, gastric aspirate, enema fluid, swabs, wound aspirates and suspected food contents should be sent in an anaerobic transport medium, ideally before initiation of the antitoxin treatment, to the concerned public health authorities. Early growth of Gram-positive bacillus with oval-shaped subterminal spores and β-hemolytic activity on the anaerobic culture media confirms the diagnosis.[15] The other tests include mouse bioassay (most sensitive), ELISA and PCR.

The electromyography (EMG) findings include small M-wave amplitudes. Repeated nerve stimulation at low frequency (3 Hz) shows decremental response whereas at high frequency of 20–50 Hz shows incremental response in M-wave amplitude (as compared to progressive decline in action potential in case of myasthenia gravis).[16] Meanwhile awaiting the culture reports imaging studies that include computed tomography (CT) scan and

Table 2: Differential diagnosis of botulism.

Condition	Clinical features	Diagnostic studies
Myasthenia gravis	Bilateral ptosis, bulbar palsies without sensory findings	Single fiber electromyography, edrophonium (Tensilon) testing (often falsely positive in botulism as well), acetylcholine receptor antibodies
Miller Fisher variant of GBS	History of fever, ocular muscular weakness, ataxia, descending paralysis	CSF study (albumin cytological dissociation, nerve conduction studies, anti GQ1b antibodies
Poliomyelitis	History of fever, asymmetric paralysis	Isolation of virus (culture)
Tick paralysis	Proximal large group of muscles involved, loss of DTR, ascending type of paralysis	Travel history, evidence or history of tick bite (transmitting tick may still be found attached to the body)
Lambert-Eaton syndrome	Autonomic symptoms (salivation, erectile dysfunction), repetitive muscle contraction on electromyography shows improvement in the muscle weakness	Electromyography, nerve conduction studies
Shell fish poisoning	Perioral numbness, paresthesia, respiratory failure	History of ingestion (<1 hour of incubation period)
Stroke syndromes	Motor weakness, altered conscious may be present	Imaging (CT scan, MRI)

(CT: computed tomography; CSF: cerebrospinal fluid; DTR: deep tendon reflexes; GBS: Guillain-Barré syndrome; MRI: magnetic resonance imaging)

magnetic resonance imaging (MRI) can be performed to rule out any cerebrovascular accident, bleed, space occupying lesions or brainstem lesion. A lumbar puncture may be performed in suspicions of infective etiology and Guillain-Barré syndrome (high cerebrospinal fluid protein counts).

TREATMENT

All the patients presenting with suspected signs and symptoms of botulism should be hospitalized and kept under observation for monitoring signs of impending respiratory failure. Treatment consists of general supportive measures and antitoxin administration. Collection of ABG samples, repeated monitoring of pulmonary vital capacity and clinical evaluation of upper airway integrity will predict for the need of intubation and mechanical ventilation. Other tests which may aid in predicting the need for mechanical ventilation include pulse oximetry, negative inspiratory force and end tidal capnography.

Although botulinum antitoxin cannot reverse the paralysis, early administration (as early as possible) of the antitoxin plays a crucial role in halting the progression of disease. In case of strong clinical suspicion, antitoxin administration should not be delayed, awaiting results of diagnostic tests. The antitoxin acts by binding with the neurotoxin and preventing its action on the neuromuscular junction. Two formulations of the toxin, trivalent, and heptavalent are available for use. Currently, CDC recommends the use of trivalent antitoxin [containing 7,500 international units (IU) type A, 5,500 IU type B, and 8,500 IU type E antitoxins] in a single 10 mL vial, diluted to 1:10 in normal saline and administered as slow intravenous infusion over 30 minutes.[3] For adults and children more than 1 year of age, equine serum antitoxin is used which carries a risk of allergic reactions and anaphylaxis, therefore a slow and diluted administration is advocated. For infants botulism, a human derived immunoglobulin (BabyBIG) is available as an intravenous preparation. HBAT (heptavalent botulinum antitoxin, antitoxin under investigation) may eventually replace the other available antitoxins since it is effective for all known toxin types. It has been shown to shorten the course of illness and reduce mortality in some studies.[9]

No antibiotics are recommended for foodborne or infant botulism. Their use is restricted for treatment of secondary infections amongst which aminoglycosides and clindamycin are contraindicated because of the potential to exacerbate the neuromuscular blockade.[3] Antibiotic use may be recommended in case of wound botulism (although not proven by clinical trials so far). Recommended antibiotics include penicillin G (3 million units intravenous 4th hourly) or metronidazole (500 mg intravenous 8th hourly).[17] Wound care and surgical debridement is strongly recommended in cases of wound botulism.

Intensive Care Unit

Intensive care unit (ICU) admission is required for airway protection, mechanical ventilatory support, fluid and nutritional support till the normal muscle functions return. At the time of ICU admission first step is the assessment and securing of airway, breathing, and circulation. Patients with impending respiratory failure need intensive care monitoring of respiratory rate, pulse oximetry, ABGs with serial measurements of forced vital capacity (FVC <15 mL/kg may need respiratory support, FVC < 12 mL/kg has high chance of needing mechanical ventilation).[6] Activated charcoal may be administered, if there are no contraindications otherwise. Activated charcoal can absorb serotype toxin A and may even be given after some time delay to act on the remnant bacteria and spores in the gut.

Ventilator dependence is high, weaning in these patients may be slow and these patients may often require tracheostomy. Even after years of recovery, diminished respiratory functions may persist in some patients.[14] Physical rehabilitation with rigorous limb physiotherapy and muscle strengthening exercises play a crucial role in early recovery.[9]

PROGNOSIS

Certain factors are associated with poorer outcomes, these include delay in administration of antitoxin (more than 24 hours), advanced age (above 60 years), and type A toxin. These patients may have a longer hospital stay, increased need for mechanical ventilation, and higher mortality rates.[9,18,19]

PREVENTION

There is no pre-exposure or postexposure prophylaxis (for asymptomatic individuals) available for the public.[3] The best method for killing the spores is heating the food

CNS Toxins

to 121°C under a pressure of 15–20 lb/in² for 20 minutes, however the toxin can be destroyed by standard heating to 80°C for 30 minutes, or 100°C for 10 minutes.[9]

CONCLUSION

Although rare, the disease is potentially fatal and can mimic other illnesses making the diagnosis difficult. Critical care and emergency specialists should familiarize themselves with the disease as many of these patients can present with respiratory failure and need for mechanical ventilation and an early recognition and administration of treatment can considerably improve the outcome and prognosis.

KEY POINTS

- Early clinical diagnosis on the basis of history and physical examination plays a crucial role.
- Classical presentation of botulism includes acute flaccid symmetric descending paralysis with cranial nerves involvement and sparing of cognitive and sensory functions. Disease marks the absence of any inflammatory evidence (fever, leukocytosis usually not seen).
- Early administration of the antitoxin on the basis of clinical suspicion is advocated to halt the progression of the disease (paralysis) in the early stages. Antitoxin does not release the toxin already bound to the presynaptic receptors therefore cannot reverse the paralysis that has already occurred.
- Antibiotics play a role only in cases of wound botulism.

REFERENCES

1. Arnon SS, Schechter R, Inglesby TV, et al. Botulism toxin as a biological weapon: medical and public health management. JAMA. 2001;285(8):1059-70.
2. Mohanty SD, Chaudhry R. Botulism: An update. J Med Microbiol. 2001;19(2):35-43.
3. CDC. (2008). Botulism: Information and Guidance for Clinicians. Centers for Disease Control and Prevention. https://www.sfcdcp.org/wp-content/uploads/2018/01/Botulism-Binder-Chapter.2008.FINAL-id312.pdf

4. Chaudhry R. Botulism: a diagnostic challenge. Ind J Med Res. 2011;134(1):10-2.
5. Shapiro RL, Hatheway CL, Swerdlow DL. Botulism in the United States: a clinical and epidemiologic review. Ann Intern Med. 1998;129(3):221-8.
6. Wenham T, Cohen A. Botulism. Continuing Education in Anaesthesia. Crit Care Pain. 2008;8(1):21-5.
7. Dowell VR. Botulism and tetanus: selected epidemiologic and microbiologic aspects. Rev Infect Dis. 1984;6 Suppl 1:S202-7.
8. Simpson LL. Identification of the major steps in botulinum toxin action. Annu Rev Pharmacol Toxicol. 2004;44: 167-93.
9. Horowitz BZ. Botulinum toxin. Crit Care Clin. 2005;21(4):825-39.
10. Thwaites CL. Botulism and tetanus. Medicine. 2014;42(1): 11-3.
11. Werner SB, Passaro D, McGee J, et al. Wound botulism in California, 1951-1998: recent epidemic in heroin injectors. Clin Infect Dis. 2000;31(4):1018-24.
12. Arnon SS. Infant botulism. In: Rudolph AM, Hoffman JIE, Rudolph CD (Eds). Rudolph's Pediatrics, 20th edition. New York: Appleton & Lange; 1996. pp. 555-8.
13. Arnon SS, Midura TF, Clay SA, et al. Infant botulism: epidemiological, clinical, and laboratory aspects. JAMA. 1977;237:1946-51.
14. Wilcox PG, Andolfatto G, Fairbarn MS, et al. Long-term follow-up of symptoms, pulmonary function, respiratory muscle strength, and exercise performance after botulism. Am Rev Respir Dis. 1989;139(1):157-63.
15. Caya JG, Agni R, Miller JE. *Clostridium botulinum* and the clinical laboratorian: a detailed review, including biologic warfare ramifications of botulinum toxin. Arch Path Lab Med. 2004;128(6):653-62.
16. Padua L, Aprile I, Monaco ML, et al. Neurophysiological assessment in the diagnosis of botulism: usefulness of single-fiber EMG. Muscle Nerve. 1999;22(10):1388-92.
17. American Academy of Pediatrics. Botulism and infant botulism (*Clostridium botulinum*). In: Kimberlin DW, Brady MT, Jackson MA, Long SS (Eds). Red Book: 2015 Report of the Committee on Infectious Diseases, 30th edition. American Academy of Pediatrics, Elk Grove Village, IL; 2015. p. 294.
18. Tacket CO, Shandera WX, Mann JM, et al. Equine antitoxin use and other factors that predict outcome in type A foodborne botulism. Am J Med. 1984;76(5): 794-8.
19. Woodruff BA, Griffin PM, McCroskey LM, et al. Clinical and laboratory comparison of botulism from toxin types A, B, and E in the United States 1975-1988. J Infect Dis. 1992;166(6):1281-3.

14 CHAPTER

Anticonvulsant Overdose

Rohit Yadav, Deven Juneja

INTRODUCTION

Antiepileptics/anticonvulsants are group of drugs used to prevent seizure activity. In between 1939 and 1980 first-generation of antiepileptic drugs were developed. Second- and third- generations of antiepileptic drugs were developed after 1993, with a better safety profile.[1] Most of the antiepileptic drugs exhibit their anticonvulsant effect by acting on sodium channels, calcium channels, and potassium channels; or by affecting gamma-aminobutyric acid (GABA) activity. Mechanism of action of the few of the newer antiepileptic drugs is not well known. The first-generation antiepileptic drugs have well established serum levels that correlate with acute toxicity and may help in guiding treatment. Second- and third-generation drugs do not have established serum levels and serum levels are not useful to guide therapy.

Newer drugs have better safety profile compared to old antiepileptic drugs and very few cases of serious complications or death are reported in the published human data. Despite of narrow therapeutic window and drug interactions due to enzyme induction, older antiepileptic drugs are still used as monotherapy or as first-line drugs because of their better potency.

Most of the cases of anticonvulsant overdose are not serious, and present with altered mental status, requiring supportive care and monitoring for a few hours with special attention to airway protection. Serious cases are due to major central nervous system (CNS) depression requiring mechanical ventilation, cardiotoxicity of sodium channel blocking drugs and seizure induced by anticonvulsant drugs.

CLASSIFICATION

Antiepileptic drugs are subdivided as per generations, with newer generations having fewer drug interactions and a better safety profile (Table 1). These drugs are also classified into different groups, as given in Table 2.

Table 1: Classification of antiepileptic drugs as per different generations of drugs.

First-generation	Second-generation	Third-generation
Phenobarbital	Oxcarbazepine	Eslicarbazepine
Phenytoin	Lamotrigine	Lacosamide
Primidone	Gabapentin	Retigabine
Carbamazepine	Pregabalin	
Valproic acid	Vigabatrin	
Ethosuximide	Topiramate	
	Tiagabine	
	Zonisamide	
	Levetiracetam	
	Rufinamide	
	Felbamate	

CNS Toxins

Table 2: Classification as per groups.

Barbiturates	Phenobarbitone
Deoxybarbiturate	Primidone
Hydantoin	Phenytoin Fosphenytoin
Iminostilbene	Carbamazepine Oxcarbazepine
Succinimide	Ethosuximide
Aliphatic carboxylic	Valproic acid Divalproex
Benzodiazepines	Clonazepam Diazepam Lorazepam Clobazam
Phenyltriazine	Lamotrigine
Cyclic GABA analog	Gabapentin
Newer drugs	Vigabatrin Topiramate Tiagabine Zonisamide Levetiracetam

(GABA: gamma-aminobutyric acid)

MANAGEMENT OF ANTIEPILEPTIC DRUGS OVERDOSE BASED ON MECHANISM OF ACTION

Drugs that Act on Voltage-dependent Sodium Channels

Carbamazepine

Carbamazepine (CBZ) is used in the management of simple and complex partial seizures, trigeminal neuralgia and bipolar disorders. CBZ act by inhibiting voltage-gated sodium channels (prolonging inactivated state) like phenytoin. It also shows lithium like effects, hence, it is used in management of bipolar disorders. CBZ is more CNS depressant then phenytoin. FDA recommends screening of HLA-B*1502 allele before starting therapy in patients of Asian ancestry in view of increased risk of Stevens–Johnson syndrome (SJS) and toxic epidermal necrolysis (TEN).[2]

Pharmacokinetics: Oral absorption is erratic as it is lipophilic drug. Peak level is achieved in 4–8 hours but may be delayed up to 24 hours. Protein binding is 75% and it is metabolized mainly in liver by oxidation to active metabolite, 10,11-epoxy CBZ and also by hydroxylation and conjugation to produce inactive metabolite. CBZ shows autoinduction mechanism during chronic use, its normal half-life of 20–40 hours is decreased to 10-20 hours, due to induction of self metabolism. Autoinduction is because of induction of cytochrome p450, which increases metabolism of other drugs also.

Clinical features of overdose: Carbamazepine overdose presents predominantly with neurologic, cardiovascular and anticholinergic symptoms. Due to erratic absorption of CBZ, initial presentation is usually with symptoms of lethargy and tachycardia. CNS effects range from drowsiness to coma depending on severity of toxicity. CBZ shows cyclical coma with fluctuating consciousness. Dysmetria and ataxia are commonly present. Tachycardia is common in CBZ overdose. Hypotension presents in severe overdose and is related to direct negative inotropic effects of CBZ. Self-limiting seizures may occur in overdose but may progress to status epilepticus. Few case reports have described myoclonus, hypotonia and hypertonia in patients with overdose.[3,4] Anticholinergic effects include hyperthermia, absent bowel sounds and urinary retention. Nystagmus and mydriasis are also frequent presenting symptoms.

Chronic use of CBZ may present with leukopenia, agranulocytosis and aplastic anemia. Hyponatremia has been associated with chronic therapy. It is usually asymptomatic and is detected as an incidental laboratory finding. One case report described CBZ-induced hyponatremia leading to seizure.[5] Hyponatremia is due to increased sensitivity of renal tubules for antidiuretic hormone, increased expression of aquaporin-2 in inner medullary collecting duct and due to alteration in sensitivity of hypothalamic osmoreceptors.[5,6] Hyponatremia related to CBZ is considered a form of syndrome of inappropriate antidiuretic hormone secretion (SIADH). Drug reaction with eosinophilia and systemic symptoms (DRESS) syndrome, SJS and TEN have also been found to be associated with chronic use.

Laboratory workup: Serum levels of CBZ well correlate with overdose. Normal therapeutic levels are between 8 and 12 mg/L, but in patients with multiple antiepileptic use, the therapeutic range may be deceased to 8–10 mg/L. CBZ overdose can be classified in four stages as per CBZ levels:[7]

1. Potentially catastrophic relapse if levels <11 mg/L
2. Disorientation and ataxia if levels >11–15 mg/L
3. Combativeness and hallucinations if levels 15–25 mg/L
4. Convulsions and coma if levels >25 mg/L.

Serum CBZ levels should be done 4th hourly in patients with severe toxicity till downward trends are observed as delayed release preparations may peak in 96 hours.[8] Liver function and renal function test should be done to ascertain any damage. Complete blood count (CBC) may reflect any adverse effect of chronic therapy (including agranulocytosis, thrombocytopenia and aplastic anemia). Hyponatremia is also not very uncommon.

Management: Management for severe toxicity starts with airway management, as CBZ is primarily a CNS depressant in high doses. Cardiovascular side effects including QT prolongation, hypotension and arrhythmias are rare, and should be managed with fluid boluses and supportive care. Gastric decontamination with activated charcoal (AC) is recommended even many hours after ingestion as CBZ has delayed absorption. Multidose-AC (MDAC) and whole bowel wash may be useful as CBZ has enterohepatic circulation and delayed absorption, but one need to be cautious in view of CNS depression associated with risk of aspiration in patients with unprotected airway and ileus due to anticholinergic effect of CBZ. Sodium bicarbonate may be useful in cardio toxicity due to sodium channel inhibition by CBZ. Hemodialysis or hemoperfusion is only indicated to improve elimination in case of persistent seizures, coma, respiratory depression requiring mechanical ventilation and in patients with hemodynamic instability. Intravenous (IV) lipid emulsion therapy (LET) has also been used successfully in a few case reports.[9] Benzodiazepines are first-line of therapy to control seizures induced by CBZ.

Eslicarbazepine

Structurally related to CBZ and oxcarbazepine, act on voltage-gated sodium channels. Used as monotherapy or as adjunctive therapy in management of partial seizures. Chronic use is associated with serious side effects like suicidal thoughts, visual impairment, hyponatremia, eosinophilia, increased transaminases, increased bilirubin, anaphylaxis, drug hypersensitivity syndrome/DRESS, SJS and angioedema. Acute toxicity profile is same as CBZ.[10]

Phenytoin

Phenytoin is a first-generation antiepileptic drug. Despite its narrow therapeutic range and significant drug interactions, it still maintains its role as an antiepileptic of choice in many disorders. It is also Vaughn–Williams class IB antidysrhythmic drug, although not used now for this purpose.

Phenytoin in therapeutic doses acts by prolonging the inactivated state of voltage sensitive neuronal Na^+ channel which inhibits high frequency discharges with no effect on low frequency discharges. At higher or toxic doses phenytoin also acts by reduction in Ca^{2+} influx, inhibition of glutamate and facilitation of GABA.

Pharmacokinetics: Phenytoin is available in both injectable and oral formulations. Absorption of oral preparation is poor as phenytoin has poor aqueous solubility. Drug is highly protein bound and is metabolized in liver by hydroxylation and glucuronide conjugation with only 5% being excreted unchanged in urine. Phenytoin follows first order kinetics (excretion of fixed percentage over fix time) but converts to zero order (excretion of fixed amount over fix time) with increase in serum levels, as metabolizing enzyme get saturated. Half-life is 12–24 hours, but progressively increases with levels higher than 10 µg/mL.

Fosphenytoin is a prodrug of phenytoin, which can be given IV/intramuscular (IM) only. Fosphenytoin has similar adverse effect profile but with less severe toxicity. Phenytoin should be given in infusion rate <50 mg/min. In older patients and patients with pre-existing cardiovascular disease, infusion should be slower than 50 mg/min. With fosphenytoin, faster delivery of drug (<150 mg/min) can be achieved.

Phenytoin toxicity may be precipitated by following risk factors:
- Excessive dose; overdose can occur either by ingestion (suicidal or accidental in children) or in hospital settings, this may be due to product labeling, as fosphenytoin dose is expressed in phenytoin equivalents, i.e. fosphenytoin 150 mg = 100 mg phenytoin)
- Unintentional toxicity in chronic users, this can be due to, change in formulation or brand; or errors in prescription or administration
- Phenytoin is highly protein bound drug. Any condition which decrease albumin levels or decrease protein bounding can increase free phenytoin levels and may precipitate toxicity, e.g. pregnancy, liver disease, malnutrition or nephrotic syndrome
- Various drug interactions also change levels of phenytoin. Cytochrome p450 inhibitors can increase levels of phenytoin by decreasing metabolism of these drugs include metronidazole, fluconazole,

cimetidine and amiodarone. Cytochrome p450 inducers (barbiturates, alcohol, rifampicin and CBZ) can decrease levels of phenytoin. Cessation of these drugs without adjusting dose of phenytoin can precipitate toxicity. Valproic acid (VPA) and sulfonylureas can precipitate phenytoin toxicity by displacing it from protein binding site.

Clinical features of overdose: Phenytoin-related poisoning is rarely fatal. Injectable phenytoin-related toxicity is mainly due to fast infusion (>50 mg/min). Severe toxicity related to tablet form is rare, but few cases of life-threatening bradycardia are reported with chronic use of phenytoin oral preparation.[11]

A review article of 32 trials and 10 case reports concluded, phenytoin cardiotoxicity is mainly related to fast IV administration, with no mortality being reported in 32 trials and mortality was only reported in a few case reports in patients with pre-existing cardiovascular comorbid conditions or metabolic derangements.[12]

With mild-to-moderate toxicity (serum levels <40 mg/L) common symptoms are nausea, vomiting, ataxia and nystagmus. Rapid IV administration is associated with bradyarrhythmia, hypotension and rarely asystole. Coexisting hyponatremia may contribute to cardiotoxic effects of phenytoin. Symptoms do not correlate with serum levels but serum levels >40 mg/L are associated with prominent CNS symptoms including coma.

Purple glove syndrome is associated with IV phenytoin administration. Patient develops blister, pain and peripheral edema of the hand receiving IV phenytoin, usually within 24 hours. Mechanism is not well understood, many proposed mechanisms correlate it with extravasation of phenytoin with irritation of soft tissues due to added propylene glycol and sodium hydroxide which could subsequently lead to vasoconstriction, microthrombus formation and edema. But in many case reports extravasation was not present and also in many cases after extravasation patients did not develop purple glove syndrome. It is suggested to use central venous access if available or large bore cannulas to avoid purple glove syndrome. Management based on few case reports includes; elevation of affected hand, application of heat, soft tissue massage, and nitroglycerine patch to local area or brachial plexus block. Surgical intervention might be required in few cases.[13]

Drug reaction with eosinophilia and systemic symptoms is associated with phenytoin treatment. It is a potentially life-threatening hypersensitivity condition with mortality of approximately 10%. DRESS usually present after 2 months of starting treatment. Few idiosyncratic reactions are also associated with phenytoin which includes TEN and SJS.[14]

Laboratory workup: Phenytoin toxicity should be suspected in any patient on oral phenytoin, presenting with dysrhythmias and having; hypoalbuminemia, hyperbilirubinemia and severe electrolyte imbalance.[7]

Laboratory workup includes serum levels of phenytoin, for confirmation of diagnosis. Normal levels are 10–20 mg/L, levels >30 mg/L are associated with clinical toxicity and levels >100 mg/L are usually lethal. Liver function test, as liver dysfunction increases duration of toxicity. Serum albumin levels, as low levels will cause increase in free fraction of the drug. As free drug levels are not measured, this reflects discrepancy in serum level and severity of toxicity. Free phenytoin reference range is 1–2.5 mg/L. Serum levels of phenytoin for hypoalbuminemia can be corrected with Sheiner–Tozer formula.[15]

Adjusted phenytoin concentration = measured total concentration/[(0.2 × albumin) + 0.1]

Serial ECG to be done as bradyarrhythmia, wide QRS complexes with ventricular dysrhythmias, atrioventricular block or sinus arrest with junctional or ventricular escape are associated with IV phenytoin.

Management: Management depends on symptoms, with severe toxicity and altered mental status, airway protection is of prime importance. Gastric decontamination with AC is recommended with dose of 1 g/kg (maximum 50 g) with recent ingestion (within few hours). MDAC is also considered by many authors in view of enterohepatic circulation of drug, even with IV toxicity.[16] Whole bowel wash or gastric lavage is not indicated.

Cardiovascular effects are usually associated with rapid injections of phenytoin. Bradyarrhythmias are rarely associated with hypotension and respond well to IV fluid boluses. If bradyarrhythmia with hypotension persists, atropine, epinephrine and dopamine are first-line therapies. Successful use of temporary transvenous pacing is also reported in cases of refractory bradycardia.[7] Other etiologies should also be ruled out in patients with persistent symptomatic bradycardia. Wide QRS and QT interval are usually self-limiting and stopping of infusion is the only treatment required in most of the patients. For wide QRS complex more than 100 ms or ventricular dysrhythmias, sodium bicarbonate 2 mmol/kg

IV repeated every 2 minute is indicated till perfusion rhythm is restored, however, multiple doses may be required. Defibrillation could be tried but is rarely helpful. Consider IV lignocaine 1.5 mg/kg, if pH more than 7.5 and patient is having dysrhythmias. Cardiovascular toxicity is thought to be associated with propylene glycol, a diluent used in IV formulation of phenytoin, as cardiac toxicity is not frequent with fosphenytoin which does not contain propylene glycol.

Seizures related to high dose phenytoin toxicity are controlled with benzodiazepines. Extracorporeal therapy to remove phenytoin is not routinely indicated but EXTRIP group recommends use of intermittent hemodialysis or hemoperfusion in selected patients with severe toxicity, coma or prolonged incapacitating ataxia.[17]

Lacosamide

Lacosamide acts on voltage-dependent sodium channels. Oral lacosamide is used as monotherapy or adjunctive therapy for focal-onset seizures. Lacosamide is available as tablet, solution and injectable formulations. Oral absorption is 100%. Excretion is renal and by biotransformation.

Fast IV administration of lacosamide is associated with bradycardia. Dose-dependent PR interval prolongation and atrial flutter and fibrillations are observed. Severe cases with third-degree heart blocks are also reported.

Management of overdose consists of gastric decontamination and sodium bicarbonate used as first-line therapy in presence of cardiovascular complications. Hemodialysis can be considered in severe toxicity.[18]

Lamotrigine

Lamotrigine is a broad spectrum antiepileptic, which act by prolonging sodium channel inactivation and also inhibit voltage gated sodium channels. Lamotrigine also acts as serotonin reuptake inhibitor, this property make patient on risk of serotonin syndrome if given with other serotonin reuptake inhibitors.[19] Initially introduced for refractory seizures but now also used as monotherapy.

Pharmacokinetics: Lamotrigine oral absorption is good with 98% bioavailability, peak concentrations reached after 1–3 hours of oral ingestion. Lamotrigine is 55% protein bound, with volume of distribution (Vd) of 0.9–1.2 L/kg. Metabolized completely in liver by glucuronidation to produce inactive 2N-glucuronide metabolite, which has complete renal excretion. Half-life is 24–30 hours,

but reduced in patients on combination therapy with phenytoin, CBZ or phenobarbitone. On the contrary, patients on VPA therapy have increased levels due to inhibition of glucuronidation.[20]

Clinical features of overdose: Lamotrigine overdose presents with prominent CNS symptoms such as oculogyric crisis, dystonia, nystagmus, ataxia, slurred speech and hypertonia. Abnormal movements like choreoathetoid movements and choreiform dyskinesia also have been described in case reports. Being a sodium channel blocker lamotrigine toxicity also presents with cardiac manifestation. This includes sinus tachycardia, wide QRS, QT prolongation, left or right bundle branch block and complete heart block.[20] Few cases of lamotrigine associated acute pancreatitis have been also reported.[21] SJS is associated with use of lamotrigine, presents early in course of treatment if patient is also taking valproate.[20]

Management: Management is mainly symptomatic, AC administration is recommended for acute intoxication. Sodium bicarbonate can be used if QRS more than 100 ms, to maintain pH 7.45–7.55. Seizures, if present, can be treated with benzodiazepines. Extracorporeal therapies are not well studied in lamotrigine toxicity. Many case reports have described effective role of LET in lamotrigine overdose-related cardiac or neurologic toxicity refractory to conventional therapy.[22]

Rufinamide

Rufinamide is a triazole derivative, which acts by prolonging inactive state of sodium channels. Used in Lennox–Gastaut syndrome. Oral absorption is slow. Chronic use is associated with few serious side effects like status epilepticus, suicidal behavior, leukopenia, drug hypersensitivity syndrome/DRESS, SJS and short QT interval. Acute overdose presents with mainly CNS symptoms, not very serious. Management is supportive only.

Zonisamide

Zonisamide acts by inhibiting voltage-gated sodium channels. Zonisamide is also a weak carbonic anhydrase inhibitor. Symptoms of overdose include diminished breathing, loss of consciousness, hypotension, electrolyte abnormality and bradycardia with wide QRS in ECG. Management includes AC, supportive care and sodium bicarbonate for wide QRS complexes more than 100 ms.

Drugs that Affect Calcium Current

Ethosuximide

Ethosuximide is a succimide derivative whose clinical effect is through thalamocortical system by suppressing T-type calcium channels. Its overdose or toxicity is not very common, as ethosuximide is prescribed only for absent seizures. Ethosuximide toxicity is mainly as coingestion.

Pharmacokinetics: Ethosuximide is very well absorbed in gastrointestinal (GI) tract and has very low protein binding and Vd of 0.67 L/kg. Metabolism is mainly hepatic with 10–20% of renal excretion.

Clinical features of overdose: Acute overdoses mainly present with nausea, vomiting and altered mental status. Coma with respiratory depression is a rare presentation. Succinimide derivative mesuximide overdose follow a biphasic profile, initial comatose state followed by improved alertness and then after 24 hours again relapse into coma. Metabolite N-desmethyl methsuximide is responsible for relapse of coma.[23] Severe toxicity is associated with CNS symptoms, respiratory depression and coma.

Laboratory work up: The therapeutic range is 40–100 mg/L, but levels do not correlate with clinical effect. Plasma concentrations are not readily available.

Management: Management starts with ABC, mainly comprise of airway protection, supportive care and monitoring. Consider AC 1 mg/kg (50 g maximum) if patient presents within 1 hour of ingestion. Gastric lavage is not recommended for patients with altered mental status. Consider intubation for airway protection in patients not able to protect airway or with respiratory depression. Benzodiazepines are indicated for seizure management. Forced diuresis or plasma exchange is not effective. In cases of serious toxicity of ethosuximide hemodialysis should be considered. For mesuximide charcoal hemoperfusion may be effective in removing N-desmethyl metabolite.[24]

Drugs that Affect Gamma-aminobutyric Acid Activity

Barbiturates—Phenobarbitone

Barbiturates are covered in detail in Chapter 7 on sedatives and hypnotics.

Benzodiazepine

Benzodiazepines are covered in detail in Chapter 7 on sedatives and hypnotics.

Vigabatrin

Vigabatrin is a newer anticonvulsant which inhibits GABA transaminase, and hence increases synaptic concentration of GABA. Its clinical use is limited due to visual impairment. Used in refractory focal seizures and infantile spasms in children with tuberous sclerosis.

Gastrointestinal absorption is 100% and it has got negligible protein binding and Vd of 1.1 L/kg. There is no hepatic metabolism and excreted 95% in urine. Peak plasma concentration is reached in 2 hours.

Retinal toxicity is a major concern for use of vigabatrin, mechanism of toxicity is unknown. Acute toxicity is rare due to limited use of this drug. Not much data is available for acute toxicity, hence symptomatic and supportive care is only warranted.

Drugs that Affect Glutamate Receptors

Perampanel

Perampanel is a noncompetitive antagonist of AMPA receptors. Used in partial seizure or as an adjunct in tonic-clonic seizure. Common features of perampanel toxicity include dysarthria, fatigue, stupor and disorientation. Symptoms may persist for 48 hours. Management is supportive only.

Drugs with Multiple Mechanism of Action

Valproate (Sodium Valproate)

Valproic acid indicated as monotherapy or adjunctive therapy for complex partial seizures, absence seizure, and many other disorders like migraine prophylaxis or bipolar mania.

Mechanism of action: Valproic acid with multiple mechanism of action consists broad clinical effectiveness: (i) Block voltage-dependent Na^+ channel, (ii) Weaker action against T-type Ca^{++} channels, and (iii) increases concentration of GABA through different mechanism. VPA indirectly increases levels of GABA in CNS by increasing glutamic acid decarboxylase (GDA) and by inhibiting GABA transaminase, this action is different from action of hypnotics-sedatives which enhance postsynaptic GABA action. Like phenytoin and CBZ, VPA also blocks voltage dependent Na channels, but this action is not thought to be important mechanism for antiepileptic activity and also not responsible for toxic effects.

Valproic acid alters fatty-acid metabolism, beta-oxidation and urea cycle. This leads to hyperammonemia, metabolic derangements, hepatitis and pancreatitis. Long-term treatment could lead to impaired reproductive functions, this could be related to oxidative stress as improvement with antioxidants demonstrated in animal studies.[25] VPA associated fatal hepatotoxicity is seen in individuals with Alpers–Huttenlocher syndrome (AHS), due to mutations in mitochondrial DNA polymerase gamma (POLG). VPA depletes carnitine level which leads to fatty liver. In therapeutic dose VPA causes minimal sedation.

Pharmacokinetics: Valproic acid comes in different preparations; syrup, capsule, enteric coated delayed release and extended release tablets. Oral preparations are rapidly absorbed from GI tract and peak serum concentrations achieved in 1–4 hours with nonenteric coated preparations. Enteric coated tablets exhibit delayed peak serum concentrations (Cmax) up to 20 hours.

Valproic acid follows first order kinetics. VPA is highly protein bound with small Vd (0.13–0.23 L/kg), most of the drug is available in extracellular space in protein bound form. Persons with hypoalbuminemia have high unbound drug concentrations despite normal total drug levels. With levels in therapeutic range VPA is 80–90% protein bound but as concentration rises, more drug is in unbound form. Only 15% fraction of VPA is protein bound, when concentration is more than 1,000 mg/L. This reflects in significant clinical toxicity and use of extracorporeal treatment in severe toxicity.

Valproic acid is primarily metabolized in the liver through glucuronide conjugation, mitochondrial β-oxidation and to lesser extent by omega-oxidation. Omega-oxidation is responsible to produce toxic metabolites. With chronic and high-dose therapy fraction of omega-oxidation increases, this increases risk of dose dependent and idiosyncratic hepatotoxicity, and metabolic and neurologic adverse effects. VPA metabolites are not measured in VPA levels. So it is possible to have ongoing VPA toxicity due to metabolites despite of normal VPA levels. Less than 5% is excreted in urine unchanged. The elimination half-life is 10–15 hours. It may be increased in neonates, liver disease and in overdose. VPA also decreases GI motility.

Clinical features of overdose: History must be taken for time of ingestion, preparation of drug (syrup, delay or extended release), any chronic therapy of VPA, any other prescribed drugs or alcohol for coingestions. Time to onset of symptoms after overdose depends on type of preparations, with nonenteric coated drugs showing fast onset of symptoms of less than 1 hour, but enteric coated tablets result in delayed symptoms onset.

Most of VPA overdose presents with only altered mental status and no other serious manifestation and follow a benign course but toxicity could range from multiorgan dysfunction, coma to even death.

Therapeutic dose is 10–15 mg/kg/day, with maximum dose up to 60 mg/kg/day, with acceptable therapeutic levels between 50 and 100 mg/L. Clinically significant toxicity rarely occurs at dose <200 mg/kg. VPA levels do not correlate well with symptoms, but many studies have described symptoms with serum levels.[26]

- With levels <450 mg/L or dose <400 mg/kg, common symptoms are only drowsiness and confusion
- Levels 450–850 mg/L or dose 400–800 mg/dL correlates with severe toxicity which includes coma
- Levels >850 mg/L or dose >1,000 mg/kg associated with life-threatening complications like, hypotension, respiratory depression requiring intubation and ventilator support, coma and metabolic acidosis.

Cerebral edema is documented with VPA toxicity within 48–72 hours. Cerebral edema is due to accumulation of the 2-EN-VPA metabolite (half-life 43 hours) in the brain and is responsible for prolonged coma. Hyperammonemia caused by VPA is not always associated with liver dysfunction and is believed due to two mechanisms; first due to propionic acid (a metabolite of VPA) and second because of relative carnitine deficiency, which favors omega-oxidation of VPA. Other manifestations are alopecia (high/chronic dose), tremors, chorea, miosis, nystagmus and rarely renal failure. Chronic therapy may be associated with non-dose-related (idiosyncratic) toxicity, which includes hepatotoxicity, hyperammonemia, pancreatitis, alopecia, thrombocytopenia, leukopenia and anemia.[27]

Laboratory workup: Laboratory findings are hypernatremia, hypocalcemia, hyperammonemia, hyperosmolality and high anion gap metabolic acidosis. VPA levels should be done every 2–4 hourly till peak is achieved and levels starts falling. CT head is not routinely indicated in VPA overdose, but to be done in patient with focal neurological deficit, persistently depressed mental

CNS Toxins

functions for more than 12 hours and high ammonia levels with encephalopathy.

Management: Management starts with ABC, consists of mainly airway protection in view of altered mental status, decontamination, supportive care and more definite therapies which include hemodialysis and hemoperfusion. Decontamination with AC single dose of 1 g/kg (maximum 50 g) is recommended if patient present within 2 hours of ingestion. AC not to be administered to patients with CNS depression and in those who are not able to protect airway.

Multidose activated charcoal is recommended by many authors in view of delayed gastric emptying by VPA and also for enteric coated delayed/extended release preparations, but based on review of literatures it is not recommended, as no clinical benefit of MDAC therapy in VPA overdose.[28] Whole bowel irrigation, gastric lavage and force diuresis are also not recommended for decontamination.

Naloxone is reported to reverse CNS depression by VPA. Naloxone can be considered in patients without history of chronic opioid use. It can be given IV/IM/SC/inhalational route; through endotracheal route it is least effective. Start with low dose of 0.04 mg IV, followed by incremental doses every 2 minutes till single dose of 2 mg achieved or reversal of symptoms, then increments of 2 mg given till reversal of symptoms or cumulative dose of 10 mg.

Carnitine is recommended in various literature for VPA induced hepatotoxicity (VHT), VPA-induced hyperammonemic encephalopathy (VHE) and levels >450 mg/L. Although there is not very strong recommendation in favor of carnitine but with good safety profile, it could be used in above mentioned conditions. It comes in oral and IV formulations. In acute toxicity IV preparations of carnitine should be used. L-carnitine is given 100 mg/kg (not more than 6 g) IV over 30 minutes, followed by 50 mg/kg (not more than 3 g) IV every 8th hourly.[29]

As in acute toxicity with high dose, unbound portion of drug increases so hemodialysis or hemoperfusion help to decease drug levels. Based on recommendations by EXTRIP work group:[30] Intermittent hemodialysis is preferred modality, if not available both hemoperfusion and CRRT are acceptable.

Topiramate

Topiramate (TPM) is used in cases of refractory cases of focal or generalized tonic-clonic seizure and also approved to be used as initial monotherapy for newly diagnosed focal or generalized tonic-clonic seizure. The FDA has approved its use in children younger than 2 years of age. TPM act by multiple mechanisms, it inhibits sodium channels like phenytoin, enhances GABA activity by postsynaptic effect and antagonizes glutamate receptors. TPM is a weak carbonic anhydrase inhibitor and can cause non-anion gap metabolic acidosis, this effect is usually clinically not significant.

Pharmacokinetics: Topiramate is rapidly absorbed orally, with half-life around 24 hours. TPM is completely excreted in urine.

Clinical features of overdose: Symptoms of acute toxicity predominantly includes drowsiness, lethargy, vertigo, agitation and confusion. Echolalia (repetition of words) and oral-buccal dyskinesia is also reported. Respiratory and CNS depression requiring intubation is rare.

Laboratory workup: Metabolic derangement may be seen within hours of ingestion which includes non-anion gap metabolic acidosis with hyperchloremia and hypokalemia (2.0–3.2 mEq/L). The metabolic acidosis may persist for days.

Management: Activated charcoal is recommended for patient presenting within 1 hour of ingestion. Electrolytes measurement with blood gas analysis is important. Hyperchloremic metabolic acidosis should be treated with IV sodium bicarbonate 1–2 mEq/kg, as sodium bicarbonate therapy may reverse antiepileptic effect of TPM, bicarbonate therapy should be given in intensive care unit only. Hemodialysis is helpful in severe neurological manifestations and metabolic abnormalities not responding to standard care.

Drugs with Other Mechanism of Action

Levetiracetam

Levetiracetam is a new antiepileptic drug, mechanism of action is not well known. Levetiracetam is used to treat partial complex seizures. Levetiracetam available in both injectable and oral formulations. Use of levetiracetam is increasing in view of fewer interactions and better safety profile.

Overdose of levetiracetam is usually not associated with serious symptoms. Common symptoms are agitation, irritability, transient leukopenia thrombocytopenia, diminished deep tendon reflex and drowsiness.

With severe toxicity it can cause respiratory depression as per few case reports.

Management consists of gastric decontamination with AC and supportive care. Few case reports suggest hemodialysis can increase rate of elimination.

Gabapentin/Pregabalin

Gabapentin/pregabalin both are GABA derivative, but do not act as GABA agonist. Gabapentin works with multiple mechanisms to enhance GABA release. Gabapentin is a first-line drug for refractory partial seizures, mostly used as an adjunctive antiepileptic drug. Also it is effective for pain due to diabetic neuropathy, postherpetic neuralgia and prophylaxis of migraine. Oral absorption is good and excreted unchanged in urine with a half-life of 6 hours.

Gabapentin/pregabalin rarely causes serious toxicity but serious outcome like coma is also reported in patient with chronic renal failure.[31] Common symptoms are myoclonus, lethargy and hypoglycemia.

Management: It includes AC and supportive care. Few case reports show faster elimination of drug with hemodialysis.[31,32]

GENERAL POINTS TO REMEMBER IN MANAGEMENT OF ANTICONVULSANTS OVERDOSE

- Most of the anticonvulsant drugs have suicidal tendency as an adverse effect
- Finger stick test for random blood sugar should be done for every patient with altered mental status. If random blood sugar <60 mg/dL, give IV thiamine 100 mg then 50 mL dextrose 50% solution
- Activated charcoal, if indicated, should only be given after ensuring a secured airway but intubation should not be done only for giving AC
- Always consider possibility of coingestion of other antiepileptic drugs, in all antiepileptic overdoses, as many of patient are on multidrug therapy.
- Urine toxicology screen should be done in all patients and pregnancy test should be done in all females of child bearing age
- During history taking always check timing of ingestion, amount of drug, formulation (delayed/extended release, useful for use of MDAC)

- Neuroimaging should be considered in patient with prolonged altered mental status, to rule out other etiologies
- Activated charcoal should be given in all antiepileptic drugs overdose presenting within 1 hour of ingestion and may be given after this period in patients with suspected overdose of CBZ, phenytoin and valproate. Dose of AC is 1 g/kg, but the dose should not exceed 50 g
- Benzodiazepines are drugs of choice in seizures due to antiepileptic overdose. IV lorazepam 0.1 mg/kg up to maximum 4 mg or IV midazolam 0.2 mg/kg up to maximum of 10 mg may be given
- Extracorporeal therapy should be considered in selected patients (covered in detail, elsewhere in the book).

CONCLUSION

In conclusion, old anticonvulsants are more potent, so despite of many drug interactions and serious side effects they still manage to be used as first-line drugs in many clinical conditions. Old anticonvulsants are widely used in monotherapy, hence effect of overdose and management is well studied. Newer antiepileptic drugs have less drug interactions and better safety profile. Serious or fatal toxicities are also rarely reported with these agents. When reported, most of the cases of these newer drugs are along with coingestion of some other drugs. Management consists of supportive care only.

KEY POINTS

- No antidote available for any anticonvulsant drugs, but few first-line therapies are well documented, like sodium bicarbonate for cardiotoxicity of sodium channel blocking drugs, benzodiazepines for antiepileptics- induced seizures, and extracorporeal therapy for selected drugs
- As most of anticonvulsants show CNS symptoms when taken in overdose, so management of airway and repeated assessment is very important.

REFERENCES

1. Tintinalli JE, Stapczynski JS, Ma OJ, et al. Tintinalli's Emergency Medicine: A Comprehensive Study Guide, 7th edition. New York: McGraw-Hill Companies; 2011. pp. 1277-82.

2. Tangamornsuksan W, Chaiyakunapruk N, Somkrua R, et al. Relationship between the HLA-B*1502 allele and carbamazepine-induced Stevens-Johnson syndrome and toxic epidermal necrolysis: a systematic review and meta-analysis. JAMA Dermatol. 2013;149:1025-32.

3. O'Neal W Jr, Whitten KM, Baumann RJ, et al. Lack of serious toxicity following carbamazepine overdosage. Clin Pharm. 1984;3:545.

4. Fisher RS, Cysyk B. A fatal overdose of carbamazepine: case report and review of literature. J Toxicol Clin Toxicol. 1988;26:477.

5. Holtschmidt-Taschner B, Soyka M. Hyponatremia-induced seizure during carbamazepine treatment. World J Biol Psychiatry. 2007;8:51-3.

6. de Braganca AC, Moyses ZP, Magaldi AJ. Carbamazepine can induce kidney water absorption by increasing aquaporin 2 expression. Nephrol DialTransplant. 2010;25:3840-5.

7. Unei H, Ikeda H, Murakami T, at al. Detoxication treatment for carbamazepine and lithium overdose. Yakugaku Zasshi. 2008;128:165-70.

8. Graudins A, Peden G, Dowsett RP. Massive overdose with controlled-release carbamazepine resulting in delayed peak serum concentrations and life-threatening toxicity. Emerg Med (Fremantle). 2002;14:89-94.

9. Baek WS. Intravenous Lipid Emulsion as an Immediate Antidote for Carbamazepine Toxicity: Tick-Tock Tick-Tock Tick-Tock! Sci J Neurol Neurosurg. 2015;1:001-002.

10. Thompson J, Powell J, Ovakim D. Intentional overdose of the novel anti-epileptic drug eslicarbazepine presenting with recurrent seizures and ventricular dysrhythmias. CJEM. 2017;1-4.

11. Su CM, Kung CT, Wang YC, et al. Life-threatening cardiotoxicity due to chronic oral phenytoin overdose. Neurol India. 2009;57:200-2.

12. Guldiken B, Rémi J, Noachtar S. Cardiovascular adverse effects of phenytoin. J Neurol. 2016;263:861-70.

13. Burneo JG, Anandan JV, Barkley GL. A prospective study of the incidence of the purple glove syndrome. Epilepsia. 2001;42:1156-9.

14. Roujeau JC. Clinical heterogeneity of drug hypersensitivity. Toxicology. 2005;209:123-9.

15. Tobler A, Hösli R, Mühlebach S, et al. Free phenytoin assessment in patients: measured versus calculated blood serum levels. Int J Clin Pharm. 2016;38(2): 303-9.

16. Skinner CG, Chang AS, Matthews AS, et al. Randomized controlled study on the use of multiple-dose activated charcoal in patients with supratherapeutic phenytoin levels. Clin Toxicol (Phila). 2012;50:764-9.

17. Anseeuw K, Mowry JB, Burdmann EA, et al. Extracorporeal Treatment in Phenytoin Poisoning: Systematic Review and Recommendations from the EXTRIP (Extracorporeal Treatments in Poisoning) Workgroup. Am J Kidney Dis. 2016;67:187-97.

18. Bauer S, David Rudd G, Mylius V, et al. Lacosamide intoxication in attempted suicide. 2010;17:549-51.

19. Kotwal A, Cutrona S. Serotonin syndrome in the setting of lamotrigine, aripiprazole, and cocaine use. Case Rep Med. 2015;2015:769531.

20. Alabi A, Todd A, Husband A, et al. Safety profile of lamotrigine in overdose. Ther Adv Psychopharmacol. 2016;6:369-81.

21. Nwogbe B, Ferié J, Smith H, et al. Significant lamotrigine overdose associated with acute pancreatitis. J R Soc Med. 2009;102:118-9.

22. Castanares-Zapatero D, Wittebole X, Huberlant V, et al. Lipid emulsion as rescue therapy in lamotrigine overdose. J Emerg Med. 2012;42:48-51.

23. Rumack BH. POISINDEX(R) Information System Micromedex, Inc., Englewood, CO, 2017; CCIS Volume 172, edition expires May, 2017. In: Hall AH, Rumack BH (Eds). TOMES(R) Information System Micromedex, Inc., Englewood, CO, 2017; CCIS Volume 172, edition expires May, 2017.

24. Thomson/Micromedex. Drug Information for the Health Care Professional. Volume 1, Greenwood Village, CO. 2007. p. 272.

25. Ourique GM, Saccol EM, Pês TS, et al. Protective effect of vitamin E on sperm motility and oxidative stress in valproic acid treated rats. Food Chem Toxicol. 2016;95:159-67.

26. Tank JE, Palmer BF. Simultaneous "in series" hemodialysis and hemoperfusion in the management of valproic acid overdose. Am J Kidney Dis. 1993;22:341-4.

27. Gram L, Bentsen KD. Valproate: an updated review. Acta Neurol Scand. 1985;72:129-39.

28. Vale J, Krenzelok EP, Barceloux VD. Position statement and practice guidelines on the use of multi-dose activated charcoal in the treatment of acute poisoning. American Academy of Clinical Toxicology; European Association of Poisons Centres and Clinical Toxicologists. J Toxicol Clin Toxicol. 1999;37:731-51.

29. Perrott J, Murphy NG, Zed PJ. L-carnitine for acute valproic acid overdose: a systematic review of published cases. Ann Pharmacother. 2010;44:1287-93.

30. Ghannoum M, Laliberté M, Nolin TD, et al. Extracorporeal treatment for valproic acid poisoning: systematic review and recommendations from the EXTRIP workgroup. Clin Toxicol (Phila). 2015;53:454-65.

31. Dogukan A, Aygen B, Berilgen MS, et al. Gabapentin-induced coma in a patient with renal failure. Hemodial Int. 2006;10:168-9.

32. Yoo L, Matalon D, Hoffman RS et al. Treatment of pregabalin toxicity by hemodialysis in a patient with kidney failure. Am J Kidney Dis. 2009;54:1127-30.

SECTION 4

Pulmonary Toxins

15. **Approach to Respiratory Failure**
    Suneel Kumar Garg, Shweta Gupta

16. **Inhalational Poisoning**
    Suneel Kumar Garg, Shweta Gupta

17. **Carbon Monoxide Poisoning**
    Ashish Bhalla, Vikas Suri, Jamshed Nayer

SECTION 4

Pulmonary Toxins

15
CHAPTER

Approach to Respiratory Failure

Suneel Kumar Garg, Shweta Gupta

INTRODUCTION

Respiratory failure is a syndrome in which the respiratory system fails to serve its function, i.e. oxygenation and/or carbon dioxide elimination, resulting in either hypoxemia (type-1), hypercarbia (type-2), or mixed respiratory failure. Poisoning and drugs overdose can present with either of these respiratory failure (Table 1). Exposure to inhalational agents (respiratory irritants, simple and chemical asphyxiants, etc.), cardiac drugs, anticancer drugs, and drug overdose predominantly lead to type-1 and type-2 respiratory failure respectively. Sometimes, the respiratory failure may be the only clue to make a diagnosis of poisoning or drug overdose in case of unknown exposure.

Mortality is very high for patients who present with poisoning or drug overdose with respiratory failure. Urgent resuscitation of these patients require rescue from the source, decontamination, oxygen, airway, and/or ventilation.

The prognosis and clinical course of these patients, who present with respiratory failure due to poisoning or drug overdose, depend largely on the quality of the care delivered in the prehospital to emergency room to intensive care unit (ICU).

PATHOGENESIS

Pathogenesis of respiratory failure is different for different substances or drugs. Human beings have an efficient pulmonary system which can be disrupted in several ways. Pulmonary injury can manifest acutely, subacutely or chronically. Respiratory irritants can cause regional pulmonary injury which includes direct cellular injury and/or destruction of type-1 and 2 pneumocytes leading to type-1 respiratory failure. Site and extent of injury to respiratory tract depends upon particle size, chemical properties and solubility of respiratory irritants. These agents cause varied extent of injury in upper and lower airways that can involve the pulmonary parenchyma, pleura, airways, pulmonary vascular system, mediastinum and the neuromuscular system leading to respiratory failure. Degree of injury also depends upon host factors and environmental factors.[1-5]

Simple asphyxiants and chemical asphyxiants can lead to displacement of oxygen from inspired air or interfere with oxygen transport to the tissues or inhibit cellular oxygen utilization respectively, leading to type-1 respiratory failure.

Combination agents can cause respiratory failure by multiple mechanisms because of mixture of multiple gases and particulate matter. Chemical warfare agents primarily affect nervous system and respiratory system and lead to bronchospasm, wheezing, muscle paralysis leading to type-1 and/or type-2 respiratory failure.

Some poisons and most of the drug overdose directly suppress the nervous system and predispose the patients to life threatening type-II respiratory failure progressing to mixed respiratory failure. Many times it is a manifestation of the aspiration pneumonia that

Table 1: Common substances and drugs causing respiratory failure (RF).

Substances/drugs	Type of RF	Comments
Respiratory irritants	type-1	Regional pulmonary injury
Simple asphyxiants	type-1	Simple displacement of oxygen from the inspired air
Chemical asphyxiants	type-1	Either interfere with oxygen transport to the tissues or inhibit cellular oxygen utilization
Combination agents	type-1	Multiple mechanism because of mixture of multiple gases and particulate matter
Chemical warfare agents	type-1 and/or type-2	Primarily affect nervous system and respiratory system
Sedatives-hypnotics	type-2/mixed	Central nervous system depression
Opioids	type-2/mixed	Central nervous system depression
Antiarrhythmic drugs	type-1	Cardiogenic pulmonary edema
Organophosphates, ACE inhibitors, cocaine, β-blockers	type-1	Bronchospasm
Anticoagulants, cocaine cyclophosphamide	type-1	Alveolar hemorrhage
Methotrexate, nitrofurantoin, hydralazine	type-1	Pleural effusion
Amiodarone, amphotericin-B, bleomycin, aspirin	type-1	Interstitial lung disease
Cocaine, bleomycin, carmustine, retinoic acid	type-1	Pneumothorax
Cyclophosphamide	type-1	Pleural thickening
Asbestos, silica, beryllium, paraquat,	type-1	Unique pulmonary toxins
Neuroparalytic snake bite	type-2/mixed	Central nervous system depression

(ACE: angiotensin converting enzyme)

results from the overdose of the drugs, but there is mixed respiratory failure. Various other drugs can affect the lung parenchyma and/or pleural space leading to type-1 respiratory failure.

APPROACH TO RESPIRATORY FAILURE

Most important steps in making diagnosis and management of poisoning and/or drug overdose are a good clinical history, physical examination, appropriate laboratory tests for identification of suspected toxin along with protocolized treatment plan (Flowchart 1).

History

As poisoning patients may be unreliable in terms of providing accurate information, especially in cases of attempted suicide or illicit drug abuse,[6,7] family members, friends, or family physician may provide actual information. A good clinical history should include information about the poison or drug, exact time, and place of ingestion or exposure and route of administration with quantity. All efforts should be made to know the intention of the poisoning or drug overdose.

Flowchart 1: Approach and management of patients with poisoning.

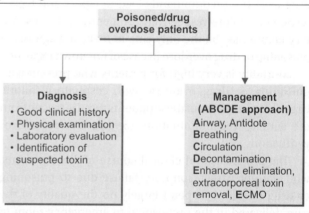

Clinical Examination

Respiratory irritants can cause inflammation of the oropharynx and upper respiratory tract leading to dyspnea, wheezing, upper airway obstruction, hoarseness of voice, laryngospasm, stridor and pulmonary edema leading to type-1 respiratory failure. These gases can also cause long-term lung damage with pulmonary fibrosis and chronic wheezing.[8-11]

Simple asphyxiants can alter oxygen delivery and lead to hypoxia and type-1 respiratory failure. There can be decrease in mental alertness, loss of consciousness, and death, with decreasing oxygen concentration.[12]

Chemical asphyxiants impair tissue oxygen delivery by shifting the oxyhemoglobin dissociation curve to the left, leading to type-1 respiratory failure. Patients can present with headache, dizziness, nausea, vomiting, altered mental status, tachypnea, and hypertension. With increasing concentration of asphyxiants, patients can become dyspneic, can have cardiac dysrhythmia, ischemia, hypotension, syncope, and seizures. Patients can even die with high concentration of asphyxiants.[13]

Smoke causes type-1 respiratory failure by causing damage to whole respiratory system as it contains multiple gases and particulate matter. Patients exposed to smoke can present with cough, shortness of breath, and hoarseness or noisy breathing.

Chemical warfare agents primarily affect nervous system and respiratory system, leading to type-1 and/or type-2 respiratory failure.[8,14] There can be varied presentation from upper and lower airway inflammation, pneumonitis, coughing, inspiratory stridor, wheezing, laryngospasm to noncardiogenic pulmonary edema.

Sedatives, hypnotics, and opioids cause respiratory depression leading to type-2 respiratory failure. Because of respiratory depression, patients can also have aspiration leading to type-1 respiratory failure.

The patient may have crackles in the case of pulmonary edema, wheezes in the case of bronchospasm, and decreased breath sounds in pleural effusion.

Laboratory Evaluation

In general, laboratory analyses are not very helpful in establishing the diagnosis of poisoning and/or drugs induced respiratory failure. Arterial blood gas (ABG) with co-oximetry [carboxyhemoglobin (carboxyHb), cyanohemoglobin (cynHb), and methemoglobinemia (MethHb)] is a valuable tool and reveals the severity of hypoxemia, type of respiratory failure and arterial oxygen saturation gap. Arterial oxygen saturation gap is classically seen with carbon monoxide (CO) poisoning and methHb. ABG will also reveal abnormally high venous oxygen saturation in poisoning with hydrogen sulfide and cyanide. Chest radiographs are typically obtained. However, high resolution computed tomography (CT) scanning is more sensitive than chest radiography for defining the radiographic abnormalities.[15]

All efforts should be made to identify the toxidrome and subsequently the offending toxin. Acute physiology and chronic health evaluation (APACHE) and simplified acute physiologic score (SAPS-II) scores are not reliable for outcome prediction in patients with poisoning. More specific scores have been developed but have not yet been thoroughly validated in the patients with poisoning, e.g. Toxscore and poisoning severity score (PPS).

Management

Patients who present with respiratory failure due to poisoning or drug overdose have poor prognosis. Prehospital and emergency room care is very important in determining the outcome of these patients. All patients presenting with respiratory failure due to poisoning or drug overdose must be admitted to the hospital. Some patients are required to admit in ICU, if they are following criteria for ICU admission (Table 2).[16]

Table 2: Criteria for ICU admission.
1. Severe/refractory hypoxemia
2. Respiratory depression ($pCO_2 > 45$ mm Hg)
3. Pulmonary edema
4. Shock
5. Cardiac arrhythmias
6. Reduced GCS/inability to protect the airway (GCS < 12)
7. Seizures
8. Worsening metabolic acidosis
9. Severe electrolyte abnormalities
10. Need for continuous infusion of antidote and its monitoring
11. Need for dialysis or hemoperfusion
12. Need for extracorporeal membrane oxygenation (ECMO)
13. Requirement for exchange transfusion

(GCS: Glasgow coma scale; ICU: intensive care unit; pCO_2: partial pressure of carbon dioxide)

Pulmonary Toxins

As with all critical patients, resuscitation should start from airway, breathing, circulation, decontamination and elimination (ABCDE). All patients presenting with type-1 respiratory failure should receive supplemental oxygen to target oxygen saturation. These patients may also require noninvasive or invasive mechanical ventilation. Patients with sedatives and hypnotics overdose usually present with type-2 respiratory failure and have high risk of aspiration. Emergency physician should keep a low threshold for airway protection for these patients. In the contrary, a high threshold of intubation should be kept in poisoning or drug exposure with short acting agents, i.e. gamma-hydroxybutyrate (GHB).[17] Oxygen therapy may actually aggravate toxicity in certain poisoning, e.g. paraquat, diquat. Special emphasis should be given to identify the toxin, where specific therapies, e.g. antidote may improve respiratory failure (Table 3).

Gastric lavage should be done within an hour in patients presenting with drug overdose. Special emphasis should be given for potential benefit versus risk of aspiration with gastric lavage.[18] Whenever indicated, activated charcoal should always be use as soon as possible after gastric lavage.[19]

Few studies suggest the possible role including prevention of early deaths with continuous venovenous hemodiafiltration with or without charcoal hemoperfusion in patients presenting with respiratory failure due to poisoning or drug overdose, e.g. paraquat poisoning. This modality has a role by promoting hemodynamic stability which is a major cause of death in paraquat poisoning.[20]

Patients with refractory hypoxemia should receive venovenous extracorporeal membrane oxygenation (ECMO) while patients with refractory shock and reversible cardiotoxicity should be given venoarterial ECMO. ECMO is most useful for poisoning with respiratory failure where the primary lung insult is reversible. There are anecdotal case reports where ECMO has been used as a rescue therapy in different poisoning with respiratory failure, e.g. organophosphorus poisoning[21] and CO poisoning, etc.

SPECIFIC MANAGEMENT

Drugs and Respiratory Failure

Specific antidote is available for cyanide, i.e. amyl nitrite, sodium nitrite, and sodium thiosulfate. Amyl nitrite is used as an emergency drug. It is available in 0.3 mL solution and used as inhalation over 15–30 seconds. It can be repeated until intravenous sodium nitrite is available. Sodium nitrite is used intravenously 300 mg or 10 mg/kg over 2–5 minutes. Dose of sodium thiosulfate is 12.5 g to be given intravenously over 10 minutes. Hydroxocobalamin is used as infusion over 15 minutes in dose of 70 mg/kg (usually 5 g).

Flumazenil is available as an antidote for benzodiazepines for reversing respiratory failure in acute overdose only. Patient with chronic overdose can have seizure after flumazenil.[22,23] Dose of flumazenil is 0.2 mg intravenous over 15–30 seconds followed by 0.3 mg over 30 seconds followed by 0.5 mg over 30 seconds at 1 minute intervals to a total dose of 3 mg/hour. Dose may be repeated at 20-minute interval, in the event of resedation; not to exceed 1 mg at any one time and no more than 3 mg/hour. Sedation is unlikely to be because of benzodiazepines, if no response to flumazenil after 5 minutes. There is no additional benefit of flumazenil dosed beyond 3 mg.[24]

Naloxone can be used for complete or partial reversal of opioid-induced sedation, hypotension, and respiratory depression.[25] Dose is 0.04–0.4 mg intravenous or intramuscular or subcutaneous initially. It can be repeated until desired response achieved. Consider other causes of respiratory depression, if desired response not observed after 0.8 mg total dose.[26]

Table 3: Antidotes for specific poison or drug.

Poison/Drug	Antidote/Intervention
Respiratory irritants	Oxygen
Carbon monoxide	100% oxygen, hyperbaric oxygen
Cyanide	Nitrites, thiosulfate, hydroxocobalamin
Chemical warfare agents	Atropine, pralidoxime, PAM autoinjectors
Benzodiazepine	Flumazenil
Opioid	Naloxone
β-blockers	Glucagon, insulin
Anticoagulants	Vitamin K1, FFP, prothrombin complex
Methotrexate	Folinic acid
Antiplatelets	Platelets transfusion
Neuroparalytic snake bite	Antisnake venom

(FFP: fresh frozen plasma; PAM: pralidoxime)

Initial antidote for chemical warfare agents is atropine. Usual dose in adults is 2–4 mg or more, to be given intravenously or intramuscularly. It is used to antagonize the excess acetylcholine that accumulates at nerve endings in the absence of functional anticholinesterase. Respiratory depression can be partially reversed, but not muscle paralysis.[27,28] Pralidoxime should be administered to complement the actions of atropine. Usual adult dose of pralidoxime is 1–2 g intravenously.[29,30] It can be repeated twice or thrice over a period of not more than 48 hours, if muscle weakness persists.

In battle situations, fast administration of antidotes becomes the main priority. This can be done by auto-injector syringes which allow the administration of the antidotes by the victim itself or by a colleague.[31,32]

Antidote for beta-blocker overdose may include glucagon which can enhance myocardial contractility, heart rate, and atrioventricular conduction. Usual dose of glucagon is 50 mg/kg intravenously loading, followed by a continuous infusion of 1–15 mg/hours titrated to patient response.[33] High-dose insulin infusion has been reported to improve outcomes in beta-blocker poisoning by promoting positive ionotropic effect. Currently, recommended regimen is a 1 U/kg bolus followed by continuous infusion of 1–10 U/kg/hour.[34]

CONCLUSION

Poisoning and drugs overdose can present with either type-1 or type-2 respiratory failure. Pathogenesis of respiratory failure is different for different substances/drugs. Good clinical history, physical examination and appropriate laboratory tests are the most important step in making diagnosis and management of poisoning and/or drug overdose. Management consist of ABCDE and specific management for particular drugs and/or poison.

KEY POINTS

- Poisoning and drugs overdose can present with either type-1 or type-2 respiratory failure.
- The prognosis and clinical course of these patients depend largely on the quality of the care delivered in the prehospital to emergency room to ICU.
- History and physical examination are the most important step in making diagnosis and management

of respiratory failure due to poisoning or drug overdose.
- Arterial blood gas (ABG) should always be done with co-oximetry.
- ABCDE remains the main stay of initial treatment and need to be modified in certain poisoning and overdose where oxygen therapy may aggravate toxicity.
- Specific therapy, i.e. antidote should be used whenever feasible as it may actually improve respiratory failure dramatically.

REFERENCES

1. Singh O, Javeri Y, Juneja D, et al. Profile and outcome of patients with acute toxicity admitted in intensive care unit: Experiences from a major corporate hospital in urban India. Indain J Anaesth. 2011;55(4):370-4.
2. Kulling P, Persson H. Role of the Intensive care unit in the management of the poisoned patient. Med Toxicol. 1986;1(5):375-86.
3. Mathru M, McDaniel LB. Primum non nocere. Is the therapy worse than the disease? Chest. 1994;105:1634-6.
4. Musshoff F, Hagemier L, Kirschbaum K, et al. Two cases of suicide by asphyxiation due to helium and argon. Forensic Sci Int. 2012;223:e27-30.
5. Dunford JV, Lucas J, Vent N, et al. Asphyxiation due to dry ice in a walk-in freezer. J Emerg Med. 2009;36:353-6.
6. Wright N. An assessment of the unreliability of the history given by self-poisoned patients. Clin Toxicol. 1980; p. 381.
7. Singh O, Nasa P. General poisoning management. In: Chawla R, Todi S (Eds). ICU Protocols. A Stepwise Approach. London: Springer; 2012.
8. ARSDR (2006). Agency for Toxic Substances and Disease Registry [online] Available from http:// www.atsdr.cdc.gov/. [Accessed November 2018].
9. Çımrın AH. İnhalasyona Bağlı Akciğer Zedelenmesi. In: Ekim N, Türktaş H (Eds). Göğüs Hastalıkları Acilleri. Ankara: Bilimsel Tıp Yayınevi; 2000. pp. 107-17.
10. Glazer CS. Acute Inhalational Injury. In: Hanley ME, Welsh CH (Eds). Current Diagnosis & Treatment in Pulmonary Medicine. International Edition. New York: Mc-Graw Hill; 2003. pp. 354-60.
11. Miller K, Chang A. Acute inhalation injury. Emerg Med Clin North Am. 2003;21:533-57.
12. DeBehnke DJ, Hilander SJ, Dobler DW, et al. The hemodynamic and arterial blood gas response to asphyxiation: a canine model of pulseless electrical activity. Resuscitation. 1995;30:169-75.
13. Gracia R, Shepherd G: Cyanide poisoning and its treatment. Pharmacotherapy 2004; 24:1358-1365.
14. Newman LS, Gottschall EB. Toxic Inhalational Lung Injury. In: Albert RK, Spiro SG, Jett JR (Eds). Clinical Respiratory Medicine. 2nd edition. Philadelphia: Mosby; 2004: pp.759-64.

15. Tamura M, Saraya T, Fujiwara M, et al. High resolution computed tomography findings for patients with drug induced pulmonary toxicity, with special reference to hypersensitivity pneumonitis like patterns in gemcitabine induced cases. Oncologist. 2013;18(4):45-49.

16. Brett AS, Rothschild N, Gray R, et al. Predicting the clinical course in intentional drug overdose: Implications for use of the intensive care unit. Arch Intern Med. 1987;147:133-7.

17. O'Connell T, Kaye L, Plosay JJ. 3d Gamma-hydroxybutyrate (GHB): A newer drug of abuse. Am Fam physician. 2000;62:2478-83.

18. Vale JA. American Academy of Clinical Toxicology, European Association of Poison Control Centres and Clinical Toxicologists. Position Statement: Gastric lavage. J Toxicol Clin Toxicol. 1997;35:711.

19. Chyka PA, Seger D. Position statement: single-dose activated charcoal. American Academy of Clinical Toxicology, European Association of Poisons Centres and Clinical Toxicologists. J Toxicol Clin Toxicol. 1997;35:721

20. Sandhu JS, Dhiman A, Mahajan R, et al. Outcome of paraquat poisoning - a five year study. Indian J Nephrol. 2003;13:64-8.

21. Yosri M, Attia AA, Abdelbary M, et al. Veno-venous Extracorporeal Membrane Oxygenation in a case of organophosphorus poisoning. Egyptian J Crit Care Med. 2016;4(1):43-6.

22. Longmire AW, Seger DL. Topics in clinical pharmacology: Flumazenil, a benzodiazepine antagonist. Am J Med Sci. 1993;306:49.

23. Mordel A, Winkler E, Almog S, et al. Seizures after flumazenil administration in a case of combined benzodiazepine and tricyclic antidepressant overdose. Crit Care Med. 1992;20:1733.

24. Spivey WH, Roberts JR, Derlet RW. A clinical trial of escalating doses of flumazenil for reversal of suspected benzodiazepine overdose in the emergency department. Ann Emerg Med. 1993;22:1813.

25. Handal KA, Schauben JL, Salamone FR. Naloxone. Ann Emerg Med. 1983;12:438.

26. Albertson TE, Dawson A, de Latorre F, et al. Tox-ACLS: Toxicologic oriented advanced cardiac life support. Ann Emerg Med. 2001;37:S78.

27. Stares JE. Medical protection against chemical-warfare agents. In: Stares J (Ed). Medical Protection Against Chemical-Warfare Agents. Stockholm: Almqvist and Wiksell International; 1976. pp. 157-66.

28. Taylor P. Anticholinesterase agents. In: Gilnan AG, Goodman LS, Gilman A (Eds). Goodman and Gilman's, The Pharmacological Basis of Therapeutics. New York: Macmillan Publishing Co. 1980. pp. 100-19.

29. Gosselin RE, Smith RP, Hodge HC, et al. Clinical Toxicology of Commercial Products, 5th edition. Williams and Willdns, Baltimore, MD, 1984. pp. I-2, II-236, III-49, III-338-40.

30. Barr SJ. Chemical warfare agents. Top Emergency Med. 1985;7(1):62-70.

31. Jokanovic M, Stojiljkovic MP. Current understanding of the application of pyridinium oximes as cholinesterase reactivators in treatment of organophosphate poisoning. Eur. J Pharmacol. 2006;553:10.

32. McDonough JH, Shih TM. In: Marrs TC, Maynard RL, Sidell FR (Eds). Chemical Warfare Agents-Toxicology and Treatment, 2nd edition. West Sussex: John Wiley & Sons Ltd. 2007. pp. 287-303.

33. Peterson CD, Leeder JS, Sterner S. Glucagon therapy for beta-blocker overdose. Drug Intell Clin Pharm. 1984;18(5):394-8.

34. Engebretsen KM, Kaczmarek KM, Morgan J, et al. High-dose insulin therapy in beta-blocker and calcium channel-blocker poisoning. Clin Toxicol (Phila). 2011;49(4):277-83.

16
CHAPTER

Inhalational Poisoning

Suneel Kumar Garg, Shweta Gupta

INTRODUCTION

Most people are at risk of inhalational exposure in their day-to-day life. They can be exposed to either household chemicals or appliances, environmental pollutants, or to industrial chemicals. Exposure can vary from suspended particles to toxic gases and fumes. The reaction to these exposures depends upon pulmonary defense mechanism, concentration, intensity, duration and chemical properties of exposed substance.

People with mild exposure and good pulmonary defense mechanism can have only vague symptoms, while people with massive exposure and poor pulmonary defense mechanism can have wide spectrum of pulmonary and systemic injuries.

Strong suspicion and knowledge are essential for making quick diagnosis and treatment, especially in case of mild exposure which is difficult to diagnose and treat. Massive exposure can be quickly diagnosed and treated because of evident history and magnitude of symptoms.

CLASSIFICATION

Historically, most inhalational substances are classified into agents causing direct pulmonary injury and agents causing systemic toxicity. Agents causing direct pulmonary injury are mainly respiratory irritants (Table 1). Exposure to direct respiratory irritants is most common among all toxic inhalations. Agents causing systemic toxicity can be further classified into simple asphyxiants (Table 2) and chemical asphyxiants (Table 3). Inhalational exposure can also be with usual combination of agents such as smoke, smog and metal fume fever.[1-5]

Agents Causing Direct Pulmonary Injury

The agents causing direct pulmonary injury are presented in Table 1.

Agents Causing Systemic Toxicity

The agents causing systemic toxicity are presented in Tables 2 and 3.

Table 1: Respiratory irritants.		
High solubility	*Intermediate solubility*	*Low solubility*
Ammonia	Chlorine	Methyl isocyanate
Hydrogen chloride	Bromine	Nitrogen mustards
Hydrogen sulfide	–	Oxides of nitrogen
Formaldehyde	–	Phosgene
Sulfur dioxide	–	Ozone
–	–	Mustard gas

Table 2: Simple asphyxiants.

Heavier than air	Lighter than air
Argon	Acetylene
Butane	Ethylene
Carbon dioxide	Methane
Ethane	Neon
Propane	Nitrogen

Table 3: Chemical asphyxiants.

Inhibiting oxygen transport	Inhibiting cellular oxygen utilization
Carbon monoxide (CO)	Acrylonitrile
Hydrogen sulfide	Cyanide (CN)
Methemoglobin (MehHb) inducer	Phosphine
Oxides of nitrogen	–

EPIDEMIOLOGY

Inhalation of household chemicals or appliances, environmental pollutants or industrial exposure may cause either irritant lung injury, or asphyxiation, or other systemic effects. Exposure can vary from accidental spills and explosions to fires. There were 5,500 and 6,000 exposures to chlorine gas in the US in 2012 and 2013 respectively. Exposures to carbon monoxide (CO) in 2012 and 2013 were 14,300 and 13,600 respectively. These data were reported by the American Association of Poison Control Centers in 2014.[6,7] In India, most of the cases are not informed or documented so incidence and prevalence as well as potential degree of the health effects produced by inhalational agents are not easy to estimate.

PATHOGENESIS

Pathogenesis is different for different inhalational substances causing direct pulmonary injury and systemic toxicity.

Respiratory irritants can cause regional pulmonary injury as pulmonary system has the greatest potential surface area of exposure. Children are more susceptible than adults because of greater concentration time exposure.[8] Water-soluble compounds can irritate the mucosal surfaces and cell barrier system from the nares to the alveoli. Injury can be exaggerated by retrograde transport of irritants by cilia lining the epithelium via an intact mucociliary action. There can also be direct cellular injury with destruction of type 1 and 2 pneumocytes leading to pulmonary edema.

Particle size, chemical properties and solubility of respiratory irritants determine the site and extent of the injury to respiratory tract. Gases with large particle size (>10 micron) and high water solubility, intermediate particle size (5–10 micron) and intermediate water solubility and small particle size (<5 micron) and low water solubility produce upper airway, middle airway and lower airway symptoms, respectively (Fig. 1).

Host factors and environmental factors also play a role in determining the degree of injury. Important host factors with worst outcome are elderly, allergic, smoker and patients with underlying lung debilitating illness. Important environmental factors with worst outcome are high concentration and long duration of exposure in a closed space.[1-4,9]

They can disrupt the gas exchange system in several ways. They can injure the alveolar epithelial cells and capillary endothelium, which can lead to reactive airway dysfunction syndrome (RADS). Interstitial airway components are also at risk. Acute exposure to airway irritants can lead to reversible bronchoconstriction, while with chronic exposure macrophage-initiated or macrophage-mediated inflammatory response plays a major role.[10]

Reactive Airway Dysfunction Syndrome

Reactive airway dysfunction syndrome often associated with exposure to high concentrations of some water-

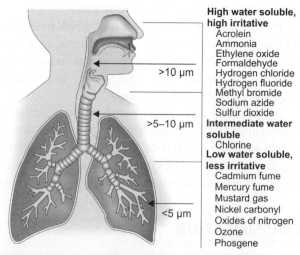

Fig. 1: Distribution of the irritant gases and the site of injury in the respiratory tract according to their particle size and water solubility.

Source: Gorguner M, Akgun M. Acute inhalation injury. Eurasian J Med. 2010;42(1):28-35.

Inhalational Poisoning

soluble airway irritants. It can be considered as a category of occupational asthma, but in contrast to asthma, it can develop abruptly without a latency period and also it is not associated with Immunoglobulin E mediated histamine release. It is provoked by exposure to small concentrations of the same agent or others. It is manifested as bronchospasm, bronchoconstriction and decreased airflow.

Most important diagnostic clue is the onset of symptoms within 24 hours of significant exposure to suspected water-soluble irritant without a competing pulmonary diagnosis.

Agents causing systemic toxicity are classified as either simple asphyxiants or chemical asphyxiants based on their mechanism of toxicity. Simple asphyxiants decrease oxygen delivery by simply displacing oxygen in inspired air, results in hypoxemia. They cause various organ dysfunctions because of hypoxemia. Chemical asphyxiants either changes oxygen affinity for hemoglobin and therefore interfere with oxygen transport system, e.g. methemoglobin (MetHb) and CO or inhibiting cellular oxygen utilization and cause tissue hypoxia, e.g. cyanide (CN).[11-13]

AGENTS CAUSING DIRECT PULMONARY INJURY

Respiratory Irritants

Respiratory irritants are the water-soluble substances, react with water at the mucosal surface of the airways generating acids, alkali or other reactive compounds, which cause direct tissue injury.

Signs and Symptoms

Signs and Symptoms depend upon concentration and duration of exposure. Soluble gases cause inflammation of the skin, oropharynx, upper respiratory tract and conjunctivitis with mild exposure. With moderate exposure, there can be burning or sometimes edema of the skin, nose and oropharynx. Individuals can have dyspnea, wheezing, chest tightness and upper airway obstruction. With severe exposure person can suffer from corneal ulceration, blindness, upper airway obstruction, hoarseness of voice, laryngospasm, stridor, pulmonary edema and burns on skin or mucous membrane of respiratory tract. Individuals often suffer residual chronic lung disease such as persistent bronchitis, bronchiectasis,

airflow obstruction, interstitial fibrosis and impaired gas exchange. The mortality rate can be up to 40% with severe exposure. Less soluble gases slowly hydrolyze in water, cause predominantly damage in lower respiratory tract. Signs and symptoms include shortness of breath, long-term lung damage with pulmonary fibrosis and chronic wheezing.[1-3,9]

Silo filler's disease is an occupational disease which mostly affects farmers and results from inhaling fumes of nitrogen dioxide given off by moist silage such as fresh corn or grains. Signs and symptoms depend upon concentration and duration of exposure. Most symptomatic exposures are mild and self-limiting as with other respiratory irritants. There can be sudden death from asphyxiation and pulmonary edema. The condition can recur 10–14 days after temporarily resolve, even without further exposure.[14]

Chemical suicide is rare but growing phenomenon. Victims often taped *Hazmat* warning signs on the window of their cars. A variety of toxic gases can be produced by mixing household chemicals and quickly reach lethal levels in the enclosed space of a car. Most common gas produced is hydrogen sulfide or disulfide. Signs and symptoms depend upon concentration and duration of exposure. Victims rapidly become unconscious and apneic, the so called "slaughterhouse sledgehammer effect". Management is mainly supportive.

Inhalation of some gases can also cause hypersensitivity pneumonitis by triggering an allergic response. In some people, inhalation over a long period of time may result in chronic bronchitis. Also, inhalation of some chemicals can be carcinogenic, e.g. arsenic compounds and hydrocarbons.

Diagnosis

Important clue to make a diagnosis is a relevant history of exposure. Signs and symptoms depend on concentration and duration of exposure. Pulse oximetry is of utmost importance. A chest X-ray can be useful to diagnose pulmonary edema or bronchiolitis. Computed tomography is especially helpful when people have symptoms with normal chest X-ray.

Treatment

Mainstay of treatment is to remove the victim from exposure followed by a primary and secondary assessment. Supportive treatment starts from decontamination, oxygen therapy, nebulized bronchodilators and inhaled or systemic steroids if needed. Irrigate the eyes with water for 15–20 minutes. Patients have to be kept in observation for need for early airway protection. Mechanical ventilation may be needed. Cricothyroidotomy may be required in more severe cases.

Prevention

Exposure to household chemicals or appliances can be prevented by keeping all household chemicals in a well-ventilated area and discontinue to use them whenever there is first sign of discomfort. Appliances should be cleaned and serviced properly. Exposure to environmental pollutants can be prevented by wearing mask while going out. Air purifier can also be used, if parts per million (ppm) of pollutants is very high. It can be helpful to prevent exposure to industrial exposure by adopting protocol for running industries.

There are numerous accidents noted in the history with release of irritant gases and its impact on masses requiring acute care (Table 4).

AGENTS CAUSING SYSTEMIC TOXICITY

Simple Asphyxiants

These substances, mostly inert gases or vapors, can alter oxygen delivery by simple displacing oxygen from the

Table 4: Historical accidents with irritant gases.

Chemical	Source	Properties	Injuries	Major incidences
Ammonia	Agriculture (mostly fertilizers), pharmaceuticals manufacturing and household cleaning products	Highly water soluble, colorless, sharp and pungent odor	Upper airways burns	Punjab, India Massive explosion in huge ammonia gas cylinder (21/02/2018) Fatalities–3, injuries–11 Punjab, India Gas tanker leak (13/06/2015) Fatalities–5, injuries–>100 Shanghai, China Leakage of anhydrous ammonia (31/08/2013) Fatalities–15, injuries–41 Minot, North Dakota Freight train derailment (18/01/2002) Fatalities–1, injuries–333 Shenxian, Shandong Province, China Spilling from a fertilizer plant (08/07/2002) Fatalities–13, injuries–11 Dakar, Senegal Explosion of ammonia tank (24/03/1992) Fatalities–116, injuries–1150 Cartagena, Colombia (09/12/1977) Fatalities–21, injuries–30 Houston, USA Rupture of ammonia tank (11/05/1976) Fatalities–6, injuries–178 Potchefstroom, Natal, South Africa Major release from a fertilizer plant (13/07/1973) Fatalities–18, injuries–65

Contd...

Chapter 16

Inhalational Poisoning

155

Contd…

Chemical	Source	Properties	Injuries	Major incidences
Chlorine	Household and hospital cleaners, bleaching agents, water or sewage disinfectant	Intermediate water solubility, dense and yellow green gas with irritating odor	Upper and lower airway inflammation, pneumonitis and noncardiogenic pulmonary edema	Southwestern Iranian province of Khuzestan Gas leak (12/08/2017) Injuries–475 Nigeria, West Africa Explosion of a chlorine gas storage tank at a water treatment plant (25/07/2015) Fatalities–8, injuries–100 Graniteville, South Carolina Freight train derailment (05/01/2005) Fatalities–9, injuries–529 Texas, USA Freight train met with an accident (28/06/2004) Fatalities–3, injuries–44 Missouri, USA Flex hose of a railroad tanker car ruptured (14/08/2002) Fatalities–67 Toulouse, France Explosion in a fertilizer plant (21/09/2001) Fatalities–30, injuries–2500 Wieltje North-east of Ypres in Belgian Flanders Used by German Army on British troops, during World War-I as chemical warfare in combination with phosgene gas (19/12/1915) Fatalities–120, injuries–1,069
Phosgene	Pesticide and other chemical manufacture	Low water solubility	Upper airway, inflammation and pneumonitis	Lake Charles, LA Leak from a chemical plant (10/09/1984) Fatalities–1, injuries–40 Wieltje North-east of Ypres in Belgian Flanders Used by German Army on British troops, during World War-I as chemical warfare in combination with phosgene gas (19/12/1915) Fatalities–120, injuries–1,069
Methyl isocyanate (MIC)	Pesticide and other chemical manufacture	Low water solubility, colorless, and tearing agent	Upper and lower airway inflammation	Bhopal, MP, India Gas leak from a pesticide plant (02/12/1984) Fatalities-19,787, injuries–55,8125

inspired air, when present in high concentrations. In low concentration, they do not have much physiological effect. Decrease oxygen availability leads to central nervous system and cardiac dysfunction.[11-13] Death occurs with very high concentration of these agents.

Signs and Symptoms

Signs and symptoms depend upon concentration and duration of exposure. Hypoxia results in autonomic stimulation and cerebral symptoms. There can be

Pulmonary Toxins

decrease mental alertness, loss of consciousness and death, when the oxygen concentration falls below 16%, 10% and 6%, respectively after the exposure to simple asphyxiants.[24]

Diagnosis

Relevant history of exposure, myriad spectrum of complaints, group of victims and rapid resolution of symptoms on removal from exposure is an important clue for diagnosis. Pulse oximetry again is of utmost importance. Radiology dose not have much importance to make a diagnosis.

Treatment

Rapid removal away from asphyxiant is as important as treatment as rescuer can become a second victim. Second most important aspect of treatment is prevention of hypoxemia.[25] Supportive treatment involves oxygen therapy and ventilation, if needed. Patients can also require fluid resuscitation, if hemodynamically unstable. All victims should be kept in close observation. Patients with prolonged hypoxia should be observed for the delayed development of posthypoxic ischemic encephalopathy.

There are accidents noted in the history with release of simple asphyxiants and its impact on masses requiring acute care (Table 5).

Chemical Asphyxiants

These are the substances, which either interfere with oxygen transport to the tissues by the red cells or inhibiting cellular oxygen utilization. Each hemoglobin tetramer has four binding sites for the oxygen. Chemical asphyxiants replace the oxygen binding site at one or more places of hemoglobin tetramer, e.g. methemoglobin (MetHb) and CO.

There are another type of chemical asphyxiants, which are mitochondrial toxins and interfere with cellular utilization of oxygen leading to abnormally high venous oxygen saturation, e.g. hydrogen sulfide, CN, etc.

Occupational exposures and fires are the most common sources of inhalational injuries. Working in confined spaces is hazardous to workers.

Signs and Symptoms

Chemical asphyxiants shift the oxyhemoglobin (OxyHb) dissociation curve to the left, impairing tissue oxygen delivery and use. Mild symptoms of asphyxia include headache, dizziness, nausea, vomiting, altered mental status, tachypnea and hypertension. More severe symptoms range from dyspnea, cardiac dysrhythmia, ischemia, hypotension, syncope, seizure and even death.[27]

Diagnosis

Pulse oximetry is unreliable in detecting carboxyhemoglobin (carboxyHb) or MetHb. Arterial blood gas with CO-oximetry is diagnostic, which shows hypoxemia, elevated carboxyHb, MetHb and metabolic acidosis. It is useful to identify the arterial oxygen saturation gap.

Treatment

All victims should be kept in close observation. Supportive treatment involves removal from exposure, administer highest concentration of available oxygen irrespective of pulse oximetry. Elective intubation and ventilation should be done in case of fire with

Table 5: Historical accident with simple asphyxiant.				
Chemical	Source	Properties	Injuries	Major incidences
Carbon dioxide	• Produced by the action of acidified water on limestone • By-product of fermentation of sugar in the brewing of beer, whisky and other alcoholic beverages • From thermal decomposition of limestone	Colorless, odorless, sharp, acidic odor at high concentration	Hypoxia by displacing oxygen in inspired air	Lake Nyos, Cameroon, Africa Limnic eruption (21/08/1986) Fatalities → 1700, Injuries—thousands of livestock up to 12 miles away

smoke inhalation. Oxygen reverses the hypoxemia and accelerates the elimination of asphyxiants. It reverses hypoxia, competes with CO for Hb binding, and promotes carboxyHb dissociation. It shortens carboxyHb half-life from 5 to 6 hours on room air to 40–90 minutes on 100% oxygen. Use of hyperbaric oxygen therapy (HBO) has been shown to be controversial, but it should be considered for severe CO poisoning. HBO further reduces the half-life of carboxyHb to 15–30 minutes. Treatment of methemoglobinemia requires methylene blue. CN toxicity requires amyl nitrite, sodium nitrite and sodium thiosulfate.

Chemical asphyxiants are also described in details in other chapter in this textbook.

COMBINATION AGENTS

Fire Smoke

Smoke has multiple toxic gases, particulate matter as well as heated gas. Smoke contains irritant gases, simple asphyxiants as well as chemical asphyxiants. Particulate matter is formed from incomplete combustion of organic material and is usually less than 0.5 μm in size. Because of its nature, smoke causes damage to whole respiratory system.[28-30] Main reason for smoke injuries is closed-space fires. Individuals who become expose to smoke in a closed space become drowsy, leading to more inhalation as they are neither able to protect themselves nor they are able to run away from the place. Damage to respiratory system is mainly because of irritant gases and heat. Thermal injuries typically limited to upper airways. Lower airway injuries are mainly because of steam inhalation. Simple asphyxiants can displace oxygen from alveoli and lead to central nervous system and cardiac dysfunction.[11-13] Chemical asphyxiants, mainly CO and CN, generated from fires are important cause of morbidity and mortality. In fact, most common source of CN poisoning in humans is from incomplete combustion of material containing nitrogen, e.g. plastic, vinyl, wool or silk.

Signs and Symptoms

Signs and symptoms depend mainly upon close versus open space, fire concentration and duration of exposure. Victims in close space are more prone for devastating injuries. They can present with cough, shortness of breath, hoarseness or noisy breathing and headache

(because of CO). Victims can also have eye damage, decrease alertness, and skin changes (pale and bluish due to lack of oxygen, bright red due to CO poisoning and burns). Seizure and coma are also possible after smoke inhalation. Clinician should be alert by looking at soot in the nose or throat.

Treatment

Treatment begins with airway, breathing, and circulation. Carboxyhb and MetHb levels are to be checked and treated accordingly. Oxygen should be providing to all victims irrespective of saturation keeping in the mind of CO poisoning and methemoglobinemia. HBO should be used to treat CO poisoning. There must be a low threshold for airway protection as with time airway can become difficult. Antibiotics may be given to treat or prevent an infection. Treatment with hydroxocobalamin and/or sodium thiosulfate is appropriate in the management of suspected CN poisoning.

Smog

Smog is mixture of smoke and fog in the air. It is a kind of air pollution. Smog results from large amounts of burning of wood and coal together especially crop in an area and the emissions from vehicles and industries. It is caused by a mixture of smoke and ozone, sulfur dioxide, nitrogen dioxide and CO. Smog is a problem in winters in India, especially in Delhi NCR. In Delhi, it was declared as a medical emergency in 2017.

Signs and Symptoms

Signs and symptoms depend mainly upon particle size in smog. Victims present with shortness of breath, pain when inhaling deeply, wheezing, coughing and acute respiratory distress. Special risk groups are patients having pre-existing obstructive lung disease or any other respiratory diseases. There is also increased cardiovascular mortality because of increased incidences of acute coronary syndrome.[31,32] Victims also become more susceptible to infection as there is drying of mucous membrane of nose and throat.

Treatment

The best treatment is prevention by wearing mask and not to get exposed to the affected area. Some victims can require oxygen and other supportive treatment. Hospital

Pulmonary Toxins

admissions and deaths increase with increasing levels of ozone.

Metal Fume Fever

Also known as Monday morning fever, is classically associated with inhalation of zinc oxide, aluminum oxide and magnesium oxide, which are produced as by products in the fumes that result when certain metals are heated. Welders are commonly exposed to the metal fumes. Cadmium fumes inhalation under poor ventilation is typical during welding or metal smelting operations. Mercury inhalation risk is mainly with metal reclamation processes. Exposure to heated fluoropolymers causes polymer fume fever while exposure to high amounts of endotoxin leads to organic dust toxic syndrome.

Signs and Symptoms

Victim can present with chills, fever, malaise and myalgia. Typical onset is 4–8 hours after inhalation of fumes or dust. Victim can also present with cough or mid dyspnea. Symptoms of a more severe metal toxicity may also include a burning sensation in the body, shock, oliguria, seizures, vomiting, watery or bloody diarrhea. It requires a prompt medical attention. Metal fume fever is very characteristic in terms of lessening of symptoms with ongoing exposure. Symptoms reappear after a period of time away from exposure. This is classically described as Monday morning fever.[33]

Diagnosis

It is essential to take good environmental and/or occupational exposure history to make the correct diagnosis as victims usually present with vague complaints. The diagnosis is based primarily upon a history of exposure to metal oxide fumes. Physical symptoms vary among persons exposed. Patients may present with respiratory findings on examination, e.g. wheezing or crackles. Chest X-ray abnormalities may also be present. White blood cell counts are usually elevated. Urine, blood and skin zinc levels may be elevated.

In 2006, approximately 700 metal fume exposures were reported to the United States Poison control center.

Treatment

This is a self-limited disease. Clinical manifestations resolve spontaneously within 12–48 hours. Bed rest, hydration and symptomatic treatment with analgesics may be needed.

CHEMICAL WARFARE AND RIOT CONTROL AGENTS

Chemical Warfare and Riot Control Agents are called as weapons of mass destruction. This is one of the curse used by mankind against humanity. These are synthetic chemicals, which can be used in any form, especially gas, liquid or aerosol. These agents are extremely toxic. Initial agents used were primarily gases, such as mustard gas, phosgene and chloropicrin, but later on organophosphate pesticides based systemic toxins also have been used.

Classification

There are many ways to classify the chemical warfare agents. Based on physiological effects on human beings, they are classified as follows:

- Nerve agents, e.g. sarin, soman and tabun
- Vesicants (blistering agents), e.g. mustards and arsenicals
- Bloods agents (cyanogenic agents), e.g. CNs
- Choking agents (pulmonary agents), e.g. chlorine, phosgene and diphosgene
- Riot control agents (tear gases), e.g. 1-chloroacetophenone (CN), 2-chlorobenzylidene malononitrile (CS) and dibenz [b, f]-1,4-oxazepine (CR)
- Psychotomimetic agents, e.g. lysergic acid diethylamide (LSD) and marijuana.

Signs and Symptoms

They primarily affect nervous system and respiratory system.[1,4] Signs and symptoms are described in Table 6 with individual historical chemical warfare agents.

Riot control agents (crowd control agents and tear gases) are different as compared to chemical warfare agents. These agents cause immediate mucous membrane irritation. Chloroacetophenone and ortho-chlorobenzamalonitrile are the most common agents worldwide.

Treatment

Treatment depends upon type of chemical warfare agent. Nerve agents are organophosphorus group and require

Inhalational Poisoning

Table 6: Historical incidences with chemical warfare agents.

Chemical	Source	Clinical findings	Management	Major incidences
Nerve agents: • Cyclosarin • Sarin • Soman • Tabun	Organophosphorus	Fasciculations, coma, sudden collapse, paralysis and apnea	• Mild effects: Atropine • Moderate effects: Atropine and pralidoxime • Severe effects: Atropine, pralidoxime, and a benzodiazepine • PAM Auto injectors (if available)	Syria war (2013)
Mustard compounds (e.g. nitrogen mustards and sulfur mustards)	Respiratory irritant	Upper and lower airway inflammation pneumonitis	• Decontamination is the key to treatment • 100% oxygen and ventilator management	World War-1 Iran Iraq war (1979-1988)
Hydrogen chloride and hydrogen fluoride	Noncardiogenic pulmonary edema	Coughing, inspiratory stridor, wheezing and laryngospasm	• Fresh air • Provide humidified oxygen • Inhaled epinephrine for stridor or upper airway obstruction • Pulmonary toilet • Bronchoscopy for severe upper airway obstruction	World war-1
Phosgene	Respiratory irritant or noncardiogenic pulmonary edema	Upper airway inflammation and pneumonitis	• Fresh air • Provide humidified oxygen	As chemical warfare in combination with chlorine gas (19/12/1915) Fatalities–120, injuries–1069 Wieltje Northeast of Ypres in Belgian Flanders Used by German Army on British troops, during World War-I
Chlorine	Respiratory irritant	Upper and lower airway inflammation, pneumonitis and noncardiogenic pulmonary edema	• Fresh air • Provide humidified oxygen	In Syria (2014) Kafr Zita chemical attack Used several times by insurgents in the Iraqi insurgency (2003-11) Wieltje north-east of Ypres in Belgian Flanders Used by German Army on British troops, during World War-I as chemical warfare in combination with phosgene gas (19/12/1915) fatalaties–120, injuries–1069

Chapter 16

Pulmonary Toxins

atropine for mild effect, atropine and pralidoxime (PAM) for moderate effect and atropine, PAM, and a benzodiazepine for severe effects. There is emergency role of PAM auto-injectors also, if available.

Mustard compounds, hydrogen chloride, hydrogen fluoride, and phosgene are respiratory irritant and require removal of exposure, decontamination, and oxygen therapy. Mechanical ventilation can also be required.

Chemical warfare and riot control agents are also described in details in other chapter in this textbook.

CONCLUSION

Most people are at risk of inhalation exposure in their day to day life. Most inhalation substances are classified into agents causing direct pulmonary injury and systemic toxicity. In India, most of the cases are not informed or documented. Pathogenesis is different for different inhalation substances causing direct pulmonary injury and systemic toxicity. Strong suspicion and knowledge is essential for making quick diagnosis and treatment.

KEY POINTS

- Exposure to inhalation substances is not unusual in day-to-day life
- Strong suspicion and vast knowledge are needed for making a quick diagnosis and treatment
- Diagnosis is straightforward in the setting of a history of exposure
- Treatment is mainly symptomatic
- When history of exposure is not clear or it is difficult to identify the agent, treatment should be focused on presenting symptoms and signs referable to a particular airway component
- An assessment should be made to identify the substance based on history and clinical presentation, e.g. respiratory irritants, simple asphyxiants, chemical asphyxiants, combination agents, etc.
- Once an assessment or differential diagnosis is made, treatment should focus on supportive care and particular organ dysfunction.

REFERENCES

1. Agency for Toxic Substances and Disease Registry. (2018) Agency for Toxic Substances and Disease Registry. [online] Available from: http:// www.atsdr.cdc.gov/ [Accessed October, 2018].

2. Çımrın AH. İnhalasyona Bağlı Akciğer Zedelenmesi. In: Ekim N, Türktaş H (Eds). Göğüs Hastalıkları Acilleri. Ankara: Bilimsel Tıp Yayınevi; 2000. pp. 107-17.

3. Glazer CS. Acute Inhalational Injury. In: Hanley ME, Welsh CH (Eds). Current Diagnosis & Treatment in Pulmonary Medicine, International Ed. New York: McGraw Hill; 2003. pp. 354-60.

4. Newman LS, Gottschall EB. Toxic Inhalational Lung Injury. In: Albert RK, Spiro SG, Jett JR (Eds). Clinical Respiratory Medicine second Edition. Philadelphia: Mosby; 2004: pp. 759-64.

5. Rosenstock L. Acute inhalational injury. In: Textbook of Clinical Occupational and Environmental Medicine. Philadelphia: WB Saunders Co;1994. pp. 236-7.

6. Mowry JB, Spyker DA, Brooks DE, et al. 2014 Annual Report of the American Association of Poison Control Centers' National Poison Data System (NPDS): 32nd Annual Report. Clin Toxicol. 2015;53(10):962-1147.

7. Mowry JB, Spyker DA, Cantilena LR Jr, et al. 2013 Annual Report of the American Association of Poison Control Centers' National Poison Data System (NPDS): 31st Annual Report. Clin Toxicol. 2014;52(10):1032-283.

8. Burri PH. Structural aspects of postnatal lung development–alveolar formation and growth. Biol Neonate. 2006;89:313-22.

9. Miller K, Chang A. Acute inhalation injury. Emerg Med Clin North Am. 2003;21:533-57.

10. Hashimoto D, Chow A, Noizat C, et al. Tissue-resident macrophages self-maintain locally throughout adult life with minimal contribution from circulating monocytes. Immunity. 2013;38:792-804.

11. Musshoff F, Hagemier L, Kirschbaum K, et al. Two cases of suicide by asphyxiation due to helium and argon. Forensic Sci Int. 2012;223:e27-30.

12. Dunford JV, Lucas J, Vent N, et al. Asphyxiation due to dry ice in a walk-in freezer. J Emerg Med. 2009;36:353-6.

13. Gill JR, Ely SF, Hua Z. Environmental gas displacement: three accidental deaths in the workplace. Am J Forensic Med Pathol. 2002;23:26-30.

14. Douglas WW, Hepper NGG, Colby TV. Silo-filler's disease. Mayo Clin Proc. 1989;64:291-304.

15. OGP. (2010). Risk assessment data directory. Report No. 434-17. [online] Available from: http://www.ogp.org.uk/pubs/434-17.pdf [Accessed October, 2018].

16. National Transportation Safety Board. (2002). Derailment of Canadian Pacific railway freight train 292-16 and subsequent release of anhydrous ammonia near Minot, North Dakota. Railroad accident report NTSB/RAR-04/01. Washington, DC: National Transportation Safety Board; 2002. [online] Available from: http://www.ntsb.gov/doclib/reports/2004/RAR0401. pdf [Accessed October, 2018].

17. The Times of India. (2015). Five dead, 100 injured in Punjab ammonia gas tanker leak. [online] Available from: http://timesofindia.indiatimes.com/india/Five-dead-100-injured-in-Punjab-ammonia-gas-tanker-leak/articleshow/47651388.cms [Accessed October, 2018].

18. Wikipedia. (2018). German Phosgene attack (19 December 1915). [online] Available from: https://en.wikipedia.org/wiki/ First_German_phosgene_attack_on_British_troops [Accessed October, 2018].

19. The 100 largest losses 1972-2011. (2011) Large property damage losses in hydrocarbon industry, 22nd edition. [online] Available from: https://usa.marsh.com/Portals/9/Documents/100_Largest_Losses2011.pdf [Accessed October, 2018].

20. National Transportation Safety Board. (2005) Collision of Norfolk Southern freight train 192 with standing Norfolk Southern local train P22 with subsequent hazardous materials release: Graniteville, South Carolina January 6, 2005. Railroad accident report NTSB/RAR-05/04. Washington, DC: National Transportation Safety Board; 2005. [online] Available from: https://www.ntsb.gov/doclib/reports/2005/RAR0504. pdf [Accessed October, 2018].

21. Occupational Safety & Health Administration (OSHA). (2013). Accident: 14259261–inhalation of phosgene gas. Report ID: 0625700 – event date: 09/10/1984. Washington, DC: US Department of Labor, Occupational Safety & Health Administration. [online] Available from: https://www.osha.gov/pls/imis/accidentsearch.accident_detail?id514259261 [Accessed October, 2018].

22. EPA air toxics Web site. (2013). Methyl isocyanate. Environmental Protection Agency. [online] Available from: http://www.epa.gov/ttnatw01/hlthef/methylis.html [Accessed October, 2018].

23. Dhara VR, Dhara R. The Union Carbide disaster in Bhopal: a review of health effects. Arch Environ Health. 2002;57:391-404.

24. DeBehnke DJ, Hilander SJ, Dobler DW, et al. The hemodynamic and arterial blood gas response to asphyxiation: a canine model of pulseless electrical activity. Resuscitation. 1995;30:169-75.

25. Rorison DG, McPherson SJ. Acute toxic inhalations. Emerg Med Clin North Am. 1992;10:409-35.

26. Baxter PF, Kapila M, Mfonfu D. Lake Nyos disaster, Cameroon, 1986: the medical effects of large scale emission of carbon dioxide. BMJ. 1989;298:1437-41.

27. Gracia R, Shepherd G. Cyanide poisoning and its treatment. Pharmacotherapy. 2004;24:1358-65.

28. Ainsile G. Inhalational injuries produced by smoke and nitrogen dioxide. Respir Med. 1993;87:169-74.

29. Gu TL, Liou SH, Hsu CH, et al. Acute health hazards of fire fighters after fighting a department store fire. Indust Health. 1996;34:13-23.

30. Alarie Y. Toxicity of fire smoke. Crit Rev Toxicol. 2002;32:259-89.

31. Samoli E, Nastos PT, Paliatsos AG, et al. Acute effects of air pollution on pediatric asthma exacerbation: evidence of association and effect modification. Environ Res. 2011;111:418-24.

32. Raaschou-Nielsen O, Andersen ZJ, Jensen SS, et al. Traffic air pollution and mortality from cardiovascular disease and all causes: a Danish cohort study. Environ Health. 2012;11:60.

33. Wong A, Greene S, Robinson J. Metal fume fever: a case review of calls made to the Victorian Poisons Information Centre. Aust Fam Physician. 2012;41:141-4.

17

CHAPTER

Carbon Monoxide Poisoning

Ashish Bhalla, Vikas Suri, Jamshed Nayer

INTRODUCTION

Carbon monoxide (CO) is a colorless, tasteless clear gas, with a density of 0.97 that of air.

SOURCES OF CARBON MONOXIDE

Sources include burning fuel, engine exhaust, gas/coal-heater emissions, smoke from accidental fires and fumes, steel foundries, pulp paper mills/formaldehyde-producing plants. Indoor burning of charcoal/animal dung produces accidental CO intoxication.[1] Incomplete combustion in gas geysers installed in bathrooms have emerged as another important cause. Poisoning can also result from inhaling solvents, and paint removers.

MECHANISM OF CARBON MONOXIDE TOXICITY

Carbon monoxide has 250 times greater affinity for binding to hemoglobin as compared to oxygen. It displaces oxygen from oxyhemoglobin (HbO_2) and transforms it into carboxyhemoglobin (HbCO). There is resultant decreased in oxygen carrying capacity. It shifts the oxygen dissociation curve to left. This results in oxygen nonavailability to the tissues.[2] At cellular level, it acts as tissue poison as it competes with oxygen for other hemoproteins such as myoglobin, peroxidase, catalase and cytochromes. Thus oxygen dependent organs, like brain and heart, become dysfunctional from CO intoxication. It activates inflammatory processes resulting in neurological damage. They contribute to the development of systemic inflammatory response syndrome (SIRS) and delayed neurological sequelae (DNS).[3]

CLINICAL FEATURES

The clinical presentation is due to hypoxic damage to the heart and brain. The extent is dependent on concentration, duration of exposure and the level of activity of the victim at the time of exposure.

Acute Poisoning

Headache is the earliest symptom of mild to moderate toxicity. This is followed by dizziness, nausea, dyspnea and loss of muscle control. Severely intoxicated patient will have cherry pink color of the skin, nails and mucosa. Cherry red discoloration is rare and found only in severe CO poisoning, it heralds poor outcome.[4] Bright red retinal veins, flame shaped retinal hemorrhages or papilledema on fundoscopy examination can be seen. In severe cases hypotension, bradycardia, bradypnea and noncardiogenic pulmonary edema may develop.[5]

Carbon Monoxide Poisoning | 163

Table 1: Symptoms of acute CO poisoning based on blood carboxyhemoglobin levels.

Carboxyhemoglobin level	Clinical features
< 10%	Very few mainly headache
10–20%	Dyspnea on exertion, lethargy, nausea, chest pain, tightness around forehead
20–30%	Headache, irritability, fatigue, nausea, vomiting, disturbed judgment, vision and vertigo
40–50%	Severe headache, confusion and collapse
50–60%	Same as above + syncope, Cheyne-Stroke breathing, fits
60–70%	Coma, seizures, respiratory failures and death, weak, thready pulse and slow breathing
80%	Rapidly fatal

Neurologic symptoms include fatigue, malaise, or flulike symptoms, nausea, vomiting, lethargy, somnolence, difficulty in concentration, and memory, emotional liability, dizziness, paresthesias and weakness. Severe symptoms are stroke, coma, seizure, and respiratory arrest.

Cardiovascular symptoms include ischemic chest pain, palpitations from dysrhythmias, mottled skin, poor capillary refill, hypotension, and cardiac arrest (Table 1).[6]

The symptoms and signs of CO toxicity are exacerbated by circumstances that increase neurologic and myocardial oxygen demand.

Subacute Poisoning

Secondary injury from ischemia imposed by CO poisoning leads to various symptoms which manifest within a few days of exposure. These include peripheral neuropathy, skin lesions (bullae and purpuric spots), rhabdomyolysis, renal failure, non-cardiogenic pulmonary edema, multiorgan failure, disseminated intravascular coagulation, circulatory shock and renal damage in addition to above mentioned features of acute toxicity. Glycosuria and albuminuria are often present.

About 40% patients with significant CO exposure, may experience DNS after apparent recovery. DNS is more frequently seen in patients with prolonged exposure, old age and in patients who initially presented with severe symptoms like coma. Chronic headache, generalized weakness, aphasia, apraxia, disorientation, hallucinations,

extra-pyramidal syndrome, gait disturbances and incontinence are important delayed manifestations.[7] Chronic long-term low dose exposure to CO can result in development of atherosclerosis and polycythemia.

DIAGNOSIS

Diagnosis of acute CO poisoning is usually based on suggestive history supported by relevant clinical examination. The diagnosis of chronic CO intoxication and related sequelae is difficult.

Standard pulse oximetry is not adequate screening tool for CO exposure, as it does not differentiate HbCO from HbO_2. A normal PaO_2 value in venous blood in presence of hypoxia will suggest the diagnosis.[8]

Eight-wavelength pulse oximeters capable of measuring HbCO and methemoglobin are being developed. HbCO is estimated by spectrophotometry bit this facility may be available in select laboratories only.

A useful bedside test for HbCO can be performed by taking 10 mL of distilled water + 1 mL of 5% NaOH and adding 1 mL of patient's blood. Straw yellow color indicates HbCO less than 20%. If the color remains pink, it indicates HbCO is greater than 20%.

Signs and symptoms of CO injury correlate reasonably well with on the scene CO-oximetry determination of HbCO levels. However, in the emergency department (ED) predictive value of HbCO measured by CO-oximetry levels falls considerably. American College of Emergency Physicians (ACEP) recommends against using pulse CO-oximetry to diagnose CO toxicity in patients with suspected acute CO poisoning.[9]

One must perform blood counts, renal functions, metabolic profile, urinalysis, lactate, creatine kinase, ECG, cardiac enzymes and coagulation profile at the time of presentation to estimate organ damage. Imaging studies like chest radiography, CT and MRI scans may be done to assess brain damage.

TREATMENT

Prehospital Care

Secure airway, breathing, and circulation in all the seriously ill or injured victim with presumed CO intoxication. The patient should be removed promptly from the source of carbon monoxide exposure. The rescuers must take proper precautions before trying to rescue victims, especially from burning buildings, as they are also at risk.

Hospital Care

Patients with mild symptoms (nausea, headache, weakness, or flu-like malaise) should receive 100 percent oxygen for a period of about 4 hours. they should be periodically assessed for complications. The half-life of HbCO is approximately 3–4 hours while breathing room air, 60 min wile breathing 100% NBO, and 15–23 min with 100% hyperbaric oxygen (HBO) at 2.5–2.8 atmospheres of pressure.[10]

A routine patient with mild symptoms will require oxygen for 4–6 hours or until HbCO level becomes less than 5%. Noninvasive continuous positive airway pressure (CPAP) ventilation using a tight mask and an inspired fraction of oxygen (FiO$_2$) of 100% can be effective in moderate to severe CO poisoning.[11] Although there is insufficient evidence to support the use of hyperbaric oxygen for treatment of patients with carbon monoxide poisoning, but it should be tried in severe cases and in patients not showing signs of clinical improvement after 4 hours of normobaric oxygen (NBO) therapy.[12] Major symptoms (any history of loss of consciousness, profound dip in blood pressure, amnesia, or myocardial ischemia) are indications for initial HBO treatment. Dramatic improvement is usually noted in symptoms and signs. However, it is important to use high flow 100% oxygen if HBO is not available. If the patients need to be referred to an institute with HBO facility, make sure that the patient receives 100% oxygen during transit.

Coexisting cyanide toxicity should be suspected in patients rescued from burning buildings without nay response to conventional therapy.

CONCLUSION

Carbon monoxide (CO) is a colorless, odorless gas, so the exposure may not be noted by the victim. Diagnosis should be suspected in unconscious patients with possible exposure to vehicle exhausts or gas/coal/wood fires, especially in enclosed spaces. Removal of patient from the scene, 100% oxygen and/or hyperbaric oxygen will help. Patients surviving the acute insult may end up with residual neurological sequel.

KEY POINTS

- Headache is the earliest symptom, followed by dizziness, nausea, dyspnea and loss of muscle control. In severe cases hypotension, bradycardia, bradypnea and noncardiogenic pulmonary edema may develop.
- Cherry red discoloration is rare and found only in severe CO poisoning, it heralds poor outcome.
- Pulse CO-oximetry is not reliable and should not be used to diagnose CO toxicity in patients with suspected acute CO poisoning.
- Noninvasive CPAP ventilation with FiO$_2$ of 100% can be effective in moderate to severe CO poisoning.
- Hyperbaric oxygen can be tried in severe cases and in patients not showing signs of clinical improvement after 4 hours of normobaric oxygen therapy.
- Delayed neurological sequelae is more frequently seen in patients with prolonged exposure, old age and those presenting with severe symptoms like coma.

REFERENCES

1. Raub JA, Mathieu-Nolf M, Hampson NB, et al. Carbon monoxide poisoning – a public health perspective. Toxicology. 2000;145:1-14.
2. Piantadosi C. Diagnosis and treatment of carbon monoxide poisoning. Resp Care Clin North Am. 1999;5:183-202.
3. Hardy KR, Thom SR. Pathophysiology and treatment of carbon monoxide poisoning. J Toxicol Clin Toxicol. 1994;32:613-29.
4. Hampson NB, Piantadosi CA, Thom SR, et al. Practice recommendations in the diagnosis, management, and prevention of carbon monoxide poisoning. Am J Respir Crit Care Med. 2012;186:1095-101.
5. Burney RE, Wu SC, Nemiroff MJ. Mass carbon monoxide poisonings: clinical effects and results of treatment in 184 victims. Ann Emerg Med. 1982;11:394-9.
6. Penney DG. Hemodynamic response to carbon monoxide. Environ Health Perspec. 1988;77:121-30.
7. Smith JS, Brandon S. Morbidity from acute carbon monoxide poisoning at three-year follow-up. BMJ. 1973;1:318-21.
8. Hampson NB. Pulse oximetry in severe carbon monoxide poisoning. Chest. 1998;114:1036-41.
9. Wolf SJ, Maloney GE, Shih RD, et al. Clinical Policy: Critical Issues in the Evaluation and Management of Adult Patients Presenting to the Emergency Department with Acute Carbon Monoxide Poisoning. Ann Emerg Med. 2017; 69:98-107.e6.
10. Pace N, Stajman E, Walker EL. Acceleration of carbon monoxide elimination in man by high pressure oxygen. Science 1950; 111:652-4.
11. Roth D, Mayer J, Schreiber W, et al. Acute carbon monoxide poisoning treatment by non-invasive CPAP-ventilation, and by reservoir face mask: Two simultaneous cases. Am J Emerg Med. 2018 36 (9):1718.
12. Buckley NA, Juurlink DN, Isbister G, et al. Hyperbaric oxygen for carbon monoxide poisoning. Cochrane Database Syst Rev. 2011;CD002041.

SECTION 5

Cardiac Toxins

18. **Poisoning Induced Circulatory Failure**
Omender Singh, Desh Deepak

19. **Aluminum Phosphide Poisoning**
Ashish Bhalla

20. **Beta-blocker and Calcium Channel Blocker Overdose**
Saswati Sinha, Subhash Kumar Todi

21. **Sodium Channel Blockers**
Deven Juneja, Omender Singh

22. **Digoxin and Other Cardiac Glycosides**
Supradip Ghosh

18
CHAPTER

Poisoning Induced Circulatory Failure

Omender Singh, Desh Deepak

INTRODUCTION

Intensive care physicians managing critically ill poisoning patients with circulatory shock is a challenging scenario as most part of the management is derived from other guidelines of hemodynamic resuscitation and surviving sepsis campaign.[1] As contrast to well researched recommendations in surviving sepsis campaign for management of sepsis and septic shock, management of poisoning patients follows the general principles of shock management with special emphasis on toxin identification, decontamination, prescription of antidote and enhancing toxin or drug elimination along with other supportive management.[2] Most data guiding management of poisoning is biased with positive case reports and series often favoring unconventional treatment modalities.[2]

EPIDEMIOLOGY

Arrhythmias, cardiogenic shock and cardiac arrest are often the presenting and persisting symptoms with exposure of certain toxins such as cardiovascular drugs. Epidemiology of these events is varying and unpredictable, but some studies have suggested up to 17% incidence in hospitalized toxicology patients.[3] Of the cardiovascular drugs induced causes of poisoning, β-blockers and calcium channel blockers (CCBs) are the leading culprits with high mortality rates of up to 60%.[4]

List of poison or drugs associated with cardiovascular instability is exhaustive, not inclusive (Boxes 1 and 2).

PATHOPHYSIOLOGY

Poisoning patients are acted upon by variety of overlapping mechanisms leading to cardiogenic, hypovolemic or distributive shock. Oxygen supply and demand mismatch causing myocardial depression or injury is often induced by excessive central or peripheral receptors stimulation leading to intense tachyarrhythmias, hypertension, agitation, hyperthermia and inhibition of oxidative phosphorylation. Beta-adrenergic antagonism and calcium channel blockade causes decrease in cardiac contractility and systemic vascular resistance (SVR) and very often various arrhythmias leading to

---

Box 1: Agents that may lead to bradycardia.

- Beta-receptor blockers
- Calcium channel blockers
- Alpha 2-receptor agonists (e.g. clonidine, dexmedetomidine)
- Cardioactive glycosides (e.g. digoxin, fox glow, yellow oleander)
- Cholinergic agents (e.g. organophosphate compounds, carbamates)
- Potassium channel blockers (type III antiarrhythmics) (e.g. sotalol, amiodarone)
- Others like aluminum phosphide

Cardiac Toxins

Box 2: Agents that may lead to tachycardia.[5]

- Sodium channel blockers such as tricyclic antidepressants, type 1 antiarrhythmics, local anesthetics, chloroquine, quinine
- Other pharmaceuticals (e.g. theophylline)
- Drugs of abuse (e.g. amphetamines, cocaine)
- Cardioactive glycosides (e.g. digoxin, fox glow, yellow oleander)
- Natural toxins (e.g. aconitine, night-shadow plants)
- Potassium channel blockers (type III antiarrhythmics) (e.g. sotalol, amiodarone)
- Noradrenaline reuptake inhibitors (e.g. venlafaxine)
- Antiepileptics (carbamazepine, phenytoin)
- Phenothiazines (thioridazine)

decrease in cardiac output (CO). Often patient can have normal to high CO with low SVR. Several toxins have arrhythmogenic properties due to acquired QT prolongation, potassium channel blockade, and altered calcium influx or efflux. In addition, there can be relative or substantial third spacing leading to hypovolemic shock.[5]

MANAGEMENT

History and physical examination is similar to any other critically ill patients with special emphasis on revisiting the history again from relatives, previous medical records and circumstantial evidence. Follow standard airway, breathing and circulation approach of emergency management. Specific antidotes are available for very few agents, but if available, they must be administered. Poisoning patient often requires unconventional therapeutic modalities which are mostly suggested based on case reports and case series in the absence of strong data based on randomized controlled trials (RCTs).[6] Specific antidotes have been discussed in other chapters.

Attending intensive care physicians should contact toxicologist or toxicology nodal center as soon as possible in all suspected or confirmed cases of poisoning, especially if patients presents with hemodynamic instability or otherwise.

Cardiopulmonary Resuscitation

Cardiac arrest is to be managed as per Advanced Cardiac Life Support (ACLS) guidelines. But these patients often require prolonged efforts with special consideration to possible toxins.[6,7] Current research is citing some role of automated mechanical compression devices (like auto pulse) in cardiac arrest situations and it may be particularly helpful in poisoning patients where neurological outcome is expectedly good such as coexisting hypothermia. No general recommendations can be made as of now but it may be worth trying as there has been good outcome with prolonged resuscitation efforts in few case reports often with extracorporeal life support (ECLS).[8,9]

Fluid Management

As derived from sepsis guidelines, start rapid administration of 30 mL/kg intravenous crystalloids for hypotension. After fluid administration, start vasopressors to keep a mean arterial pressure (MAP) 65 mm Hg for persistent hypotension. Continued fluid therapy is guided by improvement in dynamic parameters with fluid challenges while safe guarding against the fluid overload. Assessment by echocardiography to assess type of shock is an essential step, especially if patient does not respond to initial therapy. Current literature favors use of dynamic indices such as passive leg raising, institution of prespecified fluid boluses with measurement of stroke volume (SV) or CO increase by 10–15% from baseline or improvement in indices of stroke volume variation (SVV), or pulse pressure variation (PPV), due to respiratory variation in chest cavity with mechanical ventilation.[1,10]

Vasopressors

There is no evidence to suggest one vasopressor over other in case of poisoning, unlike in sepsis patients. There is some evidence from series of case reports which suggest beneficial outcomes with norepinephrine in patients with tricyclic antidepressant (TCA) overdose.[11] Adrenergic agonist agents, despite being potent vasopressors, may be insufficient to treat hypotension in certain scenarios such as β-blocker overdose, due to overwhelming blockade of β-adrenergic receptors. Same has been observed with CCBs toxicity. At present, there is insufficient evidence to support high dose vasopressors because of the potential adverse effect with high doses.[6] The 4-aminopyridine and metaraminol have been successfully used in CCB poisonings suggesting importance of understanding physiological effects of poisons in rationalizing the appropriate supportive therapy.[12] Vasopressin or analogs acting through v1 receptors decrease norepinephrine dosages while avoiding side effects. However, they themselves can affect

Poisoning Induced Circulatory Failure

poor skin and splanchnic perfusion with thrombogenic complications. There is an evidence of benefit in severe vasodilatory shock induced by CCBs and angiotensin receptor antagonist overdosage or toxicity.[12]

Adjunctive Therapies

Hemodynamically unstable and cardiac arrested poisoning patient requires unconventional or adjunctive therapies along with standard resuscitative protocols. Such measures may include supportive medications bypassing the blocked receptors (glucagon) or supporting the depressed organ till toxin is eliminated or metabolized (extracorporeal therapies).[13] Though basic principles remain same but therapies have variation depending on whether patient's predominant presenting symptom is bradycardia or tachycardia, with or without hypotension.

Therapies for Patients Presenting with Bradyarrhythmia

Bradycardia algorithm of ACLS guidelines is a useful guide in most scenarios. In this section, we will discuss some other therapies which have resulted in good outcomes as per anecdotal reports. It is suggested to consider these along with standard algorithm of resuscitation.[6]

Atropine is standard inclusion of bradycardia treatment. It is a drug of choice to reverse bradycardia induced by organ phosphorus poisoning. But bradycardia induced by CCBs or β-blocker is seldom responsive to atropine alone. More often, it is considered as temporizing measure followed by epinephrine infusion, dopamine infusion and transvenous or transcutaneous pacing.[6,13]

Calcium chloride should be given to patients with hypotension and bradycardia due to suspected CCB or β-blocker poisoning. Calcium chloride in boluses of 20 mL (10%) every 2–5 minutes is given to achieve stable heart rate and blood pressure.[13]

Glucagon

Glucagon increases the myocardial contractility by increasing intracellular calcium pool by β-adrenergic receptors independent mechanism. It has been used successfully in β-blocker and CCBs poisoning. Till date, there is no substantial evidence in the form of RCTs

barring few case reports.[14] It is given in dose of 3–10 mg intravenously (or 0.05–0.15 mg/kg) bolus followed by an infusion of 3–5 mg/h (or 0.05–0.1 mg/kg/h); infusion is titrated to achieve adequate clinical response.[6]

It has been incorporated in several algorithms as it is a useful agent in drug-induced severe bradycardia or anaphylaxis refractory to epinephrine in patients who are on chronic β-blocker therapy.[15]

High-dose Insulin Euglycemia Therapy

High-dose insulin therapy is consistent with improved hemodynamics in calcium channel and β-blockers toxicity compared to glucagon with whom both success and failures have been reported. There is no head-to-head comparison of insulin versus glucagon. Beta-blockers and CCBs cause direct myocardial depression and their effect is pronounced with metabolic derangements of hyperglycemia, insulin deficiency and acidotic state. Insulin supplementation counters β-blocker and CCB mediated insulin deficiency improves inotropic state of myocardium and overall perfusion.[5] Point worth to note is that there is no RCT, but it has shown consistent effects in toxin-induced cardiac depression.[16] Various regimens have been tried with common mode is of giving high-dose insulin with continuous concentrated dextrose solution to maintain euglycemia with simultaneous monitoring to avoid hypoglycemia and electrolyte disturbances (Box 3).[5,17]

Lipid Emulsion Infusion

Twenty percent emulsion of free fatty acids mixture is standard treatment for local anesthetics bupivacaine

---

Box 3: High dose insulin euglycemia regimen.[5]

- Bolus of 1 U/kg of regular human insulin
- Give 0.5 g/kg of dextrose IV if blood glucose is >300–400 mg/dL (16.6–22.2 mmol/L); the dextrose bolus is withheld
- An infusion of regular insulin should follow the bolus, starting at 1 U/kg/h and titrated up to 2 U/kg/h or higher if no improvement is evident after 15–30 min
- A continuous dextrose infusion beginning at 0.5 g/kg/h should also be started
- Glucose should be monitored every half hour for the first 4-h, then 1–2 hourly. It is titrated to maintain euglycemia
- Monitor electrolytes especially potassium at least 8–12 hourly

(IV: intravenous)

toxicity. Over the period, it is being recognized as rescue for several other lipophilic cardiotoxic drugs including β-blocker and CCB.[5,18]

It is postulated that lipid emulsion traps the lipophilic toxin making them unavailable to produce end organ toxic effects.[13,19] Other mechanism cited is antagonizing calcium channels blockade and providing free fatty acid as energy source in insulin deficiency state induced by β-blocker and CCB.[5]

When indicated, a proposed regimen in cardiac arrest includes a 1.5 mL/kg bolus of 20% lipid emulsion followed by a 0.25–0.5 mL/kg/min infusion[5] (Box 4).

Currently 20% lipid emulsion is accepted as rescue therapy in patients of refractory hypotension induced by cardiotoxic drugs (Box 4).[5]

Therapies for Patients Presenting with Tachyarrhythmia

Toxicology patients presenting with tachycardia management is guided as ACLS algorithm. Therapy is mainly supportive with correction of electrolytes, correction of fluid deficits, support of blood pressure often requiring cardioversion, and defibrillation with and without antiarrhythmic agents.

Hypertonic Sodium Bicarbonate

It is considered as first choice in patients presenting with wide complex tachyarrhythmia with or without hypotension in case of suspected drug overdose or poisoning causing sodium channel block such as TCAs. Direct competitive antagonism of sodium channel blockade, serum alkalization increases drug binding to plasma proteins and decreased binding at end receptors hence resulting in controlling the toxicity and hypotension. It is given in aliquots of 1–2 mmol/kg intravenously in

---

Box 4: Lipid emulsion regimen.[5]

- Bolus of 1.5 mg/kg ideal body weight of 20% ILE to be infused over 1 min followed by an infusion of 0.25 mL/kg/min
- The bolus dose can be repeated up to two times for refractory cardiovascular collapse and the infusion dose can be doubled to 0.5 mL/kg/min for persistent hypotension
- The infusion should be continued for 10 min after stabilization of hemodynamics. The maximum dose should not exceed 10 mL/kg over the first 30 min

(ILE: intravenous lipid emulsion)

---

repeated doses to achieve stable blood pressure and rhythm is achieved. Care should be taken to avoid severe alkalemic pH of >7.5 as it compromises perfusion.[13,20,21]

Severe toxicity often warrants extracorporeal therapies to augment toxin removal by various forms of renal replacement therapy such as hemodialysis, continuous renal replacement therapies and hemadsorption often with extracorporeal membrane oxygenation (ECMO) and intra-aortic balloon pump (IABP). These are applicable for any patients of cardiovascular failure presenting with bradyarrhythmia or tachyarrhythmias with compromised perfusion.[13] Renal replacement therapies have been discussed elsewhere.

Mechanical Supportive Devices

Cardiac assist devices, cardiac pacing, IABP, cardiopulmonary bypass and ECMO should be considered in refractory hypotension depending upon local availability and expertise. Experts recommend above said therapies in toxicology patients as most toxin are likely to be eliminated from the body with supportive therapy. Optimizing perfusion in such cases by means of these supportive therapies may ultimately lead to reversal of severe cardiovascular depression and hence improved outcomes. Extracorporeal support therapies are often combined with hemodialysis, plasmapheresis and other potential techniques for enhanced removal of toxins.[12,13,22]

Intra-aortic Balloon Pump

Intra-aortic balloon pump has been used as adjunct to augment CO in overdose with quinidine, propranolol, dextropropoxyphene, antihistamines, verapamil, atenolol, and organophosphate poisoning.[12] It is not recommended in ACLS algorithms of cardiac arrest as IABP does not augment CO in no flow situations.[21] Indication to use IABP is refractory shock of cardiogenic origin without any significant rhythm disturbances. Shock trial established the role of IABP in case of acute myocardial infarction, but in recent years its use has declined in view of early institution of revascularization therapy but it still holds promise in poisoning settings where other advance supportive such as ECMO is unavailable.[21]

Cardiopulmonary Pulmonary Bypass

It is a highly invasive and labor-intensive procedure which requires opening the chest cavity and major vessels cannulation with potential complications of hemorrhage and pericardial tamponade, etc. It is possible only in operating room unlike ECMO, IABP, or cardiac pacing which are possible at bedside in intensive care units. It has also been used in few cases of aconitine, diltiazem, and verapamil poisoning.[12,22]

Extracorporeal Life Support

Currently, ECMO is considered much safer technique compared to cardiopulmonary bypass as it involves arterial and venous cannulation without any sternotomy though it is not without complications like vessel injuries, hemorrhage and risk of limb ischemia are the important ones to note from several enlisted in the literature. Major advantage of ECMO is provision of blood flows in range of 1.5 to 6 liter per minute which is adequate to maintain perfusion in all kind of hemodynamically unstable patients. There are case reports of successful use of ECMO in imipramine, desipramine, carbamazepine, propranolol, acebutolol, disopyramide, quinidine, flecainide, verapamil, diltiazem, carbamate, paroxetine, digoxin and chloroquine poisoning.[12,21]

In a retrospective cohort analysis, patients of severe shock or cardiac arrest due to poisoning were analyzed for use of ECLS versus with patients who were treated with conventional treatment. Patient treated with ECLS had significant lesser mortality compared to conventional modalities even after adjusting for confounders in multivariate analysis. Surviving of ECLS-treated patients (12/14; 86%) was significantly higher compared to the conventionally treated group (23/48; 48%).[23] Growing body of evidence points toward better survival of cardiac arrest patient in ECLS support treated patients.[24]

Though it is difficult to make recommendations, but it seems to be a good tool in experts hands in patients of severe poisoning where organ support is immensely important to rescue patient.

FUTURE THERAPIES

Biventricular Devices

There is a case report where biventricular assist device was placed in a case of refractory myocardial dysfunction in scombroid poisoning. Its role in resource poor settings seems to be uncertain especially in acute setting. But with advent of percutaneously placed ventricular device, we may see change in management suggestions.

Methylene Blue

Methylene blue is rescue drug which may be used in persistent vasodilatory shock in cases of sepsis and anaphylaxis. There have been reports of its successful use in CCBs toxicity by inhibition of nitric oxide release by inhibiting cyclic guanosine monophosphate (cGMP) production since methylene blue is a cGMP inhibitor. At present dose, indications and potential side effects in this population is unclear. Therefore, it is used in same doses as in anaphylaxis and vasopressors resistant septic shock. It is given as 1 mg/kg intravenously of 1% solution as bolus. It can be repeated once more. In future, it may add to armamentarium against CCB toxicity.[25]

Terlipressin

Terlipressin is a potent synthetic vasopressin analog which can be used as intermittent dosing pattern of 6-hour duration. It is currently accepted therapy for variceal bleed and hepatorenal syndrome. Since its action is independent of adrenergic receptors, it has been used in several cases of CCB, angiotensin converting enzyme inhibitor and TCA poisoning where normal vasopressors were ineffective. It is used in dosage of 1–2 mg intravenously as bolus then repeated dosage 4–6 hourly.[26-28] It can be considered as rescue to maintain hemodynamics in appropriate settings.

High-dose Insulin Therapy

An observational retrospective study done over 3-year period studied high-dose insulin as primary intervention with an attempt to avoid vasopressors. They included 12 patients of β-blocker, CCB, coingestions, polyingestions and TCAs. They concluded vasopressors are ineffective and often harmful in cardiotoxic shock. They also concluded that insulin act as inotrope and vasodilator. Concept of high-dose insulin as preferential therapy needs further evaluation to come to conclusions as current retrospective study was too small, heterogeneous and several therapies were instituted together making it unreliable to draw any significant conclusions.[29]

High-dose Insulin and Intravenous Lipid Emulsion Therapy

Combination of these two modalities for calcium channel and β-blocker toxicity was instituted in two heterogeneous cases with several confounding factors. Since both agents act differently, it seems worth consideration in poisoning agents of high lipid solubility. Lipids sequester the toxin while high dose of insulin provide inotropic support. Further lipids and free fatty acids act as substrate for high-dose insulin.[30]

Since medicine is ever expanding branch with new challenges in toxicology, clinical medicine innovative technique consideration while supporting with rescue therapies is current rationalized approach in poisoning patients.

CONCLUSION

Management of the hypotensive critically ill poisoning patient requires vigilant and aggressive supportive therapy to support hemodynamics often requiring extreme measures to maximize improved patient outcome. Above mentioned therapies should be considered in cases of refractory hypotension in poisoning patients.

KEY POINTS

- Start with standard resuscitation approach
- In cardiac arrest, ACLS algorithm is to be followed with special concern for toxins
- Once patients remains unresponsive to initial therapy, emergency physician should get in touch with toxicologist and intensive care physician at earliest
- Institute adjunctive therapies based on patient presenting symptoms of tachycardia with hypotension or bradycardia with hypotension along with history and examination
- If patient remains hypotensive but have probability of good outcome, offer them extracorporeal therapies especially ECMO as it will give time to decide and search for appropriate antidote or elimination agent or technique.

REFERENCES

1. Rhodes A, Evans LE, Alhazzani W, et al. Surviving Sepsis Campaign: International Guidelines for Management of Sepsis and Septic Shock: 2016. Intensive Care Med. 2017;43(3):304-77.
2. Levine M, Brooks DE, Truitt CA, et al. Toxicology in the ICU: part 1: general overview and approach to treatment. Chest. 2011;140(3):795-806.

3. Manini AF, Nelson LS, Stimmel B, et al. Incidence of adverse cardiovascular events in adults following drug overdose. Acad Emerg Med. 2012;19(7):843-9.
4. DeWitt CR, Waksman JC. Pharmacology, pathophysiology and management of calcium channel blocker and beta-blocker toxicity. Toxicol Rev. 2004;23(4):223-38.
5. Jang DH, Spyres MB, Fox L, et al. Toxin-induced cardio-vascular failure. Emerg Med Clin N Am. 2014;32:79-102
6. Vanden Hoek, Morrison LJ, Shuster M, et al. Part 12: Cardiac arrest in special situations. Circulation. 2010;2:S852-861.
7. Givens ML, O'Connell E. Toxicologic issues during cardiopulmonary resuscitation. Curr Opin Crit Care. 2007;13(3):287-93.
8. Piacentini A, Volonte' M, Rigamonti M, et al. Successful prolonged mechanical CPR in a severely poisoned hypothermic patient: a case report. Case Rep Emerg Med. 2012;2012:381798.
9. Gillart T, Loiseau S, Azarnoush K, et al. Resuscitation after three hours of cardiac arrest with severe hypothermia following a toxic coma. Ann Fr Anesth Reanim. 2008;27(6):510-3.
10. Levy MM, Evans LE, Rhodes A, et al. The Surviving Sepsis Campaign Bundle: 2018 Update. Crit Care Med. 2018;46(6):925-92.
11. Teba L, Schiebel F, Dedhia HV, et al. Beneficial effect of norepinephrine in the treatment of circulatory shock caused by tricyclic antidepressant overdose. Am J Emerg Med. 1988;6(6):566-8.
12. Eyer F. Hypotension and shock in the poisoned patient. In: Brent J, McMartin K, Phillips S (Eds). Critical Care Toxicology. Switzerland: Springer International Publishing; 2015.
13. Gunja N, Graudins A. Management of cardiac arrest following poisoning. Emerg Med Australas. 2011;23(1): 16-22.
14. Bailey B. Glucagon in beta-blocker and calcium channel blocker overdoses: a systematic review. J Toxicol Clin Toxicol. 2003;41:595-602.
15. Love JN, Sachdeva DK, Bessman ES, et al. A potential role for glucagon in the treatment of drug-induced symptomatic bradycardia. Chest. 1998;114(1):323-6.
16. Holger JS, Stellpflug SJ, Cole JB, et al. High-dose insulin: a consecutive case series in toxin-induced cardiogenic shock. Clin Toxicol (Phila). 2011;49:653-8.
17. Holger JS, Engebretsen KM, Marini JJ. High dose insulin in toxic cardiogenic shock. Clin Toxicol (Phila). 2009;47:303-7.
18. Geib AJ, Liebelt E, Manini AF. Clinical experience with intravenous lipid emulsion for drug-induced cardiovascular collapse. J Med Toxicol. 2012;8:10-4.
19. Sirianni AJ, Osterhoudt KC, Calello DP, et al. Use of lipid emulsion in the resuscitation of a patient with prolonged cardiovascular collapse after overdose of bupropion and lamotrigine. Ann Emerg Med. 2008;51:412-5, 15 e1.
20. Jamaty C, Bailey B, Larocque A, et al. Lipid emulsions in the treatment of acute poisoning: a systematic review

of human and animal studies. Clin Toxicol (Phila). 2010;48(1):1-27.

21. Baud FJ, Megarbane B, Deye N, et al. Clinical review: aggressive management and extracorporeal support for drug-induced cardiotoxicity. Crit Care. 2007;11(2):207.

22. Massetti M, Bruno P, Babatasi G, et al. Cardiopulmonary bypass and severe drug intoxication. J Thorac Cardiovasc Surg. 2000;120(2):424-5.

23. Masson R, Colas V, Parienti JJ, et al. A comparison of survival with and without extracorporeal life support treatment for severe poisoning due to drug intoxication. Resuscitation. 2012;83(11):1413-7.

24. Daubin C, Lehoux P, Ivascau C, et al. Extracorporeal life support in severe drug intoxication: a retrospective cohort study of seventeen cases. Crit Care. 2009;13(4):R138.

25. Jang DH, Nelson LS, Hoffman RS, et al. Methylene blue for distributive shock: A potential new use of an old antidote. J Med Toxicol. 2013;9:242-9.

26. Moolenaar DL, van der Oord BM, Manten A. Use of terlipressin in amitriptyline overdose. Neth J Crit Care. 2011;15(2):72-80.

27. Ragot C, Gerbaud E, Boyer A. Terlipressin in refractory shock induced by diltiazem poisoning . Am J Emerg Med. 2017;35(7):1032.e1-1032.e2.

28. Samanta S, Samanta S, Baronia AK, et al. Ramipril poisoning rescued by naloxone and terlipressin. Saudi J Anaesth. 2014;8(2):311-2.

29. Holger JS, Stellpflug SJ, Cole JB, et al. High-dose insulin: A consecutive case series in toxin-induced cardiogenic shock. Clin Toxicol. 2011;49:653-8.

30. Doepker B, Healy W, Cortez E, et al. High-dose insulin and intravenous lipid emulsion therapy for cardiogenic shock induced by intentional calcium-channel blocker and beta-blocker overdose: A case series. J Emerg Med. 2014;46:486-90.

19
CHAPTER

Aluminum Phosphide Poisoning

Ashish Bhalla

INTRODUCTION

Phosphides (aluminum, zinc, calcium and magnesium) are used worldwide as grain fumigants and are highly efficacious. Low cost, easy availability and practically no residue makes them ideal grain fumigants. On the contrary, easy availability has led to them being misused as agents of self-harm.

Aluminum phosphide (AlP) is available as greenish gray tablet of 3 g which contains 56% AlP and 44% ammonium carbonate. Each tablet is capable of liberating 1 g of phosphine gas when it comes in contact with moisture. It is also formulated in India as pellets and granules. Change in the formulation as granulated powder in pouches (10 g) is one of the important reasons for marked decrease in the mortality after overdose.

The release of phosphine (PH_3) after contact of the tablet or granules with moisture or gastric acid results in toxicity. Pure phosphine is a colorless and odorless gas. Garlicky odor is attributed to impurities such as substituted phosphines, diphosphines and arsine phosphine.[1]

PATHOPHYSIOLOGY AND TOXICODYNAMICS[2-4]

Phosphine gas is liberated when metal phosphides come in contact with water in the mucosal membranes and/or gastric acid in the stomach.

$$AlP + 3H_2O = Al\,(OH)_3 + PH_3$$
$$AlP + 3HCl = AlCl_3 + PH_3$$

There is rapid absorption from mucosa and alveolar lining. Symptoms usually appear within 30 minutes after ingestion. Nontoxic residues like phosphate and hypophosphite are excreted and can be detected in urine or feces.

Phosphine is a cellular toxin, like cyanide. The exact mechanism is not clear, but evidence suggests that it inhibits mitochondrial respiration by inhibiting mitochondrial respiratory chain. This clinically manifests as tissue hypoxia and resultant metabolic acidosis.

Phosphine causes generation of highly reactive free radicals which result is widespread damage to cellular membranes. This interferes with protein synthesis and enzymatic function leading to cell death and organ failure.

Toxic Dose

A concentration of 50 ppm can lead to immediate threat to life, and exposure over 600 ppm for 30 minutes is generally fatal. Accidental exposure to higher concentrations has been reported in grain silos, ship hulls and warehouses. Death has been reported following ingestion of as little as 4 g of zinc phosphide or 500 mg of AlP.

CLINICAL PRESENTATION[1,5-9]

The clinical features depend on the route, the dose and the interval between ingestion and presentation. Toxicity following inhalation is difficult to diagnose clinically. The exposure may not be evident but the smell of rotten eggs or a garlic-like odor may be noted by patients. After exposure to gas cough and breathlessness are generally reported, gastrointestinal (GI) symptoms like nausea and vomiting are common. Chest tightness, dizziness, diplopia, weakness, paresthesias and tremors are also reported after ingestion but may be observed after large exposure to phosphine gas. Some patients may report hematemesis at presentation due to ulceration in esophagus. These patients can go on to develop esophageal strictures later.

In severe poisoning, GI manifestations are severe, and refractory hypotension, tachypnea and shock invariably develops faster. Oliguria and adult respiratory distress syndrome are common in severely hypotensive patients. Cardiac dysrhythmias are a hallmark and all kinds of rhythm disturbances may be noted. If the patient survives the acute phase, signs of capillary leak may develop. Other complications like disseminated intravascular coagulation, intravascular hemolysis, fulminant hepatic and heart failure have been reported.

The majority of deaths occur within the first 12–24 hours after ingestion. Refractory cardiogenic shock and dysrhythmias are responsible for mortality. Deaths after 24 hours after exposure are likely related to acute respiratory distress syndrome (ARDS), liver failure, renal failure or other complications.

DIAGNOSIS

The diagnosis of toxicity is mainly clinical. High index of suspicion with history of ingestion is important. The classic triad of hypotension, severe metabolic acidosis, and cardiac arrhythmia should raise the suspicion of phosphine toxicity. Garlicky odor on the breath is hallmark but may be difficult to appreciate.

The diagnosis can be confirmed by detection of phosphine in exhaled air or stomach aspirate using the silver nitrate test. Phosphine in breath can be detected using phosphine detector tubes and gas chromatography but is technically challenging and expensive.

LABORATORY WORKUP

Severe metabolic acidosis on arterial blood gas (ABG), in the presence of hypotension and arrhythmia should raise suspicion of the poisoning. ABG analysis reveals metabolic acidosis with respiratory alkalosis.

Investigations are aimed at detecting organ system dysfunction. Chest X-ray, electrocardiogram (ECG) and routine biochemistry is ordered to rule out ARDS, aspiration pneumonitis, dysrhythmias, electrolyte abnormality and acute kidney injury. In patients with moderate to severe toxicity arrhythmia can be observed on cardiac monitor. ECG findings of diffuse ST-segment elevation/depression are suggestive of toxic myocarditis.[10] Arrhythmias are evident in 10–20% patients. Conduction blocks at the level of sinus node, atrioventricular node, bundle of His or ventricle are common.[10] Bed side echocardiography can be particularly useful in detecting hypokinesia of left ventricle (LV), LV dilatation and low ejection fraction.

Serum electrolytes, blood sugar, liver, and kidney function tests are done at baseline and need to be repeated periodically. Hypokalemia can be dangerous and may potentiate arrhythmia.

Magnesium levels are variable and do not help in guiding the clinical management.

TREATMENT

Early recognition and management of poisoning is essential. Young patients presenting with severe metabolic acidosis and hypotension with high central venous pressure (CVP) should be suspected of having significant toxicity. The aim of therapy is to reverse metabolic acidosis and treat shock to maintain organ perfusion.

Gastric Decontamination

With Potassium permanganate (1:10,000), is known to oxidize phosphine and may be beneficial if done within the first hour of ingestion. However, there is no evidence that gastric lavage improves outcome in poisoned patients. Lavage may be associated with complications including in an agitated or obtunded patient and should be carefully planned after securing the airway.

It is difficult to retard phosphine absorption by any means. Administration of activated charcoal has not shown any benefit, although a theoretical possibility of phosphine adsorption is strong.

Administration of coconut oil/paraffin is potentially a risk factor for aspiration in an agitated/comatose patient, it cannot be recommended.

In the absence of any specific antidote, management remains largely supportive. Ventilation for respiratory distress, management of electrolyte abnormalities and

Cardiac Toxins

recognition/management of hypoglycemia is important. Severe acidosis is an important cause of significant myocardial depression and needs to be reversed.

The primary aim is early recognition and aggressive treatment of shock. Administration of fluids has not improved outcomes and should be avoided. One must use intravenous fluids judiciously under strict monitoring of CVP or inferior vena cava (IVC) diameter. Norepinephrine and vasopressin help maintain blood pressure and improve peripheral perfusion. Dopamine or dobutamine administration is not recommended as they may induce cardiac dysrhythmias.

Administration of steroids does not result in improved mortality and is not recommended.

Magnesium sulfate has been used in to prevent dysrhythmias and has antioxidant effects to combat free radical mediated injury. Although dysrhythmia improves yet, mortality is not affected. Amiodarone has been tried but causes severe hypotension, therefore should be avoided.

Early and effective management of metabolic acidosis can be accomplished with the administration of sodium bicarbonate infusion. Aim is to maintain serum bicarbonate level at 18–20 mmol/L and pH more than 7.1. In refractory acidosis, hemodialysis can be initiated, however, it may worsen the hypotension. Continuous venovenous hemofiltration (CVVH) may result in lesser hemodynamic compromise, thus can be used.

N-acetylcysteine (NAC) has shown conflicting results in two different human studies hence, presently cannot be recommended.[11,12] Glucose-insulin and potassium (GIK) infusion administered to produce hyperinsulinemic euglycemia has shown encouraging results. It benefits poisoned patients by providing energy, restoring calcium influx and increasing myocardial contractility. It is a promising new intervention and has shown no significant adverse effects.

Hemodynamic support to failing heart with an intra-aortic balloon pump and extracorporeal membrane oxygenation (ECMO) has shown benefit. These therapies have significant drawbacks, including high cost, limited availability. If available, these modalities may be tried.

In the case of an inhalational exposure to phosphine gas, removal from the source and administration of oxygen has been sufficient therapy in the majority of the cases. The remainder of treatment is guided by the clinical condition of the patient.

PROGNOSIS

Mortality is variable, ranging between 37% and 100%, depending on the severity.[5,8,9,11] Consumption of fresh tablet, severe metabolic acidosis, refractory hypotension, and ARDS are associated with increased mortality in ALP poisoning. A large number of clinical, biochemical parameters and a critical care scoring systems have been evaluated as predictors of mortality in AlP poisoning. However, low arterial pH (<7.2), low sodium bicarbonate levels, hypotension (systolic blood pressure <90 mm Hg) and altered mental status have been observed by many authors as predictors of poor prognosis.

CONCLUSION

Aluminum phosphide poisoning remains a major cause of mortality in patients attempting self harm in India. The diagnosis is clinical and management is generally supportive. Recently, insulin euglycemia and extracorporeal membrane oxygenation (ECMO) has shown promising results. However, lack of conclusive evidence and high cost are important deterrents in recommending these interventions as standard of care.

KEY POINTS

- Aluminum phsophide is an excellent, safe and cheap rhodenticide
- It is very effective in getting rid of pests as phosphine leaves no toxic residue on grain
- It is an important agent used by patients contemplating self harm. Easy availability and low cost makes it as one of the most sought after agent for self harm
- Ingestion is the commonest mode but increasingly inhalation of toxic gas is being reported worldwide.
- Diagnosis is mainly clinical. Gastrointestinal symptoms followed by hypotension and metabolic acidosis are classical symptoms
- Treatment is mainly aimed at supporting the failing heart along with other supportive treatment. Magnesium sulfate, sodium bicarbonate and inotropic support for heart are the mainstay of treatment. Insulin euglycemia and ECMO are important emerging therapies.

REFERENCES

1. Gupta S, Ahlawat SK. Aluminium phosphide poisoning: a review. J Toxicol Clin Toxicol. 1995;33:19-24.
2. Chugh SN, Mittal A, Seth S, et al. Lipid peroxidation in acute aluminium poisoning. J Assoc Physicians India. 1995;43:265-6.
3. Dua R, Gill KD. Aluminum phosphide exposure: implications on rat brain lipid peroxidation and

anti-oxidant defence system. Pharmacol Toxicol. 2001;89:315-9.

4. Dua R, Gill KD. Effect of aluminium phosphide exposure on kinetic properties of cytochrome oxidase and mitochondrial energy metabolism in rat brain. Biochim Biophys Acta. 2004;1674:4-11.

5. Murali R, Bhalla A, Singh D, et al. Acute poisoning: 15 year experience of a large north-west Indian hospital. Clin Toxicol (Phila). 2009;47:35-8.

6. Singh S, Dilawari JB, Vashist R, et al. Aluminium phosphide ingestion. Br Med J. 1985;290:1110-1.

7. Singh S, Bhalla A, Verma SK et al. Cytochrome-c oxidase inhibition in 26 aluminum phosphide poisoned patients. Clin Toxicol. 2006:44(2):155-8.

8. Siwach SB, Yadav DR, Arora B, et al. Acute aluminium phosphide poisoning. An epidemiological, clinical and histopathological study. J Assoc Physc India. 1988;36:594-6.

9. Shadnia S, Mehrpour O, Soltaninejad S. A simplified acute physiology score in the prediction of acute aluminum phosphide poisoning outcome. Indian J Medical Sci. 2010;64:532-5.

10. Chugh SN, Chugh K, Ram S, et al. Electrocardiographic abnormalities in aluminium phosphide poisoning with special reference to its incidence, pathogenesis, mortality and histopathology. J Indian Med Assoc. 1991; 89:32-5.

11. Bhalla A, Jyotinath P, Singh S, et al. Antioxidant therapy in patients with severe aluminium phosphide poisoning—a pilot study. Indian J Crit Care Med. 2017;21(12): 836-40.

12. Tehrani H, Halvaie Z, Shadnia S, et al. Protective effects of N acetyl cysteine on aluminium phosphide induced oxidative stress in acute human poisoning. Clin Toxicol (Phila). 2013;51(1):23-8.

20 CHAPTER

Beta-blocker and Calcium Channel Blocker Overdose

Saswati Sinha, Subhash Kumar Todi

INTRODUCTION

Beta-blockers (BBs) and calcium channel blockers (CCB) are widely used for a myriad of conditions such as hypertension, ischemic heart disease, arrhythmias and several other disorders. Although overdose with these drugs form a minority of all poisonings, these often cause severe systemic toxicity and a high mortality.[1] They often present as bradycardia, hypotension, and myocardial depression and some CCBs cause profound vasodilatory shock. Management follows the similar principles and requires a multimodal approach guided by careful hemodynamic assessment to ascertain the pathophysiology thereby guiding choice of the most appropriate therapy.

PHARMACOLOGY

Beta-blockers

There are three types of beta receptors:
1. *Beta 1:* It is primarily found in cardiac muscle and activation mediates increase in heart rate, atrioventricular (AV) conduction, contractility and decreases refractoriness of AV node
2. *Beta 2:* It is present in bronchial and peripheral smooth muscles predominantly and activation causes bronchodilation and vasodilation. They are also found in cardiac muscle

3. *Beta 3:* It is found in the heart and adipose tissue and activation causes depressed contractility and mediates thermogenesis.[2]

Calcium Channel Blockers

There are two major categories of CCBs.
1. *Dihydropyridines*: Block L-type calcium channels in peripheral vasculature, e.g. nifedipine, amlodipine, felodipine, nicardipine and isradipine which are potent vasodilators but have negligible effect on cardiac contractility or AV conduction.
2. *Nondihydropyridines*: Block L-type calcium channels in myocardium, e.g. verapamil and diltiazem and depress cardiac contractility and also affect conduction and pacemaker cells but are weak vasodilators (Table 1).

CLINICAL FEATURES

History

It should include:
- The agent—immediate or sustained release
- Possibility of coingestion of other drugs
- Timing of ingestion
- Pre-existing cardiac disorder.

Identification of overdose with sustained-release pre-parations will help decide the role of gastrointestinal (GI)

Beta-blocker and Calcium Channel Blocker Overdose

Table 1: Common clinical effects in calcium channel blocker and beta-blocker toxicity.

	Heart rate	AV conduction	QRS duration	Cardiac contractility	Systemic vascular resistance	Side effects
Beta-blocker	Decreased	Slow 1st, 2nd, 3rd degree AV block	Unchanged	Decreased	Unchanged or increased	Seizures, coma, hypoglycemia
BB with MSA	Decreased	Same as BB	Unchanged or increased	Decreased	Same as BB	Same as BB
Verapamil/diltiazem	Decreased	Asystole	Unchanged	Decreased	Increased or decreased	Hyperglycemia
Dihydropyridine CCB	Unchanged or increased	Uncommon	Unchanged	Unchanged or increased	Decreased	Seizures, lactic acidosis

(AV: atrioventricular; BB: beta-blocker; CCB: calcium channel blocker; MSA: membrane stabilizing activity)

decontamination. Specific agents like membrane-stabilizing agents may predict certain dysrhythmias like ventricular arrhythmias, e.g. propranolol, sotalol.

Physical Examination

Most common features include hypotension and bradycardia except in case of dihydropyridine CCBs like nifedipine, which might cause reflex tachycardia. However in severe overdose, even nifedipine might cause hypotension with bradycardia progressing to cardiogenic shock.

Mental status often remains clear even in the face of profound hypotension especially in CCB overdose likely due to their neuroprotective effect. However in case of severe shock, mental status impairment might occur leading to seizures, delirium and coma, especially with lipid soluble drugs like propranolol which diffuse readily across the blood brain barrier.

Beta-blockers overdose might present with hypoglycemia and bronchospasm. CCB overdose might present with hyperglycemia due to inhibition of calcium mediated insulin release.

Laboratory Evaluation

- *Electrocardiography (ECG):* Findings are bradycardia, PR prolongation, and tachycardia in dihydropyridine CCB; QRS prolongation in membrane-stabilizing agents; and QTc prolongation in case of sotalol. In severe poisoning, ECG may show severe dysrhythmia and may progress to systole

- *Capillary blood glucose:* Hypoglycemia in BB, hyperglycemia in CCBs
- *Biochemistry:* Blood urea, creatinine, electrolytes, calcium
- Chest X-ray in case of clinical features of pulmonary edema
- Serum lactate predict life-threatening poisoning (>3 mmol/L—poor prognosis).[3]

MANAGEMENT PRINCIPLES

Patients with BB or CCB overdose who present in shock need to be managed in the intensive care unit. Overdose with sustained-release preparations often have delayed toxicity and will need to be observed in a monitored unit for a period of 24 hours, even if asymptomatic on admission.

Gastrointestinal Decontamination

Gastrointestinal decontamination should be instituted in all patients with overdose of immediate-release preparations. Patients should receive one dose of activated charcoal (50 g; 1 g/kg in children) within 4 hours of ingestion. In case of depressed mental status, activated charcoal should be avoided to prevent aspiration unless the airway is protected.

If the overdose involves confirmed or suspected sustained-release preparations, whole bowel irrigation (WBI) using polyethylene glycol-based preparations[4] at the rate of 2 L/h (500 mL/h in children) until rectal effluent is clear[5,6] should be used before symptom onset as

Cardiac Toxins

hypotension and bradycardia coincides with depressed GI function and ileus and WBI should be avoided at this stage.

Initial Treatment and Resuscitation

As for all critically ill patients, initial assessment and stabilization of the airway and breathing is the priority. In hypotensive patients, initial fluid resuscitation of 1–2 L of crystalloid bolus may be administered, examining closely for volume overload.

If patient has symptomatic bradycardia or conduction disturbances, intravenous (IV) atropine maybe administered 0.5 mg every 3–5 minutes (total dose—3 mg). It may not be effective but can be tried as it is readily available and inexpensive.[7,8]

Emergent point of care echocardiography should be performed to try and ascertain the underlying mechanism of shock. Invasive assessment of cardiac output and hemodynamic parameters using pulmonary artery catheter or pulse contour cardiac output (PiCCO) measurement maybe indicated in patients with shock. This will usually guide the choice of the most appropriate vasoactive agent.

Specific Therapeutic Interventions

Although several specific interventions exist and can be implemented serially and next intervention can be chosen based on the response, often the severely poisoned are so unstable that several interventions might need to be instituted simultaneously.

The interventions include:
- Intravenous glucagon
- Intravenous calcium
- Intravenous high-dose insulin—dextrose
- Vasopressors
- Intravenous lipid emulsion (ILE)
- Pacemaker
- Extracorporeal therapies.

Intravenous Glucagon

Glucagon produces positive inotropic and chronotropic actions on cardiac muscle mediated through glucagon receptor which increases cyclic adenosine monophosphate (cAMP) independent of beta-adrenergic receptors. It improves the heart rate but has no significant effect on blood pressure.[9]

Onset of action takes a few minutes and persists for 10–15 minutes.[10] Due to the short half-life, an infusion need to be started following a loading dose. The recommended loading dose is 5–10 mg followed by 1–10 mg/h. Adverse effects include nausea, vomiting, and tachyphylaxis. Glucagon might not be available in sufficient amounts and is expensive. Hence, other agents like high-dose Insulin therapy and vasopressors are preferred over glucagon.

Intravenous Calcium

Intravenous calcium is recommended as a first-line agent in CCB and also BB toxicity based on improvement in blood pressure and cardiac output in case series.[11-14] It does not affect the heart rate. Both calcium chloride and calcium gluconate may be used.

Calcium chloride: About 10 mL of a 10% solution (1 g) should be administered via a central venous catheter. It may be repeated every 10–20 minutes to a total of 3 gram or an infusion of 0.2–0.4 mL/kg/h.

Calcium gluconate: It can be administered via a secure peripheral vein. Initial dose of 30 mL of 10% solution (3 g) followed by infusion of 0.6–1.2 mL/kg/h.[11]

Serial monitoring of serum calcium concentrations is advised to prevent iatrogenic severe hypercalcemia.

Calcium infusions alone are often insufficient and require combination with high-dose insulin therapy and vasopressors to improve the hemodynamics.

High-dose Insulin Euglycemic Therapy

High-dose insulin euglycemic therapy (HIET) is an exciting development in the treatment of severe CCB and BB overdose. There are several postulated mechanisms by which insulin improves cardiac contractility.

Under normal conditions, myocardial cells primarily derive energy from free fatty acid oxidation. However, in shock the energy substrate changes to carbohydrate metabolism.[15,16] In CCB induced shock, the cardiac myocytes cannot utilize carbohydrates due to hypoinsulinemia (inhibition of calcium-mediated insulin secretion) and an acquired insulin resistance.[17]

Moreover, the low cardiac output reduces further the delivery of glucose and insulin which potentiates the cycle of hypodynamic shock.[18] Hence, the shock is not only due to calcium channel antagonism but is also due to deranged carbohydrate metabolism.[19]

High-dose insulin euglycemic therapy increases the transport of glucose, lactate, and oxygen into the myocardial cells.[19] Insulin also increases inotropy mediated by phosphatidylinositol 3-kinase (PI3K).[20] It increases endothelial nitric oxide (NO) synthase activity thereby causing vasodilatation of peripheral arterioles in coronary, systemic and pulmonary vasculature and improves overall microcirculatory flow.[21]

High-dose insulin euglycemic therapy has become a first-line intervention in severely poisoned patient especially if the patient has myocardial dysfunction (depressed contractility on echocardiography or cardiac index is less than 2.2 L/min/m²). The onset of effect usually takes 15–60 minutes and failure of this effect in case series has been seen when it is instituted late. Hence, it should be started early when a large poisoning is suspected even before the hemodynamic instability is profound.[22,23]

A wide variation of dosage has been used. A bolus dose of 1 unit/kg followed by an infusion of 0.5 unit/kg/h has shown to improve hemodynamics.[20,24] Uptitration of dose up to 10 units/kg/h have demonstrated benefit. The dose needs to be titrated to a systolic BP of more than or equal to 100 mm Hg. Supplementation of IV dextrose (10–50%) is needed to maintain euglycemia. If no response is seen in 30–60 minutes, the dose needs to be increased. However, the glucose requirement does not necessarily increase with increased doses of insulin.

While preparing insulin infusion, the concentration should be prepared at 10 units/mL in order to avoid fluid overload due to high doses required.

Side effects of HIET include hypoglycemia and hypokalemia and blood glucose monitoring (every 15–30 min) for initial 4 hours until the blood glucose has stabilized between 100 and 200 mg/dL for at least 4 hours and then hourly thereafter is recommended. Serum potassium should be monitored every hour for the first 6 hours and then 4–6 hourly with a target serum potassium more than 3 mEq/L. Magnesium and phosphorus levels also need to be monitored.

There are no standardized guidelines to guide the duration of therapy and it has been used up to 96 hours. Blood glucose levels need to be monitored closely for 24 hours after stopping the insulin infusion as the insulin levels might remain high even after the infusion has ceased.[25]

Vasopressor Therapy

Vasopressor selection is guided by the type of shock. Shock in BB poisoning can be due to direct cardiac toxicity from bradyarrhythmias, conduction delays and negative inotropy, while in CCB it can be due to direct cardiac toxicity and/or vasodilatation. Identification of the predominant pathophysiology should guide the choice of vasopressor or inotropic agent.

In BB and CCB poisoning, the doses required might be very high and response might be unpredictable.[26-28] No single catecholamine has been found to be superior.[28] The goal should be to improve tissue perfusion and not just achieve a blood pressure target. Norepinephrine seems the most rational initial choice due to its strong alpha1 agonist (increase systemic vascular resistance) and moderate beta1 agonist (increase contractility) activity. Adrenaline infusion has both positive chronotropic and inotropic effects but in large doses can cause hyperglycemia, lactic acidosis and insulin resistance without improving tissue perfusion thereby worsening tissue ischemia.[19] Dobutamine, dopamine, and isoproterenol are associated with risk of paradoxical hypotension due to vasodilatation due to beta2 receptor stimulation. Vasopressin use in isolation has been discouraged due to its lack of efficacy and worsening survival in animal studies.[29] Vasopressin can cause reduced cardiac output and limb ischemia and should never be used in doses exceeding 0.04 IU/min. It may be used as adjunct in severe vasodilatory shock unresponsive to other catecholamine.[30]

Other Therapies

Phosphodiesterase inhibitors: These agents (amrinone, milrinone and enoximone) increase intracellular cAMP independent of beta-adrenergic receptors thereby improving inotropy. However, they also act on vascular smooth muscle causing vasodilatation and hypotension.[30] Due to limited experience in poisoning, these can be considered as third-line agents.

Levosimendan: It sensitizes myocardial troponin C to calcium and improves contractility. In animal models, it has improved cardiac output but does not increase blood pressure.[31] There is no clinical evidence to support its use, yet in BB and CCB overdose.

Intravenous Lipid Emulsion

Intravenous lipid emulsion was used initially in the management of local anesthetic associated systemic toxicity which was later found to be effective in cases of intoxication with other lipophilic drugs.[32,33] It has been recommended more as a rescue therapy for CCB and BB toxicity. A positive hemodynamic response might be evident within an hour of administration or even after several hours of therapy.

Although the exact mechanism of how ILE is effective in drug toxicity is unclear, several possibilities include "lipid sink" which is intravascular sequestration of the toxic drug to a intravascular lipid phase thereby decreasing the free blood concentration of the drug. This leads to redistribution of the drug from the tissues thereby reducing the drug concentration in the target tissues.[34] ILE might also provide a source of energy for the cardiac myocytes. They may also improve the contractility by increasing intracellular calcium levels. ILE has also been shown to alleviate ischemia reperfusion injury.

The dose suggested is 1.5 mL/kg of a 20% lipid emulsion followed by 0.25 mL/kg/min for 30-60 minutes with US Food and Drug Administration (FDA) recommending the maximum dose at 12.5 mL/kg in 24 hours.[35] Adverse effects include pancreatitis, lung injury, lipemic serum interfering with biochemical tests and possibility of paradoxically increasing absorption of toxic drugs from the GI tract.

Pacemaker

Pacing may be considered if there is unstable bradycardia or high-grade conduction disturbances if shock persists after the institution of first-line therapies like calcium, vasopressors and high-dose insulin therapies. Due to ease and ready availability, transcutaneous pacing might be attempted first and converted to transvenous later if effective.

Methylene Blue

Methylene blue has been used as rescue in the treatment of recalcitrant vasodilatory shock—the proposed mechanism being inhibition of NO–cyclic guanosine monophosphate (GMP) pathway and inhibiting NO synthesis which might be of benefit as certain CCBs like amlodipine enhance NO synthesis. The dose is 1–2 mg/kg as a single injection. Adverse effects include vomiting, hemolytic anemia in higher doses, and serotonin toxicity in case of coingestion of serotonergic drugs.[36] But, latest expert recommendations do not recommend this treatment (Table 2).

Table 2: Dosing recommendations for specific agents in calcium channel blocker and beta-blocker toxicity.

Agent	Recommended dosing	Remarks
Glucagon	• Loading dose: 5–10 mg (50 µg/kg in children) • Infusion: 1–10 mg/h	• Monitor glucose levels • Might cause nausea and vomiting
Calcium	• Calcium chloride 10%: 10 mL may be repeated every 10–20 minutes to total 3 g or infusion 0.2–0.4 mL/kg/hour • Calcium gluconate 10%: 30 mL or infusion 0.6–1.2 mL/kg/h	• Administer slowly • Keep ionized calcium upper level of normal • Calcium chloride only through central vein
Insulin—dextrose	• Initial bolus 1 unit/kg followed by infusion 0.5 units/kg/h. Start 10–50% dextrose 0.5 g/kg/hour. Insulin dose can be increased till 10 units/kg/h	• Target systolic blood pressure of 100 mm Hg • Regular monitoring of blood glucose (initially q 30 min) • Target sugar: 100–200 mg/dL • Monitor electrolytes
Vasopressors	• Norepinephrine most suitable initial choice • Vasopressin: Dose not more than 0.04 units/min	• Very high doses may be needed
Intravenous lipid emulsion	• 1.5 mL/kg of 20% lipid emulsion over 1 min followed by 0.25 mL/kg/min infusion. Two more boluses of 1.5 mL/kg or increasing infusion to 0.5 mL/kg/min (maximum dose 10 mL/kg)	• Look for response within 5 min
Methylene blue	• 1–2 mg/kg single dose	• Vomiting and hemolytic anemia are adverse effects

Extracorporeal Therapies (Extracorporeal Life Support)

Severe CCB and BB overdose account for around two-thirds of all deaths due to overdose with cardiotoxic medications. A small subset of patients who develop shock refractory to conventional therapies might benefit from extracorporeal therapies.[37] Extracorporeal therapies allow time for drugs to be redistributed or metabolized till the heart function recovers but are ineffective in refractory vasodilatory shock. Isolated case reports of successful management of severely poisoned cases with continuous venovenous hemodiafiltration (CVVHDF) with charcoal hemoperfusion have been reported.[38]

Expert recommendations now have recognized the utility of venoarterial–extracorporeal membrane oxygenation (ECMO) in the management of severely poisoned patients who are in cardiogenic shock or mixed shock with a significant cardiogenic component.[39] Complications include local bleeding, limb ischemia and issues related to nuances of the procedure. However, as expertise and familiarity with ECMO increases, timely initiation has shown to provide a survival benefit especially in patients refractory to maximal medical therapy.[40]

CONCLUSION

Management of life-threatening overdose with CCB and BBs is challenging. Since the pathophysiology of shock which occurs could be multifactorial, a multimodal approach to management is required based on careful hemodynamic assessment. Therapy must be individualized and multiple simultaneous interventions might be required to achieve the best possible outcome. The key lies in timely identification of nonresponders and institute extracorporeal therapies as salvage before organ failure and cardiac arrest sets in.

KEY POINTS

- Severe cases of BB and CCB overdose carry risk of high mortality especially in sustained-release ingestions when the peak toxicity might be delayed and need monitoring for at least 24 hours, even if asymptomatic at presentation
- Decontamination should be considered in patients who present within an hour of presentation making sure there is no risk of aspiration
- Shock due to these ingestions is multifactorial with varying degrees of myocardial depression, dysrhythmias and vasodilatation. Careful hemodynamic monitoring is the key to guide therapy
- High-dose insulin euglycemia therapy is recommended as a first-line therapy to be instituted early when myocardial depression is suspected. Norepinephrine is the usual first-line vasopressor
- Intravenous calcium, glucagon can confer some beneficial effects but are insufficient by themselves
- Pacemaker should be considered in case of unstable bradycardia or high-grade AV block
- Intravenous lipid emulsions should be considered as a rescue therapy in patients refractory to first-line therapies like calcium, vasopressors and high-dose insulin therapy
- Timely identification of shock refractory to maximal medical therapy especially with a cardiogenic component should be considered for timely initiation of VA-ECMO.

REFERENCES

1. DeWitt CR, Waksman JC. Pharmacology, pathophysiology and management of calcium channel blocker and b-blocker toxicity. Toxicol Rev. 2004;23:223-38.
2. Love JN, Howell JM, Litovitz TL, et al. Acute beta blocker overdose: factor associated with the development of cardiovascular morbidity. J Toxicol Clin Toxicol. 2000;38(3):275-81.
3. Mégarbane B, Deye N, Malissin I, et al. Usefulness of the serum lactate concentration for predicting mortality in acute beta-blocker poisoning. Clin Toxicol (Phila). 2010;48(10):974-8.
4. Thanacoody R, Caravati EM, Troutman B, et al. Position paper update: whole bowel irrigation for gastrointestinal decontamination of overdose patients. Clin Toxicol (Phila). 2015;53(1):5-12.
5. Tenenbein M. Position statement: whole bowel irrigation. American Academy of Clinical Toxicology; European Association of Poisons Centres and Clinical Toxicologists. J Toxicol Clin Toxicol. 1997;35(7):753-62.
6. Tenenbein M, Cohen S, Sitar DS. Whole bowel irrigation as a decontamination procedure after acute drug overdose. Arch Intern Med. 1987;147(5):905-7.
7. Gay R, Algeo S, Lee R, et al. Treatment of verapamil toxicity in intact dogs. J Clin Invest. 1986;77:1805-11.
8. Strubelt O. Antidotal treatment of the acute cardiovascular toxicity of verapamil. Acta Pharmacol Toxicol (Copenh). 1984;55:231-7.
9. Bailey B. Glucagon in beta-blocker and calcium channel blocker overdoses: a systematic review. J Toxicol Clin Toxicol. 2003;41:595-602.

10. Parmley WW, Glick G, Sonnenblick EH. Cardiovascular effects of glucagon in man. N Engl J Med. 1968;279:12-7.
11. Konca C, Yildizdas RD, Sari MY, et al. Evaluation of children poisoned with calcium channel blocker or beta blocker drugs. Turk Arch Ped. 2013;138-144.
12. Howarth DM, Dawson AH, Smith AJ, et al. Calcium channel blocking drug overdose: An Australian series. Hum Exp Toxicol. 1994;13:161-6.
13. Ramoska EA, Spiller HA, Winter M, et al. A one-year evaluation of calcium channel blocker overdoses: Toxicity and treatment. Ann Emerg Med. 1993;22:196-200.
14. Henry M, Kay MM, Viccellio P. Cardiogenic shock associated with calcium-channel and beta blockers: Reversal with intravenous calcium chloride. Am J Emerg Med. 1985;3:334-6.
15. Enyeart JJ, Price WA, Hoffman DA, et al. Profound hyperglycemia and metabolic acidosis after verapamil overdose. J Am Coll Cardiol. 1983;2:1228-31.
16. Kline JA, Leonova E, Raymond RM. Beneficial myocardial metabolic effects of insulin during verapamil toxicity in the anesthetized canine. Crit Care Med. 1995;23:1251-63.
17. Devis G, Somers G, Ban Obberghan E, et al. Calcium antagonists and islet function: inhibition of insulin release by verapamil. Diabetes. 1975;24:547-51.
18. Kern R. Are we ready to utilize insulin-glucose as routine therapy for calcium channel blocker toxicity? Int J Med Toxicol. 1998;1:23-7.
19. Kline JA, Leonova E, Williams TC, et al. Myocardial metabolism during graded intraportal verapamil infusion in awake dogs. J Cardiovasc Pharmacol. 1996;27:719-26.
20. Lewinski von D, Bruns S, Walther S, et al. Insulin causes $[Ca^{2+}]i$-dependent and $[Ca^{2+}]i$- independent positive inotropic effects in failing human myocardium. Circulation. 2005;111:2588-95.
21. Bechtel LK, Haverstick DM, Holstege CP. Verapamil toxicity dysregulates the phosphatidylinositol 3-kinase pathway. Acad Emerg Med. 2008;15:368-74.
22. Engebretsen KM, Kaczmarek KM, Morgan J, et al. High-dose insulin therapy in beta-blocker and calcium channel-blocker poisoning. Clin Toxicol (Phila). 2011;49:277-83.
23. Espinoza TR, Bryant SM, Aks SE. Hyperinsulin therapy for calcium channel antagonist poisoning: a seven-year retrospective study. Am J Ther. 2013;20:29-31.
24. Greene SL, Gawarammana I, Wood DM, et al. Relative safety of hyperinsulinaemia/euglycaemia therapy in the management of calcium channel blocker overdose: a prospective observational study. Intensive Care Med. 2007;33:2019-24.
25. Birnbaum K, Olson KR, Anderson IB, et al. Poisoning & Drug Overdose, 5th edition. New York, NY: McGraw-Hill; 2007. pp. 461-3.
26. Palatnick W, Jelic T. Emergency department management of calcium-channel blocker, beta blocker, and digoxin toxicity. Emerg Med Pract. 2014;16:1-19.
27. Levine M, Curry SC, Padilla-Jones A, et al. Critical care management of verapamil and diltiazem overdose with a focus on vasopressors: a 25-year experience at a single center. Ann Emerg Med. 2013;62:252-8
28. Kerns W. Management of beta-adrenergic blocker and calcium channel antagonist toxicity. Emerg Med Clin North Am. 2007;25:309-31.
29. Barry JD, Durkovich D, Cantrell L, et al: Vasopressin treatment of verapamil toxicity in the porcine model. J Med Toxicol. 2005;1:3-10.
30. Hollenberg SM. Vasoactive drugs in circulatory shock. Am J Respir Crit Care Med. 2011;183:847-55.
31. Ajiro Y, Hagiwara N, Katsube Y, et al. Levosimendan increases L-type Ca(2+) current via phosphodiesterase-3 inhibition in human cardiac myocytes. Eur J Pharmacol. 2002;435:27-33.
32. Cave G, Harvey M. Intravenous lipid emulsion as antidote beyond local anesthetic toxicity: a systematic review. Acad Emerg Med. 2009;16:815-24.
33. Ozcan MS, Weinberg G. Intravenous lipid emulsion for the treatment of drug toxicity. J Intensive Care Med. 2014;29:59-70.
34. Weinberg G. Lipid rescue resuscitation from local anaesthetic cardiac toxicity. Toxicol Rev. 2006;25:139-45.
35. Neal JM, Bernards CM, Butterworth JF, et al. ASRA practice advisory on local anesthetic systemic toxicity. Reg Anesth Pain Med. 2010;35:152-61.
36. Ramsay RR, Dunford C, Gillman PK. Methylene blue and serotonin toxicity: inhibition of monoamine oxidase A (MAO A) confirms a theoretical prediction. Br J Pharmacol. 2007;152:946-51.
37. Albertson TE, Dawson A, de Latorre F, et al. TOX-ACLS: Toxicologic-oriented advanced cardiac life support. Ann Emerg Med. 2001(4 Suppl);37:S78-90.
38. Nasa P, Singh A, Juneja D, et al. Continuous venovenous hemodiafiltration along WITH Charcoal hemoperfusion for the management of life threatening lercanidipine and amlodipine overdose. Saudi J Kidney Dis Transpl. 2014;25(6):1255-8.
39. St-Onge M, Anseeuw K, Cantrell FL, et al. Experts consensus recommendations for the management of calcium channel blocker poisoning in adults. Crit Care Med. 2017;45:e306-e315.
40. Vignesh C, Kumar M, Venkataraman R, et al. Extracorporeal membrane oxygenation in drug overdose: A clinical case series. Indian J Crit Care Med. 2018;22:111-5.

21
CHAPTER

Sodium Channel Blockers

Deven Juneja, Omender Singh

INTRODUCTION

Sodium-channel blockers (SCBs) are drugs which act by slowing the influx of sodium through the voltage-gated channels into the myocytes. Many substances have been shown to be having these sodium-channel blocking properties and several other agents may exhibit this property in overdose (Table 1).[1-3] Among these substances, tricyclic antidepressants (TCAs) and antiarrhythmic drugs belonging to the Vaughan Williams class IC are most commonly implicated agents in SCB poisoning.[4]

The voltage-gated sodium channels cause depolarization of the sodium-dependent myocardial cells located in the atria, ventricles, and His-Purkinje fibers. This causes a conformational change leading to rapid opening of the channel and the subsequent massive sodium influx termed as "phase 0". The SCBs bind to these transmembrane channels and reduce their availability for depolarization, causing a delay in the "phase 0" and slowing in the conduction of atria, ventricles, and His-Purkinje fibers. This has been termed as "quinidine-like effect".[5,6] In the calcium-dependent cells, these SCBs cause slowing of depolarization during the phase 4 although at high doses, some SCBs like lidocaine and quinidine may cause direct blockade of the calcium channels.[1,7]

The toxicity of SCBs can be potentially life-threatening and these patients may present with a varied clinical presentation which depends on the involved

Table 1: Sodium channel blocking agents.

- Tricyclic antidepressants (most common)
- Local anesthetics (bupivacaine, ropivacaine)
- Anti-arrhythmics
  - Type IA (quinidine, procainamide)
  - Type IC (flecainide, encainide)
  - Type II (propranolol)
  - Type IV (diltiazem and verapamil)
- Antimalarials (chloroquine, hydroxychloroquine, quinine)
- Antihistamines (diphenhydramine)
- Antipsychotics (phenothiazines)
- Cocaine
- Carbamazepine (in very high doses)
- Dextropropoxyphene
- Thioridazine
- Insecticides: indoxacarb and metaflumizone
- Toxins: saxitoxin and tetrodotoxin

pharmaceutical agent.[1,8] However, the basic management principles remain the same and treatment is largely symptomatic.

TRICYCLIC ANTIDEPRESSANTS

Tricyclic antidepressants have been used clinically to manage depression since the 1950s. With the

Cardiac Toxins

development of newer antidepressants, their use has reduced over the years. However, these agents are still being used in the management of several other clinical conditions like chronic or neuropathic pain, major depressive disorder, obsessive-compulsive disorders (OCDs), attention deficit hyperactivity disorder (ADHD), and nocturnal enuresis.[9-11] Commonly used TCAs are given in Table 2.

Their antidepressant effect is due to inhibition of presynaptic serotonin reuptake and norepinephrine. There is also competitive inhibition of muscarinic and alpha-adrenergic receptors along with histamine inhibition, along with antagonism of the gamma-aminobutyric acid type A (GABA$_A$) receptors. TCAs also have type IA antiarrhythmic properties secondary to blockade of cardiac sodium channels.

Tricyclic antidepressants have been recognized as one of the most common agents ingested in cases of self-poisoning. Rather, they have been shown to be the second most common cause of fatal drug overdose, after analgesics.[12,13] Among the various TCAs, dothiepin and amitriptyline have comparatively higher toxicity and are most commonly involved in fatal overdoses and dothiepin, is more like to cause seizures as compared to other TCAs.[14,15]

Toxicokinetics

Tricyclic antidepressants have a narrow therapeutic index and hence toxicity is common. Even though TCAs are absorbed rapidly from the gastrointestinal tract (GIT), the time to achieve peak drug level is delayed because TCAs cause decreased GIT motility due to their anticholinergic effects.[16] TCAs have a large volume of distribution (Vd) and are highly protein bound. They achieve high

Table 2: Commonly used tricyclic antidepressants.

Amitriptyline
Amoxapine
Clomipramine
Desipramine
Dothiepin
Doxepin
Imipramine
Maprotiline
Nortriptyline
Protriptyline
Trimipramine

concentration, up to 40–200 times more than the plasma, in the myocardium and the brain.[17] TCAs also have a high endogenous clearance, and undergo first-pass metabolism in the liver producing metabolites which are ultimately excreted in the urine.[17,18] The primary drug and its active metabolites, both undergo enterohepatic recirculation, which also prolongs the elimination time.

Clinical Features

There is a significant morbidity and mortality associated with TCA overdose. TCAs are responsible for more than 50% mortality associated with antidepressant overdose.[19] The clinical features associated with TCA toxicity may be classically divided into anticholinergic, cardiovascular and central nervous system effects (Table 3).

Anticholinergic Effects

These effects are common in TCA toxicity and can even aid in making a diagnosis. These effects are generally

Table 3: Clinical features of tricyclic antidepressant toxicity.

Anticholinergic effects	Blurred vision Dilated pupils Dry flushed skin Dry mouth Hyperthermia Ileus Mydriasis Myoclonic twitching Toxic megacolon Urinary retention
Cardiovascular system	Asystole Cardiogenic shock Heart block Hypotension Prolonged PR/QRS/QT Sinus tachycardia ST/T wave changes Tachycardia Vasodilatation Ventricular fibrillation/tachycardia
Central nervous system	Agitation Coma Delirium Drowsiness Ophthalmoplegia Pyramidal signs Respiratory depression Rigidity Seizures

Sodium Channel Blockers

mild but potentially serious complications like toxic megacolon and intestinal perforation have been also been reported.[20,21]

Due to its antihistaminic and anticholinergic properties, patients with TCA overdose may develop altered mental status which may present as agitation, sedation, delirium, or coma. Other anticholinergic symptoms include tachycardia, dry flushed skin, hyperthermia, mydriasis, ileus, and urinary retention. Patients may also develop seizures due to anticholinergic and $GABA_A$ antagonism.

Cardiovascular Effects

Cardiovascular effects like tachycardia, hypotension, and peripheral vasodilation are secondary to muscarinic and alpha-adrenergic blockade. Among the cardiovascular effects, sinus tachycardia is most commonly reported. It may be secondary to inhibition of norepinephrine reuptake or due to the anticholinergic properties of TCA.

The TCAs inhibit the sodium current leading to slowing of depolarization of the cardiac action potential. This further causes delay in propagation of depolarization through the myocardium, as well as the conducting tissue, leading to prolongation of the QRS complex and the PR/QT intervals predisposing the patient to development of cardiac arrhythmias.[22] This sodium channel inhibition in the myocardial cells may cause depressed contractility[23,24] which along with reduction in peripheral resistance, may contribute to hypotension. The reported incidence of serious arrhythmias is low[25] but hypotension may occur in up to 50% of the patients.[26]

Death is generally secondary to cardiac complications like AV conduction disturbances, wide complex arrhythmias, and myocardial depression. Death generally occurs within the first few hours of consumption and many patients die even before they reach the hospital.[27,28]

Central Nervous System Effects

Coma is common in these patients and may be present in up to 17%[29] of patients. Incidence of coma is more than 50% among patients with fatal outcomes.[27] Seizures are relatively rare complications and the reported incidence of seizures among TCA toxicity patients admitted in intensive care units (ICUs) is 6.2%.[30]

Diagnosis

There is no specific toxidrome to aid in diagnosis of TCA toxicity. Apart from the basic laboratory tests including complete blood counts, liver and kidney function tests, other tests may also be required, especially the electrocardiogram (ECG) and the arterial blood gas (ABG) analysis.

Among the metabolic complications, acidosis is most commonly present. Hypotension leading to reduced tissue perfusion and hyperlactatemia, along with respiratory depression, contribute to acidosis which is mixed acidosis having both respiratory and metabolic components.[31] Hypokalemia may also be present in several patients.[32]

Electrocardiography

On obtaining an ECG, hallmarks of TCA sodium channel blockade may be identified. The principal change in the ECG is widening of the QRS complex. The QRS complexes may rarely take the pattern of bundle branch blocks.[33] In cases of severe toxicity, the widening of QRS may become profound making it difficult to differentiate it from supraventricular and ventricular rhythms.

The common ECG changes associated with SCBs toxicity are given in Table 4.[34] Even though sinus tachycardia is more common because of anticholinergic

Table 4: Electrocardiogram changes associated with sodium channel blockade.
Sinus tachycardia
Interventricular conduction delay—prolonged QRS >100 ms in lead II
Right axis deviation of the terminal QRS: • Terminal R wave > 3 mm in aVR • R/S ratio > 0.7 in aVR
Tall R wave in aVR
Intraventricular conduction delay
QT prolongation
Abnormal QRS morphology (deep slurred S wave in I and aVL)
Brugada pattern • *Type 1:* Coved ST-segment elevation more than 2 mm in more than 1 of V1–V3 followed by a negative T wave • *Type 2:* Saddleback ST-segment elevated by >1 mm • *Type 3:* ST-segment elevated by >1 mm
Sinus bradycardia

Cardiac Toxins

and/or adrenergic effects of TCAs, sinus bradycardia may also occur due to the slowing of depolarization in the sinoatrial (SA) node. Presence of bradycardia is an indicator of severe sodium channel blockade which overshadows the chronotropic response secondary to muscarinic antagonism.[1] Other SCB agents like class IC antiarrhythmic drugs, which do not have these antimuscarinic effects, are more likely to cause bradyarrhythmias, including junctional or ventricular escape rhythms and may ultimately cause asystole.[35,36]

Treatment

Presence of arrhythmias, seizures, hypotension or altered mental status will require ICU admission. Among these symptoms, life-threatening arrhythmias are rare findings, but seizures, coma, and hypotension may frequently complicate clinical picture.[18,25,31] However, it may be challenging to predict which patient may have a poor outcome. Even though, a dose of 5–20 mg/kg is considered to be a toxic dose, it may not correlate with clinical outcomes.[28,37] In addition, predictors of poor outcomes are not clearly defined. Even serum concentrations do not correlate with the ECG findings.

Electrocardiogram changes have been shown to be better predictor of clinical outcomes than serum TCA concentration. In particular, duration of QRS or an R wave of more than 3 mm in aVR can predict development of ventricular arrhythmia and seizures.[38,39] Duration of QRS more than 100 ms has been shown to be predictive of seizures and duration more than 160 ms predictive of ventricular tachycardia.[39]

Most of the major complications of TCA toxicity occur within 6 hours of its consumption[40,41] and late complications are rare.[42,43]

General Measures

Gastric lavage or aspiration can be attempted if the patient presents within 1 hour of consumption of TCAs. Activated charcoal may be useful in decreasing the GIT absorption of TCAs and should be attempted after ensuring airway protection. Multiple-dose activated charcoal (MDAC) has also been shown to be effective as the GIT absorption of TCAs may be slow and there may be significant enterohepatic recirculation in cases of overdose.[44,45]

Sodium Bicarbonate

Sodium bicarbonate is indicated in the treatment of TCA toxicity. Sodium bicarbonate may be effective in resolving hypotension and QRS prolongation in majority of patients.[46] It may improve hypotension by volume and sodium loading and it also improves conduction of the myocardium by sodium loading and induction of alkalosis.[47] Alkalosis may potentially benefit by increasing the protein binding of the drug, thereby reducing its effective concentration and may also alter the charge of the TCA-receptor complex.[48,49]

Similarly, in patients on mechanical ventilation, alkalosis by hyperventilation may also be effective in reversing hypotension and improving myocardial conduction.[50] However, combined use of hyperventilation and sodium bicarbonate can lead to profound alkalosis and result in poorer outcomes, and hence should be avoided.[51]

Sodium bicarbonate is effective even in the absence of acidosis[52] and hence, it remains the mainstay of treatment in patients with TCA toxicity, especially those who present with life-threatening complications like fluid-unresponsive hypotension, seizures or ECG findings of prolonged QRS (>100 ms), prominent R waves in aVR or ventricular arrhythmias.[53] However, there are certain adverse effects associated with prolonged sodium bicarbonate treatment which include, fluid overload, hypocalcemia, hypokalemia and impairment of oxygen delivery by leftward shifting of the oxyhemoglobin dissociation curve.

The exact dose and length of therapy with hypertonic saline is not well-defined. However, it is generally accepted to administer a bolus dose of 1 mEq/kg of hypertonic sodium bicarbonate followed by an infusion of 15–20 mEq/hr. This dose may be effective in obtaining and maintaining a target pH of 7.50–7.60, without causing any significant rise in serum sodium levels. Caution must be exercised if this therapy is combined with hyperventilation, and it is imperative to avoid severe alkalemia (serum pH >7.60).[54]

Antiarrhythmic Treatment

Specific antiarrhythmic drugs should be avoided as correction of acidosis and hypotension is sufficient to reduce the cardiotoxic effects of TCAs in most patients. Even when they are required, certain antiarrhythmic drugs should not be used as they may exacerbate cardiotoxic effects of TCAs.

Sodium Channel Blockers

Drugs belonging to class 1A like quinidine, procainamide, and disopyramide and class 1C like flecainide also prolong cardiac depolarization similar to TCAs. Similarly, drugs belonging to class 3 like bretylium and amiodarone, which also prolong the QT interval, should be avoided, as they may also predispose to arrhythmias.

Lignocaine (lidocaine) has been shown to be effective in the management of frequent ventricular ectopics secondary to TCA overdose.[26] Phenytoin, which is a class 1B antiarrhythmic agent, is another drug which has shown some efficacy in management of ventricular arrhythmias in TCA toxicity.[55]

Alpha-blockers have also been shown to be useful in managing these arrhythmias. As they reduce myocardial contractility, they may precipitate hypotension and hence should be used with caution.[56]

Even cardioversion and defibrillation may not be successful in managing refractory ventricular arrhythmias with hemodynamic compromise. Other drugs which have been tried, with varying success rates, include glucagon,[57] magnesium sulfate,[58] and physostigmine.[59]

Hypotension

Hypotension may be secondary to reduced vascular resistance, myocardial depression or arrhythmias. Inotropic agents may be indicated if hypotensive is not responding to aggressive fluid therapy. Ideally, a pure alpha receptor agonist ought to be used to prevent the unopposed alpha stimulation caused by TCAs.[60] Noradrenaline has been shown to be superior to dopamine for management of shock in these patients, and is commended as the agent of choice.[61]

In patients with profound or persistent hypotension "rescue" measures like glucagon therapy,[62] lidocaine and magnesium sulfate,[58] intra-aortic balloon pump (IABP), extracorporeal life support,[63] and lipid emulsion therapy (LET),[64] may all be tried.

Central Nervous System Complications

Seizures are common but are mostly self-limiting. benzodiazepines may be given to control seizures.[37] However, flumazenil should not be used in patients with altered mental status as it may precipitate seizures.

Intubation and Mechanical Ventilation

Reduced consciousness or respiratory depression may require intubation for airway protection. Before intubation, it is vital to obtain an ECG to check for signs of severe toxicity. In patients with widened QRS, large terminal R wave in aVR and prolonged QT, sodium bicarbonate 1–2 mmol/kg should be given before attempting intubation, as intubation may worsen acidosis, exacerbating TCA toxicity. Post-intubation, patient should be hyperventilated to achieve alkalosis and once pH is above 7.5, sodium bicarbonate may no longer be required.

Cardiac Arrest

Patients who have severe toxicity may develop cardiac arrest. Resuscitative attempts should not be stopped until the patient is intubated, sodium bicarbonate is given and a target pH of more than 7.5 is achieved. Recovery has been reported even after prolonged resuscitation lasting for 3–5 hours after cardiac arrest.[65,66] This may be explained by the fact that there is redistribution of TCA during this time, which reduces its effective concentration and effect on the myocardium. This same rationale may also be applicable when LET is used in patients with refractory cardiac arrest, not responding to standard measures. As rescue therapy, external cardiac pacing may be attempted if heart rate is below 50/min and IABP may be tried if there is cardiogenic shock without any rhythm disturbances.[67]

Specific Antibody Fragments

Specific antibody fragments have been devised for TCAs and studied in animal models.[68] However, their clinical utility is limited due to requirement for large amounts, high cost, and renal toxicity.

Extracorporeal Therapies

Owning to their small molecular mass (between 200 Da and 400 Da), TCAs were considered to be easily dialyzable. However, their large volume of distribution, high protein binding, and good intrinsic clearance make extracorporeal therapies (ECT) less viable for managing TCA poisoning. ECT like hemodialysis, hemoperfusion, and plasmapheresis have all been tried for severely poisoned TCA patients, with varying results.[69-72] However, ECTs are currently not indicated in the management of any patient with TCA toxicity.[73]

ANTIHISTAMINE (DIPHENHYDRAMINE)

Diphenhydramine is a first generation antihistaminic agent acting on the H1 receptors. It also has anticholinergic properties. Other modes of action for diphenhydramine include potentiation of opioid receptors, increasing the dopamine concentration, and modulation of serotonin function.[74]

Diphenhydramine is commonly used to treat allergies. Its other uses include management of common cold, insomnia, tremor in parkinsonism, and nausea. It is generally taken orally but injectable preparations are also available. Overdose with diphenhydramine is relatively common because of its easy availability as an over-the-counter drug. Accidental overdose is especially common among the elderly and children.

Toxicokinetics

In general, antihistamines are highly lipid soluble and protein bound (98%). They also exhibit large Vd, up to 30 L/kg. Peak effect occurs after 2 hours of oral consumption and the effects may last up to 7 hours. They are primarily metabolized in the liver, except for drugs like cetirizine, levocetirizine and fexofenadine, which are excreted and eliminated by the kidneys.

Clinical Features

Patients with diphenhydramine toxicity generally present with classical features of anticholinergic toxicity. In cases of mild diphenhydramine overdose, the primary symptoms are typical of antimuscarinic toxidrome and patient may present with tachycardia, urinary retention, dry skin and mucosa, mydriasis, and reduced bowel sounds. Patients with moderate-to-severe overdose, may also have central antimuscarinic features including agitation, delirium, hallucinations, altered mental status or coma.[75]

Sodium channel blockade may occur in cases of severe poisoning and these patients may present with cardiovascular symptoms, secondary to delay in intraventricular conduction, similar to Vaughan Williams 1A anti-arrhythmics.[6,76] Sodium channel blockade may also cause neurological symptoms like seizures. Diphenhydramine toxicity has also been shown to be associated with rhabdomyolysis.[77-79]

Acute severe poisoning with diphenhydramine may prove to be fatal within 2–18 hours of consumption. Death generally occurs because of cardiovascular complications secondary to sodium channel blockade.[80]

Diagnosis

Diagnosis is based on history and clinical presentation as utility of serum levels is limited. ECG may show features of sodium channel blockade. QT interval may be prolonged and patients may develop cardiac arrhythmias including torsades de pointes.[81] ECG may also show wide complex tachycardia[6,82] and rarely patients may also develop the Brugada pattern.[83,84]

Rapid urine toxicology screens are unable to detect diphenhydramine, but may show false positive test for methadone.[85] Diphenhydramine can be detected in the body fluids like blood, plasma, or serum by using techniques like gas chromatography-mass spectrometry (GC-MS).[86] However, clinical utility of this test is limited because it is expensive and not widely available, but may be employed for legal investigations.

Treatment

Any patient with suspected or proven overdose of diphenhydramine, above 7.5 mg/kg in children under 6 years or 300 mg for older children and adults, should be managed in hospital. Treatment is generally symptomatic as there is no specific antidote.

Anticholinergic symptoms, like severe delirium and tachycardia, may be managed with physostigmine.[87] However, physostigmine may be contraindicated in patients with asthma or other pulmonary diseases, seizures, and in those with intraventricular conduction delay (widened QRS, bradycardia).[88,89]

Benzodiazepines may be required to manage seizures, agitation or psychosis. For management of symptoms secondary to sodium channel blockade, sodium bicarbonate remains the mainstay of therapy. Patients with severe poisoning, not responding to standard measures may be managed with LET.[90]

Several factors may influence the outcomes of these patients. These include underlying comorbid conditions, total dose ingested and any co-ingestion. Most of the patients show full recovery but patients at extremes of age may develop multiorgan failure if a large dose is consumed and may have poor outcomes.

CONCLUSION

Toxicity with SCB agents especially TCAs is common and may be potentially life-threatening. Cardiac complications are the common causes of morbidity and mortality among these patients. Most of the complications occur in the first few hours of ingestion, and hence it is imperative to make a prompt diagnosis and institute an early aggressive care. Sodium bicarbonate therapy is indicated along with fluid resuscitation and other supportive measures to improve patient outcomes. In patients on mechanical ventilation, hyperventilation should be done to achieve the target pH of around 7.50. Presently, there is no role for ECT in management of TCA overdose.

KEY POINTS

- Toxicity with SCB agents is common and may be potentially life threatening.
- Most of the complications occur in the first few hours of ingestion.
- Sodium bicarbonate therapy is indicated along with fluid resuscitation and other supportive measures.
- Hyperventitation must be done in patients on mechanical ventilation to achieve alkalosis but target pH should be maintained around 7.50.
- Death is generally due to cardiac complications.

REFERENCES

1. Kolecki PF, Curry SC. Poisoning by sodium channel blocking agents. Crit Care Clin. 1997;13:829-48.
2. Silver K, Dong K, Zhorov BS. Molecular Mechanism of Action and Selectivity of Sodium Channel Blocker Insecticides. Curr Med Chem. 2017;24(27):2912-24.
3. Pratheepa V, Vasconcelos V. Binding and Pharmacokinetics of the Sodium Channel Blocking Toxins (Saxitoxin and the Tetrodotoxins). Mini Rev Med Chem. 2017;17(4):320-7.
4. Brubacher J. Bicarbonate therapy for unstable propafenone-induced wide complex tachycardia. CJEM. 2004;5:349-56.
5. Kyle DJ, Ilyin VI. Sodium channel blockers. J Med Chem. 2007;50(11):2583-8.
6. Sharma AN, Hexdall AH, Chang EK, et al. Diphenhydramine-induced wide complex dysrhythmia responds to treatment with sodium bicarbonate. Am J Emerg Med. 2003; 21(3):212-5.
7. Létienne R, Vié B, Le Grand B. Pharmacological characterisation of sodium channels in sinoatrial node pacemaking in the rat heart. Eur J Pharmacol. 2006;530(3):243-9.
8. Henry JA, Cassidy SL. Membrane stabilising activity: a major cause of fatal poisoning. Lancet 1986;1(8495):1414-7.
9. Koszewska I, Rybakowski JK. Antidepressant-induced mood conversions in bipolar disorder: a retrospective study of tricyclic versus non-tricyclic antidepressant drugs. Neuropsychobiology. 2009;59(1):12-6.

10. Gillman PK. Tricyclic antidepressant pharmacology and therapeutic drug interactions updated. Br J Pharmacol. 2007;151(6):737-48.
11. Hejazi RA, Reddymasu SC, Namin F, et al. Efficacy of tricyclic antidepressant therapy in adults with cyclic vomiting syndrome: a two-year follow-up study. J Clin Gastroenterol. 2010;44(1):18-21.
12. Obafunwa JO, Busuttil A. Deaths from substance overdose in the Lothian and Borders region of Scotland (1983-1991). Hum Exp Toxicol. 1994;13:401-6.
13. Coleridge J, Cameron PA, Drummer OH, et al. Survey of drug related deaths in Victoria. Med J Aust. 1992;157(7):459-62.
14. Henry JA, Alexander CA, Sener EK. Relative mortality from overdose of antidepressants. BMJ 1995;310(6974):221-4.
15. Buckley NA, Dawson AH, Whyte IM, et al. Greater toxicity in overdose of dothiepin than of other tricyclic antidepressants. Lancet 1994;343(8890):159-62.
16. Jarvis MR. Clinical pharmacokinetics of tricyclic antidepressant overdose. Psychopharmacol Bull. 1991;27(4): 541-50.
17. Krishel S, Jackimczyk K. Cyclic antidepressants, lithium, and neuroleptic agents. Pharmacology and toxicology. Emerg Med Clin North Am. 1991;9(1):53-86.
18. Kerr GW, McGuffie AC, Wilkie S. Tricyclic antidepressant overdose: a review. Emerg Med J. 2001;18(4):236-241.
19. Mowry JB, Spyker DA, Cantilena LR Jr, et al. 2012 Annual Report of the American Association of Poison Control Centers' National Poison Data System (NPDS): 30th Annual Report. Clin Toxicol (Phila). 2013;51:949-1229.
20. McMahon AJ. Amitriptyline overdose complicated by intestinal pseudo-obstruction and caecal perforation. Postgrad Med J. 1989;65(770):948-9.
21. Ross JP, Small TR, Lepage PA. Imipramine overdose complicated by toxic megacolon. Am Surg. 1998;64(3):242-4.
22. Brennan FJ. Electrophysiological effects of imipramine and doxepin on normal and depressed cardiac purkinje fibers. Am J Cardiol. 1980;46(4):599-606.
23. Marshall JB, Forker AD. Cardiovascular effects of tricyclic antidepressant drugs: therapeutic usage, overdose, and management of complications. Am Heart J. 1982;103(3):401-14.
24. Taylor DJ, Braithwaite RA. Cardiac effects of tricyclic antidepressant medication: a preliminary study of nortriptyline. Br Heart J. 1978;40:1005-9.
25. Hulten BA, Heath A. Clinical aspects of tricyclic poisoning. Acta Med Scand. 1983; 213(4):275-8.
26. Langou RA, Van Dyke C, Tahan SR, et al. Cardiovascular manifestations of tricyclic antidepressant overdose. Am Heart J. 1980;100(4):458-64.
27. Callaham M, Kassel D. Epidemiology of fatal tricyclic antidepressant ingestion: implications for management. Ann Emerg Med. 1985;14(1):1-9.
28. Woolf AD, Erdman AR, Nelson LS, et al. Tricyclic antidepressant poisoning: an evidence based consensus guideline for out-of-hospital management. Clin Toxicol (Phila). 2007;45(3):203-33.

29. Starkey IR, Lawson AA. Poisoning with tricyclic and related antidepressants—a ten year review. Q J Med. 1980; 49(193):33-49.
30. Lipper B, Bell A, Gaynor B. Recurrent hypotension immediately after seizures in nortriptyline overdose. Am J Emerg Med. 1994;12(4):452-3.
31. Thorstrand C. Clinical features in poisonings by tricyclic antidepressants with special reference to the ECG. Acta Med Scand. 1976;199(5):337-44.
32. Strom J, Sloth Madsen P, Nygaard Nielsen N, et al. Acute self-poisoning with tricyclic antidepressants in 295 consecutive patients treated in an ICU. Acta Anaesthesiol Scand. 1984;28(6):666-70.
33. Snider RD. Case report: Left bundle branch blockade: rare complication of citalopram overdose. J S C Med Assoc. 2001;97(9):380-2.
34. Mehta N, Alexandrou N. Tricyclic Antidepressant Overdose and Electrocardiographic Changes. J of Emergency Medicine. 2000;18(4): 463-4.
35. Koppel C, Oberdisse U, Heinemeyer G. Clinical course and outcome in class IC antiarrhythmic overdose. J Toxicol Clin Toxicol. 1990;28(4):433-44.
36. Kim SY, Benowitz NL. Poisoning due to class 1A antiarrhythmic drugs. Quinidine, procainamide and disopyramide. Drug Saf. 1990;5(6):393-420.
37. Crome P. Poisoning due to tricyclic antidepressant overdosage: clinical presentation and treatment. Med Toxicol. 1986;1(4):261-85.
38. Boehnert MT, Lovejoy FH, Jr. Value of the QRS duration versus the serum drug level in predicting seizures and ventricular arrhythmias after an acute overdose of tricyclic antidepressants. N Engl J Med. 1985;313(8):474-9.
39. Liebelt EL, Francis PD, Woolf AD. ECG lead aVR versus QRS interval in predicting seizures and arrhythmias in acute tricyclic antidepressant toxicity. Ann Emerg Med. 1995; 26(2):195-201.
40. Tokarski GF, Young MJ. Criteria for admitting patients with tricyclic antidepressant overdosage. J Emerg Med. 1988;6(2):121-4.
41. Banahan BF Jr, Schelkun PH. Tricyclic antidepressant overdosage: conservative management in a community hospital with cost-saving implications. J Emerg Med. 1990;8(4):451-4.
42. Pentel P, Sioris L. Incidence of late arrhythmias following TCA overdose. Clin Toxicol. 1981;18(5):543-8.
43. Fasoli RA, Glauser FL. Cardiac arrhythmias and ECG abnormalities in TCA overdose. Clin Toxicol. 1981;18(2):155-63.
44. Crome P, Dawling S, Braithwaite RA, et al. Effect of activated charcoal on absorption of nortriptyline. Lancet. 1977;2(8050):1203-5.
45. Swartz C, Sherman A. The treatment of tricyclic antidepressant overdose with repeated charcoal. J Clin Psychopharmacol. 1984;4(6):336-40.
46. Hoffman JR, Votey SR, Bayer M, et al. Effect of hypertonic sodium bicarbonate in the treatment of moderate to severe cyclic antidepressant overdose. Am J Emerg Med. 1993;11(4):336-41.

47. Blackman K, Brown SG, Wilkes GJ. Plasma alkalinization for tricyclic antidepressant toxicity: a systematic review. Emerg Med. 2001;13(2):204-10.
48. Bradberry SM, Thanacoody HK, Watt BE, et al. Management of the cardiovascular complications of tricyclic antidepressant poisoning: role of sodium bicarbonate. Toxicol Rev. 2005;24(3):195-204.
49. Hagerman GA, Hanashiro PK. Reversal of tricyclic-anti depressant induced cardiac conduction abnormalities by phenytoin. Ann Emerg Med. 1981;10(2):82-6.
50. Kingston ME. Hyperventilation in tricyclic antidepressant poisoning. Crit Care Med. 1979;7(12):550-1.
51. Wrenn K, Smith BA, Slovis CM. Profound alkalemia during treatment of tricyclic antidepressant overdose: a potential hazard of combined hyperventilation and intravenous bicarbonate. Am J Emerg Med. 1992;10(6):553-5.
52. Brown TC. Sodium bicarbonate and tricyclic antidepressant poisoning. Lancet. 1977;1(8007):375.
53. Albertson TE, Dawson A, de Latorre F, et al. International Liaison Committee on R: TOX-ACLS: toxicologic-oriented advanced cardiac life support. Ann Emerg Med. 2001;37(4 Suppl): S78-90.
54. Di Grande A, Giuffrida C, Narbone G, et al. Management of sodium-channel blocker poisoning: the role of hypertonic sodium salts. Eur Rev Med Pharmacol Sci. 2010;14(1): 25-30.
55. Boehnert M, Lovejoy F. The effect of phenytoin on cardiac conduction and ventricular arrhythmias in acute tricyclic antidepressant overdose. Vet Hum Toxicol. 1985;28:297.
56. Freeman JW, Mundy GR, Beattie RR, et al. Cardiac abnormalities in poisoning with tricyclic antidepressant. Br Med J. 1969;2(5657):610-1.
57. Sener EK, Gabe S, Henry J. Response to glucagon in imipramine overdose. J Toxicol Clin Toxicol. 1995;33(1): 51-3.
58. Knudsen K, Heath A. Effects of self poisoning with maprotiline. Br Med J (Clin Res Ed). 1984;288 (6417): 601-3.
59. Buchman AL, Dauer J, Geiderman J. The use of vasoactive agents in the treatment of refractory hypotension seen in tricyclic antidepressant overdose. J Clin Psychopharmacol. 1990;10:409-13.
60. Teba L, Scheibel F, Dedhia H, et al. Beneficial effect of norepinephrine in the treatment of circulatory shock caused by tricyclic antidepressant overdose. Am J Emerg Med. 1988;6(6):566-8.
61. Boyd R, Ghosh A. Towards evidence based emergency medicine: best BETS from the Manchester General Infirmary. Glucagon in tricyclic overdose. Emerg Med J. 2003;20(3):266-7.
62. Knudsen K, Abrahamsson J. Magnesium sulphate in the treatment of ventricular fibrillation in amitriptyline poisoning. Eur Heart J. 1997;18(5):881-2.
63. Daubin C, Quentin C, Goulle JP, et al. Refractory shock and asystole related to tramadol overdose. Clin Toxicol. 2007;45(8):961-4.
64. Jamaty C, Bailey B, Larocque A, et al. Lipid emulsions in the treatment of acute poisoning: a systematic review

65. Orr DA, Bramble MG. Tricyclic antidepressant poisoning and prolonged external cardiac massage during asystole. Br Med J (Clin Res Ed). 1981. 24;283(6299):1107-8.

66. Baud FJ, Megarbane B, Deye N, et al. Clinical review: aggressive management and extracorporeal support for drug-induced cardiotoxicity. Crit Care. 2007;11(2):207.

67. Southall DP, Kilpatrick SM. Imipramine poisoning: survival of a child after prolonged cardiac massage. Br Med J. 1974;4 (5943):508.

68. Pentel PR, Scarlett W, Ross CA, et al. Reduction of desipramine cardiotoxicity and prolongation of survival in rats using polyclonal drug specific antibody Fab fragments. Ann Emerg Med. 1995;126(3):334-41.

69. Ozayar E, Degerli S, Gulec H. Hemodiafiltration: a novel approach for treating severe amitriptyline intoxication. Toxicol Int. 2012;19(3):319-21.

70. Sari I, Turkcuer I, Erurker T, et al. Therapeutic plasma exchange in amitriptyline intoxication: case report and review of the literature. Transfus Apher Sci. 2011;45(2):183-5.

71. Mutlu M, Karaguzel G, Bahat E, et al. Charcoal hemoperfusion in an infant with supraventricular tachycardia and seizures secondary to amitriptyline intoxication. Hum Exp Toxicol. 2011;30(3):254-6.

72. Winchester JF, Boldur A, Oleru C, Kitiyakara C. Use of dialysis and hemoperfusion in treatment of poisoning. In: Daugirdas JT, Blake PG, Ing TS (Eds). Handbook of Dialysis. Philadelphia, PA: Lippincott Williams & Wilkins; 2007: 300-20.

73. Yates C, Galvao T, Sowinski KM, et al. EXTRIP workgroup. Extracorporeal treatment for tricyclic antidepressant poisoning: recommendations from the EXTRIP Workgroup. Semin Dial. 2014;27(4):381-9.

74. Rollstin AD, Seifert SA. Acetaminophen/diphenhydramine overdose in profound hypothermia. Clin Toxicol (Phila). 2013;51(1):50-3.

75. Levine M, Brooks DE, Truitt CA, et al. Toxicology in the ICU: Part 1: general overview and approach to treatment. Chest. 2011;140(3):795-806.

76. Kuo CC, Huang RC, Lou BS. Inhibition of Na(+) current by diphenhydramine and other diphenyl compounds: molecular determinants of selective binding to the inactive channels. Mol Pharmacol. 2000;57(1):135-43.

77. Ramchandran K, Sirop P. Rare complications of diphenhydramine toxicity. Conn Med. 2008;72(2):79-82.

78. Coco TJ, Klasner AE. Drug-induced rhabdomyolysis. Curr Opin Pediatr. 2004;16(2):206-10.

79. Emadian SM, Caravati EM, Herr RD. Rhabdomyolysis: a rare adverse effect of diphenhydramine overdose. Am J Emerg Med. 1996;14(6):574-6.

80. Brunton L, Chabner B, Knollmann B. Chapter 32: Histamine, Bradykinin, and Their Antagonists. In: Brunton L (Ed). Goodman & Gilman's The Pharmacological Basis of Therapeutics, 12th edition. New York City: McGraw Hill; 2011. pp. 242-5.

81. Khalifa M, Drolet B, Daleau P, et al. Block of potassium currents in guinea pig ventricular myocytes and lengthening of cardiac repolarization in man by the histamine H1 receptor antagonist diphenhydramine. J Pharmacol Exp Ther. 1999;288(2):858-65.

82. Cole JB, Stellpflug SJ, Gross EA, et al. Wide complex tachycardia in a pediatric diphenhydramine overdose treated with sodium bicarbonate. Pediatr Emerg Care. 2011;27(12):1175-7.

83. Lopez-Barbeito B, Lluis M, Delgado V, et al. Diphenhydramine overdose and Brugada sign. Pacing Clin Electrophsiol. 2005;28(7):730-2.

84. Levine M, Lovecchio F. Diphenhydramine-induced Brugada pattern. Resuscitation. 2010;81(4):503-4.

85. Rogers SC, Pruitt CW, Crouch DJ, et al. Rapid urine drug screens: diphenhydramine and methadone cross-reactivity. Pediatr Emerg Care. 2010;26(9):665-6.

86. Pragst F. Chapter 13: High performance liquid chromatography in forensic toxicological analysis. In: Smith RK, Bogusz MJ (Eds). Forensic Science (Handbook of Analytical Separations), 2nd edition. Amsterdam: Elsevier Science; 2007; 6:471.

87. Manning B. Chapter 18: Antihistamines. In: Olson K (Ed). Poisoning & Drug Overdose, 6th edition. New York City: McGraw-Hill; 2012.

88. Gao M, Sato M, Ikegaya Y. Machine Learning-based Prediction of Seizure-inducing Action as an Adverse Drug Effect. Yakugaku Zasshi. 2018;138(6):809-13.

89. Leybishkis B, Fasseas P, Ryan KF. Doxylamine overdose as a potential cause of rhabdomyolysis. Am J Med Sci. 2001;322(1):48-9.

90. Abdi A, Rose E, Levine M. Diphenhydramine overdose with intraventricular conduction delay treated with hypertonic sodium bicarbonate and iv lipid emulsion. West J Emerg Med. 2014;15(7):855-8.

22 CHAPTER

Digoxin and Other Cardiac Glycosides

Supradip Ghosh

INTRODUCTION

Cardiac glycosides are naturally occurring compounds found in a variety of plants and animal species distributed widely across the world. Structurally, they consist of a steroid ring with a carbohydrate chain linked by an oxygen bridge to the third carbon of the A-ring of the steroid moiety (hence glycoside).[1] Best known cardiac glycoside is digoxin, extracted originally from foxglove plant (*Digitalis purpurea* and *Digitalis lanata*). Digoxin is used clinically in the management of patients with congestive cardiac failure (CHF) and to control the ventricular rate in patients with atrial fibrillation (AF). Other cardiac glycosides are identified from various sources. Common among them are neriifolin and thevetins A/B from yellow oleander (*Thevetia peruviana*), neriine, and oleandrin from common oleander (*Nerium oleander*), ouabain from *Strophanthus gratus*, and cerberin neriifolin and diacetyl tanghinin from sea mango (*Cerbera manghas*). Many of these plant extracts are used in herbal remedies for a large number of conditions ranging from heart disease to cancer and also as an abortifacient.[2]

Poisoning due to cardiac glycoside is common across the world, largely due to once wide-spread medicinal use of digoxin with its narrow therapeutic window (recommended range for CHF 0.5–0.9 ng/mL) and extensive drug interaction.[3] Digoxin toxicity may be accidental following prescription or dispensing errors and sometimes due to intentional overdose. In many areas of South-East Asia especially Sri Lanka and India, yellow oleander and common oleander poisoning are major public health concerns due to their easy availability.[4,5] Ingestion of seeds (yellow oleander) or oleander leaves have been shown to be associated with severe toxicity and may even be fatal. Seeds of sea mango tree, also called the suicide tree or pong-pong tree, are commonly used for suicidal intention in some rural regions of South Asia especially India and Sri Lanka.[6] Treatment of cardiac glycoside poisoning following ingestion of plant products is complicated because of their variable absorption, wide variation in toxicity threshold, limited availability of diagnostic tests, requirement for intensive care, interhospital transfer overburdening the limited health-care resources available in resource limited setting, and nonavailability of effective and inexpensive treatments.

CARDIAC GLYCOSIDES: PHARMACOLOGY

The mechanism of action for all cardiac glycosides is same with digoxin being the prototype. They act by inhibiting the Na^+/K^+-ATPase on cardiomyocytes and other cells, causing retention of Na^+ intracellularly that in turn increases the intracellular Ca^{2+} concentrations via Na^+/Ca^{2+} exchanger.[7] The elevated intracellular Ca^{2+} concentration increases cardiac contractility.

Digoxin and Other Cardiac Glycosides

Accumulation of Na^+ and Ca^{2+} in the intracellular space causes partial membrane depolarization that may increase automaticity and risk of tachyarrhythmias. Digoxin may also increase the vagal tone, reducing the activity of sinus node and prolong the conduction in the atrioventricular (AV) node which may lead to bradycardia. Several other mechanisms of action have also been reported, including endocytosis of Na^+/K^+-ATPase (adenosine triphosphatase), blockage of voltage-gated Na^+ channels, and intracellular signal transduction activation. Subtle differences may be observed between different cardiac glycosides that can affect their toxicity and response to therapy. For example, insulin seems to inhibit the effect of digoxin on Na^+/K^+-ATPase in the rat model but has no effect on ouabain, possibly explained by their different binding region.[8]

Depending upon the type of formulation, absorption of digoxin is variable and after absorption distribution to tissues takes up to 6 hours. These variability in absorption, time taken for distribution and also time-dependent binding to Na^+/K^+-ATPase explain the delayed onset of digoxin's effect. In addition, digoxin undergoes extensive enterohepatic circulation resulting in mean elimination half-life as long as 7.5 days.[7] Digoxin is mainly eliminated from the body by renal clearance. Hence, a higher serum digoxin levels, for a given dose, may be seen in individuals with kidney dysfunction. Serum digoxin concentration, when measured postdistribution (after at least 6 hours of acute poisoning) does reflect the likelihood of toxicity. Digoxin is a substrate for P-glycoprotein which is located in various body organs like the bile ducts, small intestine, and the kidneys. Amiodarone, clarithromycin, quinidine, and verapamil, which are potent inhibitors of P-glycoprotein, may decrease renal tubular secretion and also increase gastrointestinal (GI) absorption of digoxin which may cause increased serum digoxin levels.[7] In addition to digoxin concentration, certain other conditions like hypokalemia, hypomagnesemia, hypercalcemia, acid-base disturbances, and myocardial ischemia may increase the sensitivity to digoxin.[3]

Pharmacological data on other cardiac glycosides are limited. Pharmacological effects of cardiac glycosides following yellow oleander seeds are variable because of the erratic absorption (which may extend to more than 50 hours after ingestion) and depends on whether the seed was crushed or was taken as a whole.[4,7] The severity of cardiotoxicity, does not correlate well with the number of seeds ingested or area under the concentration-time curve, which suggests that there might be variability in bioavailability.[9]

CLINICAL FEATURES

Clinical features of cardiac glycosides poisoning are often nonspecific and include GI symptoms like nausea, vomiting, pain abdomen, diarrhea, or generalized weakness or drowsiness. More specific symptoms like visual changes, like green or yellow discoloration is reported only rarely that too after chronic digoxin toxicity. Cardiac toxicities account for most deaths and may present with almost any type of arrhythmias with the notable exception of atrial tachyarrhythmias with fast ventricular rate (FVR).[3] Sinus bradycardia, ventricular premature complexes (VPCs), and AV block are the most common arrhythmias described. With more severe toxicity potentially fatal arrhythmias like ventricular tachycardia (sometimes characteristic bidirectional ventricular tachycardia), ventricular fibrillation, advanced heart block, and asystole may ensue. Interestingly "Reverse Tick Sign" seen commonly in patients on digoxin is not a feature of toxicity.[3] Another characteristic finding in severe digoxin poisoning is refractory hyperkalemia.

In a prospective trial including 79 patients, admitted to a district hospital in Sri Lanka following deliberate self-ingestion of yellow oleander, the most common reported symptoms were abdominal pain and vomiting.[4] Most patients with abnormal electrocardiogram presented with bradyarrhythmia, mostly sinus bradycardia, AV node dysfunction, and sinus arrest or exit block. Forty-three percent of patients presented or developed second or third degree AV block. The time taken for progression and resolution of cardiotoxicity was not uniform, reflecting the variable pharmacokinetics. Like a patient had sinus rhythm for initial 3 days after which he developed second degree heart block. In a retrospective study from the Indian state of Kerala, 57.8% of patients admitted with sea mango seed intoxication, had bradyarrhythmias including Mobitz type 2 block and complete AV block.[6]

MANAGEMENT

Given the similarity in structure, mechanism of action and toxicity profile between different cardiac glycosides and in the absence of large data from other cardiac glycosides, treatments of cardiac glycosides poisoning are frequently extrapolated from the literature which is available for digoxin poisoning. However, recently an increasing number of clinical trials are being reported which have assessed the effects of various treatment modalities in yellow oleander poisoning.

When feasible, all patients acutely poisoned with cardiac glycosides should be admitted to an intensive care unit (ICU) for continuous cardiac monitoring. Serum digoxin concentration should be measured and a higher serum level correlates with a more severe poisoning. However, the correlation between digoxin concentration and severity of clinical manifestations is poor, reflecting the distribution kinetics of digoxin. As most digoxin assays are based on enzyme-linked immunosorbent assay (ELISA) platform with potential for crossreactivity with other cardiac glycosides, this can also be used for detecting the presence of nondigoxin cardiac glycosides (e.g. from oleander).[9] Serum K^+, Mg^{2+}, and Ca^{2+} levels must be measured initially and repeated periodically.

Toxic symptoms secondary to digoxin poisoning generally manifests inside 6 hours of last dose for both acute and chronic toxicity. If a patient remains asymptomatic during this period, electrocardiogram does not show any brady- or tachyarrhythmia, serum K^+ is within normal range, and serum digoxin level is less than 2 ng/mL, patient may be discharged home.[7] However, patients may develop a delayed onset of toxicity from yellow oleander; it is recommended to monitor these patients in a hospital setup for at least 72 hours after ingestion.[4,7]

General Management

A single dose of activated charcoal (50–100 g) must be given to all patients with suspected or proven acute ingestion of a potentially toxic exposure, irrespective of the time of exposure.[7] Multiple-dose activated charcoal (MDAC) is also recommended as it can potentially enhance the elimination of digoxin by interrupting enterohepatic circulation. In a retrospective review of 39 patients with serum digoxin level more than 2.5 ng/mL, treatment with MDAC was found to enhance digoxin elimination by 78% compared to nontreated patients.[10] In a study from Sri Lanka, 401 patients of yellow oleander toxicity were administered a single dose of activated charcoal at the time of admission and were then divided randomly to either 50 g of activated charcoal every 6 hourly for a period of 3 days or placebo groups.[11] Treatment with MDAC could significantly reduce the mortality rate at discharge compared to placebo [2.5% vs. 8%; 95%

confidence interval (CI) 0.6–10.3; coefficient of correlation (p) = 0.025]. MDAC was also found to be safe and well tolerated. However, in a subsequent larger randomized controlled trial (RCT) of 4,632 patients from Sri Lanka, MDAC was compared against single-dose activated charcoal or no activated charcoal, in patients presenting with all types of self-poisoning including 1,647 patients of yellow oleander toxicity.[12] Mortality rate was not different between single-dose activated charcoal group, MDAC group, and no charcoal group; this effect was found to be irrespective of the type of poison ingested. Considering its safety and tolerability found in all studies and possible benefit, MDAC should be considered in every patient presenting with cardiac glycoside poisoning, unless it is contraindicated because of the presence of repeated vomiting or paralytic ileus.

Correction of Electrolytes

Hypokalemia is corrected with supplemental potassium until a level of more than 4 mEq/L is achieved. Hyperkalemia is corrected by using insulin-glucose, bicarbonate, or exchange resins and hemodialysis in refractory cases or in the presence of renal failure. Use of calcium salts should be avoided because of the theoretical risk of inducing asystole or malignant arrhythmias (as intracellular calcium is already very high).[7,13] Beta-agonists should be avoided for the correction of hyperkalemia as they may precipitate tachyarrhythmias.[13] There are controversies regarding correction of hypocalcemia and better avoided in cases of cardiac glycoside poisoning.[13] Hypomagnesemia is common in chronic poisoning, most likely due to the frequent use of diuretics in these patients. Correction of magnesium level may reduce myocardial irritability and improves conduction.

Management of Bradyarrhythmias

Atropine antagonizes vagal inhibition produced by cardiac glycosides, increasing heart rate and is used as the first-line agent for symptomatic bradycardia with hypotension.[7] Usual dose is 0.6–1 mg; however, doses up to 2–3 mg have also been used. Higher doses may produce delirium and hyperthermia especially in hot tropical climate.

Temporary cardiac pacing may be an option in symptomatic bradyarrhythmias especially when antidigoxin Fab is not available. Pacing may be associated with complications including precipitating ventricular fibrillation and death.[7] In an older study, the rate of complication was as high as 36% with a fatality rate of 13%. Pacing failed to prevent life-threatening arrhythmias in 23% of cases, in comparison to 8% in patients where antidigoxin Fab was used.[14] Use of temporary pacing is also limited by logistical issues, including the need for procedural expertize and advanced facilities for monitoring which are seldom available in rural regions and in many developing countries.

Management of Tachyarrhythmias

In symptomatic supraventricular tachycardia, intravenous (IV) phenytoin can be used (100 mg bolus may be repeated in 5 minutes).[13] In rare patients with AF or flutter with rapid ventricular response following cardiac glycoside poisoning, phenytoin will not be useful and in them esmolol may be considered. The recommended dose is a bolus of 0.5 mg/kg IV to be given over 1 minute which should be followed by a continuous infusion at the rate of 0.05 mg/kg/min.[13]

In ventricular arrhythmias, lidocaine in a dose of 1.5 mg/kg IV bolus, to be followed by a continuous infusion at the rate of 2.5–4 mg/min in adults and 50 µg/kg/min in children, or phenytoin (100 mg IV bolus every 5 minutes, until the arrhythmia gets controlled or up to a maximum of 1 g in adults or 20 mg/kg in children) may be used especially when antidigoxin Fab is not available.[13] Both of these drugs are able to reduce ventricular excitability without worsening AV conduction. In selected cases refractory to lidocaine or phenytoin, IV amiodarone may be considered.[13] Beta-blockers may precipitate complete AV block and should be used with extreme caution in ventricular tachyarrhythmias. If used, IV esmolol with a short elimination half-life of 9 minutes is possible choice.[13] Magnesium (1.5 g administered intravenously over 20 minutes) may be useful in some refractory cases.[13]

Electrical cardioversion is generally ineffective in cardiac glycoside poisoning and may precipitate irreversible cardiac arrest. Cardioversion should be reserved for patients who develop ventricular dysrhythmias refractory to other treatments. Cardioversion, if required, should be done using low energy levels (20–100 J).[7,13]

Antidigoxin Fab

Antidigoxin Fab exhibits high affinity for binding digoxin and can remove it from its binding site on Na^+/K^+-ATPase.

It was first used by Smith and colleagues in 1976, for successfully treating a patient with a history of ingestion of 22.5 mg digoxin, after all conventional treatment failed.[15] Since then antidigoxin Fab (Fab) has come into wide use for treating both acute and chronic poisoning with digoxin. Because Fab can bind to other cardiac glycosides also, it has been used in the management of poisonings with other nondigoxin cardiac glycosides, especially yellow oleander.[16] The biggest deterrent to its extensive use is the high cost (~US$750 per 40 mg vial) and nonavailability of the drug in many countries including India.

In a recent systemic review, use of Fab has been shown to be both safe and efficacious in treatment of digoxin poisoning.[17] The antibody is utilized more often in the management of acute rather than chronic digoxin toxicity. It has been shown that the levels of free digoxin rapidly become negligible within a few minutes after Fab administration, with a time to reversal of digoxin toxicity within 30–45 minutes. Overall the response to digoxin Fab has varied from 80–90% to 50% with better success rate in acute poisoning. A possible explanation for this apparent poor efficacy of the antibody in chronic digoxin poisoning could be substantial comorbid illnesses like cardiac or renal dysfunction and coprescription of medications like angiotensin converting enzyme inhibitors, calcium-channel blockers, beta-blockers, or aldosterone antagonists.[18] Indications for prescribing antidigoxin Fab are in patients with life-threatening brady-/tachyarrhythmias, hyperkalemia (serum potassium levels above 6 mmol/L), or absence of hemodynamic stability with an increased serum digoxin levels (>2 ng/L or 2.6 nmol/L).[17] Suggested dosage of antidigoxin Fab is 40 mg (1 vial) as bolus, to be repeated after 1 hour if the patient continues to remain symptomatic or sooner if the patient becomes clinically unstable. Usually 40–120 mg (1–3 vials) is adequate for reverting the toxicity.[17]

In a single-center study from Sri Lanka, 66 patients of yellow oleander poisoning with significant cardiac toxicity were randomized to receive either 1,200 mg of Fab or placebo.[18] Reversal of arrhythmias, increase in heart rate, and reduction in serum K^+ level was significantly higher in antibody treated patients. Dose of antibody in yellow oleander toxicity is generally higher partly due to failure to quantify the toxin burden from history and in vitro assays and also due to lower crossreactivity between Fab and other cardiac glycosides.

Extracorporeal Treatment

Because of its high volume of distribution (Vd), hemodialysis (HD) is not effective in the treatment of digoxin toxicities. However, successful use of extracorporeal treatment like resin hemoperfusion is reported as anecdotal case reports in the literature.[19] Extracorporeal Treatments in Poisoning (EXTRIP) workgroup has recently reviewed the efficacy of extracorporeal treatment in digoxin toxicity and concluded that digoxin is only slightly dialyzable and extracorporeal treatment is not likely to improve the prognosis of patients with digoxin poisoning irrespective of the use of Fab.[20] The workgroup recommended against the use of extracorporeal treatment even in patients with severe digoxin toxicity irrespective of availability or administration of Fab.[20]

CONCLUSION

Cardiac glycosides poisoning is common especially in resource limited rural areas of South-East Asia. Despite availability of effective treatment, nonavailability of antidigoxin Fab and high treatment cost is the biggest barrier to the delivery of this therapy.[21] In future, availability of affordable treatment for poisoned patients including cardiac glycosides should be the priority for health care agencies and delivery systems.

KEY POINTS

- Cardiac glycosides poisoning is common and includes digoxin and various widely available plant toxins
- Classic manifestations of cardiac glycosides poisoning include GI/visual disturbances, potentially life-threatening brady-/tachyarrhythmias, and hyperkalemia
- The MDAC should be considered in all patients presenting with cardiac glycoside poisoning to interrupt enterohepatic circulation
- Antidigoxin Fab is the treatment of choice for all potentially life-threatening toxic manifestations including dysrhythmias, hyperkalemia, and hemodynamic instability with high serum digoxin levels, but limited by cost and nonavailability in many countries including India
- Other supportive measures include cautious use of selective antiarrhythmic drugs and correction of dyselectrolytemia especially hypo- and hyperkalemia.

IV calcium gluconate should be avoided because of the theoretical risk of precipitating arrhythmias
- As of today, extracorporeal treatment is not indicated in the management of cardiac glycoside poisoning.

REFERENCES

1. Kanji S, MacLean RD. Cardiac glycoside toxicity: more than 200 years and counting. Crit Care Clin. 2012;28:527-35.
2. Prasad A, Krishnaveni K, Neha KA, et al. A review on management of common oleander and yellow oleander poisoning. World J Pharm Pharm Sci. 2016;5:493-503.
3. Pincus M. Management of digoxin toxicity. Aust Prescr. 2016;39:18-20.
4. Eddleston M, Ariaratnam CA, Meyer WP, et al. Epidemic of self-poisoning with seeds of the yellow oleander tree (*Thevetia peruviana*) in northern Sri Lanka. Trop Med Int Health. 1999;4:266-73.
5. Bose TK, Basu RK, Biswas B, et al. Cardiovascular effects of yellow oleander ingestion. J Indian Med Assoc. 1999;97:407-10.
6. Renymol B, Sasidharan PD, Ambili NR. Study on clinical profile and predictors of mortality in *Cerbera odollam* poisoning. Indian J Crit Care Med. 2018;22:431-4.
7. Roberts DM, Gallapatthy G, Dunuwille A, et al. Pharmacological treatment of cardiac glycoside poisoning. Br J Clin Pharmacol. 2016;81:488-95.
8. Oubaassine R, Weckering M, Kessler L, et al. Insulin interacts directly with Na(+)/K(+)ATPase and protects from digoxin toxicity. Toxicology. 2012;299:1-9.
9. Roberts DM, Southcott E, Potter JM, et al. Pharmacokinetics of digoxin cross-reacting substances in patients with acute yellow oleander (*Thevetia peruviana*) poisoning, including the effect of activated charcoal. Ther Drug Monit. 2006;28:784-92.
10. Ibanez C, Carcas AJ, Frias J, et al. Activated charcoal increases digoxin elimination in patients. Int J Cardiol. 1995;48:27-30.
11. de Silva HA, Fonseka MMD, Pathmeswaran A, et al. Multiple-dose activated charcoal for treatment of yellow oleander poisoning: a single-blind, randomized, placebo-controlled trial. Lancet. 2003;361:1935-8.
12. Eddleston M, Juszczak E, Buckley NA, et al. Ox-Col Poisoning Study collaborators. Multiple-dose activated charcoal in acute self-poisoning: a randomised controlled trial. Lancet. 2008;371:579-87.
13. Nogué S, Cino J, Civeira E, et al. Digitalis poisoning: the basis for treatment with antidigoxin antibodies. Emergencias. 2012;24:462-75.
14. Taboulet P, Baud FJ, Bismuth C, et al. Acute digitalis intoxication—is pacing still appropriate? J Toxicol Clin Toxicol. 1993;31:261-73.

15. Smith TW, Haber E, Yeatman L, et al. Reversal of advanced digoxin intoxication with Fab fragments of digoxin-specific antibodies. N Engl J Med.1976;294:797-800.

16. Chan BSH, Buckley NA. Digoxin-specific antibody fragments in the treatment of digoxin toxicity. Clin Toxicol. 2014;52:824-36.

17. Chan BS, Isbister GK, O'Leary M, et al. Efficacy and effectiveness of anti-digoxin antibodies in chronic digoxin poisonings from the DORA study (ATOM-1). Clin Toxicol. 2016;54:488-94.

18. Eddleston M, Rajapakse S, Rajakanthan K, et al. Anti-digoxin Fab fragments in cardiotoxicity induced by ingestion of yellow oleander: a randomised controlled trial. Lancet. 2000;355:967-71.

19. Juneja D, Singh O, Bhasin A, et al. Severe suicidal digoxin toxicity managed with resin hemoperfusion: A case report. Indian J Crit Care Med. 2012;16:231-3.

20. Mowry JB, Burdmann EA, Anseeuw K, et al. Extracorporeal treatment for digoxin poisoning: systematic review and recommendations from the EXTRIP Workgroup. Clin Toxicol. 2016;(2):103-14.

21. Eddleston M, Senarathna L, Mohamed F, et al. Deaths due to absence of an affordable antitoxin for plant poisoning. Lancet. 2003;362:1041-4.

SECTION 6

Gastrointestinal and Liver Toxins

23. **Acetaminophen (Paracetamol) Poisoning**
    Anish Gupta, Deven Juneja

24. **NSAID Overdose**
    Anish Gupta, Omender Singh

25. **Corrosive Ingestion: Acids and Alkalis**
    Desh Deepak

SECTION 6

Gastrointestinal and Liver Toxins

23
CHAPTER

Acetaminophen (Paracetamol) Poisoning

Anish Gupta, Deven Juneja

INTRODUCTION/EPIDEMIOLOGY

Acetaminophen (paracetamol) is one of the most commonly prescribed and used analgesic, antipyretic drug worldwide. It was first synthesized in 1878 by Harmon Northrop Morse. Brodie and Axelrod were the first to correlate the analgesic effect of acetanilide to its metabolite paracetamol.[1] Paracetamol was first manufactured commercially by McNeil laboratories by the brand name Tylenol.

Acetaminophen is one of the most common causes of drug-induced liver injury (DILI).[2-4] Though the exact incidence of acetaminophen-induced liver failure in India is not known, it is the most common cause of acute liver failure (ALF) in the United States. About 20% of liver transplant cases in United States are secondary to acetaminophen poisoning.[5-8]

PHARMACOLOGY

Acetaminophen or paracetamol is the active metabolite of phenacetin. The chemical composition of acetaminophen is N-acetyl-p-aminophenol (APAP). It is a nonopioid analgesic and is available as both immediate-release and sustained-release formulations. APAP is almost completely absorbed from the gastrointestinal tract with a peak serum concentration in about 1–2 hours. Therapeutic concentrations range from 10 to 20 µg/L. Metabolism is by first order kinetics with a half-life ($t_{1/2}$) of 2–4 hours. Elimination is slower in infants, children, elderly, coingestion with certain drugs (opiates and anticholinergics), and pre-existing liver dysfunction.[9-12]

TOXICOLOGY

The therapeutic dose is 10–15 mg/kg per dose in children and up to 1,000 mg per dose in adults, given at 4–6 hourly intervals. The maximum recommended daily dose is 80 mg/kg in children and 4 g in adults.

The minimum toxic dose for a single ingestion is more than 150 mg/kg in children overall, more than 200 mg/kg in children aged 1–6 years, and greater than 7.5–10 grams in adults.[13]

At therapeutic doses, about 90% of APAP is metabolized by hepatic conjugation (sulfation or glucuronidation) to form inactive metabolites (Flowhart 1). These metabolites are nontoxic and freely excreted by the kidneys. In adults, glucuronidation is the predominant route of metabolism while in children and infants, sulfation is the primary pathway. Less than 5% of the drug is excreted unchanged in urine. The remaining 5% undergoes oxidation by cytochrome P450 oxidase system (CYP2E1) to form a highly toxic product called N-acetyl-p-benzoquinoneimine (NAPQI).[14-16] NAPQI is detoxified by glutathione (GSH) to form nontoxic

Gastrointestinal and Liver Toxins

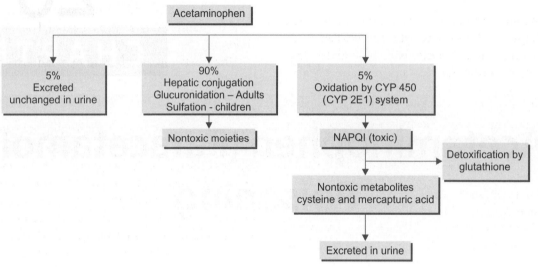

Flowchart 1: Normal metabolism of acetaminophen/paracetamol.

(CYP2E1: cytochrome P450 oxidase system; NAPQI: N-acetyl-p-benzoquinoneimine)

compounds (cysteine and mercapturic acid conjugates), which are excreted in urine.

In cases of overdose, metabolism of APAP by hepatic conjugation pathways is saturated and hence, metabolism by cytochrome P450 pathways increases leading to increased production of NAPQI.[17,18] As a result, there is increased utilization of GSH with depletion of its stores. When regeneration of GSH is inadequate to meet the increase in demand, NAPQI accumulates and irreversibly binds to hepatocyte mitochondrial proteins leading to hepatocellular injury and death (Flowchart 2). Hepatocellular necrosis is predominantly centrilobular as the maximum CYP2E1 activity is seen in these areas. Animal studies have shown that hepatocellular injury occurs when GSH stores are reduced to less than 30% of normal levels.[19]

The exact dose leading to toxic effects is unknown and may vary between individuals. Differences in existing GSH stores, rate of GSH regeneration, and CYP2E1 activity modulates the dose leading to hepatocellular injury. Other factors which influence toxicity include advanced age, chronic alcoholism, chronic liver disease, chronic tobacco use, and malnutrition.

CLINICAL FEATURES

Depending upon the time interval after ingestion, acetaminophen-induced liver injury can be divided into four stages.[13,20]

Flowchart 2: Metabolism of acetaminophen/paracetamol in overdose.

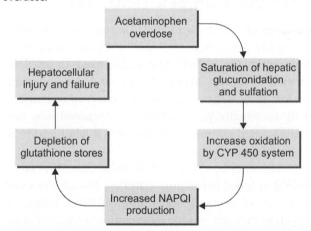

(CYP 450: cytochrome P450; NAPQI: Nacetyl-p-benzoquinoneimine)

Stage 1

It is the latent period lasting for up to 24 hours postingestion. Depending on the dose ingested, patients may be asymptomatic or rarely present with coma and metabolic acidosis. Most cases present with nausea, vomiting, malaise, weakness, pallor, and sweating. Liver function tests (bilirubin, transaminase levels, and prothrombin time) may be completely normal at this stage. Only gamma-glutamyl transferase (GGT) may be elevated and is a subtle indicator for liver injury.

Stage 2

This stage signifies the onset of liver injury with features typical of hepatitis. It typically extends between 24 to 48 hours postingestion. Symptoms include abdominal pain, nausea, vomiting, fatigue, and malaise. Clinical examination may reveal hepatomegaly with right upper quadrant tenderness. Liver function tests reveal elevated aminotransferase levels. Serum bilirubin levels and prothrombin time may be normal or slightly elevated. Although not commonly seen, depending on the extent of hepatocellular injury patients may present with signs and symptoms of liver cell failure (encephalopathy, coagulopathy, hypoglycemia, and acidosis). Renal dysfunction can occur in more than 50% cases of hepatic failure and is secondary to acute tubular necrosis.[21,22] The overall incidence of acute kidney injury is approximately 2% in all cases of acetaminophen poisoning. It manifests as an increase in creatinine and blood urea nitrogen levels and recovers spontaneously within 4 weeks.

Stage 3

This stage extends from the 3rd to 4th day postingestion. Aminotransferase levels peak at this stage signifying the stage of maximal hepatocellular injury. Most patients (irrespective of aminotransferase levels) progress to recovery with treatment. Maximal deaths occur during this stage. This is secondary to refractory metabolic acidosis, coagulopathy, cerebral edema, arrhythmias, and renal failure.

Stage 4

This is the stage of recovery and extends from day 4 to up to 2 weeks. Patients with mild toxicity commonly recover by 5th or 6th day of ingestion while more serious cases may take some weeks for recovery. Irrespective of the level of toxicity and the time taken for revival, patients who survive usually regain normal liver function. At present, there are no known cases with persistent abnormal liver function after paracetamol poisoning.

DIAGNOSIS

A detailed history should be taken with respect to the dose of drug taken, the duration of time between ingestion and presentation to a medical facility, and the reason for ingestion (suicidal, accidental). It is important to emphasize whether the drug was taken as a single large dose or multiple doses were consumed over a period of time.

The risk of hepatotoxicity can be predicted by correlating the time of ingestion to the serum acetaminophen concentration. Studies have failed to show a correlation between amount of drug ingested and its serum concentration and hence is not used to predict the risk of hepatotoxicity.[23,24] All patients with history of acetaminophen overdose should get serum acetaminophen level measured 4 hours after the time of ingestion. In situations when the exact history of time of ingestion is not available, a serum APAP level should be measured on admission and repeated 4 hours later. The serum APAP levels help predict toxicity after acute drug ingestion. The modified Rumack–Matthew nomogram is used to assess for the risk of toxicity (Fig. 1).

If the APAP value between 4 to 24 hours of ingestion falls on or above the nomogram line, then the patient is at risk of hepatotoxicity and is a candidate for antidotal therapy. It is important to note that if the value falls just below the nomogram line, there is no need for antidote to be given as the risk for liver injury is minimal.[25]

The treatment line in the modified nomogram has a 25% safety margin as compared to the original nomogram. This safety margin helps eliminate variations in acetaminophen measurements by different techniques or laboratories.[25]

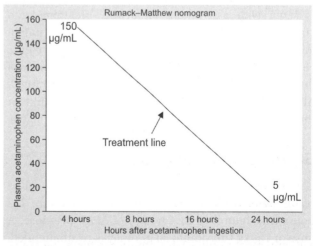

Fig. 1: Rumack–Matthew nomogram (diagrammatic representation, values are not to scale).

Drawbacks of Rumack–Matthew Nomogram

It can be used only for acute ingestions and has no role for chronic drug consumptions. If the exact time of ingestion is not known, it could be misleading and the worst value should be considered to decide on therapy. The role of nomogram in predicting risk following acute overdose of sustained release preparations in unclear. In cases when the patient presents after 24 hours and the APAP level is below the nomogram line, the risk of hepatotoxicity cannot be ruled out.

Role of Repeat Testing of N-acetyl Para-aminophenol Levels

There is no routine need for serial measurements of APAP levels. A single APAP level is sufficient to plan therapy. However, in certain exceptional cases a repeat measurement may be warranted viz exact time of ingestion unknown, ingestion of an extended release (ER) formula, and high levels of APAP at baseline with possibility of detectable levels on completion of therapy.

MANAGEMENT

A two-pronged approach is used for treating acetaminophen overdose namely, general care (gastric decontamination and organ support) and specific therapy (antidotal treatment).

General Care

The general approach to all toxicities and poisonings is same with assessment of airway, breathing, and circulation. Patients should be evaluated for a patent airway with adequate breathing and oxygenation. Hemodynamic assessment with optimization of intravascular volume status and circulation is warranted. All patients should be admitted in a critical care unit for monitoring of vital parameters and hemodynamic status.

Gastric Decontamination

Gastric decontamination with activated charcoal is recommended for all patients who present within 1–2 hours (maximum up to 4 hours) of APAP overdose. A dose of 1 g/kg (maximum 50 g) orally is recommended. Studies have shown that patients who received activated charcoal prior to N-acetyl cysteine (NAC) therapy had lesser chances of liver injury.[26,27]

Specific Therapy (Antidote)

The basis of antidote therapy is regeneration of GSH as its depletion leads to liver injury. At present, NAC is used for treatment of APAP overdose.

There are various mechanisms by which NAC helps to prevent hepatotoxicity.

N-acetyl cysteine is converted to cysteine intracellularly, which is a GSH precursor and increases GSH stores. NAC has sulfhydryl groups which can directly detoxify APAP. It increases APAP metabolism by the sulfation pathway and has a direct antioxidant effect reducing radical species mediated cellular injury and destruction.

There are two approved treatment protocols [oral and intravenous (IV)] of NAC therapy.

Oral N-acetyl Cysteine Protocol[28]

This is a 72-hour course. NAC is given as 140 mg/kg loading dose followed by 70 mg/kg every 4 hours for 17 doses. NAC can induce vomiting and hence is given with cold juices, soft drinks, or as a chilled solution. Alternatively, it can be diluted to form a 10% liquid. If vomiting occurs within 1 hour of any dose, a repeat dose needs to be given. Most patients who present within 8–10 hours of ingestion are adequately treated with oral NAC therapy.

Intravenous Therapy

3 bag regimen: This regimen consists of a loading dose of NAC at 150 mg/kg over 15 minutes. This is followed by infusion of 50 mg/kg over 4 hours and then 100 mg/kg over 16 hours. A total of 300 mg/kg is administered over a period of 20–21 hours.[29] NAC is dissolved in 5% dextrose to be administered as an infusion.

2 bag regimen: This regimen was introduced as it is said to reduce the risk of anaphylactoid reactions. In this regimen, NAC is administered at 50 mg/kg/hour over 4 hours (total 200 mg/kg) followed by an infusion of 6.25 mg/kg/hour for 16 hours (total 100 mg/kg over 16 hours).

There are no differences with respect to efficacy of oral or IV therapy.[30,31] Intravenous therapy is preferred in those with severe vomiting, hepatic failure, and contraindication to oral therapy (ileus).

Indications of N-acetyl Cysteine Therapy

- Serum APAP concentration measured at 4 hours or more, after an acute drug overdose, is above the treatment line in the modified Rumack–Matthew nomogram.

- Unknown time of ingestion
- History of acetaminophen ingestion with evidence of liver injury
- Delayed presentation, i.e. more than 24 hours after ingestion, with biochemical evidence of liver injury.

Adverse Effects of N-acetyl Cysteine

Vomiting and anaphylaxis are the most common adverse effects of oral and IV NAC, respectively. Vomiting is predominantly related to the palatability of NAC. This is managed by diluting it in juice, cola, or covering the cup. Antiemetics can be given to prevent vomiting.

Anaphylaxis is seen in 10–15% cases of patients receiving IV NAC therapy. Presentation varies from flushing, pruritis, urticaria and angioedema, and anaphylactic shock. It is advisable to stop NAC infusion in cases of hypersensitivity reactions and to restart when the reaction subsides. Antihistaminics (diphenhydramine), glucocorticoids, and epinephrine (intramuscular) may be needed in cases of systemic anaphylaxis. In some cases, patients may need to be switched to oral NAC therapy.

Duration of Therapy

The United States Food and Drug Administration (USFDA) has approved two protocols which are time based (20–21 hours for IV therapy and 72 hours for oral therapy).

Extracorporeal Therapy

Acetaminophen can be removed by hemodialysis. However, there is no routine role for hemodialysis in the treatment of acetaminophen poisoning. Some experts recommend hemodialysis in addition to NAC therapy for patients with massive drug ingestion and lactic acidosis.[32] This is not supported by any randomized controlled trials. Also, hemodialysis removes NAC and hence,

some are of the opinion that the dose of NAC should be doubled in such cases. However, in either case if the need arises early initiation of hemodialysis is recommended. The indications of extracorporeal therapy in patients with paracetamol poisoning are discussed in a separate chapter.

Liver Transplant

About 20% cases of liver transplant in United States are secondary to acetaminophen overdose. Acetaminophen overdose can lead to fulminant hepatic failure, defined as hepatic encephalopathy and coagulopathy with jaundice in patients without pre-existing liver disease.[33] The commonly used criteria for liver transplantation in cases of fulminant hepatic failure include, the United Network for Organ Sharing (UNOS) criteria and King's College criteria (Table 1).[34,35]

The UNOS criteria[34] for liver transplant in cases of acetaminophen-induced liver failure includes the following parameters—age of patient, life expectancy without transplant, presence of fulminant hepatic failure without pre-existing liver disease, coagulopathy, mechanical ventilatory support, and need for dialysis.

The King's College criteria[35] for liver transplant in acetaminophen-induced ALF includes the following parameters, i.e. arterial lactate level, serum creatinine, coagulopathy, acidosis, and presence of hepatic encephalopathy.

Cimetidine

Cimetidine was once considered as a treatment option for acetaminophen poisoning as it inhibits cytochrome P450 activity. Even though animal studies supported the role of high dose cimetidine in APAP poisoning, there are no trials at present supporting its role in humans.[36]

Table 1: The United Network for Organ Sharing (UNOS) and King's College criteria for liver transplantation in acetaminophen-induced liver failure.	
UNOS criteria	King's College criteria
Age > 18 years	Strong consideration for orthotopic liver transplant (OLT)
Life expectancy <7 days without transplant	Arterial lactate >3.5 mmol/L after early fluid resuscitation
Fulminant hepatic failure without pre-existing liver disease and one of the following: Mechanical ventilatory support, Dialysis, Continuous venovenous hemofiltration (CVVH), Continuous venovenous hemodiafiltration (CVVHDF), INR > 2	List for OLT: • pH <7.3, or • Arterial lactate >3 after adequate fluid resuscitation
	List for OLT if within 24 hours all of the following are present: • Creatinine >3.4 mg/dL • INR >6.5 • Hepatic encephalopathy (grade 3 or 4)

SPECIAL CASES

Hepatic failure

Only IV NAC therapy is recommended for patients with hepatic failure. The dosing regimen is same as previously mentioned. The only exception is that the final infusion of 100 mg/kg over 16 hours (6.25 mg/kg/h) is continued till hepatic encephalopathy resolves, international normalized ratio (INR) is less than 2, or the patient undergoes liver transplant.[37,38]

Pregnancy

Acetaminophen readily crosses the placenta and maternal overdose can lead to fetal hepatic necrosis and death.[39,40] The treatment protocols for NAC therapy are same as previously mentioned except that IV therapy is preferred so as to reduce the risk of vomiting. Early NAC therapy also helps prevent miscarriage and fetal demise.[39] In rare cases when fetus is delivered in a poisoned patient, IV NAC therapy should be administered to both the mother and the fetus.[41]

PROGNOSIS/OUTCOME

The prognosis and outcome after acetaminophen overdose are usually good if NAC is administered within 8 hours of ingestion irrespective of the serum acetaminophen concentration.[42,43] Studies are ongoing to identify biomarkers which may help identify those at risk of hepatocellular injury following acetaminophen overdose.[33,44,45]

CONCLUSION

Acetaminophen is one of the most common causes of acute liver failure in the world. Even though N-acetyl-cysteine is an available antidote for acetaminophen induced liver failure, a substantial portion of the cases may need liver transplantation. The conventional regimens of NAC are suitable for most cases but some may need longer therapy. A patient tailored approach is recommended for all patients. Since acetaminophen is available as an over the counter (OTC) medication, strict rules and regulations should be imposed by the government to limit access to individuals.

KEY POINTS

- The minimum toxic dose for a single large ingestion is more than 150 mg/kg in children, more than 200 mg/kg in children aged 1–6 years, and greater than 7.5–10 g in adults
- The risk of toxicity is assessed by measuring acetaminophen levels at 4 hours postingestion and plotting it on the Rumack–Matthew nomogram
- The Rumack–Matthew nomogram is not useful in all cases and exceptions are unknown time of ingestion, multiple drug consumptions, overdose with extended or sustained release formulations, and patients presenting 24 hours after ingestion
- The only antidote for acetaminophen toxicity is NAC. Both oral and intravenous routes have equal efficacy. Patients who receive NAC within 8 hours of ingestion usually have a good outcome irrespective of the serum acetaminophen concentration
- Patients not improving with NAC therapy may need liver transplant. The UNOS and King's college criteria are commonly used for the same.

REFERENCES

1. Brodie BB, Axelrod J. The fate of acetophenetidin (phenacetin) in man and methods for the estimation of acetophenetidin and its metabolites in biological material. J Pharmacol Exp Ther. 1949;97:58-67.
2. Bunchorntavakul C, Reddy KR. Acetaminophen-related hepatotoxicity. Clin Liver Dis. 2013;17(4):587-607.
3. Clark R, Fisher JE, Sketris IS, et al. Population prevalence of high dose paracetamol in dispensed paracetamol/opioid prescription combinations: an observational study. BMC Clin Pharmacol. 2012;12:11.
4. Yoon E, Babar A, Choudhary M, et al. Acetaminophen-induced hepatotoxicity: a comprehensive update. J Clin Transl Hepatol. 2016;4(2):131-42.
5. Watson WA, Litovitz TL, Klein-Schwartz W, et al. 2003 annual report of the American Association of Poison Control Centers Toxic Exposure Surveillance System. Am J Emerg Med. 2004;22(5):335-404.
6. Lee WM. Acetaminophen and the United States Acute Liver Failure Study Group: lowering the risks of hepatic failure. Hepatology. 2004;40(1):6-9.
7. Ostapowicz G, Fontana RJ, Schiødt FV, et al. Results of a prospective study of acute liver failure at 17 tertiary care centers in the United States. Ann Intern Med. 2002;137(12):947-54.
8. Lee WM. Acute liver failure in the United States. Semin Liver Dis. 2003;23(3):217-26.
9. Burke A, Smyth E, Fitzgerald GA. Analgesic-antipyretic and antiinflammatory agents; pharmacotherapy of gout. In: Brunton LL, Lazo JS, Parker KL (Eds). Goodman and Gilman's The Pharmacological Basis of Therapeutics. 11th edition. New York: McGraw Hill; 2006.
10. Linden CH, Rumack BH. Acetaminophen overdose. Emerg Med Clin North Am. 1984;2(1):103-19.
11. Peterson RG, Rumack BH. Pharmacokinetics of acetaminophen in children. Pediatrics. 1978;62:877-9.

12. Andreasen PB, Hutters L. Paracetamol (acetaminophen) clearance in patients with cirrhosis of the liver. Acta Med Scand Suppl. 1979;624:99-105.

13. Prescott LF. Paracetamol overdosage. Pharmacological considerations and clinical management. Drugs. 1983;25(3):290-314.

14. Corcoran GB, Mitchell JR, Vaishnav YN, et al. Evidence that acetaminophen and N-hydroxyacetaminophen form a common arylating intermediate, N-acetyl-p benzoquinoneimine. Mol Pharmacol. 1980;18(3):536-42.

15. McGill MR, Jaeschke H. Metabolism and disposition of acetaminophen: recent advances in relation to hepatotoxicity and diagnosis. Pharm Res. 2013;30(9):2174-87.

16. Manyike PT, Kharasch ED, Kalhorn TF, et al. Contribution of CYP2E1 and CYP3A to acetaminophen reactive metabolite formation. Clin Pharmacol Ther. 2000;67(3):275-82.

17. Slattery JT, Wilson JM, Kalhorn TF, et al. Dose-dependent pharmacokinetics of acetaminophen: evidence of glutathione depletion in humans. Clin Pharmacol Ther. 1987;41(4):413-8.

18. Jaeschke H, Williams CD, Ramachandran A, et al. Acetaminophen hepatotoxicity and repair: the role of sterile inflammation and innate immunity. Liver Int. 2012;32(1):8-20.

19. Mitchell JR, Thorgeirsson SS, Potter WZ, et al. Acetaminophen-induced hepatic injury: protective role of glutathione in man and rationale for therapy. Clin Pharmacol Ther. 1974;16(4):676-84.

20. McBride PV, Rumack BH. Acetaminophen intoxication. Semin Dial. 1992;5:292.

21. Mazer M, Perrone J. Acetaminophen-induced nephrotoxicity: pathophysiology, clinical manifestations, and management. J Med Toxicol. 2008;4(1):2-6.

22. Wilkinson SP, Moodie H, Arroyo VA, et al. Frequency of renal impairment in paracetamol overdose compared with other causes of acute liver damage. J Clin Pathol. 1977;30:141-3.

23. Read RB, Tredger JM, Williams R. Analysis of factors responsible for continuing mortality after paracetamol overdose. Hum Toxicol. 1986;5:201-6.

24. Ambre J, Alexander M. Liver toxicity after acetaminophen ingestion. Inadequacy of the dose estimate as an index of risk. JAMA. 1977;238:500-1.

25. Rumack BH, Matthew H. Acetaminophen poisoning and toxicity. Pediatrics. 1975;55(6):871-6.

26. Spiller HA, Krenzelok EP, Grande GA, et al. A prospective evaluation of the effect of activated charcoal before oral N-acetylcysteine in acetaminophen overdose. Ann Emerg Med. 1994;23(3):519-23.

27. Buckley NA, Whyte IM, O'Connell DL, et al. Activated charcoal reduces the need for N-acetylcysteine treatment after acetaminophen (paracetamol) overdose. J Toxicol Clin Toxicol. 1999;37(6):753-7.

28. Rumack BH, Peterson RC, Koch GG, et al. Acetaminophen overdose. 662 cases with evaluation of oral acetylcysteine treatment. Arch Intern Med. 1981;141(3 Spec No):380-5.

29. Prescott LF, Park J, Ballantyne A, et al. Treatment of paracetamol (acetaminophen) poisoning with N-acetylcysteine. Lancet. 1977;2(8035):432-4.

30. Schwarz E, Cohn B. Is intravenous acetylcysteine more effective than oral administration for the prevention of hepatotoxicity in acetaminophen overdose? Ann Emerg Med. 2014;63(1):79-80.

31. Green JL, Heard KJ, Reynolds KM, et al. Oral and intravenous acetylcysteine for treatment of acetaminophen toxicity: A systematic review and meta-analysis. West J Emerg Med. 2013;14(3):218-26.

32. Antoine DJ, Dear JW, Lewis PS, et al. Mechanistic biomarkers provide early and sensitive detection of acetaminophen-induced acute liver injury at first presentation to hospital. Hepatology. 2013;58(2):777-87.

33. Lee WM, Stravitz RT, Larson AM. Introduction to the revised American Association for the Study of Liver Diseases Position Paper on acute liver failure 2011. Hepatology. 2012;55(3):965-7.

34. Organ procurement and transplantation network. Policies. [online] Available from https://optn.transplant.hrsa.gov/governance/policies. [Accessed September, 2018].

35. O'Grady JG, Alexander GJM, Hayllar KM, et al. Early indicators of prognosis in fulminant hepatic failure. Gastroenterology. 1989;97(2):439-45.

36. Burkhart KK, Janco N, Kulig KW, et al. Cimetidine as adjunctive treatment for acetaminophen overdose. Hum Exp Toxicol. 1995;14:299.

37. Fontana RJ. Acute liver failure including acetaminophen overdose. Med Clin North Am. 2008;92(4):761-94.

38. Keays R, Harrison PM, Wendon JA, et al. Intravenous acetylcysteine in paracetamol induced fulminant hepatic failure: a prospective controlled trial. BMJ. 1991;303(6809):1026-9.

39. Riggs BS, Bronstein AC, Kulig K, et al. Acute acetaminophen overdose during pregnancy. Obstet Gynecol. 1989;74(2):247-53.

40. Haibach H, Akhter JE, Muscato MS, et al. Acetaminophen overdose with fetal demise. Am J Clin Pathol. 1984;82(2):240-2.

41. Wang PH, Yang MJ, Lee WL, et al. Acetaminophen poisoning in late pregnancy. A case report. J Reprod Med. 1997;42:367-71.

42. Smilkstein MJ, Bronstein AC, Linden C, et al. Acetaminophen overdose: a 48-hour intravenous N-acetylcysteine treatment protocol. Ann Emerg Med. 1991;20(10):1058-63.

43. Smilkstein MJ, Knapp GL, Kulig KW, et al. Efficacy of oral N-acetylcysteine in the treatment of acetaminophen overdose. Analysis of the national multicenter study (1976 to 1985). N Engl J Med. 1988;319(24):1557-62.

44. Wong A, Graudins A. Risk prediction of hepatotoxicity in paracetamol poisoning. Clin Toxicol (Phila). 2017;55(8):879-92.

45. Wong A, Sivilotti ML, Graudins A. Accuracy of the paracetamol aminotransferase multiplication product to predict hepatotoxicity in modified release paracetamol overdose. Clin Toxicol (Phila). 2017;55(5):346-351.

CHAPTER 24

NSAID Overdose

Anish Gupta, Omender Singh

INTRODUCTION

Nonsteroidal anti-inflammatory drugs (NSAIDs) are commonly prescribed for their analgesic, antipyretic and anti-inflammatory properties. With its growing use, especially in elderly, the number of patients presenting to the emergency department (ED) after acute overdoses has increased. Hence, emergency and critical care specialists should be well versed with the potential adverse effects of these drugs for efficient management of such cases.

PHARMACOLOGY[1]

Nonsteroidal anti-inflammatory drugs inhibit synthesis of prostaglandin and thromboxane by competitively inhibiting the enzyme cyclooxygenase (COX). There are two isoforms of the enzyme cyclooxygenase—(1) COX 1 and (2) COX 2.[2] COX 1 is constitutively expressed in various cells and tissues (platelets, endothelial cells, gastric mucosa, and kidneys) and regulates platelet function and renal blood flow, while COX 2 is an inducible enzyme which increases with pain and inflammation and is induced by inflammatory mediators such as cytokines, endotoxins, etc. Non-selective NSAIDs inhibit both these isoforms while there are selective drugs which only inhibit the COX-2 isoform (Flowchart 1).

Nonsteroidal anti-inflammatory drugs are well absorbed orally with plasma concentrations peaking in 1–2 hours. The plasma half-life is around 8 hours for most NSAIDs. They are highly protein bound (99%) with low volumes of distribution. They are metabolized by the liver and excreted by kidneys.

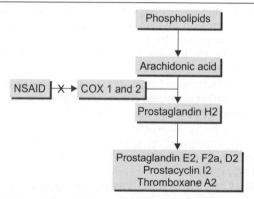

Flowchart 1: Mechanism of action of nonsteroidal anti-inflammatory drugs (NSAIDs). (COX: cyclooxygenase)

CLASSIFICATION

Nonsteroidal anti-inflammatory drugs are classified into two broad groups, i.e. non-selective COX inhibitors and selective COX-2 inhibitors (Table 1).

TOXIC DOSES

The exact toxic doses are not known. Generally, doses of less than 100 mg/kg for most NSAIDs (except mefenamic

NSAID Overdose

Table 1: Classification of nonsteroidal anti-inflammatory drugs (NSAIDs) on the basis of mechanism of action.

Non-selective COX inhibitors	• Salicylates: Aspirin • Acetic acid derivatives: Diclofenac, Etodolac, Sulindac, Indomethacin • Propionic acid derivatives: Naproxen, Ibuprofen, Ketoprofen, Fenoprofen • Fenamate derivatives: Mefenamic acid • Naphthylalkanone derivatives: Nabumetone • Enolic acid derivatives: Piroxicam
Selective COX 2 inhibitors	Celecoxib, Rofecoxib, Valdecoxib

(COX: cyclooxygenase)

acid and phenylbutazone) do not cause toxicity while doses greater than 400 mg/kg are associated with significant toxicity.[3]

TOXIC FEATURES

Always try to elicit a history of the name of drug, dose ingested, time since ingestion and whether any other drugs were coingested.

Acute overdose of NSAIDs is usually well tolerated and does not cause serious adverse effects. Patients may be asymptomatic or present with non-specific symptoms. The most common complaints are nausea, vomiting, abdominal pain, drowsiness, blurred vision, and giddiness.[4]

The various adverse effects of overdose are mentioned in Table 2.

DIAGNOSIS

Diagnosis is based mainly by eliciting a positive history of drug ingestion. Routine workup consisting of CBC, renal function tests, blood glucose levels and ECG should be done. All women of child bearing age should undergo a pregnancy test. Measuring NSAID levels in blood has no role in management as symptoms correlate poorly with blood concentration.[12]

MANAGEMENT

As in any case of drug overdose or poisoning it is important to ensure a patent airway and optimize breathing and circulation. However, respiratory depression and hypotension are not commonly seen with

Table 2: Adverse effects of nonsteroidal anti-inflammatory drugs (NSAIDs).

System	Symptoms and signs
Gastrointestinal	Nausea, vomiting, abdominal pain, dyspepsia, bleeding, peptic ulcer disease
Renal[5,6]	Acute kidney injury, renal papillary necrosis (rare), accelerated hypertension
Cardiovascular	Hypotension, cardiovascular collapse myocardial infarction, arrhythmias
Neurological[7,8]	Headaches, disorientation, drowsiness, ataxia, nystagmus, seizures, coma, psychosis, aseptic meningitis
Hematological[9,10]	Aplastic anemia, agranulocytosis bleeding
Respiratory[11]	Bronchospasm, pulmonary infiltrates with eosinophilia
Allergies/ anaphylaxis	Urticaria, angioedema, pruritus, anaphylactic shock
Acid base abnormalities	High anion gap metabolic acidosis

NSAID overdose. It is advisable to monitor all acute cases of poisoning in a critical care unit. Asymptomatic cases with ingestions of less than 100 mg/kg can be discharged under the supervision of a caregiver and if follow-up is possible. This is not valid for ingestions with mefenamic acid and phenylbutazone as their exact toxic doses are unknown and they can lead to seizures or a host of other adverse effects. Hence, such patients should be admitted and monitored for at least 24 hours.

Gastrointestinal decontamination with activated charcoal for patients presenting within 2 hours of ingestion is suggested. Dose of charcoal is 1 g/kg. NSAIDs have a low enterohepatic circulation and multiple doses of activated charcoal (MDAC) may be ineffective in such cases. Studies have not shown a beneficial effect of MDAC in acute overdose, and it is not recommended.[13]

There is no specific antidote for NSAIDs. Treatment is mainly symptomatic and supportive. Fluids should be administered to maintain intravascular volume. Crystalloids are recommended for the same. Metabolic acidosis should be corrected. Role of sodium bicarbonate for correction of acidosis is not clear and is not recommended.[3,12] Benzodiazepines are used to treat seizures. Hypothermia should be corrected with active warming techniques.

Role of Extracorporeal Therapy

Nonsteroidal anti-inflammatory drugs are highly protein bound and hence hemodialysis (HD) may be ineffective for acute toxicity. There are case reports wherein plasmapheresis was used to treat a patient with phenylbutazone overdose and ECMO was used for ibuprofen ingestion. However, the exact role of plasmapheresis and extracorporeal membrane oxygenation in cases of NSAID overdose is not clear and should be individualized.[14,15]

SALICYLATES

Salicylates are compounds found in various over the counter (OTC) medications such as aspirin, antacids, ointments, salicylic acid, oil of wintergreen, etc. Salicylates belong to the group of NSAIDs and are non-selective inhibitors of the enzyme COX. They are available in various formulations such as oral tablets, rectal suppositories, and topical preparations. We will be discussing salicylate toxicity with aspirin as the prototype drug.

Aspirin acts at various cellular sites and centers producing multiple systemic effects. Aspirin inhibits COX with consequent decrease in production of prostaglandins and thromboxanes leading to platelet dysfunction and gastric mucosal injury.[16,17] It stimulates the medullary respiratory center and the chemoreceptor trigger zone leading to tachypnea and respiratory alkalosis and nausea and vomiting respectively. It also uncouples oxidative phosphorylation leading to metabolic and lactic acidosis.[18,19]

Pharmacology

Aspirin is a weak acid and at standard therapeutic doses aspirin is rapidly absorbed from the gut with serum levels peaking within 1 hour (except in cases of delayed gastric emptying such as pylorospasm, ingestion of enteric coated and sustained or delayed release tablets or use of suppositories).[1,20,21] Aspirin is rapidly converted to salicylic acid in the body. About 90% is protein bound and is mainly metabolized by glycination (75%) in the liver to produce salicyluric acid, salicylphenolic glucuronide, salicyl acyl glucuronide, and gentisic acid. Salicyluric acid is less toxic than salicylic acid and is excreted in urine. A small amount of aspirin (10%) is excreted unchanged in urine.

Toxicity

Ingestion of large quantities of aspirin leads to saturation of the metabolic pathways and overwhelms the normal protective mechanisms against salicylates.[22] As protein binding sites and hepatic detoxification mechanisms get saturated, the free drug levels rise in the body leading to toxic side effects.

Fatal dose is considered 10–30 g in adults and 3 g in children. There is poor correlation between serum salicylate concentrations and signs and symptoms of toxicity. The normal therapeutic range for salicylates is 10–30 mg/dL.[18,19]

Toxic Manifestations

Initial presentation is nonspecific. Patients present with tachycardia, tachypnea, and hyperthermia. Nausea, vomiting, tinnitus, vertigo, and diarrhea are commonly observed in the early stages. Aspirin causes nausea and vomiting by stimulating the medullary chemoreceptor trigger zone, direct irritation of the gastric mucosa and disruption of the mucosal layer. Tinnitus is commonly seen and can be accompanied with altered sound perception and transient hearing loss.[23] These symptoms can occur at therapeutic concentrations and tend to resolve spontaneously.

Neurological

The common manifestations are lethargy, agitation, restlessness, and confusion. Some patients may present with seizures. Coma is a rare manifestation and is seen in severe cases. The CNS effects of salicylates are secondary to direct toxicity, neuroglycopenia and cerebral edema.[24,25] Salicylates specifically lower CNS glucose concentrations and neuroglycopenia can occur despite normal serum glucose concentrations.[24,25]

Acid Base Disorders

Salicylates stimulate the medullary respiratory center leading to tachypnea, hyperpnea and hyperventilation with consequent respiratory alkalosis.[19,26] Both the rate and depth of respiration are increased. Hyperpnea is an early sign of salicylate intoxication that may help establish a diagnosis.

Salicylic acid, being a weak acid does not directly alter the pH. Uncoupling of oxidative phosphorylation leads to accumulation of organic acids (lactic acid, ketoacids) causing metabolic acidosis.[26] A high anion gap metabolic acidosis is commonly observed. Thus, patients with salicylate intoxication present commonly with a primary respiratory alkalosis or a mixed acid base disorder (respiratory alkalosis and metabolic acidosis). Respiratory acidosis and pure metabolic acidosis are uncommon findings and when present should prompt suspicion of other coingestants. The severity of salicylate poisoning can be graded into three categories based on the serum pH levels and acid base abnormality. Mild poisoning is characterized by a pH more than 7.45 and a pure respiratory alkalosis, moderate poisoning is characterized by a normal pH (7.35–7.45) and a mixed acid base disorder (respiratory alkalosis and metabolic acidosis) while severe poisoning is depicted by a subnormal pH (< 7.35) and metabolic acidosis ± respiratory alkalosis.

Others

Salicylates can lead to noncardiogenic pulmonary edema and acute lung injury especially in elderly and with chronic intoxications.

Arrhythmias are common and are secondary to fluid and electrolyte derangements and direct effect on membrane permeability of cardiac myocytes.[27] Hypotension is secondary to hypovolemia caused by poor intake, hyperthermia, vomiting, and diuresis.[28] Thrombocytopenia may be seen but is not of clinical significance.[29] Hemorrhage is a rare manifestation. Large doses can lead to hepatotoxicity with signs and symptoms of liver failure and coagulopathy.

Investigations

Serum Salicylate Levels

The serum salicylate levels are measured using spectrophotometric analysis.[30] Serum lipids interfere with spectrophotometry and ultracentrifugation should be performed prior to testing the sample.[31] Therapeutic concentrations range between 10 mg/dL to 30 mg/dL. There is no correlation between serum levels and toxic manifestations, but values above 40 mg/dL are associated with toxicity. In patients with clinical signs of toxicity, serum salicylate levels should be measured every 2 hours, till two successive measurements show a decreasing trend or the value reaches below 40 mg/dL or the patient shows improvement in clinical condition.

Earlier the *Done nomogram* was used to predict the risk of toxicity depending on the serum salicylate concentrations. The nomogram is no longer used as it had a low predictive value.[32]

It is important to understand that in some cases (pylorospasm, ingestion of extended release formulations) the serum salicylate levels may not rise for a couple of hours and laboratory values should be interpreted with caution in patients fitting the clinical picture.[33,34] Always interpret the serum salicylate values in the context of patient's clinical status and acid base status (pH levels).

Ferric Chloride Spot Test

The ferric chloride helps detect salicylate in urine.[35] A 10% solution of ferric chloride is used and it turns urine purple in presence of salicylate. However, the test has limitations as a positive result only signifies exposure to salicylate and does not imply overdose. False positive results are seen with acetoacetic acid, phenylpyruvic acid, phenothiazines and phenylbutazone.

Serum Electrolytes

Alkalinization can lead to hypokalemia and hence, potassium levels should be monitored frequently and corrected aggressively. Hypokalemia leads to absorption of potassium via H^+/K^+ exchanger in the distal tubule. The secretion of H^+ ion interferes with urinary alkalinization which is an important aspect of therapy.

Renal Function Tests

Aspirin is excreted by the kidneys; creatinine and blood urea nitrogen levels should be measured at baseline and repeated daily. Acute kidney injury and renal failure may prompt need for dialysis in such patients.

ABG

The most common primary acid base abnormality is respiratory alkalosis. A primary respiratory alkalosis and metabolic acidosis can also be seen. A high anion gap acidosis is commonly observed. However, a normal anion gap acidosis does not rule out salicylate toxicity. Isolated metabolic acidosis is rare and should prompt evaluation of other causes of poisoning. Hyperlactatemia is a common finding as salicylates uncouple oxidative phosphorylation and increase anaerobic metabolism leading to increase in lactate production.

Liver Function Tests and Coagulation Parameters

In rare cases of salicylate poisoning, transaminitis (elevated AST and ALT) and coagulopathy (raised prothrombin time and raised international normalized ratio) may be present.

Diagnosis

The diagnosis is established on the basis of history, clinical findings, acid base abnormalities, and elevated serum salicylate levels. Always interpret the serum salicylate values in context to the blood pH and patients' clinical condition. Decreasing values are not always indicative of improvement especially if patient shows clinical deterioration.

Management

The management of salicylate poisoning is plagued with complexities. Since, there is no specific antidote for salicylate poisoning treatment is mainly supportive. Management begins with stabilizing and optimizing the ABCs (airway, breathing and circulation).

Airway and Breathing

Oxygen should be administered to all patients to maintain saturation above 92%. Endotracheal intubation in an aspirin poisoned patient is dangerous and has resulted in worsening of clinical condition and in severe cases even death.[36,37] It should be done only in cases of hypoventilation, respiratory failure (as determined by ABG), acute respiratory distress syndrome, and deteriorating neurological status. Aspirin stimulates the respiratory center in the medulla causing an increase in minute ventilation by increasing both the respiratory rate (RR) and tidal volume (TV). Increase in minute ventilation leads to respiratory alkalosis by decreasing carbon dioxide levels ($PaCO_2$) which acts as a protective mechanism and traps the salicylate ions in the blood. During endotracheal intubation, the administration of sedative and neuromuscular blockers leads to apnea with resultant respiratory acidosis. This effect blunts the protective effect of alkalosis leading to redistribution and crossover of nonionized salicylate into the brain. As a result, there is increase concentration of salicylate in the brain with consequent increase in toxicity. Some schools of thought advise sodium bicarbonate administration prior to intubation so as to maintain an alkalotic pH (7.45–7.5).

The ventilatory settings should be adjusted to maintain a high minute ventilation either by maintaining a high respiratory rate (preferably patients pre-intubation rate) or/and a high tidal volume.

Circulation

Hypotension is a common finding in salicylate toxicity. Hypotension occurs secondary to increased insensible fluid losses (fever, respiratory losses from tachypnea), vomiting, natriuresis and systemic vasodilatation.[38] Aggressive fluid resuscitation should be instituted early in the absence of contraindications. Vasopressors may be added in fluid unresponsive patients. No specific vasopressor is recommended.

Gastrointestinal Decontamination

Activated charcoal (AC) should be given to all patients who present within 2 hours of ingestion. The dose is 1 g/kg (maximum 50 gram). AC can be administered beyond 2 hours in patients with ingestion of enteric coated tablets, delayed gastric emptying (pylorospasm) and bezoar formation. Multiple dose activated charcoal (MDAC) and whole bowel irrigation has shown to decrease salicylate levels in patients who have ingested enteric coated tablets or sustained release preparations.[39,40]

Supplemental Glucose

All patients with altered mental status should receive supplemental glucose irrespective of serum glucose concentrations. Neuroglycopenia is seen in aspirin poisoned patients despite normal serum glucose levels.[25,41] At present there is no robust evidence as to what level the blood glucose should be maintained. However, it is preferable to maintain serum glucose levels in the high normal range. Serum glucose levels should be monitored frequently (every 1–2 hours) till patient shows clinical progress.

Alkalinization of Serum and Urine

Urine and serum alkalinization are central to the management of patients with salicylate or aspirin poisoning.[42,43] Salicylic acid is a weak acid and at steady state it exists in equilibrium as shown.

$$\text{Salicylic acid} \leftrightarrow \text{Salicylate ion} + H^+$$

Increase in the systemic pH (alkalemia) helps reduce toxicity by two mechanisms. As pH rises the equation shifts to the right, thus causing salicylic acid to diffuse down the concentration gradient from the CNS into the blood stream. As a result, the CNS concentration of salicylic acid decreases. This leads to a leftward shift of the equation with increased formation of salicylic acid in the CNS. This further leads to diffusion of the acid into the blood stream thus alleviating the toxic effects of aspirin.

Sodium bicarbonate is administered as an intravenous bolus dose of 1–2 mEq/kg followed by an infusion at the rate of 25–50 mEq/hour. A typical preparation consists of 150 mEq of sodium bicarbonate in 1 liter of 5% dextrose solution. Potassium chloride (20–40 mEq/L) can be added to this preparation as alkalinization leads to intracellular shift of potassium leading to hypokalemia. The infusion is titrated to target a urine pH of 7.5–8 and a urine output of 2–3 mL/kg/hour. Urinary alkalinization in turn increases salicylate excretion by more than ten-fold. Salicylate ion is excreted in the proximal convoluted tubule. Similar to the mechanism stated earlier, alkaline urine also causes dissociation of salicylic acid to salicylate ion thereby preventing back diffusion into the systemic circulation and increasing elimination.

During alkalinization therapy serum potassium should be monitored frequently and maintained in the high normal range as reclamation of potassium in the kidneys in exchange for hydrogen ions may hamper urinary alkalinization.

Alkalinization therapy is not a contraindication despite a primary respiratory alkalosis.[42] In salicylate poisoning, respiratory alkalosis leads to bicarbonaturia. Bicarbonate deficit also occurs secondary to high anion gap metabolic acidosis seen in salicylate poisoning. Hence, alkalinization therapy is administered irrespective of alkalemia. There is no specific target serum pH to be achieved but it is advisable to maintain serum pH less than 7.6. Urine pH should be maintained between 7.5 and 8.

Fluids

Intravenous fluids are administered to maintain adequate intravascular volume and urine output. Urine output is usually targeted in the high normal range, between 1 mL/kg/hour to 2 mL/kg/hour.[28] There is no routine role of diuretics to induce forced diuresis as salicylate excretion depends upon pH and not urinary flow rate.[42]

Carbonic Anhydrase Inhibitor

Carbonic anhydrase inhibitors (acetazolamide) alkalinize urine by reducing bicarbonate reabsorption and thus increases salicylate excretion. However, bicarbonate loss reduces serum pH which in turn potentiates salicylate movement into the CNS and exacerbates toxicity. At present there is no recommendation for the use of acetazolamide in salicylate poisoning.[44]

Hemodialysis

Hemodialysis is an effective modality to remove salicylate from blood. In earlier days charcoal hemoperfusion was used for salicylate removal but with the use of HD its need has reduced. Hemodialysis is a better modality as it not only removes salicylate but also corrects electrolyte, acid-base and fluid abnormalities. It is important to note that continuous renal replacement therapy (CRRT) is considered inferior to hemodialysis for removal of salicylic acid and is not routinely recommended.[45-47] Hemodialysis achieves faster clearance of salicylic acid and correction of fluid, electrolyte and acid base disorder as compared to CRRT. It is preferable to use a high bicarbonate dialysate solution for HD. Peritoneal dialysis is also not effective at removal of salicylate and is seldom used. The indications of dialysis[18,45] are summarized in Box 1.

There are no absolute cut-off serum salicylate values for the initiation of hemodialysis. However, in patients with acute toxicity and serum salicylate levels greater than 100 mg/dL and in patients with chronic toxicity along with signs and symptoms of toxicity and values of 40 mg/dL or greater, consideration of dialysis is warranted. The need for dialysis is in principle governed by the patients' clinical condition. It is always advisable to initiate dialysis early so as to improve outcome.

> **Box 1:** Indications for hemodialysis.
>
> - Altered mental status, coma, seizures, cerebral edema
> - Pulmonary edema, acute respiratory distress syndrome
> - Acute kidney injury
> - Refractory acidosis (pH < 7.2)
> - Markedly elevated serum salicylate concentrations
> - Hyperthermia
> - Deteriorating clinical condition despite alkalinization therapy
> - Contraindication to sodium bicarbonate (renal failure, pulmonary edema)

Glycine

Glycine or N-glycylglycine can be administered orally to poisoned patients. Since approximately 75% of salicylic acid is metabolized by glycination to non-toxic metabolites (salicyluric acid), theoretically supplemental glycine may help reduce salicylic acid levels.[47] At present there is limited data to support its role for treatment of salicylate poisoning.

Prognosis

Salicylates are one of the most commonly prescribed and used drugs worldwide. As per data from the American Association of Poison Control Center, National Poison Data System (NPDS),[48] analgesics were the most commonly abused substances in adults more than 20 years old with approximately 24% deaths due to intoxication with aspirin or aspirin-combination drugs. Overall, the mortality from acute overdose is about 1% while in those with chromic intoxication it is higher to the tune of 25%.

CONCLUSION

NSAIDs' are amongst the most common class of drugs prescribed to treat pain and inflammation. Over the counter availability and chronic abuse have made it a significant contender for drug overdose and toxicity. Since, there is no specific antidote available, management is mainly symptomatic and supportive. Patients should be educated about the side effects and toxicity of NSAIDs as self overdosing is the common cause of toxicity. Government should frame laws regarding over the counter availability of such drugs to limit its widespread abuse.

KEY POINTS

- The exact toxic doses are unknown. As a norm doses less than 100 mg/kg (except mefenamic acid and phenylbutazone) are not considered to be associated with toxicity and doses more than 400 mg/kg are always associated with toxicity
- There is no specific antidote for NSAID poisoning and even MDAC is ineffective for NSAIDs
- In salicylates toxicity, the primary acid base abnormality is respiratory alkalosis as it stimulates the respiratory center in the medulla. A high anion gap metabolic acidosis is commonly observed
- Alkalinization of serum and urine are the mainstays for management of salicylate poisoning. Target urine pH of 7.5–8. Respiratory alkalosis is not a contraindication to alkalinization therapy
- Keep a high threshold for endotracheal intubation as it blunts the protective effect of respiratory alkalosis and can increase mortality.

REFERENCES

1. Hoffman RS, Howland MA, Lewin NA, et al. Goldfrank's Toxicologic Emergencies, 10th edition. New York: McGraw-Hill; 2014.
2. Parente L, Perretti M. Advances in the pathophysiology of constitutive and inducible cyclooxygenases: two enzymes in the spotlight. Biochem Pharmacol. 2003;65(2):153-9.
3. Volans G, Monaghan J, Colbridge M. Ibuprofen overdose. Int J Clin Pract. 2003;(135):54-60.
4. Smolinske SC, Hall AH, Vandenberg SA, et al. Toxic effects of nonsteroidal anti-inflammatory drugs in overdose. An overview of recent evidence on clinical effects and dose-response relationships. Drug Saf. 1990;5(4):252-74.
5. Gambaro G, Perazella MA. Adverse renal effects of anti-inflammatory agents: evaluation of selective and nonselective cyclooxygenase inhibitors. J Intern Med. 2003;253(6):643-52.
6. Griffin MR, Yared A, Ray WA. Nonsteroidal antiinflammatory drugs and acute renal failure in elderly persons. Am J Epidemiol. 2000;151(5):488-96.
7. Sánchez-Hernandez MC, Delgado J, Navarro AM, et al. Seizures induced by NSAID. Allergy. 1999;54(1):90-1.
8. Vale JA, Meredith TJ. Acute poisoning due to non-steroidal anti-inflammatory drugs. Clinical features and management. Med Toxicol. 1986;1(1):12-31.
9. Risks of agranulocytosis and aplastic anemia. A first report of their relation to drug use with special reference to analgesics. The International Agranulocytosis and Aplastic Anemia Study. JAMA. 1986;256(13):1749-57.
10. Nelson L, Shih R, Hoffman R. Aplastic anemia induced by an adulterated herbal medication. J Toxicol Clin Toxicol. 1995;33(5):467-70.
11. Goodwin SD, Glenny RW. Nonsteroidal anti-inflammatory drug-associated pulmonary infiltrates with eosinophilia. Review of the literature and Food and Drug Administration Adverse Drug Reaction reports. Arch Intern Med. 1992;152(7):1521-4.
12. Hall AH, Smolinske SC, Stover B, et al. Ibuprofen overdose in adults. J Toxicol Clin Toxicol. 1992;30(1):23-37.
13. Position statement and practice guidelines on the use of multi-dose activated charcoal in the treatment of acute poisoning. American Academy of Clinical Toxicology; European Association of Poisons Centres and Clinical Toxicologists. J Toxicol Clin Toxicol. 1999;37(6): 731-51.
14. Marciniak KE, Thomas IH, Brogan TV, et al. Massive ibuprofen overdose requiring extracorporeal membrane oxygenation for cardiovascular support. Pediatr Crit Care Med. 2007;8(2):180-2.

15. Geith S, Renner B, Rabe C, et al. Ibuprofen plasma concentration profile in deliberate ibuprofen overdose with circulatory depression treated with therapeutic plasma exchange: a case report. BMC Pharmacol Toxicol. 2017;18(1):81

16. Vane JR, Botting RM. The mechanism of action of aspirin. Thromb Res. 2003;110(5-6):255-8.

17. Cadavid AP. Aspirin: the Mechanism of Action Revisited in the Context of Pregnancy Complications. Front Immunol. 2017;8:261.

18. O'Malley GF. Emergency department management of the salicylate-poisoned patient. Emerg Med Clin North Am. 2007;25(2):333-46.

19. Hill JB. Salicylate intoxication. N Engl J Med. 1973;288(21):1110-3.

20. Pierce RP, Gazewood J, Blake RL Jr. Salicylate poisoning from enteric-coated aspirin. Delayed absorption may complicate management. Postgrad Med. 1991;89(5):61-4.

21. Wortzman DJ, Grunfeld A. Delayed absorption following enteric-coated aspirin overdose. Ann Emerg Med 1987:434-36.

22. Garella S. Extracorporeal techniques in the treatment of exogenous intoxications. Kidney Int. 1988:735-54.

23. Cazals Y. Auditory sensori-neural alterations induced by salicylate. Prog Neurobiol. 2000;62(6):583-631.

24. Rauschka H, Aboul-Enein F, Bauer J, et al. Acute cerebral white matter damage in lethal salicylate intoxication. Neurotoxicology. 2006;28(1):33-7

25. Thurston JH, Pollock PG, Warren SK, et al. Reduced brain glucose with normal plasma glucose in salicylate poisoning. J Clin Invest. 1970;49(11):2139-45.

26. Gabow PA, Anderson RJ, Potts DE, et al. Acid-Base Disturbances in the Salicylate-Intoxicated Adult. Arch Intern Med. 1978;138(10):1481-4.

27. Kent K, Ganetsky M, Cohen J, et al. Non-fatal ventricular dysrhythmias associated with severe salicylate toxicity. Clin Toxicol (Phila). 2008;46(4):297-9.

28. Temple AR. Acute and chronic effects of aspirin toxicity and their treatment. Arch Intern Med. 1981;141(3):364-9.

29. Visentin GP, Liu CY. Drug Induced Thrombocytopenia. Hematol Oncol Clin North Am. 2007;21(4):685.

30. Okuno S, Wada Y. Measurement of serum salicylate levels by solid-phase extraction and desorption/ionization on silicon mass spectrometry. J Mass Spectrom. 2005;40(8):1000-4.

31. Charlton NP, Lawrence DT, Wallace KL. Falsely elevated salicylate levels. J Med Toxicol. 2008;4(4):310-1.

32. Dugandzic RM, Tierney MG, Dickinson GE, et al. Evaluation of the validity of the Done nomogram in the management of acute salicylate intoxication. Ann Emerg Med. 1989;18(11):1186-90.

33. Rivera W, Kleinschmidt KC, Velez LI, et al. Delayed salicylate toxicity at 35 hours without early manifestations following a single salicylate ingestion. Ann Pharmacother. 2004;38:1186.

34. Drummond R, Kadri N, St-Cyr J. Delayed salicylate toxicity following enteric-coated acetylsalicylic acid overdose: a case report and review of the literature. CJEM. 2001;3:44.

35. Hoffman RJ, Nelson LS, Hoffman RS. Use of ferric chloride to identify salicylate-containing poisons. J Toxicol Clin Toxicol. 2002;40(5):547-9.

36. Greenberg MI, Hendrickson RG, Hoffman M. Deleterious effects of endotracheal intubation in salicylate poisoning. Ann Emerg Med. 2003;41(4):583-4.

37. Stolbach AI, Hoffman RS, Nelson LS. Mechanical ventilation was associated with acidemia in a case series of salicylate-poisoned patients. Acad Emerg Med. 2008;15(9):866-9.

38. Leatherman JW, Schmitz PG. Fever, hyperdynamic shock, and multiple-system organ failure. A pseudo-sepsis syndrome associated with chronic salicylate intoxication. Chest. 1991;100(5):1391-6.

39. Kirshenbaum LA, Mathews SC, Sitar DS, et al. Does Multiple-Dose Charcoal Therapy Enhance Salicylate Excretion? Arch Intern Med. 1990;150(6):1281-3.

40. Kirshenbaum LA, Mathews SC, Sitar DS, et al. Whole-bowel irrigation versus activated charcoal in sorbitol for the ingestion of modified-release pharmaceuticals. Clin Pharmacol Ther. 1989;46(3):264-71.

41. Kuzak N, Brubacher JR, Kennedy JR. Reversal of salicylate-induced euglycemic delirium with dextrose. Clin Toxicol (Phila). 2007;45(5):526-9.

42. Proudfoot AT, Krenzelok EP, Vale JA. Position Paper on urine alkalinization. J Toxicol Clin Toxicol. 2004;42(1):1-26.

43. Prescott LF, Balali-Mood M, Critchley JA, et al. Diuresis or urinary alkalinisation for salicylate poisoning? Br Med J (Clin Res Ed). 1982;285(6352):1383-6.

44. Sweeney KR, Chapron DJ, Brandt JL, et al. Toxic interaction between acetazolamide and salicylate: case reports and a pharmacokinetic explanation. Clin Pharmacol Ther. 1986;40(5):518-24.

45. Juurlink DN, Gosselin S, Kielstein JT, et al. Extracorporeal Treatment for Salicylate Poisoning: Systematic Review and Recommendations From the EXTRIP Workgroup. Ann Emerg Med. 2015;66(2):165-81.

46. Goodman JW, Goldfarb DS. The role of continuous renal replacement therapy in the treatment of poisoning. Semin Dial. 2006;19(5):402-7.

47. Patel DK, Ogunbona A, Notarianni LJ, et al. Depletion of plasma glycine and effect of glycine by mouth on salicylate metabolism during aspirin overdose. Hum Exp Toxicol. 1990;9(6):389-95.

48. Mowry JB, Spyker DA, Brooks DE, et al. 2014 Annual Report of the American Association of Poison Control Centers' National Poison Data System (NPDS): 32nd Annual Report. Clin Toxicol (Phila). 2015;53(10):962-1147.

25 CHAPTER

Corrosive Ingestion: Acids and Alkalis

Desh Deepak

INTRODUCTION

Ingestion of corrosives acids and alkalis can cause mild-to-severe local tissue injury to gastrointestinal (GI) tract, respiratory tract, skin and eyes, and systemic complications depending upon the route of exposure. The severity of tissue damage and inflammatory response depends upon, but not limited to, the type of agent (acid/alkali), the chemical nature (pH <2 or >11), titratable acid or alkaline reserve (TAR), amount ingested, physical form (solid/liquid), and concentration and duration of contact of the corrosive with the mucosa. Presence of food can also alter the extent of injury.[1-4]

EPIDEMIOLOGY

The acid and alkalis exposure can be either intentional or accidental; however, the true epidemiology from India cannot be elucidated due to variable reporting and insufficient data from very few Indian case series. In Indian perspective, the disease burden varies significantly (13–44.6%), wherein most of the poisoning is due to ingestion of household corrosive agents.[5,6] Results of a prospective long-term study from the All India Institute of Medical Sciences, New Delhi concluded that corrosive substances were responsible for 13.6% of all cases of fatal poisoning presenting to the tertiary center. Domestic cleaning products caused 39.6% cases of corrosive poisoning; however, in more than half of cases

(56.26%) an exact cause could not be identified. Sulfuric acid was ingested in 68.75% of all identifiable cases of corrosive agent. In 87.5% cases, the intent was concluded to be suicidal.[7] Western data has estimated a prevalence of 2.5–5% with corrosive ingestion, with high morbidity and mortality rates of 50% and 13%, respectively.[8] In United States of America, children form the majority patients of corrosive ingestion, while the rest comprise of psychotic, suicidal, and alcoholic adult patients.[9] But one must be aware that though less in number, adult cases have more grievous injuries resulting in high mortality and morbidity which may be related to excess volume of exposure and frequent coingestions.[8]

CAUSATIVE AGENTS

- *Strong alkali*: Sodium or potassium hydroxide, bleach (hypochlorite) are few examples, often found in drain cleaner and household cleaning products.[4]
- *Concentrated acids*: Hydrochloric acid, sulfuric acid, nitric acid, and phosphoric acid are few examples of acids, commonly found in toilet bowl or swimming pool cleaners, antirust compounds, or in battery fluid. Phenol is a common ingredient of antiseptic/disinfectant solutions.[4]

Pathogenesis

The mechanism of injury in alkali ingestion is liquefaction necrosis, while in case of acids it is coagulation necrosis.[10]

Alkali such as ammonia or sodium hydroxide causes rapidly progressive damage extending through the layers of tissues, till it is buffered by tissue fluids. Ninety to hundred percent of alkali injury cases involve esophagus and gastrium. In up to 30% cases, duodenal involvement has been observed.[11] In acute phase (first 3–4 days), tissues are very fragile and friable with frequent ulcers and slough formation. In the next phase (up to 2 weeks), granulation tissue and fibrosis sets in and eventually healing occurs in 4–12 weeks, often requiring intervention to prevent stricture formations.[10,12]

Acid injury usually causes limited damage due to coagulation of superficial tissue protein and blood vessels forming a protective layer limiting the progression. Nonetheless, tissue damage can still be extensive if volume of ingestion is high or if liquid preparations are ingested. Acids cause instantaneous superficial damage with tissue reaction and hence, they are extremely painful. Being painful, they are deterrent for further ingestion. An injury caused by acid usually heals by an eschar formation.[12,13]

Sweeping generalizations that alkali causes more injury than acid is not accurate, as corrosive injury depends upon several physiochemical properties of the chemical and its variable interaction with the human body. In an isolated study, which compared one particular acid ingestion (glacial acetic acid) versus alkali ingestion, it was found that patients who have ingested glacial acetic acid were sicker, developed more complications like perforation and sepsis, eventually requiring intensive care support and had worst outcome. Early endoscopy graded extent of injury was the best predictor of anticipated complication and mortality.[14] Grading systems Kikendall and Zargar classification similar to burns grading system are used which are based on early endoscopic evaluation.[9,11]

Clinical Presentation[3,10,12,15]

Initial signs and symptoms can be very deceptive; hence, all patients need observation for at least 24 hours. Severe signs and symptoms suggest presence of severe injury.

Central Nervous System

- Altered sensorium (especially with coingestion of alcohol)

Cardiovascular System

Hypotension due to hypovolemia is common due to repeated vomiting, third space losses, and rarely hemorrhage. Sepsis secondary to perforation peritonitis, mediastinal perforation, and mediastinitis can also cause hemodynamic instability.

Gastrointestinal Tract

Severe pain can occur due to ulcers on lips, oropharynx, and esophagus along with diffuse gastritis. Patients can present with complaints of dysphagia/odynophagia, retrosternal chest pain, epigastric pain, retching, and emesis.

Initial presentation can be of acute abdomen due to GI perforation and/or peritonitis.

Respiratory Tract

- Excessive salivation, hoarseness, expectoration, hematemesis
- Dyspnea due to laryngospasm, chemical pneumonitis, pulmonary edema, esophageal perforation causing pneumomediastinum.

Skin

- Pain, erythema, vesicle formation

Eye and Adnexa

- Acutely, eye involvement may present as severe pain, epiphora, foreign body sensation, blurred vision, corneal epithelial defects, conjunctival congestion
- Limbal ischemia leads to corneal opacity, severe dry eye, symblepharon, etc.

Complications[12]

Early

- Necrosis of tissue with initial contact of corrosive agents causing intense pain. Airway edema and obstruction is a deadly complication associated with oropharyngeal injury often involving upper respiratory tract
- First 24–72 hours is the crucial period where perforation and ulceration can happen
- Fibrosis and scarring set in around 14–21 days postexposure

Gastrointestinal and Liver Toxins

- *Other acute complications*: Shock, renal failure, sepsis, disseminated intravascular coagulation, acute respiratory distress syndrome.

Late

- Strictures start forming in few weeks postexposure
- Esophageal and gastric carcinoma formation take few years to decades to develop following injury
- Skin scars
- Corneal opacity, dry eye, symblepharon.

Investigations

See Box 1.

Management[3,9,10,12]

Management of corrosive injury is not well studied in the randomized controlled trials. Most of its guidance comes from standard textbooks, few case series, and animal data.

Triaging

Based on detailed clinical history and examination, patient should be triaged either to ward or intensive care unit.

Ward or emergency room: Asymptomatic patients where history is very reliable need observation for at least 24 hours and an early endoscopy to assess the severity of injury.[14]

Intensive care unit: Patients with large amounts of corrosive ingestion or the ones with endoscopic esophageal damage with grades 2B or greater (Zargar classification) should always be admitted in an intensive care unit to avoid/manage acute life-threatening conditions. The cases in which reliable history is in question, patient should be hospitalized, and an early endoscopy needs to be done.[14]

General Management[3,9,10,12]

Basic management should be started simultaneously with ABCD (airway, breathing, circulation, disability evaluation, and decontamination) approach.

- *Airway protection*: In the presence of hypoxemia with altered sensorium, especially with signs and symptoms of upper airway obstruction, an airway should be secured (especially in view of planned endoscopy). Severely symptomatic patient with respiratory distress/stridor/hoarse voice should be intubated early. Always consider rapid sequence intubation and use short-acting agents. If time permits, take samples of serum and urine beforehand, for toxicology screening, to avoid confusion with anesthetic agent used in intubation
- Breathing should be optimized with appropriate supportive devices of oxygen delivery such as nasal cannula or face mask to maintain a SpO_2 of more than 95%. Avoid noninvasive ventilation, as there is a high risk of conversion of minor injury to perforation. If required, go for invasive ventilation
- Monitor consciousness, heart rate, electrocardiography (ECG) rhythm, blood pressure, plethysmographic saturation, respiratory rate, and urinary output. Obtain peripheral venous access and start guided fluid therapy. Patient may need arterial line or central line placement and monitoring of advanced parameters
- Keep patient nil by mouth until evaluation has been done by endoscopy to grade the injury and delineate the management plan. Never insert nasoenteric tube blindly
- Local lesions of skin and eye should be irrigation with copious amount of sterile water for at least 5 minutes. Details have been discussed at the end of this chapter

---

Box 1: Investigations to be done in case of corrosive agents poisoning.

Investigations[3,10,12]

- Complete blood count
- Renal function test, liver function test, serum electrolytes
- Coagulation profile, blood grouping
- Arterial blood gas, anion gap, serum osmolality, osmolar gap, lactate
- Serum/urine toxicology screen
- ECG, chest X-ray, abdominal X-ray, ultrasound abdomen
- CT thorax and abdomen*
- Endoscopic ultrasound†
- Barium studies‡

* Sensitivity and specificity of CT has been found to be more than that of endoscopic grading system in predicting the development of esophageal strictures.[16]
† May be helpful in predicting stricture formation.[17]
‡ Not indicated in acute settings, but in late presentations they can be used to assess strictures.[10]
(CT: computed tomography; ECG: electrocardiography)

- Do not use emetics agents (they can cause more harm than benefit by inducing perforation)
- Do not use neutralizing agents. Theoretically, it may help but neutralization produces heat, which can be damaging by itself. Currently, there are no general recommendations for neutralization[18]
- Oral pharyngeal examination to be done. Even if the oropharynx is clear of any burns, it does not guarantee an absence of perforation or injury in other areas of GI tract[12]
- Upper GI endoscopy should be performed early (with in first 24–48 hours) in all cases, to evaluate the extent of damage and plan further management[14]
- In the presence of perforation, surgical management is imperative. Severe caustic injuries causing tracheobronchial injury or severe esophageal injuries may even require emergency surgeries.[19]

Upper Gastrointestinal Endoscopy

The indications and contraindications of upper GI endoscopy are given in Table 1.[10,12]

Complications of endoscopy are rare, but they include perforation, ulceration, bleeding, and infection.

Endoscopic Classification

Classifications given by Zargar and Kikendall are currently being followed to grade esophageal injury which help in prediction of subsequent clinical progression.[9,11] To keep discussion simple, only Zargar system is presented in Table 2.

Upper Gastrointestinal Endoscopy-guided Management

- Endoscopy should be done to evaluate severity of lesions according to the Zargar grading system.
- In grade 1 or 2A lesions, start liquid diet early and then switch patients to a regular soft diet based on acceptance, gradually, by the end of 10th day.[10]
- Place endoscopic-guided nasoenteric feeding tube in grade 2B or 3 lesions. After 48 hours of observation in grade 2B, oral liquids can be started cautiously only if the patient can swallow saliva and should further be observed for any signs of leak.[10]
- Grade 3 lesions require close monitoring for any signs of perforation. They require long-term support with tube feedings (naso-oroenteric, gastrostomy, and jejunostomy). These patients need follow-up for screening and treatment for strictures.[10]
- Give proton pump inhibitor or H_2 blocker.
- Nutritional management is an important aspect of corrosive ingestion as it directly affects GI tract. As discussed above, based on endoscopy, an appropriate route for feeds and type of diet can be decided based on severity of lesions. Surgical cases require gastrostomy/jejunostomy for nutritional management.
- Role of systemic steroids to prevent stricture formations is debatable. With current evidence it is not recommended.[20]
- No role of prophylactic antibiotics. But should be administered in case of GI perforation.

Table 1: Indications and contraindications of upper gastrointestinal endoscopy.

Indications	Absolute contraindications
All patients within first 24 hours of corrosive exposure, as sometimes sign and symptoms appear late	Gastrointestinal perforation
Delayed endoscopy to be done 3 weeks after exposure for evaluation and stricture dilation, if needed	Hemodynamic instability (stabilize the patient first, then perform endoscopy)
	Respiratory distress or suggestive of glottic edema. Intubate the patient first, then continue with endoscopy
	Relative contraindications
	Between 72 hours to 3 weeks of corrosive exposure (risk > benefit)
	Uncorrected coagulopathy (unless severe and obvious bleeding patient)

Gastrointestinal and Liver Toxins

Table 2: Zargar classification.[11]

Grade 0	Normal mucosa
Grade 1	Edema and erythema of the mucosa
Grade 2a	Hemorrhage, erosions, blisters, superficial ulcers
Grade 2b	Circumferential lesions
Grade 3a	Focal deep-gray or brownish-black ulcers
Grade 3b	Extensive deep-gray or brownish-black ulcers
Grade 4	Perforation

- *Experimental/newer techniques*: Prophylactic esophageal stenting is not recommended.[21] Although with the currently available self-expanding plastic stents which are easily retrievable and cause less tissue reactions, options have increased.[22] In a pediatric study of severe caustic esophageal injury, the use of early (prophylactic) dilatation did not eliminate stricture formation completely, but strictures resolved more easily with early bougienage.[23]

Surgical Management

- Patients in intensive care having signs and symptoms of severe abdominal pain, abdominal hypertension, respiratory distress, ascites, pleural effusion, metabolic acidosis in blood gas analysis with hyperlactemia should be evaluated for perforation peritonitis or mediastinitis necessitating emergency surgical intervention, involving thoracic, abdominal, or combined approach with or without laparoscopy. Procedures range from stenting, esophagectomy, leakage repair to gastric or colonic interposition.[12,24]
- *Stricture management*: Strictures which failed to resolve with endoscopic dilation and medical management need surgical repair with resection and anastomosis with or without repair.[24]

COMMON CORROSIVE AGENTS

Hydrofluoric Acid

It is present in home rust removers, metal cleaners, and electronic manufacturing.

Solutions of concentrations varying from 5% to 50% exposure cause deep burns as compared to small area of exposure. Inhalation exposure with fumes can also cause acute lung injury. Fluoride ions penetrate and precipitate magnesium and calcium insoluble salts causing hypocalcemia, and hypomagnesia. Electrolyte imbalance and direct cardiotoxicity by fluoride ions causes arrhythmias which can result in death. Initial treatment involves copious irrigation with water followed by local calcium gluconate 2.5% gel application. Aggressive supportive therapy along with intravenous calcium and magnesium replacement is the mainstay of treatment.[25,26]

Phenol (Phenyl)

Exposure can be oral and dermal. From mild symptoms ranging from nausea, vomiting, diarrhea and abdominal pain; these patients can have severe corrosive injury to the mouth, throat, esophagus, and stomach with bleeding, perforation, scarring, or stricture formation as potential sequelae. These patients can have agitation, seizures, or coma with hypotension or dysrhythmia due to free plasma concentration of phenol. Decontamination with removal of clothing, flushing body with water, then brushing ethyl alcohol for dermal exposure is an important consideration. Treatment is mainly supportive.[27]

White Phosphorus (Fire Crackers)

Exposure can cause dermal burns by combined oxidative and thermal injury. Post burns, these patients are likely to have life-threatening electrolyte abnormalities, i.e. hypocalcemia, hyperphosphatemia, and often hepatic necrosis requiring supportive intensive care management. Calcium and phosphorus levels should be monitored frequently in first 72 hours for appropriate management. Dermal wounds should be thoroughly washed with water and then wrapped in saline-soaked gauzes. Visible particles should be picked up cleanly with forceps. These patients often require repeated surgical debridement to remove all particles. Surgical management is continued following the principles of burns management.[28]

Hydrochloric Acid (Toilet Cleaner)

Accidental oral exposure of undiluted hydrochloric acid in large quantity results in diffuse upper GI damage. Dermal exposure needs flushing with copious amount of water while oral ingestion requires urgent endoscopy within 12 hours to ascertain the damage and manage the complications. Aggressive intensive care support and surgical intervention is needed in case of complications of perforation in thoracic or abdominal cavity.[29]

Anhydrous Ammonia (Agriculture Fertilizers and Industrial Refrigerant)

Injury is mainly after inhalation exposure, but it often follows ingestion. Patient can have symptoms of oropharyngeal, epigastric, and retrosternal discomfort. Even GI perforations have been reported up to 48 hours after ingestion. Due to its extreme water solubility, it can cause widespread pulmonary damage often requiring intubation and ventilation. Decontaminate with copious water irrigation. Rinse mouth thoroughly with water. Arrange for endoscopic evaluation with supportive management.[30]

List of alkalis and acids causing systemic toxicity is exhaustive; therefore, one should get in touch with toxicology centers to guide treatment in individual exposures. Agency for toxic substances and disease registry guidelines can be used to guide management in individual corrosive exposures.[31]

Irrigation/Decontamination

There are no set recommendations, but in acute presentations irrigation with copious amount of water is suggested. Alkali injury may require longer duration of irrigation. In case of eye involvement, 15–30 minutes of irrigation is suggested. For irrigation, generally sterile water is suggested.

Exception to Irrigation with Water

- *Dry lime*: Contains calcium oxide which reacts with water to form calcium hydroxide which is a stronger alkali. Brushing off solid particles to be done
- *Metals*: React with water to form hazardous by-products. Remove solid particles with dry forceps. Repeated application of mineral oil to be done to remove smaller particles
- *Phenol*: Not soluble in water. Polyethylene glycol sponging is needed for its removal.

Follow-up

- Explain the need for regular follow-up to the patient and be on a look out for the sequelae and plan their management. Printed material for patient education may provide significant help
- Long-term follow-up by gastroenterologist, dermatology, and ophthalmology is often required.

CONCLUSION

Corrosive injury is common problem with varied presentations where timely management with early endoscopy, grade assessment, nutritional support and early involvement of gastroenterologist to plan long-term management is prudent.

KEY POINTS

- Perform early endoscopy in first 24 hours, as initial signs and symptoms are often misleading
- Absence of oropharyngeal injury does not rule out esophageal or gastric involvement
- Hemodynamic stability and secure airway is a priority over upper GI endoscopy
- Always contact designated regional poison control center for guidance on treatment
- Moderate-to-severe injury patients should be observed, evaluated, and managed in intensive care units with advanced monitoring capabilities, along with round the clock back up of gastroenterologist, surgical, and intervention specialties.

REFERENCES

1. Goldman LP, Weigert JM. Corrosive substance ingestion: a review. Am J Gastroenterol. 1984;79:85-90.
2. Wasserman RL, Ginsburg CM. Caustic substance injuries. J Pediatr. 1985;107(2):169-74.
3. Brent J, Burkhart K, Dargan P. Critical Care Toxicology: Diagnosis and Management of the Critically Poisoned Patient, 1st edition. St Louis: Mosby: 2005. pp. 1035-44.
4. Goldfrank LR. Caustics. Goldfrank's Toxicologic Emergencies, 8th edition. New York: McGraw-Hill; 2006.
5. Patil A, Peddawad R, Verma V, et al. Profile of acute poisoning cases treated in a tertiary care hospital: a study in Navi Mumbai. APJMT. 2014;3(1):36-40.
6. Singh O, Javeri Y, Juneja D, et al. Profile and outcome of patients with acute toxicity admitted in intensive care unit: Experiences from a major corporate hospital in urban India. Indian J Anaes. 2011;55:370-4.
7. Swain R, Behera C, Gupta S. Fatal corrosive ingestion: A study from South and South-East Delhi, India (2005-2014). Medicine, Science and Law. 2016;56(4):252-7.
8. Contini S, Scarpignato C. Caustic injury of the upper gastrointestinal tract: a comprehensive review. World J Gastroenterol. 2013;19(25):3918-30.
9. Kikendall JW. Caustic ingestion injuries. Gastroenterol Clin North Am. 1991;20(4):847-57.
10. Chibishev A, Pereska Z, Chibisheva V, et al. Corrosive poisonings in adults. Materia Socio Medica. 2012;24(2):125-30.

11. Zargar SA, Kochhar R, Nagi B, et al. Ingestion of strong corrosive alkalis: spectrum of injury to upper gastrointestinal tract and natural history. Am J Gastroenterol.1992;87(3):337-41.

12. Raghu R, Naik R, Vadivelan M. Corrosive poisoning. Indian Journal of Clinical Practice. 2012;23(3):131-4.

13. Fisher RA, Eckhauser ML, Radivoyevitch M. Acid ingestion in an experimental model. Surg Gynecol Obstet. 1985;161(1):91-9.

14. Poley JW, Steyerberg EW, Kuipers EJ, et al. Ingestion of acid and alkaline agents: outcome and prognostic value of early upper endoscopy. Gastrointest Endosc. 2004;60(3):372-7.

15. Gaudreault P, Parent M, McGuigan MA, et al. Predictability of esophageal injury from signs and symptoms: a study of caustic ingestion in 378 children. Pediatrics. 1983;71(5):767-70.

16. Ryu HH, Jeung KW, Lee BK, et al. Caustic injury: can CT grading system enable prediction of esophageal stricture? Clin Toxicol (Phila). 2010;48(2):137-42.

17. Kamijo Y, Kondo I, Kokuto M, et al. Miniprobe ultrasonography for determining prognosis in corrosive esophagitis. Am J Gastroenterol. 2004;99(5):851-4.

18. Penner GE. Acid ingestion: toxicology and treatment. Ann Emerg Med.1980;9(7):374-9.

19. Chirica M, Resche-Rigon M, Bongrand NM, et al. Surgery for caustic injuries of the upper gastrointestinal tract. Ann Surg. 2012;256(6):994-1001.

20. Fulton JA, Hoffman RS. Steroids in second degree caustic burns of the esophagus: a systematic pooled analysis of fifty years of human data: 1956-2006. Clin Toxicol (Phila). 2007;45(4):402-8.

21. Mills LJ, Estrera AS, Platt MR. Avoidance of esophageal stricture following severe caustic burns by the use of an intraluminal stent. Ann Thorac Surg. 1979;28:60-5.

22. Evrard S, Le Moine O, Lazaraki G, et al. Self-expanding plastic stents for benign esophageal lesions. Gastrointest Endosc. 2004;60(6):894-900.

23. Tiryaki T, Livanelioğlu Z, Atayurt H. Early bougienage for relief of stricture formation following caustic esophageal burns. Pediatr Surg Int. 2005;21(2):78-80.

24. Zhou JH, Jiang YG, Wang RW, et al. Management of corrosive esophageal burns in 149 cases. J Thorac Cardiovasc Surg. 2005;130:449-55.

25. Sanz-Gallén P, Nogué S, Munné P, et al. Hypocalcaemia and hypomagnesaemia due to hydrofluoric acid. Occup Med. 2001;51:294-5.

26. Yamaura K, Kao B, Limori E, et al. Recurrent ventricular tachyarrhythmias associated with QT prolongation following hydrofluoric acid burns. J Toxicol Clin Toxicol. 1997;35(3):311-3.

27. Spiller HA, Quadrani-Kushner DA, Cleveland P. A five year evaluation of acute exposures to phenol disinfectant (26%). J Toxicol Clin Toxicol. 1993;3192:307-13.

28. Barillo DJ, Cancio LC, Goodwin CW. Treatment of white phosphorus and other chemical burn injuries at one burn center over a 51-year period. Burns. 2004;30(5):448-52.

29. Koschny R, Herceg M, Stremmel W, et al. Fatal course of a suicidal intoxication with hydrochloric acid. Case Rep Gastroenterol. 2013;7(1):89-96.

30. Amshel CE, Fealk MH, Phillips BJ, et al. Anhydrous ammonia burns case report and review of the literature. Burns. 2000;26:493.

31. https://www.atsdr.cdc.gov/ [Assessed June, 2018].

SECTION 7

Hematological Toxins

26. **Warfarin and Superwarfarin Toxicity**
    Mohit Mathur

27. **Overdose of Newer Anticoagulants**
    Pravin Amin, Vinay Amin

28. **Dyshemoglobinemias**
    Jeetendra Sharma, Shivangi Khanna

SECTION 7

Hematological Toxins

26 CHAPTER

Warfarin and Superwarfarin Toxicity

Mohit Mathur

INTRODUCTION

Derivatives of coumarin have broad ranging applications, therapeutically as anticoagulants and commercially as rodenticides. In this chapter, we will be discussing various aspects of toxicity due to warfarin and their longer acting version superwarfarins. Toxicity due to warfarin, which has been one of the most widely used oral anticoagulant agent, can occur due to intentional overdose but can also occur unintentionally in patients already on warfarin with increased serum drug levels due to factors like change in diet, liver dysfunction, initial dosing phase, and most importantly because of drug interactions with agents (e.g. propranolol, piroxicam, amiodarone, erythromycin, omeprazole, and fluconazole) which displace warfarin from their protein binding sites.[1] Superwarfarins are used commercially as rodenticides and toxicity because of their use is almost always intentional.[2,3] The United States Environmental Protection Agency in its label review manual for pesticides has categorized (on the basis of lethal dose 50) anticoagulant rodenticide poisons which include warfarin and superwarfarins as "less toxic" with signal word "caution" to be mentioned on the product label.[4]

BRIEF HISTORY OF WARFARIN AND SUPERWARFARINS

Bishydroxycoumarin (dicoumarol) was identified in 1939 as the agent responsible for the deaths in cattle due to

a sudden hemorrhagic disorder that resulted from the ingestion of spoiled silage from sweet clover.[5] Sweet clover contains a harmless ingredient coumarin which upon getting spoiled/spoilt gets converted to dicoumarol. Nine years later, warfarin was introduced as a more powerful and synthetic derivative of bishydroxycoumarin. Warfarin was an acronym for *Wisconsin Alumni Research Foundation*, (which helped the research and obtained the patent) with the suffix *"arin"* derived from its parent molecule coumarin. It was developed to be used as a rodenticide only and its therapeutic potential as an anticoagulant was realized after an army inductee survived suicidal ingestion of massive amounts of it in the year 1952. Interestingly, it was abused even before its therapeutic use was realized. The United States Food and Drug Administration approved it in the year 1954 and its earliest recipient was the then US President Eisenhower who received it when he had myocardial infarction in the year 1955.[6]

After nearly 20 years of rampant use of warfarin as a very successful rodenticide, rodent strains started to acquire resistance to warfarin by the way of mutations in *VKORC1* gene, which resulted in decreased binding to warfarin. This led to the search for more powerful derivatives and as a result superwarfarins were developed by attaching phenyl rings to the 4-hydroxycoumarin moiety which increases their hydrophobicity and resultant tissue accumulation plus retention. *Examples of superwarfarins include* bromadiolone, brodifacoum, diphenadione, chlorphacinone, and pindone out of which difenacoum and brodifacoum are most commonly available.[7] Difenacoum was commercially available in United Kingdom in 1970s. Some of the available rodenticide brands in India containing superwarfarins are racumin sure from Bayer (contains bromadiolone) and D-con (contains brodifacoum). Superwarfarins are also referred to as second generation warfarins or long-acting anticoagulant rodenticides (LAARs).

MECHANISM OF ACTION

As we proceed further, it is important to understand the mechanism of action of warfarin (Fig. 1). Coagulation factors II, VII, IX, and X along with anticoagulation factors proteins C and S are synthesized in liver in the inactive form. Carboxylation of the glutamic acid residues of these factors is required to convert them to their active form. The process of carboxylation is catalyzed by the enzyme gamma-glutamyl carboxylase. This process of carboxylation also requires reduced vitamin K (KH_2) which gets converted to its oxidized or epoxide form (KO) in the process. For carboxylation process to continue uninterrupted, KH_2 must be continuously regenerated from KO and this process of regeneration is catalyzed by the enzyme vitamin K_1 2,3-epoxid reductase. Warfarin inhibits this enzyme and therefore prevents regeneration of KH_2, leading to interruption in the synthesis of active form of clotting factors II, VII, IX, and X and the anticoagulant proteins C and S.[8-10]

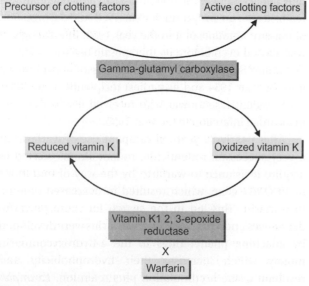

Fig. 1: Mechanism of action of warfarin.

Toxicokinetics and Toxicodynamics

When it comes to toxicokinetics of an acute overdose of these drugs, the literature is limited. Warfarin follows first order elimination and has a half-life of 21.7 hours[11] and the anticoagulant effect lasts for about 5–7 days after a single dose of warfarin.[12] In contrast, superwarfarins follow zero order saturation-dependent kinetics and have much more prolonged half-lives of greater than 20 days with anticoagulant effect lasting from weeks to months.[13] There is a case report of brodifacoum overdose where the half-life was found to be 56 days.[14] Oral bioavailability of both is nearly 100% with significantly high protein binding to the extent of 97%. Ingestion is the most common mode of toxicity, but dermal absorption is also a possible route and case reports of talcum powder contaminated with warfarin leading to fatal epidemic in neonates has been described.[15,16]

In terms of their ability to antagonize vitamin K, superwarfarins are 100 times more powerful due to their lipophilic nature causing them to be retained in liver for longer duration.[17] Because of being 100-fold stronger and having significant prolonged duration of action, superwarfarins have completely replaced warfarin as rodenticides.

Warfarin is metabolized in liver by cytochrome P-450 isoenzyme and metabolites are excreted in bile.[12,18-20] Patients with liver disease can have unpredictable half-lives and clinical effect due to varying rates of metabolism. Some of the metabolites are excreted through kidneys, hence possibility of prolonged effects in patients with renal dysfunction cannot be ruled out. The dose in which warfarin becomes toxic is very variable. A onetime ingestion in a dose as high as 10–20 mg rarely causes serious manifestations; however, repeated intake of normal doses can produce toxicity especially if taken along with drugs which interact with it or in the presence of hepatic dysfunction, low albumin states, or bleeding diathesis. On the other hand, superwarfarins by the virtue of being extremely potent can produce profound toxicity even with single ingestion of dose as small as 1 mg.

EPIDEMIOLOGY

Anticoagulant rodenticides constitute the major cause for rodenticide poisoning exposures in the developed world.[21,22] In the developing world, unintentional inadvertent ingestion of a single, small dose is very common. As per data published by American Association of Poison Control Centers (AAPCC) for the year 2016 in United States, a total of 1,532 cases of warfarin exposure were reported. Cases of unintentional exposure leading to toxicity were 1,326 (87%) and the remaining cases were of intentional toxicity. Most of the cases occurred in persons older than 19 years of age. Major outcomes were reported in only 11 cases and no mortality happened. Occupational exposure in workers exposed in the manufacturing and using of rodenticides has been reported, especially when precautions are not appropriate.[16,23]

APPROACH CONSIDERATIONS

History

As in any other poisoning, obtaining detailed and accurate history is of paramount importance. Intent of ingestion, the specific agent consumed, amount, timing, coingestion of other toxins/drugs, pre-existing diseases, and detailed medication history (medications can decrease or increase the metabolism of warfarin) are the important aspects. The product label should be sought, and the regional poison control center should be contacted to obtain more details about the product and anticipated complications. Intentional overdose is usually obvious from initial history but may need to be suspected in cases of unexplained coagulopathy. Munchausen syndrome or Munchausen syndrome by proxy in child abuse cases where in these drugs have been used are well described in literature.

CLINICAL PRESENTATION AND EVALUATION

The only major symptom of significance is bleeding which can be external but more problematic and noteworthy is internal bleeding. Intracranial hemorrhage and massive gastrointestinal (GI) hemorrhage are the two most catastrophic presentations but fortunately are not very common. Frank hematuria with abdominal or flank pain is the most common type of significant bleeding associated with warfarin overdose.[18,24-26] Major bleeding can happen in almost any site like within spinal cord, pericardium, within liver parenchyma, retroperitoneal region, pulmonary or adrenal region, but these are uncommon. Common and less threatening bleeding manifestations include superficial ecchymosis, epistaxis, bleeding from gums, subconjunctival hemorrhage, or vaginal bleeding. Those having major hemorrhage may

present with signs of shock while those with intracranial hemorrhage may present with altered sensorium with signs of raised intracranial pressure. Occult internal bleeding makes scenario even more challenging. A digital rectal examination may help in locating occult GI hemorrhage. Due to certain peculiar toxicokinetic aspects of warfarin and superwarfarins, acute ingestion poses certain clinical challenges:

- *Delay in presentation*: Prolongation of prothrombin time/international normalized ratio (PT/INR) happens after a delay of nearly 12–24 hours because previously formed and already circulating clotting factors are not affected by warfarin and these must first undergo normal catabolism before the anticoagulation becomes evident.[18] Due to varying degradation half-lives of each of these (factor II—60 hours, factor VII—4–6 hours, factor IX—24 hours, and factor X—48–72 hours), the time of onset of anticoagulation varies widely and cases of suspected or confirmed overdose should be frequently followed-up for coagulation abnormalities for a period of at least 36–48 hours from the time of ingestion. A normal PT/INR even 48–72 hours after ingestion practically rules out significant ingestion.
- Sometimes PT/INR may be prolonged as the levels of factors with short half-lives decrease below 30% (in particular factor VII), but full anticoagulant effect or bleeding is not evident for days beyond INR prolongation, due to the long half-lives of other factors (particularly factor II). No direct correlation can be drawn between any specific value of raised INR and bleeding episodes. Even with INR more than 10, major bleeding episodes are not very common.
- *Prolonged duration and rebound toxicity*: Because of their prolonged duration of action, superwarfarins can produce prolonged coagulopathy lasting for many months and recurrent bleeding is possible.[24,27] Cases have been reported wherein patients with warfarin toxicity in whom INR was normalized with vitamin K treatment, were readmitted with bleeding events and raised INR more than 3 days after discharge.
- Concurrent acute alcohol intoxication may decrease hepatic metabolism of warfarin whereas chronic alcohol use might increase the metabolism.
- Even though bleeding is the most common presentation, we should also be aware about a paradoxical sounding complication, which is thrombosis.

Warfarin produces a transient paradoxical hyperco-agulable state after beginning of treatment as it also reduces the activity of anticoagulant proteins C and S. Proteins C and S have half-lives of 8 and 30 hours approximately. Because of their shorter half-lives, balance shifts in favor of clotting in the initial phase of beginning of treatment and later as clotting factors are inhibited, anticoagulant state starts. Majority of cases of poisoning due to warfarin and superwarfarin have reported bleeding as the presentation but thrombosis has also been reported and clinicians should be aware of this uncommon presentation also.[28-30]

- *Drug and food item (including herbal products) interactions*: The list of drugs which have significant interaction with warfarin is exhaustive and the most important ones are shown in Table 1. It is important to realize that every drug which patient was taking previously or has coingested or is about to receive after ingestion for management of toxicity, should be screened for possible interaction. Warfarin due to its significant protein binding and metabolism in liver by cytochrome P-450 system has significant interactions with other drugs and many food items.

LABORATORY INVESTIGATIONS

Serum levels of warfarin are not routinely available and are not deemed necessary or useful to guide clinical management of acute overdoses. Superwarfarin qualitative screen and quantitative testing for brodifacoum and difenacoum [by normal-phase high performance liquid chromatography (HPLC) with diode array detection] are available though not in India and may be of utility only to confirm exposure where ingestion is suspicious or more importantly for estimating the duration of therapy with vitamin K. Baseline and thereafter 24–48 hourly measurements of PT and INR are the most effective manner of quantifying anticoagulation.[31] As previously discussed, PT/INR may not be prolonged until 24–48 hours postingestion. Serum levels of vitamin K—dependent clotting factors (II, VII, IX, and X) can be obtained and decreased levels are helpful in confirming suspected poisonings though their utility in clinical management is not much.[32] Measurement of vitamin K_1 and vitamin K_1 2,3-epoxide levels (by reversed-phase HPLC with postcolumn derivetization and fluorescence detection) can specify the degree of inhibition of carboxylation but are more for research purposes only. Vitamin K_1 2,3-epoxide levels also assume importance in occupational chronic exposure in workers, because they remain abnormal for many months even after cessation of exposure and can serve as long-term markers of exposure as compared to standard coagulation parameters.[23,33]

Ancillary studies may be required in those with any evidence of bleeding on examination or coagulopathy on testing. Complete blood count followed by frequent hemoglobin estimations should be done as per bleeding status. Sample for blood typing and screening (cross-matching) may be drawn in cases of intentional ingestion of toxic doses. Urine analysis for microscopic hematuria or stool for guaiac may not be of much benefit. If coingestion is suspected, then sample for acetaminophen levels and toxicology screen should also be obtained. Further evaluation including imaging and endoscopies may be performed depending on the specific site of bleeding and clinical features.

Role of mixing studies comes when there is a dilemma between anticoagulation caused by warfarin or superwarfarins and that caused by antifactory antibodies or factor inhibitor like lupus anticoagulant.[34] In case of warfarin or superwarfarin induced anticoagulation, mixing patients serum with normal serum in equal quantity will restore deranged PT to normal level.

TREATMENT

A dose of less than 1 mg of superwarfarin is considered nontoxic and does not warrant medical evaluation but in most cases of anticoagulant rodenticide ingestion, it is difficult to determine the exact amount ingested and hence amount cannot be relied upon to assess toxicity. Indications for immediate medical evaluation are intentional ingestion (e.g. self-harm, misuse, abuse, or malicious intent), symptomatic patients, or high dose/unknown amount ingestion. These patients should be admitted for observation after initial evaluation. Even though there are few small case series that document some instances of coagulopathy in children or older adults who have ingested nontoxic amounts of anticoagulant rodenticides and who are not on warfarin therapy,[35] still there is no strong evidence to suggest any laboratory assessment or observation in such patients and is not advisable because no major instances of bleeding have been found to happen with ingestion of up to one packet of anticoagulant rodenticide.[36,37]

Warfarin and Superwarfarin Toxicity

Table 1: Drugs which have significant interaction with warfarin.

	Increase INR (potentiates)	*Decrease INR (inhibits)*
Drugs	**Cardiac** • Amiodarone • Diltiazem • Quinidine • Propranolol • Propafenone • Cholesterol-lowering agents (e.g. gemfibrozil, clofibrate, fenofibrate, fluvastatin, lovastatin, rosuvastatin, simvastatin) • Sulfinpyrazone • Ropinirole	**Cardiac** • Cholestyramine • Bosentan
	Anti-inflammatory, analgesics • Phenylbutazone • Piroxicam • Acetylsalicylic acid • Acetaminophen • Celecoxib • Dextropropoxyphene • Tramadol	**Anti-inflammatory, analgesics** • Mesalamine
	GI drugs • Cimetidine • Omeprazole	**GI drugs** • Sucralfate
	CNS drugs • Alcohol with liver disease • Citalopram • Entacapone • Sertraline • Disulfiram • Chloral hydrate • Fluvoxamine • Phenytoin (biphasic with later inhibition)	**CNS drugs** • Enzyme-inducing antiepileptic drugs (e.g. carbamazepine, barbiturates, chlordiazepoxide • Phenytoin (mixed effects described)
	Antimicrobials • Amoxicillin, amoxicillin-clavulanate • Doxycycline • Cephalosporins • Fluoroquinolones (e.g. ciprofloxacin, levofloxacin, moxifloxacin, norfloxacin) • Macrolides (e.g. azithromycin, erythromycin, clarithromycin) • Metronidazole • Trimethoprim-sulfamethoxazole • Isoniazid • Azole antifungals [e.g. fluconazole, miconazole (oral), voriconazole]	**Antimicrobials** • Dicloxacillin • Griseofulvin • Nafcillin • Rifampin • Ritonavir • Ribavirin
	Chemotherapeutic agents, antimetabolites • Capecitabine, gemcitabine • Paclitaxel • Fluorouracil (5-FU) • Imatinib • Tamoxifen	**Chemotherapeutic agents, antimetabolites** • Mercaptopurine • Azathioprine
	Others • Allopurinol • Androgens (e.g. methyltestosterone, oxandrolone, testosterone) • Tolterodine • Zileuton	**Others** • Vitamin K • Raloxifene

Contd...

Hematological Toxins

Contd...

	Increase INR (potentiates)	Decrease INR (inhibits)
Food	• Cranberry juice • Alcohol • *Ginkgo biloba*, dong quai, fenugreek, chamomile (increases bleeding risk independent of PT/INR) • Mango • Grapefruit juice • Fish oil • Boldo fenugreek, guilinggao, danshen, dong quai, lycium barbarum	• Saint John's wort • Large amounts of avocado • Kale, spinach, Brussels sprouts, collards, mustard greens, chard, broccoli, asparagus • Green tea • Soymilk • Ginseng

(CNS: central nervous system; GI: gastrointestinal; INR: international normalized ratio; PT: prothrombin time)

If the patient is seeking medical attention within 1 hour of ingestion, then activated charcoal (AC) should be considered, if there is no risk for aspiration. Between 1 and 2 hours of ingestion, AC can still be considered, more so in cases of coingestion with agents which delay gastric emptying. Beyond 2 hours, AC is unlikely to prevent absorption and is not recommended. Data is not supportive of techniques like multiple-dose activated charcoal (MDAC), or hemodialysis to enhance elimination of these compounds and hence they are not recommended.[38] There are few small studies in which cholestyramine was found to enhance elimination of warfarin or superwarfarin from GI tract, but further evaluation is needed before any recommendation can be made.[39,40]

Gastric lavage is of limited utility in any poisoning more so if rapid administration of AC can be accomplished and has no role here also. Whole bowel irrigation is also not supported by evidence to be any benefit. Any other coingestion should be actively sought and treated. Also imperative is to check the possible interaction of every drug being administered to the patient as many drugs can increase or decrease the metabolism of warfarin/superwarfarins.

Assessment of hemodynamic status along with usual supportive measures become more important when the patient is presenting late (24–48 hours after ingestion) with bleeding manifestations or with signs of hemodynamic compromise implying occult bleeding. Depending on the site and severity of bleeding, relevant treatment should be instituted like airway support and antiedema measures for intracranial hemorrhage or endoscopic in consultation with relevant specialist.

Further treatment can be decided as per these three clinical situations:

1. *Absence of coagulopathy*: Patients who continue to have normal coagulation parameters even at 48 hours after ingestion are not found to be at risk for any major bleeding or coagulopathy. Case reports of rebound bleeding beyond 3 days in case of warfarin overdose are there; however, they are too few to be of any significance and these patients can be safely discharged. There is no role of prophylactic vitamin K therapy in these patients as it is not needed, and it may mask the onset of anticoagulation.

2. *Presence of coagulopathy but no active bleeding*: Varies as per the molecule:
   • *Superwarfarins*: If INR is less than 4, then only observation and serial monitoring is required. If INR is more than 4, then oral vitamin K_1 (phytomenadione or phytonadione) should be preferred over intravenous (IV) vitamin K_1, if available. Vitamin K_3 (or menadione) is not directly active as a coenzyme and therefore less effective in reversing anticoagulation. Intravenous vitamin K_1 carries significant risk of anaphylaxis and therefore should be used cautiously. If patients develop anaphylaxis, then infusion should be immediately stopped, and diphenhydramine should be administered. Intravenous vitamin K should be given slowly in infusion over 30 minutes. It should be reserved for patients with life-threatening or serious bleeding. Oral vitamin K_1 has very good bioavailability and is recommended when there is no life-threatening bleeding. Subcutaneous or intramuscular route is not preferred as it may lead to hematoma formation in anticoagulated patients. In various case reports, doses of oral vitamin K_1 varying from 15 mg/day to 600 mg/day for 30–200 days have been used but a dose of 10 mg to start

with in adults is reasonable.[20,24-26] Consultation with hematologist should be obtained for long-term dosing and monitoring. Monitoring for up to several weeks may be required.[24]

- *Acute warfarin ingestion*: If INR is less than 9, then the risk of bleeding has not been found to be very high. If no further warfarin exposure is expected, then nothing more needs to be done apart from discontinuing warfarin. If there is any other factor which makes these patients prone to high risk of bleeding, then oral vitamin K_1 in the dose of 1–2.5 mg can be given. If INR is more than 9, then give oral vitamin K_1 in the dose of 2.5–5 mg and reassess INR after 24 hours. Vitamin K therapy may need to be repeated after 24 hours, if INR remains elevated. Management of patients with toxicity due to chronic warfarin use is beyond the scope of this chapter.

3. *Presence of coagulopathy with active bleeding*: Patients presenting with life-threatening bleeding like intracranial, genitourinary, or GI hemorrhage require immediate reversal which cannot be achieved with vitamin K therapy. These patients should be managed with 4-factor prothrombin complex concentrate (PCC) in a dose of 25–50 international units/kg (maximum dose 2,000 international units).[41,43] It may be repeated after 12 hours. If 4-factor PCC is not available, then 3-factor PCC should be used. If both are not available, then fresh frozen plasma (FFP) should be infused[18,41,42] in a dose of 15–30 mL/kg (approximately 4 units in a normal adult). Historically, FFP was the first line of treatment in warfarin toxicity with severe bleeding. FFP transfusion may need to be given again as the factors in FFP are cleared from circulation more rapidly as compared to warfarin or superwarfarin remaining in the tissues. Even though utility of PCC is limited by high cost, it offers certain definite advantages over FFP. It does not require thawing or blood group typing and hence valuable time can be saved. It results in rapid reversal of coagulopathy as compared to FFP. It mitigates the risk of transfusion reactions, infectious disease transmission, and volume overload. Recombinant factor VIIa (rFVIIa) has also been found to rapidly correct INR within hours in patients of warfarin toxicity.[44-46] It may be considered in situations where PCC is not readily available. An appropriate dose is 20 μg/kg. In the few studies available, secondary end points like time to operative intervention and intracranial hematoma size reduction did improve; however, no mortality benefit could be demonstrated for either PCC or rFVIIa over FFP.[47,48] Packed red blood cell should be transfused as per blood loss. Even though vitamin K_1 does not have any immediate effect, it should be given by slow IV infusion in a dose of 10 mg. Consultation with hematologist should be sought, wherever possible.

In cases of ingestion with suicidal intent, psychiatric evaluation should be obtained, and patient should be kept under close supervision.

Long-term Follow-up

Risk of rebound toxicity should be explained at the time of discharge[49] and patients should be instructed to avoid activities which can predispose to bleeding events. In case of superwarfarin poisoning, prolonged vitamin K_1 therapy extending up to weeks may be required.[50] Patients may need to be given vitamin K_1 daily in the dose of 50–200 mg and need to complete full course must be emphasized to the patient.[49] If patient was taking warfarin previously for any medical indication, then heparin can be used if continued anticoagulation is imperative. It must be noted that if patient has received high doses of vitamin K, then they may become resistant to warfarin for several days leaving patients exposed to a procoagulant state.

CONCLUSION

Most of the times, warfarin and superwarfarin toxicity lead to minor clinical manifestations and do not require reversal with vitamin K therapy. It is important to be aware about the indications for reversal therapy either immediately with PCC, rFVIIa, or FFP or gradually with vitamin K. A thorough understanding of the mechanism of action and interactions with other drugs is also imperative to better manage the toxicity. Need for long-term follow-up with coagulation studies is also a derivation of this thorough understanding.

KEY POINTS

- Vitamin K is a cofactor for the synthesis of active form of clotting factors II, IV, IX, and X, and warfarin acts as a vitamin K antagonist thereby producing anticoagulation

Hematological Toxins

- Superwarfarins are longer acting and more powerful versions of warfarin. Because of these attributes, they have replaced warfarin as the anticoagulant rodenticide
- Life-threatening bleeding complications include intracranial, genitourinary, or GI hemorrhage and should be managed with urgent reversal of anticoagulation
- In most of the situations without life-threatening bleeding, reversal using vitamin K is adequate
- Risk of rebound toxicity in case of warfarin and prolonged need for vitamin K therapy in superwarfarin toxicity should always be contemplated.

REFERENCES

1. Haemostasis and Thrombosis Task Force for the British Committee for standards in Haematology. Guidelines on oral anticoagulation; 3rd edition. Br J Haematol. 1998;101:374-87.
2. Anderson IB. Warfarin and related rodenticides. In: Olson KR (Ed). Poisoning and Drug Overdose, 6th edition. New York: The McGraw-Hill Companies; 2012. pp. 409-11.
3. Chen BC, Su M. Antithrombotics. In: Hoffman RS, Howland MA, Lewin NA, Nelson LS, Goldfrank LR (Eds). Goldfrank's Toxicologic Emergencies, 10th edition. New York,: McGraw-Hill Education; 2015.
4. United States Environmental Protection Agency. Label review manual, Office of Pesticide Programs (Chapter 7: Precautionary statements). New York: United States Environmental Protection Agency; 2018.
5. Hogg K. Blood coagulation and anticoagulant, fibrinolytic, and antiplatelet drugs. Goodman & Gilman's: The Pharmacological Basis of Therapeutics, 13th edition. New York, NY: McGraw-Hill education; 2018.
6. Dhungat JP. Discovery of anticoagulant warfarin. J Assoc Physicians India. 2017;65(7):115.
7. Hadler MR, Shadbolt RS. Novel 4-hydroxycoumarin anticoagulants active against resistant rats. Nature. 1975;253:275-7.
8. Hanley JP. Warfarin reversal. J Clin Pathol. 2004;57: 1132-9.
9. Butler AC, Tait RC. Management of oral anticoagulant-induced intracranial haemorrhage. Blood Rev. 1998;12:35-44.
10. Pindur G, Morsdort S. The use of prothrombin complex concentrates in the treatment of hemorrhages induced by oral anticoagulation. Thromb Res. 1999;95:S57-S61.
11. Hackett LP, Ilett KF, Chester A. Plasma warfarin concentrations after a massive overdose. Med J Aust. 1985;142:642-3.
12. Yip L. Anticoagulant rodenticides. In: Dart RC, Caravati EM, McGuigan MA (Eds). Medical Toxicology. Philadelphia, PA: Lippincott Williams & Wilkins; 2004. p. 1497.

13. O'Reilly RA, Aggeler PM, Leong LS. Studies on the coumarin anticoagulant drugs: The pharmacodynamics of warfarin in man. J Clin Invest. 1963;42:1542-51.
14. Olmos V, Lopez CM. Brodifacoum poisoning with toxicokinetic data. Clin Toxicol (Phila). 2007;45(5):487-9.
15. Martin-Bouyer G, Khanh NB, Linh PD, et al. Epidemic of haemorrhagic disease in Vietnamese infants caused by warfarin-contaminated talcs. Lancet. 1983;1:230-2.
16. Spiller HA, Gallenstein GL, Murphy MJ. Dermal absorption of a liquid diphacinone rodenticide causing coagulopathy. Vet Hum Toxicol. 2003;45:313-4.
17. Gebauer M. Synthesis and structure-activity relationships of novel warfarin derivatives. Bioorg Med Chem. 2007;15:2414-20.
18. Watt BE, Proudfoot AT, Bradberry SM, et al. Anticoagulant rodenticides. Toxicol Rev. 2005;24:259-69.
19. Lai M, Ewald M. Anticoagulants. In: Shannon MW, Borron SW, Burns MJ (Eds). Haddad and Winchester's Clinical Management of Poisoning and Drug Overdose. Saunders; 2007. p. 1051.
20. Berny PJ, de Oliveira LA, Videmann B, et al. Assessment of ruminal degradation, oral bioavailability, and toxic effects of anticoagulant rodenticides in sheep. Am J Vet Res. 2006;67:363-71.
21. Dawson A, Garthwaite D. Rodenticide usage by local authorities in Great Britain. In: Department for Environment (Ed). Pesticide Usage Survey Report 185, F.a.R.A. York UK; 2001.
22. Bronstein AC, Spyker DA, Cantilena LR Jr, et al. 2011 Annual report of the American Association of Poison Control Centers' National Poison Data System (NPDS): 29th Annual Report. Clin Toxicol (Phila). 2012;50:911-1164.
23. Svendsen SW, Kolstad HA, Steesby E. Bleeding problems associated with occupational exposure to anticoagulant rodenticides. Int Arch Occup Environ Health. 2002;75: 515-7.
24. Bruno GR, Howland MA, McMeeking A, et al. Long-acting anticoagulant overdose: brodifacoum kinetics and optimal vitamin K dosing. Ann Emerg Med. 2000;36: 262-7.
25. Hollinger BR, Pastoor TP. Case management and plasma half-life in a case of brodifacoum poisoning. Arch Intern Med. 1993;153:1925-8.
26. Stanton T, Sowray P, McWaters D, et al. Prolonged anticoagulation with long-acting coumadin derivative: Case report of a brodifacoum poisoning with pharmacokinetic data. Blood. 1988;73:310a.
27. Watts RG, Castleberry RP, Sadowski JA. Accidental poisoning with a superwarfarin compound (brodifacoum) in a child. Pediatrics. 1990;86:883-7.
28. De Paula EV, Montalvao SA, Madureira PR, et al. Simultaneous bleeding and thrombosis in superwarfarin poisoning. Thromb Res. 2009;123:637-9.
29. Chua JD, Friedenberg WR. Superwarfarin poisoning. Arch Intern Med. 1998;158:1929-32.
30. Kruse JA, Carlson RW. Fatal rodenticide poisoning with brodifacoum. Ann Emerg Med. 1992;21:331-6.

31. Caravati EM, Erdman AR, Scharman EJ, et al. Long-acting anticoagulant rodenticide poisoning: an evidence-based consensus guideline for out-of-hospital management. Clin Toxicol (Phila). 2007;45(1):1-22.

32. Miller MA, Levy PD, Hile D. Rapid identification of surreptitious brodifacoum poisoning by analysis of vitamin K-dependent factor activity. Am J Emerg Med. 2006;24(3):383.

33. Fristedt B, Sterner N. Warfarin intoxication from percutaneous absorption. Arch Environ Health. 1965;11:205-8.

34. Spahr JE, Maul JS, Rodgers GM. Superwarfarin poisoning: a report of two cases and review of the literature. Am J Hematol. 2007;82(7):656-60.

35. Su M. Anticoagulants. In: Nelson LS, Lewin NA, Howland MA, Hoffman RS (Eds). Goldfrank's Toxicologic Emergencies, 9th edition. New York: McGraw HIll Medical; 2011. p. 861.

36. Watt BE, Proudfoot AT, Bradberry SM, et al. Anticoagulant rodenticides. Toxicol Rev. 2005; 24:259-69.

37. Ingels M, Lai C, Tai W, et al. A prospective study of acute, unintentional, pediatric superwarfarin ingestions managed without decontamination. Ann Emerg Med. 2002;40:73-8.

38. Lai M, Ewald M. Anticoagulants. In: Shannon MW, Borron SW, Burns MJ (Eds). Haddad and Winchester's Clinical Management of Poisoning and Drug Overdose. Saunders; 2007. pp. 1051.

39. Jähnchen E, Meinertz T, Gilfrich HJ, et al. Enhanced elimination of warfarin during treatment with cholestyramine. Br J Clin Pharmacol. 1978;5:437-40.

40. Renowden S, Westmoreland D, White JP, et al. Oral cholestyramine increases elimination of warfarin after overdose. Br Med J (Clin Res Ed). 1985;291:513-4.

41. Yasaka M, Oomura M, Ikeno K, et al. Effect of prothrombin complex concentrate on INR and blood coagulation system in emergency patients treated with warfarin overdose. Ann Hematol. 2003;82:121-3.

42. Zupancić-Salek S, Kovacević-Metelko J, Radman I. Successful reversal of anticoagulant effect of superwarfarin poisoning with recombinant activated factor VII. Blood Coagul Fibrinolysis. 2005;16:239-44.

43. Schulman S, Furie B. How I treat poisoning with vitamin K antagonists. Blood. 2015;125(3):438-42.

44. Deveras RA, Kessler CM. Reversal of warfarin-induced excessive anticoagulation with recombinant human factor VIIa. Ann Intern Med. 2002;137(11):884-8.

45. Ilyas C, Beyer GM, Dutton RP, et al. Recombinant factor VIIa for warfarin-associated intracranial bleeding. J Clin Anesth. 2008;20(4):276-9.

46. Nishijima DK, Dager WE, Schrot RJ, et al. The efficacy of factor VIIa in emergency department patients with warfarin use and traumatic intracranial hemorrhage. Acad Emerg Med. 2010;17(3):244-51.

47. Huttner HB, Schellinger PD, Hartmann M, et al. Hematoma growth and outcome in treated neurocritical care patients with intracerebral hemorrhage related to oral anticoagulant therapy: comparison of acute treatment strategies using vitamin K, fresh frozen plasma, and prothrombin complex concentrates. Stroke. 2006;37(6):1465-70.

48. Kalina M, Tinkoff G, Gbadebo A, et al. A protocol for the rapid normalization of INR in trauma patients with intracranial hemorrhage on prescribed warfarin therapy. Am Surg. 2008;74(9):858-61.

49. Berling I, Mostafa A, Grice JE, et al. Warfarin poisoning with delayed rebound toxicity. J Emerg Med. 2017;52 (2):194-6.

50. Tsutaoka BT, Miller M, Fung SM, et al. Superwarfarin and glass ingestion with prolonged coagulopathy requiring high-dose vitamin K1 therapy. Pharmacotherapy. 2003;23(9):1186-9.

CHAPTER 27

Overdose of Newer Anticoagulants

Pravin Amin, Vinay Amin

INTRODUCTION

The direct-acting oral anticoagulants (DOACs) need no monitoring as compared to warfarin and hence are presently in vogue. Direct thrombin inhibitors (DTIs) act by preventing thrombin from converting fibrinogen into fibrin by directly binding to thrombin. DTI may be parenteral (argatroban, bivalirudin, and desirudin) or oral (dabigatran etexilate, ximelagatran). By binding directly to factor Xa, the direct factor Xa inhibitors act by preventing factor Xa from converting prothrombin to thrombin. Only oral agents are currently available namely rivaroxaban, apixaban, edoxaban and betrixaban. Figure 1 illustrates the sites of action of DOACs in the coagulation pathway. The additional advantage of these newer molecules is that they have no interactions with food or other medications in contrast to warfarin.

THERAPEUTIC ROLE AND MONITORING OF DOACS

These newer molecules have been extensively studied in preventing strokes for patients with chronic non-valvular atrial fibrillation (AF) in several large well conducted studies.[1-4] Other indications for these agents are in prevention and in the therapy of venous thromboembolism.[5-8] These newer agents have a rapid onset of action within 1–3 hours of administration, this has to be taken into consideration while switching to DOACs from other anticoagulation agents. As compared to warfarin DOACs do not warrant routine anticoagulation monitoring as their pharmacodynamics and pharmacokinetic are predictable.[9] There are clear indications to monitor anticoagulation in clinical situations such as major bleeds, emergency surgery or invasive procedures in intensive care unit (ICU), renal and liver failure.[10] DOACs do have an effect on coagulation assays which can be demonstrated in Table 1.

Currently the evidence suggests that the routine coagulation tests such as thrombin time

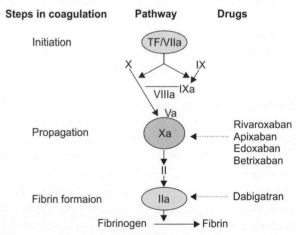

Fig. 1: Sites of action of direct-acting oral anticoagulants in the coagulation pathway.

Overdose of Newer Anticoagulants

Table 1: Comparison between different direct-acting oral anticoagulants.

	Dabigatran	Rivaroxaban	Apixaban	Edoxaban
aPTT	☑	☒	☒	?
TT, dTT	☑	☒	☒	☒
ECT	☑	☒	☒	☒
Anti-FXa assays	☒	☑	☑	☑
PT	☒	☑	☒	☑
INR	☒	☒	☒	☒

(aPTT: activated partial thromboplastin time; dTT: diluted thrombin time; ECT: ecarin clotting time; INR: international normalized ratio; PT: prothrombin time; TT: thrombin time)

(TT), prothrombin time (PT), and activated partial thromboplastin time (aPTT) should only be used to corroborate the DOACs anticoagulation effect rather than to modify the dosages. Dabigatran definitely prolongs PT-international normalized ratio (INR) but has poor sensitivity. Its correlation with aPTT is curvilinear, hence these test are not advocated as monitoring tools.[11] In the same way, PT and aPTT are also prolonged by all the factor Xa inhibitors, but at a lower sensitivity. TT may be very sensitive for the estimation of dabigatran activity but, in case the plasma is diluted, TT may be used to monitor the drug.[11] A more accurate method is to use ecarin clotting time (ECT) for dabigatran and techniques to determine antifactor Xa activity for the factor Xa inhibitors (Table 2).[11]

BLEEDING WITH DOACS

The incidence of bleeding with anticoagulants remains a major risk factor contributing to associated morbidity and mortality. In comparison to warfarin, the chances of fatal [intracerebral hemorrhage (ICH)] intracranial bleeding with DOACs are clearly lower.[12] The extent and the site of bleeding would validate the degree of response in a clinical setting. An occult bleed in the gastrointestinal (GI) tract may seem innocuous, but could progress to a life-threatening lower GI bleed. A major bleeding like GI bleed, hemoptysis, epistaxis, severe menorrhagia, retroperitoneal bleeding, etc. may need rapid interventions. A serious bleeding may be linked with substantial blood loss necessitating blood transfusion. ICH or bleeding into compartments may be life-threatening. Across various trials and meta-analysis morbidity and mortality was worse with warfarin as

Table 2: Methods to monitor direct-acting oral anticoagulants (DOACs).

DOAC	Ideal method	During crisis
Dabigatran	1. Ecarin clotting time 2. Diluted thrombin time	aPTT
Rivaroxaban	Anti-factor Xa	PT
Apixaban	Anti-factor Xa	PT
Edoxaban	Anti-factor Xa	-

(aPTT: activated partial thromboplastin time; PT: prothrombin time)

Table 3: The HAS-BLED risk criteria.

HAS-BLED risk criteria	Score
Hypertension	1
Abnormal renal or liver function (1 point each)	1 or 2
Stroke	1
Bleeding	1
Labile INR	1
Elderly (e.g. age >65 years)	1
Drugs or alcohol (1 point each)	1 or 2

(HAS-BLED: hypertension, abnormal renal/liver function, stroke, bleeding history or predisposition, labile INR, elderly, drugs/alcohol concomitantly)

compared to DOACs.[12,13] Certain risk stratification tools such as HAS-BLED score (Table 3) incorporates parameters such as age, comorbidities (e.g. renal and liver disease, hypertension, malignancy, etc.), previous bleeding, and anemia are utilized to assess the bleeding risk in patients on anticoagulants. Patients with acute

Hematological Toxins

venous thromboembolism (VTE) with an HAS-BLED score more than or equal to 3 points, have an increased risk of major bleeding.[14]

Life-threatening bleeding needs assertive interventions to prevent a catastrophe. Intervention would clearly depend on the rapidity of onset of hemorrhage, the site and the volume of blood loss. Table 4 reviews the phase 3 clinical trials of various DOACs such as apixaban, dabigatran, edoxaban and rivaroxaban in management of patients with non-valvular AF and the associated bleeding risk.[15]

An occult bleeding may be harmless initially but in due course may lead to major morbidity or mortality (e.g. retroperitoneal bleeding). Major bleeding may need an intervention for managing the crisis (e.g. surgery, interventional radiology, endoscopic therapy). A very minor bleeding may not require cessation of anticoagulation therapy. DOAC-associated bleeding seems to have better outcomes in comparison to vitamin K antagonists. In a large meta-analysis of 13 randomized controlled trials (RCTs) having 102,707 adults, the observed case-fatality rate for major bleeding in patients taking DOACs was 7.6% versus 11% for patients on warfarin.[12] For GI bleeding, two medications can be challenging, hence, all efforts should be made to avoid giving rivaroxaban and dabigatran in patients with GI intolerance. As, compared to warfarin, for GI bleeding, low-dose edoxaban or even apixaban may be a better choice. Most of the studies have shown a higher bleeding risk from anticoagulation in older patients in comparison to younger patients. This holds true even with DOACs. However, DOACs do not have any increased bleeding risk while having a head-to-head comparison with low-molecular-weight heparin (LMWH) and warfarin in a recently conducted meta-analysis. This meta-analysis had 10 RCTs which included 25,031 elderly patients.[16] DOACs are dependent on renal functions for their clearance and it is imperative to measure creatinine clearance in all patients with major, unexplained bleeding.

MANAGEMENT OF SEVERE BLEEDING WITH DOACS

Patients with life-threatening bleeding must be admitted in ICU as they may need hemodynamic support. All anticoagulant and antiplatelet drugs should be withdrawn. Transfusions to prevent severe anemia, and in the event of major blood loss, platelets and plasma may need to be replaced. The assistance of surgeon, interventional radiologist and perhaps a neurosurgeon may be sought based on the site of hemorrhage. Particularly in the event of ICH, subarachnoid hemorrhage and subdural hemorrhage in the presence of raised intracranial hypertension rapid intervention after addressing the coagulopathy may be a life-saving maneuver. In life-threatening bleeds antifibrinolytic agent (e.g. tranexamic acid, epsilon-aminocaproic acid) should be considered but may not be very effective.[17] An important feature of

	RE-LY		ROCKET-AF	ARISTOLE	ENGAGE -AF	TIMI 48
	Dabigatran 150 mg (n = 6,076)	Dabigatran 110 mg (n = 6,076)	Rivaroxaban (n = 7,111)	Apixaban (n = 9,088)	Edoxaban 60 mg	Edoxaban 30 mg
Major bleeding	3.1% per year	2.71% per year	3.6% per year	2.13% per year	2.75% per year	1.61% per year
Intracranial bleeding	0.30% per year	0.23% per year	0.5% per year	0.33% per year	0.38% per year	0.26% per year
Gastrointestinal bleeding	1.51% per year	1.21% per year	2.00% per year	0.76% per year	1.51% per year	0.82% per year

Table 4: Phase 3 trials of various direct-acting oral anticoagulants (DOACs) showing the primary safety outcomes.

Note:
1. RE-LY = Randomized Evaluation of Long-term anticoagulation therapy.[4]
2. ROCKET-AF = Rivaroxaban Once daily oral direct factor Xa inhibition Compared with vitamin K antagonism for prevention of stroke and Embolism Trial in Atrial Fibrillation.[2,15]
3. ENGAGE-AF TIMI 48 = Effective aNti-coaGulation with factor Xa next GEneration in Atrial Fibrillation—Thrombolysis in Myocardial Infarction study 48.[3]
4. ARISTOTLE = Apixaban for Reduction in STroke and Other ThromboemboLic Events in Atrial Fibrillation.[1]

Overdose of Newer Anticoagulants

Table 5: Agents used for major direct-acting oral anticoagulants (DOACs)-induced bleeding.

Agent	Factors	Dosage and route
3-factor PCC	II, IX, X	50 U/kg, IV May repeat after 12 hr
4-factor PCC	II, VII, IX, X, Proteins C and S	50 U/kg, IV; Stat dose

management in major bleeds is to try drug removal from GI tract and circulation. Oral administration of activated charcoal may be attempted in order to eliminate any unabsorbed dabigatran etexilate present in the GI tract, especially if the ingestion has taken place within the last 2 hours. Studies in patients with renal impairment have shown that hemodialysis may be used to remove active dabigatran from circulation.[18-21] In warfarin-induced bleeding, nonspecific hemostatic products such as fresh frozen plasma (FFP) and prothrombin complex concentrate (PCC) replace clotting factors and along with the addition of vitamin K.[22] As exogenous clotting factors are also inhibited by DOACs, FFP may not successfully work against DOAC-mediated anticoagulation.[23] Unactivated PCCs and activated PCCs (aPCCs) both include clotting factors filtered from human plasma and are different in their composition [e.g. 3-factor and 4-factor (Table 5)].

In a recent study, out of 84 adult patients who received a fixed dose of a 4-factor PCC (25 units/kg) for the reversal of rivaroxaban or apixaban for a major bleeding event, 69% achieved hemostasis.[24] Recombinant activated factor VII (rFVIIa) is ineffective in treating DOAC-associated bleeding.[25,26]

AGENT-SPECIFIC INTERVENTIONS FOR REVERSALS

Specific reversal agents are presently available in order to control life-threatening bleeding in DOAC-treated patients and improve outcomes. These reversal agents need to be administered during serious bleeding or due to overdosage and in the perioperative period to attain hemostasis. A monoclonal antibody fragment idarucizumab especially targets and reverses the effect of dabigatran. Studies have shown that within a few minutes of idarucizumab administration, complete reversal of the anticoagulation caused by dabigatran may occur.[27,28] Idarucizumab has approximately 350 times

more affinity than thrombin to bind dabigatran. After an intravenous dose of 5-g idarucizumab, the percentage reversal of patients diluted TT or ECT within 4 hours was 100%.[29] Andexanet has also been reported to reverse the anticoagulation secondary to apixaban and rivaroxaban use in older healthy individuals, within a few minutes of its administration, with no apparent clinical adverse effects.[30] Andexanet, administered as a 2-hour infusion, has shown to significantly decrease the activity of anti-factor Xa in patients who have life-threatening bleeds secondary to factor Xa inhibitors, and hemostasis could be achieved in 79% of these individuals.[31] In a pilot study to bind DTIs, factor Xa inhibitors using ciraparantag, heparins (including LMWH and fondaparinux), was able to reverse their anticoagulant properties.[32] FXa(I16L), has been shown to immediately restore hemostasis in case of anticoagulation secondary to use of DOAC. FXa[I16L] improved clotting and reduced blood loss after rivaroxaban therapy, and the effect of rivaroxaban and dabigatran has also been shown to get reversed in vitro.[33]

CONCLUSION

Direct oral anticoagulants reversibly inhibit coagulation factors and exhibit a half-life which is shorter than that of warfarin. Current agents available in therapeutics are DTIs like dabigatran and the direct factor Xa inhibitors which include apixaban, betrixaban, edoxaban, and rivaroxaban. The bleeding risk with DOACs is lesser than warfarin, but major serious bleeding has been documented with these newer agents. In the presence of major bleeding due to DOACs the offending drug should be withdrawn, component therapy should be transfused aptly, appropriate interventions like endoscopy, interventional radiology and surgery may need to be implemented. Specific antidotes to these newer agents such as idarucizumab and andexanet, though expensive are available and should be used to attain hemostasis.

KEY POINTS

- The DOACs need no monitoring as compared to warfarin and hence are presently in vogue
- In comparison to warfarin, the chances of fatal intracranial bleeding with DOACs are clearly lower
- In life-threatening bleeds antifibrinolytic agents like tranexamic acid, and epsilon-aminocaproic acid should be considered but may not be very effective.

Non-specific hemostatic products such as FFP and PCC may be used to replace clotting factors along with addition of vitamin K

- Hemodialysis may be used to remove active dabigatran from circulation
- Specific reversal agents, like idarucizumab and Andexanet, may be used to control life-threatening bleeding and improve outcomes.

REFERENCES

1. Granger CB, Alexander JH, McMurray JJ, et al. Apixaban versus warfarin in patients with atrial fibrillation. N Engl J Med. 2011;365(11):981-92.
2. Patel MR, Mahaffey KW, Garg J, et al. Rivaroxaban versus warfarin in nonvalvular atrial fibrillation. N Engl J Med. 2011;365(10):883-91.
3. Giugliano RP, Ruff CT, Braunwald E, et al. Edoxaban versus warfarin in patients with atrial fibrillation. N Engl J Med. 2013;369(22):2093-104.
4. Connolly SJ, Ezekowitz MD, Yusuf S, et al. Dabigatran versus warfarin in patients with atrial fibrillation. N Engl J Med. 2009;361(12):1139-51.
5. Schulman S, Kearon C, Kakkar AK, et al. Dabigatran versus warfarin in the treatment of acute venous thromboembolism. N Engl J Med. 2009;361(24):2342-52.
6. Agnelli G, Buller HR, Cohen A, et al. Oral apixaban for the treatment of acute venous thromboembolism. N Engl J Med. 2013;369(9):799-808.
7. Hokusai VT, Buller HR, Decousus H, et al. Edoxaban versus warfarin for the treatment of symptomatic venous thromboembolism. N Engl J Med. 2013;369(15):1406-15.
8. Investigators E, Bauersachs R, Berkowitz SD, et al. Oral rivaroxaban for symptomatic venous thromboembolism. N Engl J Med. 2010;363(26):2499-510.
9. Miyares MA, Davis K. Newer oral anticoagulants: a review of laboratory monitoring options and reversal agents in the hemorrhagic patient. Am J Health Syst Pharm. 2012;69(17):1473-84.
10. Favaloro EJ, Lippi G, Koutts J. Laboratory testing of anticoagulants: the present and the future. Pathology. 2011;43(7):682-92.
11. Baglin T, Keeling D, Kitchen S. Effects on routine coagulation screens and assessment of anticoagulant intensity in patients taking oral dabigatran or rivaroxaban: guidance from the British Committee for Standards in Haematology. Br J Haematol. 2012;159(4):427-9.
12. Chai-Adisaksopha C, Hillis C, Isayama T, et al. Mortality outcomes in patients receiving direct oral anticoagulants: a systematic review and meta-analysis of randomized controlled trials. J Thromb Haemost. 2015;13(11):2012-20.
13. Inohara T, Xian Y, Liang L, et al. Association of Intracerebral Hemorrhage Among Patients Taking Non-Vitamin K Antagonist vs Vitamin K Antagonist Oral Anticoagulants With In-Hospital Mortality. JAMA. 2018;319(5):463-73.

14. Kooiman J, van Hagen N, Iglesias Del Sol A, et al. The HAS-BLED Score identifies patients with acute venous thromboembolism at high risk of major bleeding complications during the first six months of anticoagulant treatment. PLoS One. 2015;10(4):e0122520.
15. Patel MR, Hellkamp AS, Fox KA. Point-of-Care Warfarin Monitoring in the ROCKET AF Trial. N Engl J Med. 2016;374(8):785-8.
16. Sardar P, Chatterjee S, Chaudhari S, et al. New oral anticoagulants in elderly adults: evidence from a meta-analysis of randomized trials. J Am Geriatr Soc. 2014;62(5):857-64.
17. Frontera JA, Lewin JJ 3rd, Rabinstein AA, et al. Guideline for Reversal of Antithrombotics in Intracranial Hemorrhage: a Statement for Healthcare Professionals from the Neurocritical Care Society and Society of Critical Care Medicine. Neurocrit Care. 2016;24(1):6-46.
18. Getta B, Muller N, Motum P, et al. Intermittent haemodialysis and continuous veno-venous dialysis are effective in mitigating major bleeding due to dabigatran. Br J Haematol. 2015;169(4):603-4.
19. Chai-Adisaksopha C, Hillis C, Lim W, et al. Hemodialysis for the treatment of dabigatran-associated bleeding: a case report and systematic review. J Thromb Haemost. 2015;13(10):1790-8.
20. Khadzhynov D, Wagner F, Formella S, et al. Effective elimination of dabigatran by haemodialysis. A phase I single-centre study in patients with end-stage renal disease. Thromb Haemost. 2013;109(4):596-605.
21. Wanek MR, Horn ET, Elapavaluru S, et al. Safe use of hemodialysis for dabigatran removal before cardiac surgery. Ann Pharmacother. 2012;46(9):e21.
22. Holbrook A, Schulman S, Witt DM, et al. Evidence-based management of anticoagulant therapy: Antithrombotic Therapy and Prevention of Thrombosis, 9th ed: American College of Chest Physicians Evidence-Based Clinical Practice Guidelines. Chest. 2012;141(2 Suppl):e152S-e84S.
23. Ageno W, Gallus AS, Wittkowsky A, et al. Oral anticoagulant therapy: Antithrombotic Therapy and Prevention of Thrombosis, 9th ed: American College of Chest Physicians Evidence-Based Clinical Practice Guidelines. Chest. 2012;141(2 Suppl):e44S-e88S.
24. Majeed A, Agren A, Holmstrom M, et al. Management of rivaroxaban- or apixaban-associated major bleeding with prothrombin complex concentrates: a cohort study. Blood. 2017;130(15):1706-12.
25. Xu Y, Schulman S, Dowlatshahi D, et al. Direct Oral Anticoagulant- or Warfarin-Related Major Bleeding: Characteristics, Reversal Strategies, and Outcomes From a Multicenter Observational Study. Chest. 2017;152(1):81-91.
26. Arellano-Rodrigo E, Lopez-Vilchez I, Galan AM, et al. Coagulation Factor Concentrates Fail to Restore Alterations in Fibrin Formation Caused by Rivaroxaban or Dabigatran in Studies With Flowing Blood From Treated Healthy Volunteers. Transfus Med Rev. 2015;29(4):242-9.

27. Pollack CV Jr, Reilly PA, Eikelboom J, et al. Idarucizumab for Dabigatran Reversal. N Engl J Med. 2015;373(6):511-20.

28. Glund S, Stangier J, Schmohl M, et al. Safety, tolerability, and efficacy of idarucizumab for the reversal of the anticoagulant effect of dabigatran in healthy male volunteers: a randomised, placebo-controlled, double-blind phase 1 trial. Lancet. 2015;386(9994):680-90.

29. Pollack CV Jr. Evidence supporting idarucizumab for the reversal of dabigatran. Am J Emerg Med. 2016;34(11S):33-8.

30. Siegal DM, Curnutte JT, Connolly SJ, et al. Andexanet Alfa for the Reversal of Factor Xa Inhibitor Activity. N Engl J Med. 2015;373(25):2413-24.

31. Connolly SJ, Milling TJ Jr, Eikelboom JW, et al. Andexanet Alfa for Acute Major Bleeding Associated with Factor Xa Inhibitors. N Engl J Med. 2016;375(12):1131-41.

32. Galliazzo S, Donadini MP, Ageno W. Antidotes for the direct oral anticoagulants: What news? Thromb Res. 2018;164(Suppl 1):S119-S23.

33. Thalji NK, Ivanciu L, Davidson R, et al. A rapid pro-hemostatic approach to overcome direct oral anticoagulants. Nat Med. 2016;22(8):924-32.

28 CHAPTER

Dyshemoglobinemias

Jeetendra Sharma, Shivangi Khanna

INTRODUCTION

Dyshemoglobinemias are a group of disorders in which the hemoglobin (Hb) molecule is functionally altered and becomes incapable of carrying oxygen. The commonly found functional alterations of Hb molecule are carboxyhemoglobin (COHb), methemoglobin, and sulfhemoglobin. COHb is formed as a result of carbon monoxide (CO) poisoning and is considered as an environmental emergency.

CARBOXYHEMOGLOBINEMIA

Approximately 50,000 people every year are affected by CO poisoning in the United States.[1] The clinical spectrum of CO poisoning ranges from headache and dizziness to coma and death.[2] Long-term neurocognitive sequelae occur in 15–40% of affected people.[1] Out of the moderately to severely affected patients, approximately one-third suffer from cardiac problems like arrhythmias, systolic dysfunction of left ventricle, and myocardial infarction (MI). Mortality rate ranges from 1% to 3% of affected individuals.[1]

Etiology and Pathogenesis

Carbon monoxide poisoning occurs as a result of routine activities, fire hazards, or large scale disasters (hurricanes, floods, or storms). Apart from sources like faulty furnaces, improperly ventilated flame-based heating sources, and automobile exhausts, endogenous sources have been suggested like sepsis and hemolytic anemia but they are rarely of clinical relevance.[3,4] The World Health Organization (WHO) holds that CO levels in excess of 6 parts-per million (ppm) can be potentially deleterious over a period of time[5] (Flowchart 1).

Carbon monoxide binds to Hb and forms COHb. Exposure to as low as 10 ppm of CO can lead to detectable COHb levels of more than 2% in blood. COHb more than 2% in nonsmokers and more than 10% in smokers is considered to be abnormal.[6]

Mechanism of Toxicity

Hemoglobin Binding

The CO binds to the ferrous heme containing proteins with high affinity. The Hb binds 250 times more avidly to CO as compared to oxygen.[7] The binding of CO to Hb leads to stabilization of the R state of the Hb molecule, thereby increasing the affinity of oxygen binding to other sites on the Hb tetramer. This leads to decreased tissue delivery of oxygen and leftward shift of oxyhemoglobin dissociation curve (Haldane effect).

Mitochondrial Dysfunction and Free Radical Generation

The CO binds to ferrous heme in the active site of cytochrome oxidase, thus the oxidative phosphorylation

Flowchart 1: Causes of carbon monoxide poisoning.

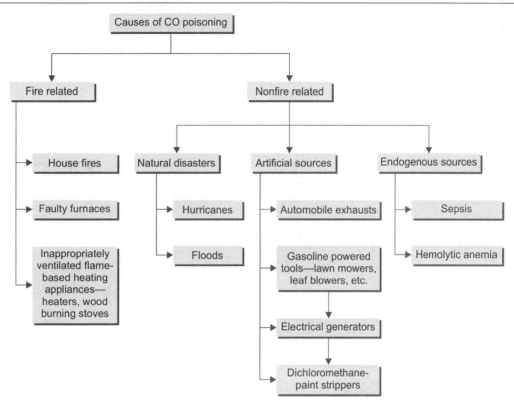

(CO: carbon monoxide)

is shut down in the mitochondria. The CO binding affinity of cytochrome oxidase is three-fold when compared to oxygen; therefore, increased binding occurs in hypoxic situations. As the oxidative phosphorylation is shut down, other electron carriers in the electron transport chain continue to shuttle electrons, leading to generation of free radicals like superoxide, leading to further damage to tissues and organs.[8-10]

Platelet Activation and Mediating Inflammation

The CO causes activation of platelets by displacement of nitric oxide (NO) from its surface. The displaced NO binds to superoxide radical leading to generation of peroxynitrite which further inhibits mitochondrial function and causes activation of more platelets.[11-13]

Activated platelets lead to degranulation of neutrophils leading to release of myeloperoxidase (MPO). This MPO then amplifies inflammation by causing activation, adhesion, and degranulation of more neutrophils and release of proteases. These proteases cause generation of reactive oxygen species (ROS) by oxidation of xanthine dehydrogenase to xanthine oxidase in the endothelium. MPO and ROS cause lipid peroxidation which forms adducts with myelin basic protein, leading to lymphocyte response and microglia activation. Thus, this mechanism of MPO activation and ROS generation is responsible for delayed neurological sequelae.

Mechanism of Brain Ischemia

Carbon monoxide poisoning leads to decrease in oxygen delivery and shut down of mitochondrial oxidative phosphorylation. This results in ischemic brain injury by excitotoxic mechanisms, ionic imbalance, depolarization, and oxidative stress. Reduction in adenosine triphosphate (ATP) production leads to activation of proteases and lipases, which further causes mitochondrial membrane depolarization, cell death, and release of neurotransmitters, especially glutamate. Glutamate activates the N-methyl, D-aspartate receptors, leading to cellular dysfunction and apoptosis[14-16] (Flowchart 2).

Hematological Toxins

Clinical Features and Diagnosis

Carbon monoxide poisoning is characteristically diagnosed by the clinical triad of symptoms consistent with CO poisoning, history of recent CO exposure, and elevated COHb levels in blood. However, these criteria are not strict as many patients are found unconscious

Flowchart 2: Pathophysiology of carbon monoxide poisoning.

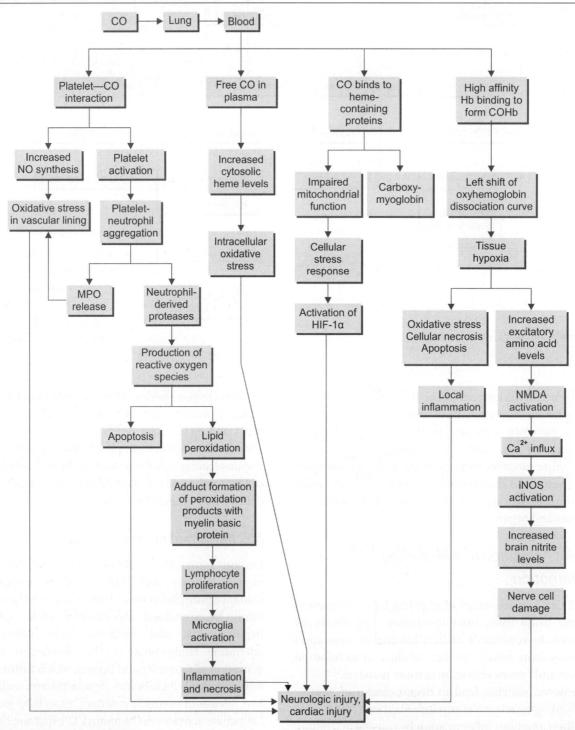

(CO: carbon monoxide; Hb: hemoglobin; HIF-1α: hypoxia-inducible factor 1-alpha; iNOS: nitric oxide synthase; MPO: myeloperoxidase; NMDA: N-methyl-D-aspartate; NO: nitric oxide)

and make history unobtainable. Also, caution should be exercised while excluding CO poisoning in areas of chronic low level exposure of CO, where measurement of ambient CO levels can aid in diagnosis. Evidence of elevated COHb levels in blood confirms the diagnosis due to suspected exposure (Flowchart 3).

Carboxyhemoglobin and Smoking

Generally, the COHb level in smokers is around 3–5%. For each pack of cigarettes smoked each day, the COHb level rises by 2.5%. In heavy smokers, especially with underlying lung pathology, the COHb levels can rarely rise to as high as 10%. A COHb level of 3–4% in nonsmokers and 10% in smokers is considered to be well above the normal expected range.[17]

The symptoms of CO poisoning range from headache, nausea, vomiting, dizziness, altered mentation, chest pain, dyspnea, and loss of consciousness. The common practice of looking for "cherry red" discoloration of skin for diagnosis of CO poisoning is not actually without downfalls. The concept as described by Hoppe in 1857,[18] was that COHb is actually a brighter shade of red when compared to oxyhemoglobin. The blood color in the capillaries determines the skin color. Therefore, it is reasonable to believe that the skin color of an individual with elevated CO levels might change to bright red. When skin color of individuals dying with CO poisoning was measured using reflectance spectrophotometry, it was seen that less than one-third actually had a "cherry red" color to their skin. Chronic lower level exposure presents as chronic fatigue, paresthesias, vertigo, abdominal pain, diarrhea, polycythemia, and recurrent infections (Table 1).

Table 1: Signs and symptoms of carbon monoxide poisoning.

Severity	Signs and symptoms
Mild	Fatigue, malaise, headache, dizziness, disorientation, confusion, blurred vision, nausea, vomiting
Moderate	Ataxia, syncope, tachypnea, dyspnea, palpitations, chest pain, rhabdomyolysis
Severe	Hypotension, arrhythmias, MI, coma, respiratory depression, seizures, cardiogenic pulmonary edema

(MI: myocardial infarction)

Cardiovascular Effects

Decreased oxygen delivery due to CO poisoning leads to compensation in the form of increased cardiac contractility and oxygen extraction until all the compensatory mechanisms are exhausted. This along with propensity of CO to cause thrombosis and direct binding of CO to myofilaments increases the risk of MI even in patients with normal cardiovascular physiology. Inhibition of oxidative phosphorylation and decreased availability of ATP alters the calcium gradients, increases intracellular calcium concentration and sensitivity of myofilaments to calcium, leading to a hyperadrenergic state. Most commonly found abnormality in CO poisoning is prolongation of QT interval. CO is also reported to increase the late component of inward sodium current by increasing NO levels. Therefore, NO synthase inhibitors like L-NAME (N omega-nitro-L-arginine methyl ester) and sodium channel inhibitor like ranolazine can be used for management of arrhythmias and prolonged QT interval in CO poisoning.[19]

Neurological Effects

Carbon monoxide poisoning can lead to development of long-term neurologic sequelae, related to brain injury. Symptoms like impairment of memory, cognitive dysfunction, anxiety, depression, and vestibular or motor effects can present within 6 weeks, more commonly in younger individuals (< 36 years) and more than 24 hours of CO exposure. Even low level of exposure is associated with long-term effects that do not resolve after the source of CO is removed, indicating brain injury. Magnetic resonance imaging (MRI) in CO poisoned patients most commonly demonstrates white matter hyperintensities

Flowchart 3: Triad for diagnosis of carbon monoxide poisoning.

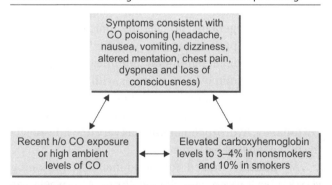

(CO: carbon monoxide; h/o: history of)

(WMH) particularly in the periventricular area and hippocampal atrophy. WMH in centrum semiovale are associated with cognitive defects. Thalamus, putamen, and caudate nucleus may also be involved, appearing as asymmetric hyperintense lesions in T2 weighted and fluid attenuation inversion recovery (FLAIR) images. Computerized tomography (CT) scans demonstrate bilateral symmetric attenuation. In very severe cases, the brainstem and cerebellum may be involved. Delayed posthypoxic leukoencephalopathy can occur in CO poisoning due to impaired cellular metabolism and direct myelotoxicity, observed as diffuse WMH in T2 weighted images. Neuronal loss and apoptosis may occur in CO poisoned patients with or without long-term sequelae, seen as sulcal widening and increased size of the ventricles, disproportionate to the patient's age.[20-22]

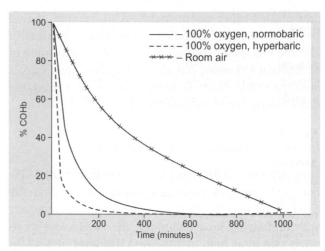

Fig. 1: Decay of carboxyhemoglobin with oxygen therapy. (COHb: carboxyhemoglobin)

Management of Carbon Monoxide Poisoning

Immediate management of a victim of CO poisoning is removal of the patient from the source of CO, administration of 100% oxygen, and transfer to a hospital where more definitive management can be done.

Carbon Monoxide Poisoning and Oxygen Therapy

Without oxygen, the elimination half time of CO is approximately 320 minutes on room air. Administration of oxygen by tight-fitting mask (normobaric oxygen therapy—NBO$_2$) decreases the elimination half-life to 74 minutes. Hyperbaric oxygen therapy (HBO$_2$) can further reduce the elimination half time to approximately 20–30 minutes (Fig. 1).[23]

The administration of NBO$_2$ should begin as soon as the patient is received to a medical facility, well before the diagnosis is confirmed. It was recommended to add carbon dioxide (CO$_2$) to oxygen (O$_2$) for increasing alveolar ventilation. However, the ventilatory response varies among individuals, so addition of CO$_2$ may be risky as it can add to the acidosis, already present in individuals who are retaining CO$_2$ due to ventilatory depression caused by CO poisoning.

The major goal of HBO$_2$ is to prevent long-term neurocognitive sequelae. In case hyperbaric oxygen is not available, normobaric 100% oxygen should be given until the COHb levels fall to less than 3% and the symptoms of CO poisoning abate, which typically takes around 6 hours. All patients should be considered as potential candidates of HBO$_2$ therapy, especially those with loss of consciousness, neurological deficits, severe metabolic acidosis, ischemic cardiac changes, and with COHb more than 25%. It is also reasonable to repeat HBO$_2$ therapy in persistently symptomatic patients. The maximum numbers of HBO$_2$ treatments are not clearly recommended, but it is considered appropriate to allow a maximum of three treatments to such patients.

If CO poisoning is believed to be intentional, a toxicology screen should be conducted in such patients. If the mental status changes appear to be disproportionate to the level of CO exposure suspected, coingestion of substances should be ruled out. Blood alcohol levels should be measured at the least in such patients.

Cyanide poisoning should be suspected in CO poisoned patients caught in house fires, especially if the arterial blood gas (ABG) shows a pH less than 7.20 and a plasma lactate of more than 10 mmol/L. Empiric management of cyanide poisoning should start in such patients at the earliest.[24] They should receive immediate parenteral administration of 5 g hydroxocobalamin over 15 minutes with repeat dosing up to 15 g. Pediatric patients should receive 70 mg/kg hydroxocobalamin, repeated twice if necessary. Fortunately, hydroxocobalamin has very few side effects in smoke inhaled patients.

All patients treated for accidental CO poisoning should be followed-up for at least 4–6 weeks as long-term neurological effects like memory disturbance, depression, anxiety, vestibular problems, and inability to calculate can develop after acute management of CO poisoning.[25] All survivors of intentional CO poisoning should be followed-up by a psychiatrist as rates of completed suicides are very high in such patients.[26]

METHEMOGLOBINEMIA

Methemoglobinemia is said to occur when the red blood cells (RBCs) contain methemoglobin levels higher than 1%. Methemoglobin has iron in the oxidized state (Fe^{+3}), rendering it useless for carrying oxygen and causing a functional state of anemia. Methemoglobin also causes leftward shift of oxyhemoglobin dissociation curve, leading to decreased delivery of oxygen to the tissues.[27,28]

Etiology and Pathogenesis

The Hb molecule is made up of four globin chains and each of these is attached to a heme group which contains iron in the form of Fe^{+2}, i.e. the reduced form. This form of iron can share an electron with oxygen, leading to formation of oxyhemoglobin. As the oxygen is released from oxyhemoglobin molecule into the tissues, the iron is again reduced to Fe^{+2} form. If the Hb molecule loses its electron and the iron atom becomes oxidized, it does not have electrons to bind to the oxygen molecule, reducing its capacity to carry oxygen. This may occur in times of oxidative stress.

Normally, methemoglobin levels are maintained to less than 1% with the help of two mechanisms, the first being the hexose monophosphate shunt pathway in the RBCs (utilizes glutathione for reduction) and the second one is through the action of diaphorase I and II enzymes. The diaphorase I and II pathways utilize NADH and NADPH, respectively to reduce methemoglobin. Diaphorase I pathway is responsible for reduction of 95–99% of normally produced methemoglobin. Cytochrome b5 reductase plays a major role in transferring electrons from NADH to methemoglobin in this pathway. The diaphorase II pathway has a minor role to play in normal individuals. It utilizes glutathione production and glucose 6 phosphate dehydrogenase (G6PD) for reduction of methemoglobin. It is a major pathway for methemoglobin reduction in patients with congenital cytochrome b5 reductase deficiency. This NADPH dependent diaphorase II pathway can be accelerated to approximately five times of normal

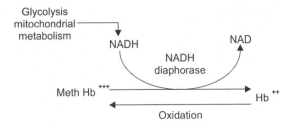

Fig. 2: Metabolic process depicting reduction of methemoglobin. (Meth Hb: methemoglobin NAD: nicotinamide adenine dinucleotide)

activity by exogenous substances like methylene blue (Fig. 2).

Classification

Congenital

- *Type I*: Cytochrome b5 reductase deficiency is detectable only in RBCs. Homozygotes are cyanotic but asymptomatic, while heterozygotes may develop symptomatic methemoglobinemia after exposure to certain drugs or toxins. It has autosomal recessive inheritance
- *Type II*: Cytochrome b5 reductase deficiency is generalized and is detectable in all tissues. It presents as severe, lethal and progressive neurological deficits like microcephaly and mental retardation along with methemoglobinemia. The affected individuals usually die at a very early age
- *Type III*: Cytochrome b5 reductase deficiency is limited only to the hematopoietic cells and clinically resembles type I
- *Type IV*: It occurs due to deficiency of a cofactor and resembles type I clinically
- *Hemoglobin M disease*: The inheritance pattern is autosomal dominant in which the tyrosine residue on the Hb molecule is replaced with histidine, which causes displacement of the heme group, thereby allowing oxidation of the ferrous iron to ferric state and forms a functionally impaired Hb. Three phenotypic variants are observed according to the globin chain affected
  o *Alpha-chain variant*: causes persistent neonatal cyanosis
  o *Beta-chain variant*: does not cause cyanosis till fetal Hb has reduced till several months after birth
  o *Gamma-chain variant*: causes transient neonatal cyanosis which resolves after the level of fetal Hb is reduced.

Hematological Toxins

- *Hemoglobin E disease (HbE)*: HbE beta thalassemia is associated with higher methemoglobin levels, especially in those patients who have undergone previous splenectomy.

Acquired

- *Occupational exposures*: Nitrates, aniline, nitrobenzene
- *Household exposures*: Shoe polishes, shoe dyes containing aniline, perfumes, flavoring essence, nitrite contamination of water
- Premature infants and infants less than 4 months are at an increased risk because NADH reductase levels are low at birth and reach adult levels at 4 months. Higher gastric pH in infants favors proliferation of bacteria leading to increased conversion of nitrate to nitrite. Acute gastroenteritis, leading to loss of stool bicarbonate, causes metabolic acidosis and further impairs the activity of NADH reductase enzyme
- Intensive care unit (ICU) hemodialysis
- *Drug exposures*: Table 2 includes drugs which can cause methemoglobinemia.

Clinical Features

Signs and symptoms of methemoglobinemia are given in Table 3.

Diagnosis

- Investigations to rule out hemolysis should be performed. These include complete blood count (CBC), reticulocyte count, peripheral smear review, lactate dehydrogenase (LDH), bilirubin, haptoglobin, and Heinz body preparation
- *Investigations to rule out organ failure*: Liver function tests, electrolytes, and renal function tests
- *Investigations for detecting hereditary cause of methemoglobinemia*: Hemoglobin electrophoresis to detect hemoglobin M (HbM) and deoxyribonucleic acid (DNA) sequencing of globin chain can be performed for diagnosis of HbM disease. Specific enzyme assays for NADH reductase and cytochrome b5 reductase levels in specific cells like platelets, fibroblasts, or granulocytes can be performed
- Measurement of blood levels of nitrite and specific toxins should be done in suspected cases. The treatment is usually started before these levels are obtained.

Table 2: Drugs causing methemoglobinemia.

Categories	Drugs
Analgesics	• Acetaminophen • Fentanyl • Phenazopyridine • Celecoxib
Anti-infective agents	
Antimicrobials	• Cotrimoxazole • Dapsone • Nitrofurantoin • Clofazimine • Phenazopyridine • Sulfonamides
Antimalarials	• Quinine • Chloroquine • Primaquine
Antimycobacterial drugs	• Rifampicin
Anticonvulsants	• Phenobarbitone • Phenytoin • Sodium valproate
Vasodilators	• Nitroglycerine • Isosorbide dinitrate • Amyl nitrite • Nitric oxide • Sodium nitroprusside
Local anesthetics	• Benzocaine • Prilocaine • Lidocaine • Bupivacaine • EMLA
Miscellaneous	• Metoclopramide • Oral hypoglycemics • Flutamide • Riluzole • Methylene blue

(EMLA: eutectic mixture of local anesthetics)

Table 3: Signs and symptoms of methemoglobinemia[29-31].

Meth Hb levels (%)	Signs and symptoms
< 3	None
3–10	Blue/slate gray skin
10–20	Cyanosis, chocolate-brown blood
20–50	Breathlessness, headache, dizziness, syncopal attacks
50–70	Tachypnea, lactic acidosis, seizures, arrhythmias, CNS depression, coma
> 70	Death

(CNS: central nervous system, Meth Hb: methemoglobin)

- *Bedside tests*: To detect if the dark blood is due to methemoglobinemia, 100% oxygen can be bubbled through it in a tube. In methemoglobinemia, the blood remains dark in spite of the oxygen exposure. Another method is to place one to two drops of blood on a white paper and blowing oxygen over it. Deoxygenated Hb changes to bright red, while methemoglobin remains brown.
- *Arterial blood gas*: Falsely elevated saturation of oxygen is observed in ABG with methemoglobinemia. Detection of a "saturation gap", i.e. difference between saturation observed by pulse oximetry and ABG is a useful clue. The PaO_2 is unaffected in methemoglobinemia.
- *Oximetry*: Pulse oximetry is unreliable in cases of methemoglobinemia as methemoglobin offers optical interference by absorbing light at both the wavelengths used for pulse oximetry, i.e. 660 and 940 nm. Therefore, the saturations observed plateau at 85%. Co-oximetry should be used wherever possible as it uses four wavelengths of light and can differentiate between methemoglobin, oxy-, and deoxyhemoglobin. The presence of methylene blue interferes with detection of methemoglobin with co-oximetry; therefore, it cannot be reliably used if treatment has already been started for methemoglobinemia.
- *Potassium cyanide (KCN) test*: This test can be used to differentiate between methemoglobin and sulfhemoglobin. Methemoglobin reacts with cyanide to form cyanmethemoglobin which has a bright red color, while sulfhemoglobin does not react with cyanide.

Management

Early establishment of diagnosis and administration of treatment is imperative. Although, it may be necessary to conduct an array of investigations to rule out cardiac and pulmonary causes of cyanosis in ambiguous cases. Once the diagnosis is confirmed, the offending agent or oxidizing substance should be withdrawn and oxygen supplementation should start at the earliest.

Patients with asymptomatic cyanosis can be discharged after an observation period of about 6 hours, only if the offending agent has been withdrawn and is not known to cause rebound methemoglobinemia. Symptomatic patients with high levels of methemoglobin should be admitted to the hospital.

As soon as the diagnosis is confirmed, a search for etiology should commence either by obtaining blood levels or by gastric lavage. Removal of the offending agent and monitoring of blood methemoglobin levels is sometimes all that is required in patients with low methemoglobin levels. Treatment is advisable in patients having methemoglobin levels 20% or higher and also at lower methemoglobin levels, if there are comorbidities present or evidence of end organ dysfunction.

Methylene blue 1–2 mg/kg (up to a total of 50 mg in adults, adolescents, and older children) as a 1% solution in intravenous (IV) saline over 3–5 minutes is recommended for symptomatic patients. Administration may be repeated at 1 mg/kg every 30 minutes as necessary to control symptoms. A maximum dose of 7 mg/kg can be given, as methylene blue at higher dose can itself cause methemoglobinemia. It is contraindicated in G6PD deficiency, as it can lead to hemolysis in absence of G6PD. It should be used with caution in patients already on serotonergic psychiatric drugs, as it can precipitate serotonergic syndrome by increasing serotonin levels in brain by monoamine oxidase-A inhibition. Methylene blue is ineffective in HbM disease, diaphorase II deficiency, and in sulfhemoglobinemia.[32-35]

Exchange transfusion or HBO_2 can be used in G6PD deficient patients who are severely symptomatic and unresponsive to methylene blue. Automated RBC exchange, also called RBC apheresis or erythrocytapheresis is preferred over exchange transfusion of whole blood if available. The patient's RBC are removed and replaced by packed red blood cell units. A bedside hemoglobinometer may be used for continuous monitoring of Hb in the patient. The advantage of RBC apheresis is that the replacement RBCs do not have to be reconstituted in AB plasma, which is an expensive blood product and is required for exchange transfusion. Hyperbaric oxygen allows oxygenation to continue through dissolved plasma oxygen, while the Hb carrier is ineffective.

Infants who have methemoglobinemia due to metabolic acidosis should be treated with fluids and bicarbonate. Dextrose-containing fluids should be preferred as NADPH dependent clearance of methemoglobin requires glucose to function.

Patients with mild chronic methemoglobinemia due to enzyme deficiencies may be treated with oral medications: methylene blue 100–300 mg/day (may produce blue urine), ascorbic acid 200–500 mg/day, and riboflavin 20 mg/day.

Cimetidine can be tried for dapsone-induced methemoglobinemia to prevent further formation of its metabolite. *N*-acetylcysteine is not currently an approved treatment for methemoglobinemia, although it is shown to reduce methemoglobin levels.

CYANIDE TOXICITY

Etiology and Pathogenesis

Accidental poisoning is caused by inhalation of hydrogen cyanide gas or absorption of cyanide containing solutions or gas through the skin. It can also result from prolonged infusions of certain drugs like sodium nitroprusside. Prolonged ingestion of certain foods containing cyanide like bitter almonds, cassava root, and apricot seeds can result in cyanide poisoning. The most common source of cyanide exposure is smoke inhalation from industrial or residential fires.[36,37]

Mechanism of Toxicity

Cyanide causes toxicity with inhibition of enzymes like cytochrome oxidase, xanthine oxidase, carbonic anhydrase, and glutamate dehydrogenase. By inhibition of the cytochrome oxidase system, cyanide inhibits the electron cytochrome chain that is responsible for production of ATP. The aerobic oxidation is thereby shut down, but production of pyruvate is continued by glycolysis, which is eventually converted to lactate. The energy production, therefore, becomes inefficient. Systemic acidosis occurs not because of the rising lactate levels, but due to overproduction of hydrogen ions by cellular production of ATP without normal balancing with oxidative phosphorylation.[38]

Cyanide toxicity affects the most ATP dependent organs first, like heart and brain. Cardiac cytochrome oxidase is particularly sensitive to cyanide. Inhibition of superoxide dismutase and glutathione reductase may further increase the injury by generation of free radicals.

Neurotoxicity is caused by stimulation of N-methyl D-aspartate receptors and release of glutamate, eventually enhancement of intracellular calcium release, leading to cell death. Cyanide also inhibits glutamate decarboxylase, the enzyme responsible for production of gamma-aminobutyric acid (GABA). Loss of GABA action leads to increased risk of seizures.[39]

Clinical Features

Clinical features of cyanide poisoning depend upon the route of exposure, type of cyanide involved, and the dose. Rapidity of onset of symptoms is maximum with gaseous exposure, followed by soluble salt, insoluble salt, and cyanogens.

Exposure to high levels of vapor can lead to (Table 4): Exposure to lower vapor concentrations and liquid exposure can cause anxiety, vertigo, weakness, trembling, headache and loss of consciousness. Cyanogen chloride exposure causes skin and mucous membrane irritation, lacrimation, rhinorrhea, bronchorrhea, cough, chest tightness, and pulmonary edema. Higher doses can cause similar systemic symptoms as HCN exposure. Another important finding is the bitter almond odor of cyanide, but unfortunately it is recognized by only 40–60% of the population. The characteristic skin color of a cyanide poisoned patient is cherry red due to reduced consumption of oxygen, leading to arterialization of venous blood, but the patient can be found cyanosed with prolonged respiratory failure and shock.

Lethal dose: Orally administered HCN to adult, lethal dose is estimated to be 50–100 mg, and for KCN, about 150–250 mg.[40]

Diagnosis

The most important diagnostic test in cyanide poisoning is an ABG analysis. High lactates and high anion gap metabolic acidosis are the two most common and universal findings in these patients. Both of these can result from various clinical effects of cyanide like seizures, respiratory failure, cardiac failure, shock, and catecholamine release. A plasma lactate concentration of more than 8 mmol/L was found to be 94% sensitive and 70% specific in predicting a blood cyanide concentration of more than 1.0 mg/L in a study conducted by Baud et al.

Table 4: Symptoms of cyanide poisoning after exposure to cyanide.

Symptoms	Duration after exposure
Hyperpnea and hypertension	15 seconds
Loss of consciousness	30 seconds
Convulsions	30–45 seconds
Respiratory arrest	3–5 minutes
Bradycardia, hypotension, and cardiac arrest	5–8 minutes

in residential fire victims and pure cyanide intoxications. Exclusion of patients treated with catecholamines increased the specificity.[41] As lactate levels can be increased in various other diseases, the lactate levels are a useful screening tool only in patients with strongly suspected cyanide exposure. Measurement of serial lactate levels can predict the need for repeat dosing and the effectiveness of antidotal therapy.

Other more specific tests include measurement of thiocyanate in urine (which is a useful marker of exposure) and whole blood cyanide concentration assay. Cyanide typically concentrates in RBCs; therefore, whole blood cyanide concentration is most commonly used as a diagnostic test. Blood cyanide concentration does correlate well with the cyanide levels (Table 5).

Postmortem measurement of tissue cyanide levels in liver and heart may be more accurate than blood cyanide levels.

Many other nonspecific findings like elevated mixed venous oxygen saturation, hyperglycemia, and ST segment shortening resulting in origin of T wave over the R wave on an electrocardiogram (ECG) can indicate toward cyanide poisoning.

Management

Prehospital care of suspected cyanide poisoning victims includes removal from the source of cyanide exposure, removal of the clothing, and decontamination with soap and water as the first step. Aggressive airway management and administration of high flow oxygen should be commenced at the earliest. Continuous cardiac monitoring should begin and advanced cardiac life support (ACLS) protocols be followed for dysrhythmias. Decontamination with activated charcoal (1 g/kg) should be done in cases of oral ingestion. The gastric aspirate can be potentially hazardous and can cause secondary contamination. Administration of cyanide antidotes should begin as soon as possible, without waiting for

Table 5: Signs and symptoms of cyanide poisoning according to blood cyanide levels.[42]

Signs and symptoms	Cyanide levels
Flushing and tachycardia	0.5–1 mg/L
Obtundation	1–2.5 mg/L
Coma	2.5–3 mg/L
Death	3 mg/L

laboratory confirmation of the diagnosis in strongly suspected cases.

Cyanide Antidotes

Cyanide antidotes are discussed in Table 6.

Delayed effects of cyanide toxicity like lung injury, acute respiratory distress syndrome (ARDS), and neurological sequelae can complicate the recovery course. Patients can develop delayed neurologic sequelae, days to months after the initial poisoning. Parkinsonian symptoms including bradykinesia, dysarthria, rigidity, and ataxia can occur with injury to the putamen and globus pallidus and the cerebral cortex and cerebellum (as seen on neuroimaging). Treatment with dopaminergic agents has yielded significant clinical improvement in some patients but is often of no benefit.

SULFHEMOGLOBINEMIA

Sulfhemoglobinemia is abnormal attachment of sulfur atom to Hb molecule, rendering it nonfunctional for oxygen transport. It is caused by exposure to sulfur containing drugs like sulfonamides, sulfasalazine, phenazopyridines, overdose of sumatriptan, dapsone, cotrimoxazole, etc. Patients usually present with cyanosis. It has been shown that less sulfhemoglob in (0.5 g/dL) is needed to cause cyanosis as compared to methemoglobin (1.5 g/dL) and deoxygenated Hb (5 g/dL). The condition usually resolves by itself as affected RBCs get destroyed after completion of their life span, but multiple blood transfusions may be required in extreme cases.[43,44]

CONCLUSION

Dyshemoglobinemias are a group of disorders caused by functional alteration of the Hb molecule, thereby reducing the oxygen carrying capacity. Prompt diagnosis and management of individual disorders is imperative for reducing morbidity and mortality and obtaining a favorable long-term neuropsychological outcome.

KEY POINTS

- Low threshold for suspicion of CO poisoning should be kept in patients at high risk of CO exposure and prompt administration of oxygen should start as soon as it is suspected

Hematological Toxins

Table 6: Cyanide antidotes.

Antidote	Mechanism of action	Administration	Adverse effects
Amyl nitrite	• Methemoglobin (eventually cyanmethemoglobin) formation • Vasodilatation (increase blood flow to liver and increased detoxification)	• Before IV access: 1 ampule (0.3 mL) of amyl nitrite broken over a handkerchief and held in front of the patient's mouth for 15 seconds and removed for 15 seconds. This is repeated till IV access can be secured and IV sodium nitrite can be given. Alternatively, it can be given through a ventilation system or in aerosolized form	• Reduced oxygen carrying capacity of blood • Hypotension
Sodium nitrite	• Methemoglobin (eventually cyanmethemoglobin) formation • Vasodilatation (increase blood flow to liver and increased detoxification)	• Adults: 300 mg (10 mL of a 3% solution) or 10 mg/kg IV for 3–5 minutes (2.5–5 mL/min) • Children: 6–8 mL/m² or 2 mL/kg (not to exceed 10 mL)	• Reduced oxygen carrying capacity of blood • Hypotension
Sodium thiosulfate	• Additional sulfur donor to facilitate cyanide metabolism by enzymes like rhodanese, 3-mercaptopyruvate sulfurtransferase, and thiosulfate reductase	• Adults: 12.5 g (1 ampule) in 50 mL NS IV over 30 minutes • Children: 7 g/m² (not to exceed 12.5 g)	• None significant
Hydroxocobalamin	• Binds cyanide intracellularly to form cyanocobalamin	• Adults: 5 g IV over 15 minutes (one dose to be repeated as needed) • Children: 70 mg/kg	• Hypertension • Transient discoloration of secretions
4-Dimethylamino-phenol	• Methemoglobin formation	• 3–5 mg/kg IV	• Reduced oxygen carrying capacity of blood • Necrosis at injection site (specially with IM injections)
Dicobalt edetate	• Directly binds cyanide	• 300 mg (in 20% dextrose, 20 mL—1 ampule) IV. To be repeated for two doses if no recovery occurs	• Cardiovascular toxicity, angioedema

(IM: intramuscular; IV: intravenous)

- All patients with CO poisoning should be followed-up for 4–6 weeks after recovery and evaluated for long-term neuropsychological complications
- Methemoglobinemia should be suspected in patients having a history of drug overdose or exposure to dyes and chemicals, presenting with nonspecific symptoms along with cyanosis
- Careful history taking and evaluation for G6PD deficiency should be done in patients who are to receive methylene blue
- Prompt initiation of exchange transfusion or RBC apheresis is a useful alternative, wherever the local facilities permit
- Cyanide poisoning should be strongly suspected in victims of residential fires and prompt resuscitation measures should be undertaken. Early administration of cyanide antidotes is lifesaving in such cases.

REFERENCES

1. Rose JJ, Wang L, Xu Q, et al. Carbon Monoxide Poisoning: Pathogenesis, Management, and Future Directions of Therapy. Am J Respir Crit Care Med. 2017;195(5):596-606.
2. Hampson NB, Dunn SL; members of the UHMS/CDC CO Poisoning Surveillance Group. Symptoms of acute carbon monoxide poisoning do not correlate with the initial carboxyhemoglobin level. Undersea Hyperb Med. 2012;39:657-65.

3. Omaye ST. Metabolic modulation of carbon monoxide toxicity. Toxicology. 2002;180(2):139-50.
4. Bauer I, Pannen BH. Bench-to-bedside review: Carbon monoxide–from mitochondrial poisoning to therapeutic use. Crit Care. 2009;13(4):220.
5. Penney D, Benignus V, Kephalopoulos S, et al. Carbon monoxide. WHO Guidelines for Indoor Air Quality: Selected Pollutants. Geneva: WHO; 2010.
6. Hampson NB, Piantadosi CA, Thom SR, et al. Practice recommendations in the diagnosis, management, and prevention of carbon monoxide poisoning. Am J Respir Crit Care Med. 2012;186:1095-101.
7. Hall J. Guyton and Hall Textbook of Medical Physiology. Philadelphia, PA: Saunders/Elsevier; 2010.
8. Gnaiger E, Lassnig B, Kuznetsov A, et al. Mitochondrial oxygen affinity, respiratory flux control and excess capacity of cytochrome c oxidase. J Exp Biol. 1998;201: 1129-39.
9. Wald G, Allen DW. The equilibrium between cytochrome oxidase and carbon monoxide. J Gen Physiol. 1957;40:593-608.
10. Lo Iacono L, Boczkowski J, Zini R, et al. A carbon monoxide–releasing molecule (CORM-3) uncouples mitochondrial respiration and modulates the production of reactive oxygen species. Free Radic Biol Med. 2011;50:1556-64.
11. Thom SR, Ohnishi ST, Ischiropoulos H. Nitric oxide released by platelets inhibits neutrophil B2 integrin function following acute carbon monoxide poisoning. Toxicol Appl Pharmacol. 1994;128:105-10.
12. Thom SR, Xu YA, Ischiropoulos H. Vascular endothelial cells generate peroxynitrite in response to carbon monoxide exposure. Chem Res Toxicol. 1997;10: 1023-31.
13. Thom SR, Bhopale VM, Han ST, et al. Intravascular neutrophil activation due to carbon monoxide poisoning. Am J Respir Crit Care Med. 2006;174:1239-48.
14. Kim I, Xu W, Reed JC. Cell death and endoplasmic reticulum stress: disease relevance and therapeutic opportunities. Nat Rev Drug Discov. 2008;7:1013-30.
15. Piantadosi CA, Zhang J, Levin ED, et al. Apoptosis and delayed neuronal damage after carbon monoxide poisoning in the rat. Exp Neurol. 1997;147:103-14.
16. Ishimaru H, Katoh A, Suzuki H, et al. Effects of N-methyl-D-aspartate receptor antagonists on carbon monoxide-induced brain damage in mice. J Pharmacol Exp Ther. 1992;261:349-52.
17. Radford EP, Drizd TA. Blood carbon monoxide levels in persons 3–74 years of age: United States, 1976–80. Advance data from Vital and Health Statistics, No. 76. DHHS Publ. No. (PHS) 82-1250. Hyattsville, MD: National Center for Health Statistics; Office of Health Research, Statistics, and Technology; Public Health Service; U.S. Department of Health and Human Services; 1982.
18. Hoppe F. Uber die Einwirkung des Kohlenoxydgases auf das Hämatoglobulin. Virchows Arch Pathol Anat Physiol Klin Med. 1857;11:288.
19. Dallas ML, Yang Z, Boyle JP, et al. Carbon monoxide induces cardiac arrhythmia via induction of the late Na1 current. Am J Respir Crit Care Med. 2012;186:648-56.
20. Mimura K, Harada M, Sumiyoshi S, et al. Long-term follow-up study on sequelae of carbon monoxide poisoning; serial investigation 33 years after poisoning [in Japanese]. Seishin Shinkeigaku Zasshi. 1999;101:592-618.
21. Weaver LK, Valentine KJ, Hopkins RO. Carbon monoxide poisoning risk factors for cognitive sequelae and the role of hyperbaric oxygen. Am J Respir Crit Care Med. 2007;176:491-7.
22. Parkinson RB, Hopkins RO, Cleavinger HB, et al. White matter hyperintensities and neuropsychological outcome following carbon monoxide poisoning. Neurology. 2002;58:1525-32.
23. Weaver LK, Hopkins RO, Chan KJ, et al. Hyperbaric oxygen for acute carbon monoxide poisoning. N Engl J Med. 2002;347:1057-67.
24. Baud FJ. Cyanide: critical issues in diagnosis and treatment. Hum Exp Toxicol. 2007;26:191-291.
25. Pages B, Planton M, Buys S, et al. Neuropsychological outcome after carbon monoxide exposure following a storm: a case–control study. BMC Neurol. 2014; 14:153.
26. Hampson NB, Hauff NM, Rudd RA. Increased long-term mortality among survivors of acute carbon monoxide poisoning. Crit Care Med. 2009;37:1941-7.
27. Mansouri A, Lurie AA. Concise review: methemoglobinemia. Am J Hematol. 1993;42(1):7-12.
28. Curry S. Methemoglobinemia. Ann Emerg Med. 1982;11(4):214-21.
29. Goldfrank's Toxicologic emergencies, 9th edition. 2010. pp. 1698-710.
30. Wright RO, Lewander WJ, Woolf AD. Methemoglobinemia: etiology, pharmacology, and clinical management Ann Emerg Med. 1999;34:646-56.
31. Trapp L, Will J. Acquired methemoglobinemia revisited. Dent Clin N Am. 2010;54:665-75.
32. Goluboff N, Wheaton R. Methylene blue induced cyanosis and acute hemolytic anemia complicating the treatment of methemoglobinemia. J Pediatr. 1961;58:86-9.
33. Price D. Methemoglobinemia. In: Goldfrank LR, Flomenbaum NE, Lewin NA, Weisman RS, Howland MA, Hoffman RS (Eds). Goldfrank's Toxicologic Emergencies, 6th edition. Old Tappan, NJ: Appleton & Lange; 1998. pp. 1507-23.
34. Harvey JW, Keitt AS. Studies of the efficacy and potential hazards of methylene blue therapy in aniline-induced methaemoglobinaemia. Br J Haematol. 1983;54:29-41.
35. Roigas H, Zoellner E, Jacobasch G, et al. Regulatory factors in methylene blue catalysis in erythrocytes. Eur J Biochem. 1970;12:24-30.
36. Gracia R, Shepherd G. Cyanide poisoning and its treatment. Pharmacotherapy. 2004;24(10):1358-65.
37. Curry SC, LoVecchio FA. Hydrogen cyanide and inorganic cyanide salts. In: Sullivan JB, Krieger GR (Eds). Clinical

Environmental Health and Toxic Exposures, 2nd edition. Philadelphia, PA: Lippincott Williams & Wilkins; 2001. pp. 705-16.

38. Curry SC, LoVecchio FA. Hydrogen cyanide and inorganic cyanide salts. In: Sullivan JB Krieger GR (Eds). Clinical Environmental Health and Toxic Exposures, 2nd edition. Philadelphia, PA: Lippincott Williams & Wilkins; 2001. pp. 705-16.

39. Tursky T, Sajter V. The influence of potassium cyanide poisoning on the gamma-aminobutyric acid level in rat brain. J Neurochem. 1962;9:519-23.

40. Ballantyne B. The forensic diagnosis of acute cyanide poisoning. In: Ballantyne B (Eds). Forensic Toxicology. Bristol: Wright Publication; 1974. pp. 99-113.

41. Baud FJ, Borron SW, Megarbane B, et al. Value of lactic acidosis in the assessment of the severity of acute cyanide poisoning. Crit Care Med. 2002;30(9): 2044-50.

42. Baskin SI, Brewer TG. Cyanide poisoning. In: Sidell FR, Takefuji ET, Franz DR (Eds). Medical Aspects of Chemical and Biological Warfare. Washington, DC: Office of the Surgeon General; 1997. pp. 271-86.

43. Gopalachar AS, Bowie VL, Bharadwaj P. Phenazopyridine-induced sulfhemoglobinemia. Ann Pharmacother. 2005;39(6):1128-30.

44. Flexman AM, Del Vicario G, Schwarz SK. Dark green blood in the operating theatre. Lancet. 2007;369(9577): 1972.

SECTION 8

Renal Toxins and Extracorporeal Therapies

29. **Approach to Toxin Induced Acute Renal Failure**
    Sahil Bagai, Dinesh Khullar

30. **Extracorporeal Therapies: General Principles**
    Deven Juneja, Omender Singh

31. **Extracorporeal Therapies: Specific Poisons**
    Deven Juneja, Omender Singh

32. **Extracorporeal Membrane Oxygenation**
    Anna L Condella, Edward W Boyer

29
CHAPTER

Approach to Toxin Induced Acute Renal Failure

Sahil Bagai, Dinesh Khullar

INTRODUCTION

Acute kidney injury (AKI) is defined by an increase of more than 0.3 mg/dL serum creatinine within 48 hours occurring as a result of an injury that causes a functional or structural change in the kidney.[1] AKI occurs in approximately 5% of hospitalized patients and about 30% of intensive care unit (ICU) patients. AKI is a frequent accompaniment in critical care patients, more so in patients with poisonings. Even modest degrees of AKI can increase death rates by approximately fivefold.[2]

Poisonings and envenomation may lead to AKI through several different mechanisms. Some of the toxins may result in hemolysis or rhabdomyolysis, which may further lead to pigment-induced AKI. Presence of other factors like hypotension or infection may further contribute to AKI.

Indian studies have shown an incidence of AKI around 5.6% in patients with poisoning and envenomation, with paraquat and snakebites as being common causes of AKI in these patients.[3]

Common poisoning causing rhabdomyolysis include opioids, benzodiazepines, and antipsychotics (Table 1).

Tubular injury often occurs from a combination of vasoconstriction affecting kidney perfusion and direct cellular toxicity or, may be of immunological origin such as in case of interstitial nephritis.[2]

Amongst common poisonings that are of interest to a critical care nephrologists are namely snake venoms,

Table 1: Common toxins associated with rhabdomyolysis.[4]
Amphetamine
Antipsychotics
Benzodiazepines
Beta-blockers
Carbon monoxide
Clonidine
Gabapentin
Methanol
Opioids
Organophosphates
Snake venom
Tricyclic antidepressants (TCA)

bee and wasp sting bite, paraphenylene diamine (PPD) and other aniline substance, organophosphorus (OP) compounds, copper sulfate, datura, aluminum phosphide, paraquat, methyl alcohol, ethyl alcohol, lithium poisoning, heavy metals, and rodenticides.

CLINICAL FEATURES

Patients with AKI who land up in ICU with history of accidental or abuse poisoning mostly present with oliguria, anuria or nonoliguric AKI and associated manifestations of poisoning, i.e. shock, tachypnea,

Renal Toxins and Extracorporeal Therapies

vomiting, pain abdomen, bleeding, etc.[5] Patients with bleeding from orifices may have fang marks on the body or may have marks of hornet bite stings. Patients with alcohol intake can have fruit like odor from mouth. These are clues which may assist in diagnosis of poisoning.

MECHANISMS OF INJURY

Most of the toxic agents directly injure S1 segment of the proximal tubules, leading to acute tubular necrosis (ATN). ATN can also be seen indirectly if S3 segment gets involved secondarily to hypotension in any critically sick patient. In some cases rhabdomyolysis, pigment cast nephropathy has been other forms of renal injury reported after poisonings.

AGENTS CAUSING ACUTE KIDNEY INJURY (TABLE 2)

Paraphenylenediamine

Hair dyes and fortified "henna" used for tattooing are common source of PPD. Contact with photocopying and printing inks can result in occupational exposure. PPD can affect gastrointestinal tract, liver, brain, and kidneys. ATN and pigment cast nephropathy are pathophysiological

mechanisms causing AKI. In 1982, two cases of PPD were reported from a center in India.[6]

Organophosphorus Poisonings

They are available as pesticides and herbicides. These toxins inhibit enzyme acetylcholine esterase, resulting in accumulation of acetylcholine in synaptic junctions. This uninhibited action of acetylcholine leads to cholinergic crises which predispose kidneys to ischemic ATN. As per one study OP poisoning was associated with a six times higher risk of AKI.[7]

Datura

It is a poison from flowering plant. Scopolamine, hyoscyamine, and atropine are active ingredients mainly in seeds and flowers. Renal injury occurs indirectly because of the cholinergic crisis which results in ischemic ATN. Interstitial edema and direct tubular insult can also occur in datura poisoning.[8]

Rodenticides

It is commonly used in the developing world for homicide purpose. Active metabolic compounds are brodifacoum,

Table 2: Poisoning causing acute kidney injury.			
Poisoning	*Active compound*	*Source*	*Mechanism of renal injury*
Paraphenylenediamine	Paraphenylenediamine	Hair dyes, fortified henna	ATN, pigment nephropathy
Methanol	Methyl alcohol	Industrial solvents	ATN
Organophosphorus	Acetylcholine	Pesticides, herbicides	Ischemic ATN
Paraquat	Superoxide radical	Herbicide	Direct cellular damage, toxic ATN
Copper sulfate	Copper sulfate	Pesticides, herbicides	ATN, pigment nephropathy
Datura	Hyoscyamine, sclopamine	Seeds	Ischemic ATN, interstitial edema
Rodenticide	Brodifacoum, diphacinone, warfarin	Rodenticide	ATN, pigment nephropathy
Benzodiazipines ingestion	Benzodiazipines ingestion	Lorazepam	Ischemia reperfusion, ATN
Snake/hornet bite	Phospholipase A2		ATN, ACN, pigment cast nephropathy
Lead poisoning	Lead	Paints	Fanconi syndrome
Arsenic	Ar^{2+}	Insecticides	Proximal RTA, CIN
Cadmium	Cd^{2+}	Batteries	Nephrolithiasis, CIN, proximal tubular injury
Lithium	Li^{2+}	Drugs	DI, CIN

(ACN: acute cortical necrosis; ATN: acute tubular necrosis; CIN: chronic interstitial nephritis; DI: diabetes insipidus)

warfarin, and bromadiolone. Rapid blood loss after coagulopathy can lead to ischemic ATN and hemoglobin pigments can also cause tubular blockade leading to AKI.[8]

Copper Sulfate (CuSO₄)

It is a blue and odorless salt used as fungicides, herbicides, and insecticides.[9] Absorption occurs via gastrointestinal tract, lungs, and skin. Neurological symptoms such as delerium, coma, convulsion, hypotension, respiratory failure, pallor or jaundice point toward systemic toxicity. Pigment nephropathy and ATN are most likely reasons for AKI.[10]

Propylene Glycol Toxicity

Lorazepam and diazepam use propylene glycol as solvent which can cause AKI. Midazolam does not require this solvent so does not cause AKI. It is also characterized by hyperosmolarity and a high anion gap metabolic acidosis. It can occur with normal doses and renal function, but it is usually associated with dosages above the recommended range of 0.1 mg/kg/h and/or renal impairment. An osmolar gap more than 10 mmoles/L suggests that the serum propylene glycol concentration is high enough to cause toxicity.[11] Treatment consists of avoiding offending agent and, if severe, dialysis.

Barbiturates

They are the agents used in ICU setting for delirious patients. Toxic serum levels of phenobarbital are greater than 3 mg/dL, and coma begins to appear at levels of 6 mg/dL. Multidose activated charcoal should be considered as first-line therapy and alkalinization of the urine may also be useful in the case of long-acting barbiturates. Hemodialysis (HD) should be contemplated when coma is prolonged, especially when complications of coma, such as pneumonia, refractory hypotension persist. There is, however, no evidence that HD will improve overall survival. Long-extended duration dialysis is recommended by a few.

Toxic Alcohols

Unexplained metabolic acidosis accompanied by increased anion and osmolal gaps is classical of toxic alcohols. Although methanol and ethyl alcohol are themselves harmless, methanol metabolite formate and ethylene metabolite glycolate, glyoxylate, and oxalate respectively, accumulate following large ingestions. Above plasma levels of approximately 20 mg/dL (approximately 6 mmol/L of methanol or 3 mmol/L of ethylene glycol), these metabolites can cause specific end-organ damage.[12] History of use of automotive coolant or antifreeze, windshield wiper fluid, solvents points to toxicity by these alcohols.

Mild central nervous system (CNS) depression can be seen as a result of any alcohol intake but coma, seizures, hyperpnea (Kussmaul-Kien respirations) and hypotension all signify intake of toxic dosages of alcohol. An afferent pupillary defect is an ominous sign of advanced methanol poisoning. Retinal sheen due to retinal edema, and hyperemia of the optic disk are the eye changes observed with methanol toxicity.

Methanol or ethylene glycol toxicity is delayed when ethanol is coingested. Ethylene glycol metabolism can lead to cranial nerve palsies in addition to oliguria and hematuria.

Paraquat Poisoning

Paraquat is a nonselective herbicide that is cheap and easily available. Paraquat gets concentrated in cells and undergoes redox cycling leading to production of superoxide radical which causes direct cellular damage or can lead to formation of other reactive oxygen species and nitrite radicals.[13] Multiorgan failure can ensue in hours or days. The organs most affected are those with high blood flow and oxygen tension, particularly the lungs, heart, kidneys, and liver.

Acute kidney injury suggests significant paraquat poisoning and may occur due to paraquat-induced ATN or volume depletion. Impaired renal function is associated with increased mortality.[14] Best extracorporeal therapy is hemoperfusion but the same is required to be done within 4 hours. Paraquat poisoning is associated with very high mortality.

HEAVY METAL POISONING AND AKI

Kidney has a unique ability to reabsorb and accumulate divalent metals making it susceptible to heavy metals. The extent of renal damage is determined the nature, dose, route, and duration of exposure.

Lead Poisoning

Acute renal manifestation of lead nephropathy is proximal tubular dysfunction (Fanconi syndrome). The lead gets reabsorbed in the proximal tubular cells and affects the renal vasculature. Proximal tubular cells when affected show presence of intranuclear inclusions composed of a lead-protein complex. Grossly kidneys appear smaller with characteristic microscopic picture of acellular interstitial nephritis. Glomeruli are spared and vessels demonstrate medial thickening and narrowing of the lumen. Immunofluorescence is negative.

Chronic lead nephropathy has presentation similar to hypertensive nephropathy but peripheral neuropathy, basophilic stippling and perivascular cerebellar calcification are features differentiating it from the latter.

Cadmium

Cadmium is used in the manufacture of glass and alloys. Most common site affected is proximal tubule. Kidney involvement occurs in the form of proximal tubular dysfunction, nephrolithiasis, and chronic interstitial nephritis. The mechanism of injury is largely unknown. History of exposure with elevated urinary beta-microglobulin and cadmium levels (> 7 µg/g creatinine) are diagnostic. Discontinuation of exposure does not seem to limit the renal progression.

Arsenic

It is used in insecticides and weed killers. It usually damages nerves and skin but rarely can affect kidneys. Proximal renal tubular acidosis (RTA) and chronic interstitial fibrosis are lesions usually seen with arsenic exposure. High urinary arsenic levels are diagnostic.

Lithium

It is a therapeutic option in cases of bipolar disorder. Lithium decreases intracellular inositol, which helps in mood stabilization. It has a good bioavailability. Lithium is handled by kidneys similar to sodium. Lithium is associated with chronic renal injury which manifests as diabetes insipidus, and chronic interstitial nephritis. The therapeutic safe range for lithium is between 0.8 mEq/L and 1.2 mEq/L and severe toxicity is seen at levels more than or equal to 3.5 mEq/L. Lithium low molecular weight, negligible protein binding and small volume of distribution makes it easily dialyzable. Therefore, HD is the treatment of choice for severe lithium toxicity.

It is recommended to use longer duration of HD to minimize the rebound in serum lithium levels.[15]

ENVENOMATION AND BITES CAUSING AKI

Snake bites account for significant morbidity and mortality in Asia and Africa. The risk of snakebite is maximum during the rainy season and after floods due to displacement of snakes from their burrows. Most venomous snakes belong to one of the two families, Elapidae and Viperidae.

Elapidae

Elapid snakes are found widely throughout tropical and subtropical regions of Asia and Africa. Common names include cobras, kraits. Shorter fangs (compared to body size), a less triangular head with a more subtle transition from head to body and a larger scale pattern on the head distinguish them from Viperidae family. They can affect kidneys by causing rhabdomyolysis or ATN.

Viperidae

Viperid snakes have a similar geographical distribution to elapid snakes. Vipers (e.g. Russell, carpet, saw-scaled) and adders are some snakes of this family. Snakes belonging to the Viperidae family typically have folding, long fangs, triangular heads with an abrupt transition to the body, and smaller numerous scales on the head. They can also cause rhabdomyolysis, and/or acute kidney injury.

Management of snakebite requires supportive treatment plus definitive treatment in the form of polyvalent antivenom. AKI can occur as a result of toxins and lead to toxic ATN or secondary to rhabdomyolysis or disseminated intravascular coagulation.[16] Independent risk factors for AKI include age less than 12 years, a delay in administering antivenom by more than 2 hours, and a elevated creatinine kinase (> 2,000 U/L).[17]

To prevent rhabdomyolysis related renal injury, it is recommended that rapid infusion of isotonic saline is done to establish urine output of 200–300 mL/h along with antisnake venom. Antivenom may prevent the development of muscle toxicity but does not appear to reverse established rhabdomyolysis.

The urine output should be monitored closely, since oliguria in patients who have been adequately volume repleted usually indicates renal failure. Short-term dialysis may be required. Rarely the renal damage may be permanent as a result of bilateral renal cortical necrosis requiring long-term management for renal failure.

Hornet Bite

Wasps and bees stings can cause multiorgan involvement. AKI can occur due to coagulopathy.[18] Toxins such as phospholipase A2 and hyaluronidase present in the venom play a pathogenic role. Patients classically present with oliguria, microhematuria, and hypertension. Intravascular hemolysis, rhabdomyolysis or shock can cause AKI. Rarely acute cortical necrosis can be seen in these patients.[19,20]

APPROACH TO AKI WITH POISONING

Management requires an extensive evaluation. It starts with confirmation of poisoning to identification of the agent, severity, and prediction of toxicity. Therapy comprises of supportive care, preventing absorption, and enhancing elimination.

Renal involvement increases the mortality in these patients and requires meticulous care.

GENERAL MANAGEMENT OF AKI

Life-threatening fluid and electrolyte abnormalities should be identified and addressed immediately. Few emergent conditions requiring aggressive management include:

- Fluid overload;
- Hyperkalemia (serum potassium > 5.5 mEq/L) or a rapidly increasing serum potassium;
- Signs of uremia, such as pericarditis, or an otherwise unexplained decline in mental status; and
- Severe metabolic acidosis (pH < 7.1).

All these listed conditions eventually would require one or other form of dialysis but in view of high mortality and morbidity associated, medical therapy must ensue until a definitive therapy can be started.

Volume Assessment

Assessment of intravascular volume in all AKI patients is pivotal for it having bearing on overall mortality. Even modest amount of fluid overload results in increased mortality.[21]

- *Volume depletion*: Patients presenting with profuse vomiting and diarrhea, hypotension, tachycardia and/or oliguria should be given liberal fluids. This fluid challenge can prevent progression of AKI. This is especially true for certain etiologies such as rhabdomyolysis. In the absence of hemorrhagic shock, all patients with poisoning should be started on intravenous crystalloids preferably normal saline rather than colloids.[22]
- *Volume overload*: This is only true indication of giving diuretics in patients with AKI, else diuretics are not recommended in patients with AKI.

Hyperkalemia

It is a common and life-threatening complication of AKI. It is especially seen more in oliguric patients who are catabolic or have evidence of active cellular breakdown, such as rhabdomyolysis. Medical management must be done in all patients to keep serum potassium levels to less than 5.5 mEq/L. Dialysis is always considered in patients who have hyperkalemia resistant to medical therapy.

Metabolic Acidosis

The excretion of acid and regeneration of bicarbonate is impaired in the setting of a low glomerular filtration rate (GFR) resulting in metabolic acidosis. Acidosis is a myocardial depressant and hence associated with increased mortality. Sodium bicarbonate and dialysis are modes to correct acidosis. In patients with volume overload and/or oligoanuria, dialysis is offered upfront as treatment for acidosis.

Nutritional Support

All patients with poisoning admitted to ICU are catabolic and have high energy and protein requirement. Protein energy wasting is common among critically ill patients with AKI and contributes to mortality. Average calorie requirement for patient with any stage of AKI is usually 20–30 Kcal/kg/day. Protein requirement increases with worsening staging of AKI. Whereas nondialysis patients with only mild to moderate illness require only 0.8–1.2 g/kg/day, critically ill patients or patients who are on dialysis generally require 1.2–1.5 g/kg/day or more.[23]

Renal Replacement Therapy

Indications where extracorporeal therapies may be helpful are:

- Ingestion of a poison whose elimination can be enhanced.
- Failure of a patient to respond to maximal supportive care.

- The clinical course is predicted to be complicated based on the nature and/or concentration of the toxin, impaired clearance of the toxin or is complicated by comorbid illness, concomitant severe electrolyte or other laboratory derangements.

Hemodialysis

Hemodialysis is rarely needed in the care of poisoned patients, although HD is most common used extracorporeal modality for poison elimination.[24]

Hemodialysis is most useful in removing toxins with the following characteristics:
- Low molecular weight (< 500 Daltons);
- Small volume of distribution (< 1 L/kg);
- Low degree of protein-binding;
- High water solubility;
- Low endogenous clearance (< 4 mL/min/kg); and
- High dialysis clearance relative to total body clearance.

Indications and techniques of extracorporeal therapy in poisoning are discussed in detail in a separate chapter.

Urinary Alkalization

The urinary excretion is enhanced by altering the urinary pH. Altering the pH converts a lipid-soluble intact acid or base into the charged salt, making diffusion into the kidney impossible.

Drugs where urinary alkalinization can be helpful:
- They are predominantly eliminated unchanged by the kidney;
- They are distributed primarily in the extracellular fluid compartment;
- They are minimally protein-bound; and
- They are weak acids.

Drugs that can be eliminated using urinary alkalinization are in Table 3.[25]

Urine alkalinization is contraindicated in patients with established or incipient renal failure, pulmonary edema, and cerebral edema.

PROGNOSIS OF PATIENTS WHO HAD AKI

Patients who develop AKI are at increased risk to develop chronic kidney disease in future. There is emerging recognition that even minor short-term changes in serum creatinine are associated with increased mortality.[26]

Table 3: Elimination of drugs using urinary alkalinization.

Sulfonamides
Fluoride
2,4-Dichlorophenoxyacetic acid (herbicide)
Chlorpropamide
Salicylates
Methotrexate
Barbiturates • Phenobarbital • Barbital

CONCLUSION

Acute kidney injury (AKI) is a common occurrence in patients with poisoning. Meticulous evaluation and early management is the need of the hour in managing critical patients who present with poisoning and AKI. Extracorporeal therapies are effective in poisoning induced AKI.

KEY POINTS

- Kidney injury due to toxins results in a sizeable number of ICU admissions.
- Vasoconstriction, direct cellular toxicity or immunological injury is the most common pathogenic mechanism implicated in toxin-related AKI.
- Patients with impaired kidney function, diabetes mellitus, cardiovascular diseases, and advanced age are at increased risk.
- Most of the cases of toxin-related AKI can be managed with meticulous management of the volume status.

REFERENCES

1. Malhotra R, Kashani KB, Macedo E, et al. A risk prediction score for acute kidney injury in the intensive care unit. Nephrol Dial Transplant. 2017;32(5):814-22.
2. Evenepoel P. Acute toxic renal failure. Best Pract Res Clin Anaesthesiol. 2004;18(1):37-52.
3. Siva Kumar DK, Karthikeyan M. Study of clinical profile and outcome of acute kidney injury in acute poisoning and envenomation. Int J Adv Med. 2018;5(2):249-56.
4. Mousavi SR, Vahabzadeh M, Mahdizadeh A, et al. Rhabdomyolysis in 114 patients with acute poisonings. J Res Med Sci. 2015;20(3):239-43.
5. Hamdouk MI, Abdelraheem MB, Taha AA, et al. Paraphenylenediamine hair dye poisoning. In: De Broe ME, Porter GA, Bennett WM, Deray G (Eds). Clinical Nephrotoxins: Renal Injury from Drugs and Chemicals, 3rd edition. New York: Springer; 2008. pp. 671-9.

6. Chugh KS, Malik GH, Singhal PC. Acute renal failure following paraphenylene diamine [hair dye] poisoning: Report of two cases. J Med. 1982;13(1-2):131-7.

7. Lee FY, Chen WK, Lin CL, et al. Organophosphate Poisoning and Subsequent Acute Kidney Injury Risk. A Nationwide Population-Based Cohort Study. Medicine. 2015;94(47):e2107.

8. Naqvi R. Acute kidney injury from different poisonous substances. World J Nephrol. 2017;6(3):162-7.

9. Oldenquist G, Salem M. Parenteral copper sulfate poisoning causing acute renal failure. Nephrol Dial Transplant. 1999;14(2):441-3.

10. Mortazavi F, Javid AJ. Acute renal failure due to copper sulfate poisoning: a case report. Iran J Pediat. 2009;19(1):75-8.

11. Barnes BJ, Gerst C, Smith JR, et al. Osmol gap as a surrogate marker for serum propylene glycol concentrations in patients receiving lorazepam for sedation. Pharmacotherapy. 2006;26(1):23-33.

12. Kerns W 2nd, Tomaszewski C, McMartin K, et al. Formate kinetics in methanol poisoning. J Toxicol Clin Toxicol. 2002;40(2):137-43.

13. Suntres ZE. Role of antioxidants in paraquat toxicity. Toxicology. 2002;180(1):65-77.

14. Pawan M. Acute kidney injury following paraquat poisoning in India. Iran J Kidney Dis. 2013;7(1):64-6.

15. Amdisen A. Clinical features and management of lithium poisoning. Med Toxicol Adverse Drug Exp. 1988;3(1): 18-32.

16. Chugh KS. Snake-bite-induced acute renal failure in India. Kidney Int. 1989;35(3):891-907.

17. Pinho FM, Zanetta DM, Burdmann EA. Acute renal failure after Crotalus durissus snakebite: a prospective survey on 100 patients. Kidney Int. 2005;67(2):659-67.

18. Barr SE. Allergy to Hymenoptera stings: a review of the world literature: 1953-1970. Ann Allergy. 1971;29(2):49-66.

19. Dhanapriya J, Dinesh kumar T, Sakthirajan R, et al. Wasp sting-induced acute kidney injury. Clin Kidney J. 2016;9(2):201-4.

20. Kim YO, Yoom SA, Kim KJ, et al. Severe rhabdomyolysis and acute renal failure due to multiple wasp stings. Nephrol Dial Transplant. 2003;18(6):1235.

21. Bellomo R, Cass A, et al. Renal Replacement Therapy Study Investigators, An observational study fluid balance and patient outcomes in the Randomized Evaluation of Normal vs. Augmented Level of Replacement Therapy trial. Crit Care Med. 2012;40(6):1753-60.

22. Finfer S, Bellomo R, Boyce N, et al. A comparison of albumin and saline for fluid resuscitation in the intensive care unit. N Engl J Med. 2004;350(22):2247-56.

23. Fouque D, Kalantar-Zadeh K, Kopple J, et al. A proposed nomenclature and diagnostic criteria for protein-energy wasting in acute and chronic kidney disease. Kidney Int. 2008;73(4):391-8.

24. Patel N, Bayliss GP. Developments in extracorporeal therapy for the poisoned patient. Adv Drug Deliv Rev. 2015;90:3-11.

25. Proudfoot AT, Krenzelok EP, Vale JA. Position paper on urine alkalinization. J Toxicol Clin Toxicol. 2004;42(1):1-26.

26. Garella S. Extracorporeal techniques in the treatment of exogenous intoxications. Kidney Int. 1988;33(3):735-54.

30
CHAPTER

Extracorporeal Therapies: General Principles

Deven Juneja, Omender Singh

INTRODUCTION

Extracorporeal removal of toxins is not a new concept. Surprisingly, extracorporeal therapies have been used in removal of exogenous substances much before they were recognized as standard therapies for the management of patients with chronic renal disease. The first published case of successful use of hemodialysis (HD) was more than 100 years ago.[1] Although this report involved an overdose of salicylate in a dog, extracorporeal toxin removal (ECTR) is being increasingly used in humans now.

The mainstay of management of patients with poisoning is general supportive care and use of antidotes, if available. Nonetheless, all attempts to reduce absorption and enhance elimination of the poison must be undertaken, to improve patient outcomes. Measures to enhance elimination may be broadly classified as corporeal and extracorporeal methods. Corporeal measures basically occur in the body and on the other hand, extracorporeal measures occur outside the body, mostly using an extracorporeal circuit. Examples of corporeal measures include multiple-dose activated charcoal (MDAC), forced diuresis and urinary alkalinization. These measures are easy to employ and are routinely used in the management of poisoned patients.

Extracorporeal toxin removal is still largely underutilized as evidenced by the fact that during a 20-year period till 2005, only 19,351 cases of use of ECTR were reported in United States.[2] Another more recent report stated that out of more than 600,000 cases of poisoning reported in various American hospitals, ECTR was employed in mere 0.1% of intoxications.[3] Its utility is not only limited by lack of availability, but also because of lack of understanding of these techniques. Hence, a better understanding of the type of poisons which can be dialyzed and the types of ECTR available, is essential to improve the utility of this mode of therapy in the management of poisoned patients.

FACTORS AFFECTING DIALYZABILITY

Understandably, not all poisons can be dialyzed. Hence, before considering ECTR for any patient with poisoning, it is imperative to assess the dialyzability of the toxin involved. Several factors have been shown to affect the dialyzability of toxins, these include—molecular weight (MW), protein binding, lipid solubility, endogenous clearance and volume of distribution (Vd).[4]

Molecular Weight

Molecular weight of the involved toxin plays an important role in determining if ECTR can be employed and if useful, which mode of ECTR may be more effective. HD removes the toxins mainly by diffusion across the semipermeable membrane. Higher MW of the toxin prevents its free passage across this membrane and adversely affects its dialyzability. Lower MW toxins (<500 D), easily diffuse through the pores and even low-flux dialysis filters may be effective in their removal. Most of the toxins have low MW and hence, HD may be employed in most of the cases. The large MW solutes (>1,000 D), are unable to pass freely through these pores, and hence, are not dialyzable using conventional filters in HD. For such toxins, high efficiency or high flux filters or convective clearance may be more effective.[4]

Protein Binding

Poisons binding to proteins are classically considered to be nondialyzable, as protein-poison complex is generally bigger than the pore size of the dialysis membranes and hence, diffusion of solute across the membranes is not possible. Even convective removal is ineffective as the poison is bound to nonultrafilterable plasma proteins. So, highly protein bound drugs are not considered for ECTR. However, in case of overdose, protein binding sites may become saturated which may increase the serum concentration of the free poison which can be dialyzed.[4] Drugs like valproate and salicylate, which are otherwise protein-bound, are therefore dialyzable in patients with overdose. Other drugs like phenytoin, which is also protein bound, has small binding constant and hence, it easily dissociates from its binding site making it available for ECTR.[5] Other factors can also influence the amount of protein binding and proportion of free drug. Hypoalbuminemia leads to reduced availability of proteins for drug binding and uremic acidosis also reduces the sites for binding of acidic toxins like phenytoin, salicylates and warfarin.[6]

Examples of highly protein-bound drugs are arsenic, calcium channel blockers (CCBs), diazepam, phenytoin and nonsteroidal anti-inflammatory drugs (NSAIDs) including salicylates, thyroxine and tricyclic antidepressants (TCAs). Examples of toxins with low protein binding include alcohols, aminoglycosides, and lithium. Alterations in protein binding may become clinically relevant in cases of drugs like lithium and digoxin, which have a narrow therapeutic index.[7]

Hemoperfusion (HP) can be effective in such cases as the charcoal or resin adsorbent can easily bind with these protein-binding toxins. In addition, plasmapheresis is also a good option for ECTR as it is effective in removal of highly protein bound drugs.

Lipid Solubility

Highly lipophilic drugs are also not ideal for ECTR removal as they tend to spread widely in the different body compartments. Hence, conventional HD might not be able to achieve adequate clearance for these drugs and HP may be a better option. As these agents are widely distributed in the body, they also have a tendency to get released in the intravascular space, leading to "rebound" increase in the serum concentrations.[8]

Endogenous Clearance

It is suggested that the extracorporeal clearance of the poison must be at least 30% of the total clearance for it to have any significant contribution in toxin removal.[9] Hence, drugs like cocaine, which otherwise has a small size and is not significantly protein bound, is not considered to be dialyzable as it has got a high endogenous clearance.

Volume of Distribution

As extracorporeal therapies only remove the poisons present in the intravascular compartment, drugs with high Vd are not considered to be dialyzable.[4] However, if the ECTR is initiated before the poison gets fully distributed into the deep compartments, it still might be able to achieve significant drug clearance (e.g. thallium).

Examples of drugs with high Vd include β-blockers, barbiturates, CCBs, chloroquine, colchicines, digoxin, phenothiazines, quinidine, strychnine and TCAs. Examples of drugs with small Vd include alcohols, aminoglycosides, lithium, paracetamol, salicylates and theophylline.

TYPES OF EXTRACORPOREAL TOXIN REMOVAL

Several extracorporeal therapies have been tried, with varied success rates, for removal of toxins. These include, intermittent HD (IHD), HP, sustained low-efficiency dialysis (SLED), intermittent hemofiltration (IHF) or hemodiafiltration, continuous renal replacement therapy (CRRT), therapeutic plasma exchange (TPE), exchange transfusion, peritoneal dialysis (PD), albumin dialysis, cerebrospinal fluid (CSF) exchange (CFE) and extracorporeal life support like extracorporeal membrane oxygenation (ECMO).[10]

Intermittent Hemodialysis

This mode of dialysis is based on the diffusion process in which the solutes move from greater to lesser concentration, across a semipermeable membrane. It was classically used in clearance of small molecules (<500 D), but with the availability of modern filters, it may be useful in removal of larger molecules also. It may also aid in rapid correction of acid–base and electrolyte abnormalities and the combined process of ultrafiltration may help in fluid removal also.

Currently, IHD is the most commonly prescribed mode of extracorporeal therapy not only for the management of patients with end-stage renal disease (ESRD), and acute kidney injury (AKI) but also for poisoning.[2] It has also been shown to be at least 30% cheaper than any other form of ECTR.[11] These properties of wide availability, ease of operation, lower rates of complications, and relatively low cost make it the most widely used mode of ECTR (Table 1).[2,11,12] Other advantages of IHD include rapid poison clearance and its ability to concomitantly treat electrolyte and acid-base abnormalities.[2]

The removal of poison depends on the dialyzer surface area, the porosity of the membrane, and the flow rates of the blood and the dialysate.[13] The drugs, which are most amenable for removal with HD are those with a low MW, small Vd, low protein binding and low lipid solubility. Examples of such drugs include ethylene glycol, methanol, salicylates and theophylline.

Table 1: Advantages and disadvantages of hemodialysis.	
Advantages	*Disadvantages*
• Widely/easily available • Easy to operate • Lower complication rates • Lower operational costs • Rapid poison clearance • Concomitantly treat metabolic disorders	• Less effective for highly protein bound poisons • Less effective for poisons with large molecular weights • Less effective for highly lipophilic poisons • May cause hemodynamic instability

Hemoperfusion

The basic principle behind this form of ECTR is use of adsorbent columns, made of activated charcoal or an ion exchange resin, to adsorb the toxins. Use of activated charcoal over charcoal, reduces hypersensitivity reactions and increases pore size and surface area for adsorption. Ion exchange resins adsorbent columns contain XAD 4 amberlite (Jafron Biomedical HA 230) which may provide better clearance as compared to the earlier columns containing XAD 2.[14] These HP cartridges may require priming with 2–3 L of normal saline or dextrose, before initiating HP and can be performed using the standard HD machines. However, it can also be done using the standard CRRT machines.[15,16]

Drug clearance in HP is dependent on several factors like type of adsorptive column (charcoal vs. resin), surface area of the filter, column's mass and its pore size, and configuration.[14] Resins columns may offer better clearance than charcoal columns for several toxins like amanita A and B, bromine, barbiturates, carbamazepine, camphor, diazepam, digoxin, metamizole, methaqualone, oxyphenbutazone, paraoxon, parathion, phenylbutazone, pine oil, procainamide, propyphenazone, selenium, TCAs, valproic acid and vasopressors.[14,17]

Charcoal HP may be better for some other drugs like acetaminophen, salicylates, chloroquine, diquat and methotrexate. However, certain other drugs like adriamycin, aminophenazone, disopyramide, mercury, paraquat and theophylline are not affected by the type of column used and have similar clearance with charcoal and resin adsorbents.[14]

Molecular-weight dose not effect toxin removal by HP and there is no absolute cut-off for MW for performing HP, unlike HD. Only clearance of poisons with very high MW, exceeding 5,000 Da, may get affected when using HP.[18] The poison elimination with HP is also not affected by the serum concentration of the poison, as the clearance is not dependent on the concentration gradient. Clearance of lipophilic toxins is favored, by HP. Resins columns exhibit even better adsorption and clearance for lipophilic drugs, as compared to charcoal columns.[14] Although being used less commonly now, HP has got some distinct advantages over HD (Table 2).[14]

The efficacy of HP is limited by the tendency of HP columns to get saturated with plasma proteins and cellular debris.[19] This may occur between 2 and 6 hours of initiating HP. Hence, it is recommended to change the

Extracorporeal Therapies: General Principles

Table 2: Advantages and disadvantages of hemoperfusion.

Advantages	Disadvantages
• More effective for highly protein bound poisons • More effective for poisons with large molecular weights • More effective for poisons with high lipid solubility • Concentration independent poison clearance • Rapid poison clearance	• Limited availability • May cause hemodynamic instability • Higher complication rates • Higher operational costs • Not effective in managing concomitant metabolic abnormalities • Saturation of columns

HP column after every 3–4 hours. However, for most of the poisons, a single session of 3–4 hours is sufficient.

The clearance efficiency of HP may be enhanced by putting multiple columns in series. Even simultaneous use of HP and HD in series has also been shown to be superior to any of these two techniques used alone.[20,21] It is generally accepted that the blood should pass through the HD filter before the HP column, as this will delay the saturation of the HP column and increase its life and efficiency.

Complications associated with HP are generally secondary to nonspecific adsorption of various biological components to the HP column. These include leukopenia, thrombocytopenia, hypocalcemia, hypophosphatemia and hypofibrinogenemia. Leukopenia and thrombocytopenia are common and HP may cause up to 50% reduction in the number of white blood cells and platelets.[22-24] Electrolyte abnormalities and hypoglycemia are generally unpredictable, hence a close watch on all these parameters have to be kept.[24] Complication rates have generally reduced after use of modern advanced columns.[25]

Intermittent Hemofiltration and Hemodiafiltration

Intermittent hemofiltration is a mode of extracorporeal therapy, which relies solely on convection only. On the other hand, intermittent hemodiafiltration (IHDF) combines the use of both convection and diffusion. In convection, the solvent and solutes move across a semipermeable membrane according to the pressure gradient, also called solvent drag.

The efficacy of toxin removal is affected by the degree of binding to proteins, pore size of the dialyzer membranes, and the ability of the solute to pass through the membrane by convection (ultrafiltration and sieving coefficients). The clearance of these convection-based techniques is similar to IHD in regard to protein-binding and Vd. However, these techniques may allow clearance of molecules of higher MW, as high as 40,000 Daltons, as compared to IHD.[26,27] This property may make these techniques more favorable in ECTR, but their clinical utility is diminshed by limited availability, higher technical requirements and lack of experience.[28] The poisons for which HF may be useful include hirudin, lithium, methanol, methotrexate, procainamide, thallium and vancomycin.[29]

Continuous Renal Replacement Therapy

Continuous renal replacement therapies may be further classified as continuous venovenous hemofiltration (CVVH), continuous venovenous HD (CVVHD) and continuous venovenous hemodiafiltration (CVVHDF). These newer modalities are generally performed in intensive care units (ICUs) in hemodynamically unstable patients who cannot tolerate high-efficiency intermittent treatments. The basic principles of dialysis and convection also apply to these CRRT techniques but these techniques remove fluid and solutes gradually over a prolonged time as the flow rates of blood and effluent are significantly lower. As a result, the clearance of poisons also occurs over a prolonged time.[30]

Continuous renal replacement therapy is generally not favored because of inferior drug clearance as compared to HD or HP, higher costs and need for expertise and special equipment. However, CRRT may have an advantage in patients who are hemodynamically unstable and in management of poisons which have a tendency to show "rebound phenomenon" like poisons with large Vd, and high tissue binding. These drugs include lithium, methotrexate and procainamide.[31] It may also be useful in patients with or at risk of developing cerebral edema. CRRT has also been tried in management of patients with paraquat, thallium and methanol toxicity.[29]

Sustained Low-efficiency Dialysis

Sustained low-efficiency dialysis, sustained low-efficiency daily dialysis (SLEDD), and prolonged intermittent renal replacement therapy (PIRRT) are all

Renal Toxins and Extracorporeal Therapies

hybrid techniques developed with an aim to combine advantages of both IHD and CRRT techniques. The duration of therapy, and dialysate (QD) and blood (QB) flow rates are also in between to that of IHD and CRRT. This technique may offer hemodynamic stability comparable to that of CRRT and clearance comparable to that of IHD. Generally, the duration of treatment is around 6–12 hours, blood flow rates of 200–300 mL/min and dialysate flow rates of 300 mL/min. Another advantage of SLED is that it can be performed using most of the modern dialysis machines used for IHD.

Small solute clearance of SLED and CRRT is also comparable.[32,33] However, CRRT may offer better middle and large molecule clearance owing to its prolonged duration and use of additional convective clearance.[33,34] Use of modern high-flux filters and using both diffusive and convective techniques by performing sustained low-efficiency diafiltration (SLED-f), the clearance of middle and large molecules may be considerably improved.[35] However, utility of SLED in managing poisoning patients is limited by lack of data and facilities to perform SLED-f are not widely available.[28,36,37] Nonetheless, SLED may be used as an alternative to IHD, especially in hemodynamically unstable patients not tolerating IHD.

Therapeutic Plasma Exchange or Plasmapheresis

The process of extracorporeal separation of plasma from the cellular components of blood is termed as TPE. In plasma exchange, plasma is replaced by fresh frozen plasma (FFP), but when other products like albumin are used for replacing plasma, it is termed plasmapheresis.

The process of plasma exchange can be performed either by centrifugation or filtration. In centrifugation, the plasma is separated from the other blood components by gravity and density, inside a centrifuge. In the filtration process, blood is made to pass through one (single) or two filters (cascade filtration) with large pores. The efficacy of both these procedures is comparable as per the amount of plasma protein cleared per unit of plasma exchanged. The blood flow rates may differ slightly in these two procedures with rates of 100–150 mL/min in centrifugation,[38] compared to 100–200 mL/min in plasmafiltration.[39] Typically, around 30 mL/min of plasma is removed in a single exchange, but with modern techniques, this may go up to 50–60 mL/min.[40,41]

Generally, one session lasts for around 2–4 hours.[42] Even though TPE can be performed using peripheral venous access, use of central catheters increases its efficacy by improving blood flows rates and clearance.[38] The number of plasma volume exchanged determines the clearance capacity of TPE.[43] However, for removal of poisons, it is generally believed that there is no additional benefit after two plasma volumes exchange. Hence, as per the American Society for Apheresis (ASFA) guidelines, it is recommended to perform one–to–two total plasma volumes exchanges per day till the resolution of clinical symptoms and the release of poison from tissues becomes insignificant.[44]

Therapeutic plasma exchange is particularly suited to remove large[45] and highly protein bound poisons[46] as it can essentially remove all substances from the plasma, even proteins. Plasmapheresis has been mostly used in the management of mushroom (Amanita phalloides) poisoning. Amanita phalloides is associated with high mortality (25–50%) and hence all attempts to reduce absorption and early elimination must be made.[47] Gastrointestinal lavage, followed by decontamination using activated charcoal and early use of ECTR, may be beneficial. As it is highly protein bound, HP and plasmapheresis may be attempted and maximum benefits may be expected, if ECTR is initiated within 36 hours of ingestion. Early removal of amatoxins using plasmapheresis has been shown to reduce mortality to as low as 4.8%.[48]

Plasmapheresis is also effective in removing L-thyroxine, which is highly protein bound, verapamil, diltiazem, carbamazepine, organophosphorus compounds and theophylline.[46,49] Plasmapheresis has been used as adjunctive therapy in addition to antidigoxin antibodies in digitalis intoxication in patients with renal failure to prevent the rebound caused by dissociation of the digoxin-antidigoxin complexes.[50] Plasmapheresis has also been shown to be effective in reducing mortality in patients with ethylene dibromide poisoning, especially, if employed within 24 hours of its ingestion.[51]

Another indication for plasmapheresis may include management of toxicities, which have been complicated by massive hemolysis (like sodium chlorate toxicity) or methemoglobinuria.

However, it has significantly lower clearance capacity as compared to IHD, IHF or HP.[43] As TPE also eliminates red blood cells (RBCs) and free hemoglobin patients may develop anemia.[52] Other associated complications are immunosuppression, bleeding, and hypersensitivity reactions secondary to replaced plasma proteins or albumin. In addition, as most of the commonly implicated poisons have small or medium molecular size, the utility of TPE is further limited. Presently, TPE is indicated only when other modes of ECTR are not available or feasible.

Peritoneal Dialysis

In this dialysis mode, the dialysate is infused in the peritoneal cavity of the patient through a peritoneal catheter. In this technique, the peritoneal membrane functions as the dialyzer and the solute moves from the blood to the dialysate based on the concentration gradient, by diffusion. The clearance capacity in PD depends on the molecular mass of the solute, dialysate flow rate, surface area of the peritoneum, and the hemodynamic status of the patient, with hypotensive patients having poorer clearance rates.[2,53]

Poison removal by PD may be improved by adding dextrose to the dialysis fluid which may increase the convective gradient and may enhance removal of larger MW compounds by ultrafiltration. In addition, by alkalinizing or acidifying the PD fluid, elimination of certain poisons may be improved by the phenomenon of ion trapping. Addition of albumin to the PD fluid has also shown to increase the removal of protein bound poisons like barbiturates.[54]

Due to its limited clearance capacity, PD is rarely used in the management of poisoned patients.[2,7,55] Presently, PD is only indicated for toxin removal in patients who are already on PD for management of ESRD, are having only mild symptoms and no other mode of ECTR is available. Other indications of PD may be in pediatric poisoning, where HD may be difficult to perform or in hemodynamically unstable patients when CRRT is not available.

Extracorporeal Liver Assist Devices

Extracorporeal liver assist device (ELAD) or albumin dialysis is a technique to replace the function of the liver in patients with severe cirrhosis or fulminant liver failure, mostly employed as a bridge to liver transplantation. There are different types of albumin dialysis, which are commercially available—molecular adsorbent recirculating system (MARS),[56] single pass albumin dialysis (SPAD)[57] and the Prometheus system.[56]

The principle behind albumin dialysis is that when albumin is added to the dialysate it leads to formation of protein-binding disequilibrium, which causes the unbound drug in the blood to cross and bind to the albumin on the dialysate side. Hence, ELAD may be advantageous in removal of protein-bound toxins.[58] However, the clearance capacity of these modes is significantly lesser than IHD and hence ELAD does not seem to offer any clinical advantage. Moreover, high cost, limited availability and unpredictable efficacy further limits its utility.[57,59]

Exchange Transfusion

Exchange transfusion is a technique in which therapeutic apheresis is performed and the patient's RBCs are separated from other components of the blood. These RBCs are replaced with colloids or normal donor RBCs or sometimes even both. A single exchange generally removes around two-thirds of the circulating RBCs. Exchange transfusion is generally indicated to remove pathogenic factors associated with RBCs and hence is useful in the management of diseases like severe malaria, sickle cell disease or babesiosis. In toxicology, it has been used in the management of severe hemolysis associated with arsine gas inhalation[60] and removal of certain drugs, which are highly bound to RBCs (cyclosporine and tacrolimus).[10] Exchange transfusion has also been used to treat methemoglobinemia associated with toxic exposure to drugs like dapsone, sodium nitrite, propranolol and aniline.[10] As it is simple to use in infants, it may be used for managing toxic overdoses of drugs like theophylline, barbiturates and salicylates in infants.

Cerebrospinal Fluid Exchange

Cerebrospinal fluid exchange has been rarely performed in the management of life-threatening neurological complications of certain toxins like methotrexate, particularly after an inadvertent intrathecal administration.[61,62] In this procedure, CSF is drained through a ventricular catheter and a sterile solution consisting of albumin and sodium chloride is inserted into the lumbar subarachnoid space as a replacement.

ISSUES WITH EXTRACORPOREAL TOXIN REMOVAL

Apart from understanding the toxicokinetics of the poison and the intricacies of the various modes of ECTR,

Renal Toxins and Extracorporeal Therapies

it is also important to understand several other issues which may affect the decision to initiate or continue ECTR.

Lack of Trials

Conducting clinical trials for poisoning patients is considered very difficult due to numerous reasons like difficult to obtain consent, heterogeneous nature of the poisons and patients, and relatively low mortality associated with poisonings.[4,63] As a result, most of the data available is from the case reports or case series.[63]

Obsolete Technology

Technology associated with extracorporeal therapies had made significant advancements. Use of high-flux and high-efficiency dialysis filters has become the norm. These membranes have much superior molecular cutoff values (10,000 Da vs. 500 Da), have larger surface areas (2.5 m^2 vs. 0.5 m^2), and have much improved ultrafiltration coefficients (50–90 vs. 5 mL/h/mm Hg), in comparison to the previously used cuprophane membranes. Use of newer catheters and better dialysis machines tolerating higher blood flows have allowed better poison clearance. However, much of the current evidence is based on studies or case reports published decades ago using older filters and obsolete technology. Basing current recommendations on these reports is not feasible.

Rebound Phenomenon

Certain toxins, especially those which have a large Vd, tend to move out of the intravascular compartment, only to return back after some time. Hence, the drug levels may rise again after some time of completion of ECTR therapy, leading to worsening of clinical symptoms, and poor outcomes. CRRT may be an option in such patients as it is performed over a prolonged period, and any toxin which diffuses back in the intravascular space overtime, will get removed.

Early End-organ Damage

Certain poisons like paraquat have all the physical characteristics, which may characterize them to be highly dialyzable. However, unless the ECTR is initiated very early after its ingestion, it cannot have any meaningful impact on outcome, because paraquat can rapidly cause severe pulmonary damage.[64,65] Hence, in the management of toxicology patients, what really matters is the removal of poison from the target organ, rather than from the plasma for example cardiac muscles for digoxin, central nervous system (CNS) for lithium and lung parenchyma for paraquat poisoning.

Withdrawal Symptoms

Overdose of certain therapeutic drugs (valproic acid, phenytoin and theophylline) will lead to high serum drug levels and toxic symptoms. However, when ECTR is applied, the drugs levels suddenly reduce, sometimes to subtherapeutic levels, leading to withdrawal symptoms.

CONCLUSION

Early resuscitation and organ support remain the mainstay of management of poisoning patients. ECTR may play a crucial role in managing certain patient subgroups with severe intoxications and may prove life-saving. However, before initiating ECTR, a thorough assessment of patient's clinical status, poison's characteristics, complexities of available modes of ECTR and risk evaluation should be done. The algorithm in Flowchart 1[65] may aid in choosing the right mode of ECTR. Hence, it is imperative to use ECTR in the correct clinical setting to optimize outcomes and minimize complications.

KEY POINTS

- Extracorporeal toxin removal is a valuable therapeutic modality for management of patients with severe poisonings
- Ideally, a toxin with low MW, protein binding, fat solubility and Vd is amenable for ECTR
- Guidelines may not be available to guide therapy in all cases
- The characteristics of the suspected poison and understanding of the intricacies of the available modes of ECTR will help in choosing the right patient and the right mode of ECTR.

Flowchart 1: Algorithm to choose the right mode of extracorporeal toxin removal.

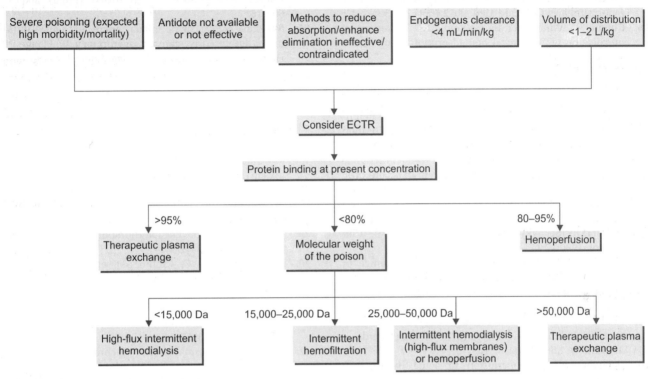

(ECTR: extracorporeal toxin removal)

REFERENCES

1. Abel JJ, Rowntree LG, Turner BB. On the removal of diffusible substances from the circulating blood by dialysis. Tans Assoc Am Physicians. 1913;58:51-4.
2. Holubek WJ, Hoffman RS, Goldfarb DS, et al. Use of hemodialysis and hemoperfusion in poisoned patients. Kidney Int. 2008;74:1327-34.
3. Mowry JB, Spyker DA, Cantilena LR Jr, et al. 2012 Annual Report of the American Association of Poison Control Centers' National Poison Data System (NPDS): 30th Annual Report. Clin Toxicol (Phila). 2013;51:949-1229.
4. Ghannoum M, Nolin TD, Lavergne V, et al; EXTRIP workgroup. Blood purification in toxicology: nephrology's ugly duckling. Adv Chronic Kidney Dis. 2011;18(3):160-6.
5. Ghannoum M, Troyanov S, Ayoub P, et al. Successful hemodialysis in a phenytoin overdose: case report and review of the literature. Clin Nephrol. 2010;74:59-64.
6. Lam YW, Banerji S, Hatfield C, et al. Principles of drug administration in renal insufficiency. Clin Pharmacokinet. 1997;32:30-57.
7. Pond SM. Extracorporeal techniques in the treatment of poisoned patients. Med J Aust. 1991;154:617-22.
8. Orlowski JM, Hou S, Leikin JB. Extracorporeal removal of drugs and toxins. In: Ford M, Delaney KA, Ling L, Erickson T. (Eds). Clinical toxicology, 1st edition. St Louis, MO: WB Saunders Company; 2001. pp. 43-50.
9. Maher JF, Schreiner GE. The dialysis of poisons and drugs. Trans Am Soc Artif Intern Organs. 1968;14:440-53.
10. Ouellet G, Bouchard J, Ghannoum M, et al. Available extracorporeal treatments for poisoning: overview and limitations. Semin Dial. 2014;27(4):342-9.
11. Bouchard J, Lavergne V, Roberts DM, et al. Availability and cost of extracorporeal treatments for poisonings and other emergency indications: a worldwide survey. Nephrol Dial Transplant. 2017;32(4):699-706.
12. Tyagi PK, Winchester JF, Feinfeld DA. Extracorporeal removal of toxins. Kidney Int. 2008;74:1231-3.
13. Winchester JF. Dialysis and hemoperfusion in poisoning. Adv Ren Replace Ther. 2002;9:26-30.
14. Ghannoum M, Bouchard J, Nolin TD, et al. Hemoperfusion for the treatment of poisoning: technology, determinants of poison clearance, and application in clinical practice. Semin Dial. 2014;27(4):350-61.
15. Nasa P, Singh A, Juneja D, et al. Continuous venovenous hemodiafiltration along with charcoal hemoperfusion for the management of life-threatening lercanidipine and amlodipine overdose. Saudi J Kidney Dis Transpl. 2014;25(6):1255-8.
16. Garg SK, Goyal PK, Kumar R, et al. Management of life-threatening calcium channel blocker overdose with continuous veno-venous hemodiafiltration with charcoal hemoperfusion. Indian J Crit Care Med. 2014;18(6): 399-401.

17. Juneja D, Singh O, Bhasin A, et al. Severe suicidal digoxin toxicity managed with resin hemoperfusion: A case report. Indian J Crit Care Med. 2012;16(4):231-3.

18. Cohan SL, Winchester JF, Gelfand MC. Treatment of intoxication with charcoal hemadsorption. Drug Metab Rev. 1982;13:681-93.

19. Hampel G, Widdop B, Goulding R. Adsorptive capacities of hemoperfusion devices in clinical use. Artif Organs. 1978;2:363-6.

20. Dehua G, Daxi J, Honglang X, et al. Sequential hemoperfusion and continuous venovenous hemofiltration in treatment of severe tetramine poisoning. Blood Purif. 2006;24:524-30.

21. Bentley C, Kjellstrand CM. The treatment of severe drug intoxication with charcoal hemoperfusion in series with hemodialysis. J Dial. 1979;3:337-48.

22. Mamdani B, Dunea G, Siemsen AW. Long-term hemoperfusion with coated activated charcoal. Clin Toxicol. 1980;17:543-6.

23. Mydlik M, Bucek J, Derzsiova K, et al. Influence of charcoal haemoperfusion on platelet count in acute poisoning and during regular dialysis treatment. Int Urol Nephrol. 1981;13:387-9.

24. Koffler A, Bernstein M, LaSette A, et al. Fixed-bed charcoal hemoperfusion. Treatment of drug overdose. Arch Intern Med. 1978;138:1691-4.

25. Haapanen EJ. Hemoperfusion in acute intoxication. Clinical experience with 48 cases. Acta Med Scand Suppl. 1982;668:76-81.

26. Ward RA, Schmidt B, Hullin J, et al. A comparison of on-line hemodiafiltration and high-flux hemodialysis: a prospective clinical study. J Am Soc Nephrol. 2000;11:2344-50.

27. Ahrenholz PG, Winkler RE, Michelsen A, et al. Dialysis membrane-dependent removal of middle molecules during hemodiafiltration: the beta2-microglobulin/albumin relationship. Clin Nephrol. 2004;62:21-8.

28. Bailey AR, Sathianathan VJ, Chiew AL, et al. Comparison of intermittent haemodialysis, prolonged intermittent renal replacement therapy and continuous renal replacement haemofiltration for lithium toxicity: a case report. Crit Care Resusc. 2011;13:120-2.

29. Mendonca S, Gupta S, Gupta A. Extracorporeal management of poisonings. Saudi J Kidney Dis Transpl. 2012;23(1):1-7.

30. Kim Z, Goldfarb DS. Continuous renal replacement therapy does not have a clear role in the treatment of poisoning. Nephron Clin Pract. 2010;115:c1-6.

31. Leblanc M, Raymond M, Bonnardeaux A, et al. Lithium poisoning treated by high-performance continuous arteriovenous and venovenous hemodiafiltration. Am J Kidney Dis. 1996;27:365-72.

32. Berbece AN, Richardson RM. Sustained low-efficiency dialysis in the ICU: cost, anticoagulation, and solute removal. Kidney Int. 2006;70:963-8.

33. Liao Z, Zhang W, Hardy PA, et al. Kinetic comparison of different acute dialysis therapies. Artif Organs. 2003;27:802-7.

34. Thanacoody RH. Extracorporeal elimination in acute valproic acid poisoning. Clin Toxicol (Phila). 2009;47:609-16.

35. Marshall MR. Dialytic management of acute kidney injury and intensive care unit nephrology. In: Floege JJR, Feehally J (Eds). Comprehensive Clinical Nephrology, 4th edition. St. Louis: Elsevier Saunders Company; 2010. pp. 843-52.

36. Fiaccadori E, Maggiore U, Parenti E, et al. Sustained low-efficiency dialysis (SLED) for acute lithium intoxication. Nephrol Dial Transplant. 2008;24:329-32.

37. Lund B, Seifert SA, Mayersohn M. Efficacy of sustained low-efficiency dialysis in the treatment of salicylate toxicity. Nephrol Dial Transplant. 2005;20:1483-84.

38. Okafor C, Kalantarinia K. Vascular access considerations for therapeutic apheresis procedures. Semin Dial. 2012;25:140-4.

39. Tan HK, Hart G. Plasma filtration. Ann Acad Med Singapore. 2005;34:615-24.

40. Ibrahim RB, Liu C, Cronin SM, et al. Drug removal by plasmapheresis: an evidence-based review. Pharmacotherapy. 2007;27:1529-49.

41. Kaplan AA, Bailey RA, Kew CE, et al. High flux plasma exchange using a modified rotating membrane system. ASAIO J. 1996;42:957-60.

42. Madore F. Plasmapheresis technical aspects and indications. Crit Care Clin. 2002;18(2):375-92.

43. Jones JS, Dougherty J. Current status of plasmapheresis in toxicology. Ann Emerg Med. 1986;15:474-82.

44. Szczepiorkowski ZM, Winters JL, Bandarenko N, et al. Apheresis Applications Committee of the American Society for A. Guidelines on the use of therapeutic apheresis in clinical practice–evidence-based approach from the Apheresis Applications Committee of the American Society for Apheresis. J Clin Apher. 2010;25:83-177.

45. Solomon A, Fahey JL. Plasmapheresis therapy in macroglobulinemia. Ann Intern Med. 1963;58:789-800.

46. Jha S, Waghdhare S, Reddi R, et al. Thyroid storm due to inappropriate administration of a compounded thyroid hormone preparation successfully treated with plasmapheresis. Thyroid. 2012;22:1283-6.

47. Nenov D, Nenov K. Therapeutic apheresis in exogenous poisoning and in myeloma. Nephrol Dial Transplant. 2001;16 (Suppl 6):101-2.

48. Jander S, Bischoff J. Treatment of Amanita phalloides poisoning: I. Retrospective evaluation of plasmapheresis in 21 patients. Ther Apher. 2000;4:303-7.

49. Nenov VD, Marinov P, Sabeva J, et al. Current applications of plasmapheresis in clinical toxicology. Nephrol Dial Transplant. 2003;18 (Suppl 5):v56-8.

50. Rabetoy GM, Price CA, Findlay JW, et al. Treatment of digoxin intoxication in a renal failure patient with digoxin specific antibody fragments and plasmapheresis. Am J Nephrol. 1990;10:518-21.

51. Pahwa N, Bharani R, Jain M, et al. Therapeutic plasma exchange: an effective treatment in ethylene dibromide poisoning cases. J Clin Apher. 2013;28(5):374-7.

52. Meert KL, Ellis J, Aronow R, et al. Acute ammonium dichromate poisoning. Ann Emerg Med. 1994;24:748-50.
53. Manley HJ, Bridwell DL, Elwell RJ, et al. Influence of peritoneal dialysate flow rate on the pharmacokinetics of cefazolin. Perit Dial Int. 2003;23:469-74.
54. Exaire E, Trevino-Becerra A, Monteon F. An overview of treatment with peritoneal dialysis in drug poisoning. Contrib Nephrol. 1979;17:39-43.
55. Lee CS, Peterson JC, Marbury TC. Comparative pharmacokinetics of theophylline in peritoneal dialysis and hemodialysis. J Clin Pharmacol. 1983;23:274-80.
56. Krisper P, Stauber RE. Technology insight: artificial extracorporeal liver support–how does Prometheus compare with MARS? Nat Clin Pract Nephrol. 2007;3:267-76.
57. Krisper P, Stadlbauer V, Stauber RE. Clearing of toxic substances: are there differences between the available liver support devices? Liver Int. 2011;31(Suppl 3):5-8.
58. Sen S, Ratnaraj N, Davies NA, et al. Treatment of phenytoin toxicity by the molecular adsorbents recirculating system (MARS). Epilepsia. 2003;44:265-7.
59. Churchwell MD, Pasko DA, Smoyer WE, et al. Enhanced clearance of highly protein-bound drugs by albumin-supplemented dialysate during modeled continuous hemodialysis. Nephrol Dial Transplant. 2009;24:231-8.
60. Romeo L, Apostoli P, Kovacic M, et al. Acute arsine intoxication as a consequence of metal burnishing operations. Am J Ind Med. 1997;32:211-6.
61. Jardine LF, Ingram LC, Bleyer WA. Intrathecal leucovorin after intrathecal methotrexate overdose. J Pediatr Hematol Oncol. 1996;18:302-4.
62. Finkelstein Y, Zevin S, Raikhlin-Eisenkraft B, et al. Intrathecal methotrexate neurotoxicity: clinical correlates and antidotal treatment. Environ Toxicol Pharmacol. 2005;19:721-5.
63. Singh O, Javeri Y, Juneja D, et al. Profile and outcome of patients with acute toxicity admitted in intensive care unit: Experiences from a major corporate hospital in urban India. Indian J Anaesth. 2011;55(4):370-4.
64. Hampson EC, Pond SM. Failure of haemoperfusion and haemodialysis to prevent death in paraquat poisoning. A retrospective review of 42 patients. Med Toxicol Adverse Drug Exp. 1988;3:64-71.
65. Ghannoum M, Hoffman RS, Gosselin S, et al. Use of extracorporeal treatments in the management of poisonings. Kidney Int. 2018;94(4):682-8.

31 CHAPTER

Extracorporeal Therapies: Specific Poisons

Deven Juneja, Omender Singh

INTRODUCTION

There is growing evidence regarding use of extracorporeal toxin removal (ECTR) in the management of acute poisonings. However, due to lack of large scale randomized control trials (RCTs), it is very difficult to formulate guidelines for any particular drug or poison. Hence, the Extracorporeal Treatments in Poisoning (EXTRIP) workgroup was formed to evaluate the clinical evidence and make recommendations for use of ECTR in the management of patients with poisonings.[1] Evidence-based recommendations for using ECTR is presently limited to only a few drugs (Table 1).[2-14] Based on the current evidence, the EXTRIP group has advised against the use of ECTR in any patient with tricyclic antidepressants (TCAs) and digoxin overdose. Here, we will be discussing the indications, choice of ECTR, and when to stop the therapy, for the drugs for which ECTR is currently recommended.

ACETAMINOPHEN

Acetaminophen is the most commonly used analgesic worldwide.[15] It is also the most commonly overdosed medicine and the leading cause of drug-induced liver failure in many western countries.[16-18] Even in patients who are administered the antidote, N-acetylcysteine (NAC), within 8 hours ingestion, mortality associated with acetaminophen overdose remains significant.[19,20]

It is argued that these deaths occur in patients who have consumed massive dosages. These patients rapidly develop signs of mitochondrial dysfunction, metabolic acidosis, and altered mental status, which may be present even at the time of presentation to the hospital.[21]

Toxicokinetics

Acetaminophen has a molecular weight 151.2 Daltons (Da) and it has good oral bioavailability of 60–90%. It exhibits

Table 1: Role of extracorporeal toxin removal as per the current Extracorporeal Treatments in Poisoning (EXTRIP) recommendations.

ECTR is recommended for:
- Acetaminophen[2]
- Barbiturates[3]
- Carbamezapine[4]
- Lithium[5]
- Metformin[6]
- Methanol[7]
- Phenytoin[8]
- Salicylic acid[9]
- Thallium[10]
- Theophylline[11]
- Valproic acid[12]

ECTR is not recommended for:
- Digoxin[13]
- Tricyclic antidepressants[14]

(ECTR: extracorporeal toxin removal)

Extracorporeal Therapies: Specific Poisons   275

low protein binding of 10–30%, which does not change even in cases of overdose.[22] Its volume of distribution (Vd) is around 0.8–1.0 L/kg and the acceptable therapeutic range is 8–20 mg/L (55–133 µmol/L).

Patients with massive ingestions (above 500 mg/kg) may develop altered consciousness and metabolic acidosis with hyperlactemia, within 12 hours of ingestion and generally before development of any biochemical or clinical evidence of liver toxicity. Serum acetaminophen levels in these patients may be much higher than the therapeutic levels, often above 750 mg/L (5,000 µmol/L).

Role of Extracorporeal Toxin Removal

N-acetylcysteine is the standard therapy which is sufficient for the management of most of the patients with acetaminophen overdose. Rarely, when NAC is not available or the serum acetaminophen levels are very high, in patients with massive ingestions, ECTR may be required. ECTR may also be useful in correcting the associated metabolic acidosis and removal of toxic metabolites like N-acetyl-p-benzoquinone imine (NAPQI). However, ECTR should not be used, only on the basis of the reported or suspected ingested dose or serum acetaminophen levels, especially if NAC is administered (Table 2).[2]

Table 2: Extracorporeal toxin removal in the management of acetaminophen toxicity.[2]
Indications for ECTR:
In the presence of any of the following: • Serum acetaminophen levels above 1,000 mg/L (6,620 µmol/L) and NAC is not administered   • Patient presenting with altered mental status, metabolic acidosis, elevated lactate, and serum acetaminophen levels above 700 mg/L (4,630 µmol/L) and NAC is not administered   • Even if NAC is administered but the patient presents with altered mental status, metabolic acidosis, elevated lactate, and serum acetaminophen levels are above 900 mg/L (5,960 µmol/L)
Cessation of extracorporeal toxin removal: • ECTR should be continued till sustained clinical improvement is apparent
Choice of ECTR: • IHD is the preferred mode of ECTR   • Intermittent hemoperfusion (HP) or continuous renal replacement therapies (CRRTs) may be used as alternatives   • Exchange transfusion may be a valid alternative in neonates

(ECTR: extracorporeal toxin removal; IHD: intermittent hemodialysis; NAC: N-acetylcysteine)

Current evidence suggests that NAC is also dialyzable and up to 50% of the drug may get removed if intermittent hemodialysis (IHD) is being performed. Hence, to maintain the same concentration of NAC, it is imperative not only to continue NAC infusion during ECTR, but to increase the dose accordingly.[23]

BARBITURATES

Barbiturates are a group of sedative-hypnotic drugs which have been used as anxiolytics, hypnotics, and anticonvulsants. However, because of their potential for addiction and overdose, they have been largely replaced by benzodiazepines in routine clinical practice. They are broadly classified as long acting (phenobarbital, mephobarbital) and short acting depending on their pharmacokinetic properties. Short-acting agents have been further classified into ultra-short (thiopental sodium, methohexital sodium), short (secobarbitone, hexobarbitone, pentobarbitone, cyclobarbitone), and intermediate-acting (allobarbital, pentohexital sodium) agents.[24]

Toxicokinetics

Short-acting agents are lipid soluble, more protein bound, and have a more rapid onset but shorter duration of action. Short-acting barbiturates are metabolized primarily by the liver.[25] On the other hand, long-acting barbiturates are less lipid soluble, less protein bound, have smaller Vd, and are mainly excreted as active drugs by the kidneys.[25]

Long-term users may develop tolerance to the sedative-hypnotic effects but respiratory depression may still develop if the serum drug concentration is high. These patients are also at risk of developing symptoms of drug withdrawal, if serum levels are rapidly reduced after ECTR.[24]

Role of Extracorporeal Toxin Removal

Extracorporeal toxin removal is recommended in patients with severe long-acting barbiturate toxicity (Table 3).[3] Because of their larger Vd and greater lipid solubility, short-acting barbiturates are cleared less effectively by ECTR. Urine alkalinization also does not increase the elimination of these short-acting barbiturates.

Extracorporeal toxin removal may also be instrumental in reducing the duration of coma, intensive

Renal Toxins and Extracorporeal Therapies

Table 3: Extracorporeal toxin removal in the management of barbiturate toxicity.[3]

Indications for ECTR:

In the presence of any of the following:
- Any symptom suggestive of severe poisoning
  - ○ Prolonged coma (present or expected)
  - ○ Shock
  - ○ Respiratory depression requiring mechanical ventilation
- Lack of clinical response to MDAC treatment
- Rising or persistently high serum barbiturate, in spite of MDAC treatment

Choice of ECTR:
- IHD is the preferred mode
- HP or CRRT are acceptable alternatives

Cessation of ECTR:
- When there is apparent clinical improvement

(CRRT: continuous renal replacement therapy; ECTR: extracorporeal toxin removal; HP: hemoperfusion; IHD: intermittent hemodialysis; MDAC: multiple-dose activated charcoal)

Table 4: Extracorporeal toxin removal in the management of carbamazepine toxicity.[4]

Indications for ECTR:

In the presence of any of the following
- Multiple seizures refractory to standard therapy
- Life-threatening dysrhythmias

ECTR should also be considered in the presence of:
- Prolonged coma or respiratory depression requiring mechanical ventilation
- Persistently high or increasing serum carbamazepine levels, in spite of MDAC and other supportive therapeutic measures

Cessation of ECTR:
- Presence of apparent clinical improvement *or*
- Serum carbamazepine levels less than 10 mg/L (42 μmol/L)

Choice of ECTR:
- IHD is the preferred mode of ECTR
- Intermittent hemoperfusion or CRRT are acceptable alternatives

(CRRT: continuous renal replacement therapy; ECTR: extracorporeal toxin removal; IHD: intermittent hemodialysis; MDAC: multiple-dose activated charcoal)

care unit (ICU) and hospital length of stay (LOS), duration on mechanical ventilation, and associated complications like pneumonia, cardiorespiratory compromise, and renal failure. However, measures like multiple-dose activated charcoal (MDAC), which may be useful in increasing elimination of barbiturates, should be continued even during ECTR.[26]

CARBAMEZAPINE

Carbamazepine is used for the management of patients with bipolar disorder, neuropathic pain, seizure disorder, and hyperactivity. It has a narrow therapeutic index; hence, chances of overdose are high. Even though the associated mortality with carbamazepine overdose is low, it is associated with high morbidity, prolonged ICU and hospital stay, and requirement for invasive mechanical ventilation.[27]

Toxicokinetics

Carbamazepine is highly protein bound; up to 70–80% and this percentage remains high even in case of overdose. It is highly lipophilic and has a low Vd of 0.8–1.4 L/kg. It is primarily metabolized by the cytochrome P450 (CYP) enzymes in the liver, and only a minor proportion (1–3%) is excreted unchanged in the urine.

The therapeutic serum levels of carbamazepine lies in the range of 4–12 mg/L (17–51 μmol/L) and clinically significant toxicity has been reported when serum levels go above 40 mg/L (169 μmol/L), but symptoms may occur at lower serum concentrations too.[27] The mortality rate associated with carbamazepine toxicity is around 13% and the reported lethal dose is around 23.6 gram.[27]

Role of Extracorporeal Toxin Removal

There is no specific antidote for carbamazepine toxicity, but most of the patients can be successfully managed with supportive care, fluid resuscitation, organ support, and treatment of seizures with benzodiazepines. MDAC has been shown to enhance elimination and improve patient outcome;[28] hence, it is recommended for managing patients with life-threatening ingestions.[26] However, its use may be limited in patients with reduced bowel motility, and those with unprotected airways.[29]

As per the current evidence, ECTR should be considered in patients with severe carbamazepine poisoning (Table 4).[4] The effect of ECTR on mortality may be unclear, but ECTR may be useful in reducing the duration of mechanical ventilation, LOS in ICU, and the related costs.[30] As the presence of seizures and dysrhythmias may signify severe toxicity and are associated with poor clinical outcomes, presence of these symptoms should be considered for initiation of ECTR.[27]

Carbamazepine is mostly protein bound; hence, hemoperfusion (HP) is considered to be the most effective mode for performing ECTR. Both resin and charcoal columns may be used for this purpose.[31,32] However, its utility may be limited by associated complications and restricted availability. Other techniques, especially IHD with modern filters may also be successful in removing carbamazepine,[33] and it is currently recommended as the modality of choice.[4] Irrespective of the ECTR modality used, MDAC should be continued even during ECTR.[4]

LITHIUM

Lithium is a commonly prescribed psychiatric medicine which is used in the management of manic phase of depressive disorders. However, it has got a narrow therapeutic index. Hence, there is always a potential for overdose. Lithium overdose may be life-threatening and there are limited treatment options to manage such patients. In addition, prolonged high serum levels increase the risk of chronic neurological damage. Hence, it becomes imperative to reduce the serum levels immediately.

Toxicokinetics

Lithium has good oral bioavailability and distributes widely in the total body water. Its initial Vd is 0.5 L/kg but it gradually increases to 0.7–0.9 L/kg.[34] It does not bind to serum proteins and is excreted entirely unchanged in the urine. Its half-life is 12–27 hours, but it may get prolonged to up to 58 hours in elderly patients or in those who take lithium chronically.[35]

Role of Extracorporeal Toxin Removal

Studies have shown that lithium is easily dialyzable and most of the reports have shown clinical improvement in patients with lithium overdose, whenever ECTR has been used. In addition, hemodialysis has shown to reduce serum lithium levels at a much higher rate than that cleared by the kidneys. The EXTRIP workgroup has recommended ECTR as a tool to manage lithium overdose as it is highly dialyzable (Table 5).[5]

The clinical decision regarding initiation of ECTR should be taken considering the serum lithium levels, renal function, pattern of lithium toxicity, clinical status of the patient, and the availability of the extracorporeal therapies. The association between serum lithium levels and clinical toxicity is controversial. However, it

Table 5: Extracorporeal toxin removal in the management of lithium toxicity.[5]

Indications for ECTR:

In the presence of any of the following:
- Impaired renal function with serum lithium levels more than 4.0 mEq/L
- Presence of life-threatening symptoms like reduced consciousness, seizures, or dysrhythmias irrespective of serum lithium levels
- Serum lithium levels more than 5.0 mEq/L
- Patient is confused
- If the expected time to reduce serum lithium levels below 1.0 mEq/L with standard management is more than 36 hours

ECTR should be stopped when:
- Serum lithium levels are reduced below 1.0 mEq/L
- There is apparent clinical improvement
- After at least 6 hours of ECTR session, if serum lithium levels are unavailable

Choice of ECTR:
- Intermittent hemodialysis is the preferred mode
- CRRT is an acceptable alternative

(CRRT: continuous renal replacement therapy; ECTR: extracorporeal toxin removal)

is generally agreed that if the serum lithium levels are above 5.0 mEq/L, ECTR should be considered as the risk of toxicity is high in such patients. In addition, lithium is more amenable for removal when serum levels are high. As kidney is the sole organ involved in lithium removal, ECTR should also be considered in patients with impaired renal function.

Charcoal HP has been shown to be useless in the treatment of patients with lithium overdose as charcoal does not adsorb lithium.[36,37] As the clearances obtained with peritoneal dialysis (PD) are very poor, it is therefore not recommended.[5]

After termination of the ECTR session, serum lithium levels should be monitored for at least next 12 hours to decide regarding the use of subsequent ECTR sessions.[5]

METFORMIN

Metformin is a commonly used biguanide oral hypoglycemic agent which is prescribed for management of patients with noninsulin dependent diabetes mellitus (NIDDM). It acts by inhibiting gluconeogenesis, facilitating cellular glucose uptake, and by decreasing insulin resistance. However, metformin overdose may lead to severe toxicity and may be associated with high mortality rates.

Toxicokinetics

Metformin is a small molecule with a molecular weight of 165 Da and is not protein bound. It has a Vd of 1–5 L/kg. Metformin is eliminated from the body largely unchanged by the kidneys. Hence, its elimination decreases with reduction in glomerular filtration rate.[38]

Metformin-associated Lactic Acidosis

Metformin-associated lactic acidosis (MALA) has been described as serum lactate levels above 5 mmol/L along with arterial pH below 7.35, associated with metformin exposure.[39]

It is further classified into two specific categories: incidental or chronic MALA and intentional or acute MALA. Chronic MALA is a result of accumulation of metformin along with alteration of production and/or clearance of lactate. On the other hand, acute MALA, also known as metformin-induced lactic acidosis (MILA), occurs after an acute overdose of metformin leading to lactic acidosis.[40-42]

As metformin is primarily eliminated by the kidneys, renal dysfunction is a major contributing factor of metformin toxicity. Other factors like hypotension, dehydration, sepsis, ischemia, and liver impairment, which lead to increased production or impaired clearance of lactates, may also contribute to lactic acidosis.

Role of Extracorporeal Toxin Removal

Aggressive resuscitation and organ support remains the mainstay of initial therapy for metformin toxicity, as there is no specific antidote. In spite of early aggressive care, the associated mortality remains high in the range of 30–50%.[43,44]

The ECTR is recommended in the management of patients with severe metformin poisoning (Table 6).[6]

Intermittent hemodialysis is preferred over continuous renal replacement therapy (CRRT) as lactate clearance may be superior with IHD. Lactate clearance may also be enhanced with use of higher effluent rates[45] and high-flux/high-efficiency dialyzers.[46] As metformin is not protein bound, HP[47] or plasma exchange[48] does not offer any advantage over IHD or CRRT, and are also not very effective in correcting acid-base abnormalities.[49]

METHANOL

Consumption of contaminated illicit or homemade alcoholic beverages is a common cause of methanol

Table 6: Extracorporeal toxin removal in the management of metformin toxicity.[6]

Indications for ECTR:

Presence of any of the following:
- Serum lactate levels above 20 mmol/L
- Blood pH ≤ 7.0
- Failure of standard therapy

ECTR should also be considered if:
- Serum lactate levels are between 15 mmol/L and 20 mmol/L
- Blood pH is between 7.0 and 7.1
- In the presence of shock, impaired renal function, liver failure, or reduced consciousness

Cessation of ECTR:
- When serum lactate levels are below 3 mmol/L and blood pH is above 7.35

Choice of ECTR:
- IHD with bicarbonate buffer is the preferred mode
- CRRT is a valid alternative

(CRRT: continuous renal replacement therapy; ECTR: extracorporeal toxin removal; IHD: intermittent hemodialysis)

poisoning and it is associated with substantial morbidity and mortality.[50,51] If the therapy is delayed or inadequate, fatality rate may exceed 40% and those who survive, may develop severe visual impairment and/or motor and cognitive disorders.[52,53]

Toxicokinetics

Hepatic alcohol dehydrogenase (ADH) first metabolizes methanol to formaldehyde and then to formic acid. Formic acid is considered to be the major toxic compound. Ethanol and fomepizole are the prescribed antidotes which are competitive inhibitors of ADH and prevent metabolism of methanol to its toxic components.

Molecular weight of methanol is 32.04 g/mol and that of formic acid is 46.03 g/mol, and they are both water soluble. Methanol has low protein binding and low Vd of 0.6–0.8 L/kg.[54] The toxic adult dose is 30 mL or 30 g,[55] and a dose of 60 mL may be lethal.[56] Serum methanol levels above 200 mg/L (9.4 mmol/L) are considered to be toxic.[57]

Role of Extracorporeal Toxin Removal

Literature suggests that use of fomepizole, in patients presenting early, with normal renal function and absence of any visual or neurological dysfunction, may

Extracorporeal Therapies: Specific Poisons

obviate the need for ECTR.[58,59] However, ECTR may be instrumental in preventing toxicity and facilitating clinical recovery, especially reversal of neurotoxicity, and hence is indicated in the treatment of patients with severe toxicity (Table 7).[7]

Both, clinical presentation and laboratory tests may aid in identifying patients which may benefit from ECTR. Presence of clinical symptoms like coma, seizures, or new vision defects signifies severe methanol toxicity.[60,61]

In addition, laboratory parameters like admission serum pH levels correlate with clinical outcomes and arterial pH below 7.0 may be associated with high mortality rates.[61] However, correction of acidemia may require large doses of sodium bicarbonate which may increase the risk of complications like hypernatremia, tetany, or volume overload.[62] Metabolic acidosis may persist in some patients in spite of bicarbonate therapy, which may suggest ingestion of massive dose of methanol,

---

Table 7: Extracorporeal toxin removal in the management of methanol toxicity.[7]

Indications for ECTR:

Presence of any of the following:
- Severe methanol poisoning, as evidenced by presence of any of the following:
  - Neurological symptoms like coma, seizures, or new vision deficits
  - Metabolic acidosis, serum pH ≤ 7.15, or persistent metabolic acidosis in spite of adequate supportive measures and antidotes or presence of high anion gap >24 mmol/L
- Serum methanol concentration
  - More than 700 mg/L (21.8 mmol/L), if fomepizole therapy is available
  - More than 600 mg/L (18.7 mmol/L), if ethanol treatment is being given
  - More than 500 mg/L (15.6 mmol/L), if ADH blocker is not being given
  - Osmolal/osmolar gap may be used, if methanol concentration is not available
- Impaired renal function

Choice of ECTR:
- IHD is the preferred mode
- CRRT may be used, if patient is hemodynamically unstable or if IHD is unavailable

Cessation of therapy:
- ECTR may be discontinued when the methanol concentration is less than 200 mg/L (6.2 mmol/L) and the patient shows clinical improvement

(CRRT: continuous renal replacement therapy; ECTR: extracorporeal toxin removal; IHD: intermittent hemodialysis)

---

or inadequate ADH inhibition secondary to insufficient dose of antidotes (ethanol or fomepizole).

As tests to measure serum methanol levels may not be widely available, other tests like osmolal/osmolar gap (OG) have also been recommended. OG correlates well with serum methanol levels and it has been shown that an OG of 20 mOsm/kg H_2O gap corresponds to methanol levels of 20 mmol/L (641 mg/L). Hence, OG levels around 25–30 mOsm/kg H_2O have been suggested as the criteria for initiating ECTR based on the current evidence.[63,64]

Further, some authors have suggested that the base deficit may better reflect the severity of metabolic acidosis, and hence a base deficit of more than 15 mmol/L should be criteria for initiating ECTR.[58]

The antidotes used in the management of methanol toxicity, ethanol, and fomepizole are also dialyzable. Hence, their levels might get reduced to subtherapeutic levels when ECTR is initiated. Therefore, it is suggested that their maintenance dosage should at least be doubled initially and then should be titrated as per the clinical response.[65] If fomepizole, is used as an antidote, it is advisable to give a loading dose of 15 mg/kg, which should be followed by an infusion at rate of 1–1.5 mg/kg/h, or to repeat the loading dose of 15 mg/kg every 4th hourly.[58]

Empirically, a duration of 8 hours for IHD and 18 hours for CRRT, has been suggested on the basis of half-life of formate. Other laboratory parameters have also been suggested as markers for cessation of ECTR therapy. These include resolution of acidemia along with an OG level below 20 mOsm/kg H_2O on two samples taken at an interval of at least 1 hour.[66]

PHENYTOIN

Phenytoin, a hydantoin derivative, is a commonly prescribed drug for treatment of tonic-clonic, psychomotor, and neurosurgery-associated seizures.[67] Overdose of phenytoin is common, although rarely fatal with a reported mortality of 3.5%.[68] Oral overdose may manifest with cerebellar and vestibular effects, like nausea, vomiting, multidirectional nystagmus, dizziness, and ataxia.[69] However, severe overdose may lead to seizures, coma, and respiratory depression.[69] Intravenous overdose produces a similar clinical picture, but cardiotoxicity can also occur which may manifest with arrhythmias, hypotension, and bradycardia.[70] However, these side effects are largely attributed to the diluent (propylene glycol) rather than the drug itself.[71]

Fosphenytoin is a prodrug of phenytoin, which is more water soluble and has reduced local side effects. Its overdose, may also present with a similar clinical picture and patients may present with seizures, drowsiness/lethargy, hypotension and ataxia. Patients may also develop cardiovascular symptoms like hypotension, bradyarrhythmias and other conduction abnormalities.[72]

Toxicokinetics

The molecular mass of phenytoin is 252 Da and it is extensively protein bound (around 90%). Even in cases of overdose, this proportion decreases only slightly to 75–80%.[73] The absorption of the oral formulation may be slow and variable; hence, the clinical effects may be unpredictable in cases of overdose.

Phenytoin has a low Vd of around 0.6–0.8 L/kg. It is primarily metabolized by the hepatic CYP enzyme system and less than 1% is excreted unchanged in the urine. The therapeutic range of phenytoin is 10–20 mg/L (39.6–79.2 mmol/L). In therapeutic doses, its half-life is 1.5–3 hours and for extended release preparations, it is around 4–12 hours. However, in case of an overdose, the half-life may become excessively prolonged even beyond 100 hours.[74] This may result in prolonged toxicity and extended hospitalization.

Role of Extracorporeal Toxin Removal

As there is no specific antidote, the management of such patients is largely supportive. Even use of MDAC is not routinely advocated in all patients.[26] As per the current recommendations, phenytoin is considered to be moderately dialyzable, and ECTR is a reasonable option in the management of selected cases of severe poisoning (Table 8).[8] As the mortality associated with phenytoin overdose is small, the primary indication of ECTR would be to reduce morbidity associated with incapacitating or prolonged ataxia, and coma. ECTR may be instrumental in rapid elimination of phenytoin from the blood, which will reduce its concentration from the cerebrospinal fluid (CSF), thereby reducing its central nervous system (CNS) toxicity. However, ECTR should not be initiated solely based on suspected dose of phenytoin ingested or serum phenytoin concentration.

As phenytoin is largely protein bound, HP and therapeutic plasma exchange are expected to be most efficient for removing phenytoin. Historically, IHD has not shown to be effective in removal of phenytoin[75,76]

Table 8: Extracorporeal toxin removal in the management of phenytoin toxicity.[8]

Indications for ECTR:

Presence of any of the following:
- Expected or present prolonged coma
- ECTR is also a reasonable option in patients with prolonged incapacitating ataxia

Cessation of ECTR:
- ECTR should be continued till there is apparent clinical improvement

Choice of ECTR:
- IHD is the preferred mode
- HP is an acceptable alternative

(ECTR: extracorporeal toxin removal; HP: hemoperfusion; IHD: intermittent hemodialysis)

but with use of modern high-efficiency filters, especially in the presence of conditions like kidney dysfunction and hypoalbuminemia, which reduce protein binding, IHD may be effective.[77] Addition of a charcoal column, in series after dialysis filter, has also been suggestive to improve phenytoin clearance.[78]

SALICYLIC ACID

Acetylsalicylic acid (aspirin) is the most commonly used salicylate but the term "salicylates" also includes other forms like methyl salicylate, sodium salicylate, and bismuth subsalicylate.

Aspirin is a common cause of overdose and every year several deaths are reported related to aspirin overdose.[16,79]

Toxicokinetics

Acetylsalicylic acid is a small organic acid which has a molecular mass of 180 Da. It is highly protein bound (90%), but the protein binding sites may get saturated and the protein binding can get reduced to as low as 30% in patients with overdose. Its Vd is low (0.2 L/kg), and the therapeutic range is between 0.4 mmol/L to 1.8 mmol/L (5–25 mg/dL). Toxic dose is considered to be above 150 mg/kg and the reported lethal dose is more than 500 mg/kg.[80,81]

Role of Extracorporeal Toxin Removal

Patients with overdose develop metabolic acidosis with hyperlactatemia. Multiple organ dysfunction may ensue,

Extracorporeal Therapies: Specific Poisons

but death typically occurs due to cerebral edema which occurs because of high salicylate levels in the CNS. CNS entry of salicylates is facilitated by low serum pH, hence, it is vital to maintain normal pH in such patients.[82,83]

Any signs or symptoms suggestive of CNS involvement may suggest severe toxicity. Patients may also develop acute respiratory distress syndrome (ARDS) due to salicylate toxicity and hence, oxygen requirement, which may be a harbinger of early ARDS, may also signify severe toxicity.

Treatment of patients with salicylate overdose is mainly supportive. However, bicarbonate therapy is an important component of therapy as it maintains normal serum pH and also causes alkaluria, which helps in urinary salicylate excretion, especially when urinary pH is above 7.5.[84]

Extracorporeal toxin removal has been recommended in the management of patients with severe salicylate poisoning (Table 9).[9] It not only rapidly reduces the concentration of the circulating salicylate but also helps in correction of acidemia, which in turn prevents entry of salicylate in the CSF. Both hemodialysis and HP provide good clearance of salicylates.[85] Although CRRT has been tried in the management of salicylate overdose, clearance of salicylate remains significantly inferior as compared to hemodialysis or HP.[86] As per the recommendations, intravenous bicarbonate should be continued even during ECTR.[9]

THALLIUM

Historically, thallium salts have been used as medicinal agents for management of ringworm infections and as rodenticides.[87,88] Presently, they are primarily used for radioactive contrast, in electric lighting, manufacture of optical lenses, and extreme cold thermometers. However, in certain parts of the world, they are still used as rodenticides and hence, poisonings are still reported.[89] Thallium is highly toxic and may lead to serious morbidity. Even a dose as low as 6 mg/kg may be fatal.[87]

Toxicokinetics

Thallium has a molecular mass of 204.4 Da (g/mol), and has a large Vd (3–10 L/kg) and extensive enterohepatic recirculation. These factors increase its half-life to 2–4 days and sometimes even up to 15 days.[90,91] It does not bind to proteins and has an excellent bioavailability of 90–100%.[90] It is mostly excreted unchanged in the bile and feces (51%) and urine (26%).[92]

Role of Extracorporeal Toxin Removal

The treatment of patients with thallium toxicity is supportive. Orogastric lavage may be done if massive ingestion is suspected and the patient presents within 1–2 hours of ingestion. Activated charcoal is indicated as it has high absorptive capacity for thallium.[93] Prussian blue has also been tried orally as an ion exchanger which may be effective in enhancing fecal elimination of thallium.[93]

Dose-effect relationship of thallium ingestion is unclear.[94] Initial symptoms, like gastrointestinal symptoms and tachycardia, are nonspecific. Other symptoms like ascending painful neuropathy and alopecia, which may suggest thallium overdose, develop later and by that time it is already late to initiate ECTR. Signs suggesting CNS involvement, like seizures, confusion, or coma, are indicators of poor overall outcome.

Based on the current evidence, ECTR is recommended for management of patients with severe thallium poisoning (Table 10).[10] However, because of its

---

Table 9: Extracorporeal toxin removal in the management of salicylate toxicity.[9]

Indications for ECTR:

Presence of any of the following:
- Serum salicylate levels above 7.2 mmol/L (100 mg/dL)
- Serum salicylate levels above 6.5 mmol/L (90 mg/dL) in the presence of impaired renal function
- Presence of clinical symptoms suggestive of severe toxicity
  - Altered mental status
  - New onset hypoxia requiring supplemental oxygen
- ECTR is also recommended, if there is failure of standard therapy in the presence of:
  - Serum salicylate levels above 6.5 mmol/L (90 mg/dL)
  - Serum salicylate levels above 5.8 mmol/L (80 mg/dL), in the presence of renal failure
  - Serum pH less than 7.2

Cessation of therapy:
- There is apparent clinical improvement and serum salicylate levels below 1.4 mmol/L (19 mg/dL) or ECTR has been conducted for at least 4–6 hours, in absence of serum salicylates levels

Choice of ECTR:
- IHD is the preferred mode
- HP or CRRT are valid alternatives
- Exchange transfusion may be tried in neonates

(CRRT: continuous renal replacement therapy; ECTR: extracorporeal toxin removal; HP: hemoperfusion; IHD: intermittent hemodialysis)

Table 10: Extracorporeal toxin removal in the management of thallium toxicity.[10]

Indications for ECTR:
- Suspected thallium exposure based on history or clinical features
- Serum thallium levels above 1.0 mg/L
- ECTR should also be considered if serum thallium levels are between 0.4 mg/L and 1.0 mg/L

Cessation of ECTR:
- ECTR should be continued till serum thallium levels have remained below 0.1 mg/L for at least 72 hours

Choice of ECTR:
- IHD is the preferred mode of ECTR
- Intermittent hemoperfusion or CRRT can be used as alternatives

(CRRT: continuous renal replacement therapy; ECTR: extracorporeal toxin removal; IHD: intermittent hemodialysis)

high Vd, thallium cannot be substantially removed from the circulation with any kind of ECTR. CNS distribution of thallium takes around 24 hours[90,91] and hence, it is reasonable that if ECTR is initiated before this time period, it may be beneficial in reducing CNS toxicity and improving outcomes. Therefore, when indicated, ECTR should preferably be started within 24–48 hours of thallium exposure. As thallium is primarily excreted by the kidneys, presence of any renal dysfunction should lower the threshold for initiating ECTR.

Traditionally, HP has been considered to be the most efficient mode of ECTR for removing thallium. However, with modern ECTR techniques and high-flux filters, even IHD may be equally efficient. Even when ECTR is initiated, other therapies aimed at enhancing elimination of thallium, like MDAC and Prussian blue, should be continued.

THEOPHYLLINE

Theophylline is a methylxanthine compound derived from the plants. It is similar to other methylxanthine compounds like caffeine, paraxanthine, and theobromine. Theophylline is commonly prescribed as a bronchodilator in the management of patients with asthma and chronic obstructive pulmonary disease (COPD). It is available in both oral and intravenous (aminophylline; 85% of anhydrous theophylline) formulations.

Toxicokinetics

Theophylline has a low molecular weight of 180 Da and is moderately protein bound (40–60%). Protein binding may be further reduced in patients with uremia and cirrhosis.[95] It has excellent oral bioavailability of up to 90% and a low Vd of approximately 0.5 L/kg.

Theophylline is primarily metabolized in the liver by the CYP enzymes and hence, its metabolism is affected by factors which induce (smoking, phenytoin, and phenobarbital) or inhibit (cimetidine and macrolides) the CYP enzymes.[96,97] Only a small proportion of theophylline (<10%) is excreted unchanged by the kidneys.[98]

The half-life of theophylline is 8–11 hours, but in patients with overdose, it exhibits zero-order elimination which markedly increases its half-life. Its therapeutic range is 5–15 mg/L (28–83 mmol/L) and toxicity may develop if serum concentration increases beyond 25 mg/L (139 mmol/L). The reported toxic dose is more than 15 mg/kg; whereas, a dose above 100 mg/kg may prove to be lethal.

Role of Extracorporeal Toxin Removal

Theophylline toxicity is a potentially life-threatening medical emergency. Even though several studies have suggested a relationship between serum theophylline levels[99,100] and clinical symptoms, especially in patients with acute poisoning, this relationship remains controversial.[101]

Presence of symptoms like shock, intractable seizures, and life-threatening dysrhythmias are suggestive of severe toxicity and are associated with high mortality.[97,102] Chronic exposure to theophylline, especially in extremes of age, is associated with more toxicity and poorer outcomes.

As there is no specific antidote, the management of patients with theophylline poisoning remains supportive. MDAC is recommended as it enhances elimination of theophylline,[26] but its utility may be limited by intractable vomiting[103] which is commonly present in these patients, especially in patients with massive overdose.[104]

Extracorporeal toxin removal is recommended in the management of patients with severe theophylline poisoning (Table 11).[11] Use of ECTR with modes like HP or hemodialysis may enhance theophylline clearance from the body by several folds[105,106] and may also augment its removal from the CNS.[107] ECTR especially hemodialysis, may also aid in correcting acidosis and hyperthermia.

Previous studies had shown that HP may provide best clearance. However, use of high-efficiency modern

Extracorporeal Therapies: Specific Poisons

Chapter 31

Table 11: Extracorporeal toxin removal in the management of theophylline toxicity.[11]

Indications of ECTR:
- Serum theophylline levels above 100 mg/L (555 µmol/L) in patients with acute exposure
- Presence of severe complications like seizures, life-threatening dysrhythmias, or shock
- Rising serum theophylline levels or clinical deterioration in spite of optimal therapy

ECTR should also be considered if:
- Serum theophylline levels are above 60 mg/L (333 µmol/L) in patients with chronic exposure
- Extremes of age (<6 months or >60 years) and serum theophylline above 50 mg/L (278 µmol/L) in presence of chronic exposure
- Contraindications/nonavailability of gastrointestinal decontamination

Cessation of ECTR:
- Apparent clinical improvement *or*
- Serum theophylline levels below 15 mg/L (83 µmol/L)

Choice of ECTR:
- IHD is the preferred mode of ECTR
- Hemoperfusion and CRRT are valid alternatives
- Exchange transfusion is an acceptable alternative in neonates

(CRRT: continuous renal replacement therapy; ECTR: extracorporeal toxin removal; IHD: intermittent hemodialysis)

filters has improved efficiency of IHD in the recent years. Further, it is suggested that use of HP and hemodialysis filters in series may provide the best clearance of theophylline.[108] It is also recommended that MDAC therapy should be continued even during ECTR as it may provide an additive effect to ECTR.[11]

VALPROIC ACID

Valproic acid is widely prescribed for the management of partial and generalized seizure disorders.

Toxicokinetics

It has a small molecular mass (144 Da) and has saturable plasma protein binding. As a result, at therapeutic doses when serum concentrations are below 100 mg/L, 94% valproic acid is protein bound. However, after an overdose when serum concentrations rise, plasma proteins get oversaturated and the concentration of free active fraction increases. When serum concentrations reach above 1,000 mg/L, less than 15% valproic acid is protein bound.

Valproic acid is largely metabolized in the liver by glucuronide conjugation and only a small proportion of it is excreted in the urine unchanged.[109] Its elimination half-life also increases dramatically to more than 30 hours after an overdose as compared to 12 hours at therapeutic concentrations.[110]

Data suggests that the serum valproic acid level correlates with severity of toxicity. Serum concentrations between 50 and 100 mg/L are considered to be in the therapeutic range. Patients may manifest clinical signs of CNS depression at levels above 200 mg/L with sedation, ataxia, and lethargy.[111] If serum levels rise beyond 400 mg/kg, patients may exhibit signs of severe valproic acid poisoning with coma, respiratory depression, cerebral edema, hemodynamic instability, and high mortality rates.[111]

Role of Extracorporeal Toxin Removal

The mainstay of treatment remains early aggressive and supportive care. L-carnitine has been commended as an antidote for management of patients with valproic acid overdose and hyperammonemic encephalopathy.[112] Studies have shown that neither urine alkalinization nor MDAC are useful in increasing elimination of valproic acid in poisoned patients and hence, these therapies are not currently recommended.[26,113]

In patients with valproic acid toxicity, ECTR may be helpful in reducing the duration of coma, reducing the need for invasive mechanical ventilation, and also prevent development of cerebral edema;[12] and hence, it is indicated in the management of severe valproic acid toxicity (Table 12).[12] IHD may also have an added advantage of correcting the associated acidemia and rapid elimination of ammonia. Hyperammonemia is often an accompanied complication of valproic acid toxicity which may contribute to cerebral edema and poor outcomes. As ammonia distributes in total body water, IHD has been shown to be the most efficient mode for ammonia removal. CRRT may be preferred in patients with suspected or documented cerebral edema, as it may have less impact on intracranial pressures.[114]

There are certain complications specific to use of ECTR in patients with valproic acid toxicity. Withdrawal seizures can occur if the serum valproic acid levels fall below the therapeutic range, in an epileptic patient.[115] Intracranial pressure may also increase during ECTR in patients with or at risk of cerebral edema.[116]

Table 12: Extracorporeal toxin removal in the management of valproic acid toxicity.[12]

Indications for ECTR:
- ECTR is indicated if *any* of the following is present:
  - Serum valproic acid levels more than 1,300 mg/L (9,000 mmol/L)
  - Cerebral edema or shock
- ECTR should also be considered in patients with valproic acid toxicity if *any* of the following is present:
  - Serum valproic acid levels more than 900 mg/L (6,250 mmol/L)
  - Need for invasive mechanical ventilation because of coma or respiratory depression
  - Acute hyperammonemia
  - Blood pH ≤ 7.10

ECTR should be stopped when:
- Apparent clinical improvement or serum valproic acid levels in therapeutic range of 50–100 mg/L (350–700 mmol/L)

Choice of ECTR:
- IHD is the preferred mode of ECTR
- HP and CRRT are valid alternatives

(CRRT: continuous renal replacement therapy; ECTR: extracorporeal toxin removal; HP: hemoperfusion; IHD: intermittent hemodialysis)

CONCLUSION

Based on the current evidence, ECTR is recommended in management of patients with severe toxicity of the following drugs: acetaminophen, barbiturates, carbamazepine, lithium, metformin, methanol, phenytoin, salicylic acid, thallium, theophylline, and valproic acid. Presently, the EXTRIP group has recommended against the use of ECTR in patients with overdose of TCAs and digoxin. However, use of ECTR is still evolving and future studies may expand its role in the management of more poisonings. Hence, it is imperative to have a clear understanding of the pharmacokinetics and pharmacodynamics of the drugs involved and the utility and shortcomings of the ECTR before it is applied in any poisoning patient. If applied in the correct clinical scenario, it may prove life-saving.

KEY POINTS

- Extracorporeal toxin removal may be clinically useful in selected patients with severe poisoning with acetaminophen, barbiturates, carbamazepine, lithium, metformin, methanol, phenytoin, salicylic acid, thallium, theophylline, and valproic acid

- Extracorporeal toxin removal is currently not recommended in any patient with TCAs and digoxin overdose
- Hemodialysis may be used as the modality of choice for performing ECTR
- Continuous renal replacement therapy may be used, as an alternative, especially in hemodynamically unstable patients
- If indicated, ECTR should be initiated as early as technically possible and preferably within 24 hours of exposure to the drug.

REFERENCES

1. Ghannoum M, Nolin TD, Lavergne V, et al.; EXTRIP workgroup. Blood purification in toxicology: nephrology's ugly duckling. Adv Chronic Kidney Dis. 2011;18(3):160-6.
2. Gosselin S, Juurlink DN, Kielstein JT, et al.; Extrip Workgroup. Extracorporeal treatment for acetaminophen poisoning: recommendations from the EXTRIP workgroup. Clin Toxicol (Phila). 2014;52(8):856-67.
3. Mactier R, Laliberté M, Mardini J, et al.; EXTRIP Workgroup. Extracorporeal treatment for barbiturate poisoning: recommendations from the EXTRIP Workgroup. Am J Kidney Dis. 2014;64(3):347-58.
4. Ghannoum M, Yates C, Galvao TF, et al.; EXTRIP workgroup. Extracorporeal treatment for carbamazepine poisoning: systematic review and recommendations from the EXTRIP workgroup. Clin Toxicol (Phila). 2014;52(10):993-1004.
5. Decker BS, Goldfarb DS, Dargan PI, et al.; EXTRIP Workgroup. extracorporeal treatment for lithium poisoning: Systematic review and recommendations from the EXTRIP Workgroup. Clin J Am Soc Nephrol. 2015;10(5):875-87.
6. Calello DP, Liu KD, Wiegand TJ, et al.; Extracorporeal Treatments in Poisoning Workgroup. Extracorporeal Treatment for Metformin Poisoning: Systematic Review and Recommendations from the Extracorporeal Treatments in Poisoning Workgroup. Crit Care Med. 2015;43(8):1716-30.
7. Roberts DM, Yates C, Megarbane B, et al.; EXTRIP Work Group. Recommendations for the role of extracorporeal treatments in the management of acute methanol poisoning: a systematic review and consensus statement. Crit Care Med. 2015;43(2):461-72.
8. Anseeuw K, Mowry JB, Burdmann EA, et al.; EXTRIP Workgroup. Extracorporeal Treatment in Phenytoin Poisoning: Systematic Review and Recommendations from the EXTRIP (Extracorporeal Treatments in Poisoning) Workgroup. Am J Kidney Dis. 2016;67(2): 187-97.
9. Juurlink DN, Gosselin S, Kielstein JT, et al.; EXTRIP Workgroup. Extracorporeal Treatment for Salicylate Poisoning: Systematic Review and Recommendations

Extracorporeal Therapies: Specific Poisons

from the EXTRIP Workgroup. Ann Emerg Med. 2015;66(2):165-81.

10. Ghannoum M, Nolin TD, Goldfarb DS, et al.; Extracorporeal Treatments in Poisoning Workgroup. Extracorporeal Treatment for Thallium Poisoning: Recommendations from the EXTRIP Workgroup. Clin J Am Soc Nephrol. 2012;7(10):1682-90.

11. Ghannoum M, Wiegand TJ, Liu KD, et al.; EXTRIP Workgroup. Extracorporeal treatment for theophylline poisoning: systematic review and recommendations from the EXTRIP workgroup. Clin Toxicol (Phila). 2015;53(4):215-29.

12. Ghannoum M, Laliberté M, Nolin TD, et al. on behalf of the EXTRIP Workgroup. Extracorporeal treatment for valproic acid poisoning: Systematic review and recommendations from the EXTRIP workgroup. Clin Toxicol. 2015;53:454-65.

13. Mowry JB, Burdmann EA, Anseeuw K, et al.; EXTRIP Workgroup. Extracorporeal treatment for digoxin poisoning: systematic review and recommendations from the EXTRIP Workgroup. Clin Toxicol (Phila). 2016;54(2):103-14.

14. Yates C, Galvao T, Sowinski KM, et al.; EXTRIP Workgroup. Extracorporeal treatment for tricyclic antidepressant poisoning: recommendations from the EXTRIP Workgroup. Semin Dial. 2014;27(4):381-9.

15. Josephy PD. The molecular toxicology of acetaminophen. Drug Metab Rev. 2005;37:581-94.

16. Mowry JB, Spyker DA, Cantilena LR Jr, et al. 2012 Annual Report of the American Association of Poison Control Centers' National Poison Data System (NPDS): 30th Annual Report. Clin Toxicol (Phila). 2013;51:949-1229.

17. Leise MD, Poterucha JJ, Talwalkar JA. Drug-induced liver injury. Mayo Clin Proc. 2014;89:95-106.

18. Lopez AM, Hendrickson RG. Toxin-induced hepatic injury. Emerg Med Clin North Am. 2014;32:103-25.

19. Bourdeaux C, Bewley J. Death from paracetamol overdose despite appropriate treatment with N-acetylcysteine. Emerg Med J. 2007;24:e31.

20. Schwartz EA, Hayes BD, Sarmiento KF. Development of hepatic failure despite use of intravenous acetylcysteine after a massive ingestion of acetaminophen and diphenhydramine. Ann Emerg Med. 2009;54:421-3.

21. Shah AD, Wood DM, Dargan PI. Understanding lactic acidosis in paracetamol (acetaminophen) poisoning. Br J Clin Pharmacol. 2011;71:20-8.

22. Milligan TP, Morris HC, Hammond PM, et al. Studies on paracetamol binding to serum proteins. Ann Clin Biochem. 1994;31:492-6.

23. Grunbaum AM, Kazim S, Ghannoum M, et al. Acetaminophen and n-acetylcysteine dialysance during hemodialysis for massive ingestion. Clin Toxicol. 2013;51:270-1.

24. Mihic S, Harris R. Chapter 17: Hypnotics and sedatives. In: Brunton LL, Chabner BA, Knollmann BC (Eds). Goodman & Gilman's The Pharmacological Basis of Therapeutics, 12th edition. New York, NY: McGraw-Hill; 2011. pp. 457-80.

25. Roberts DM, Buckley NA. Enhanced elimination in acute barbiturate poisoning—a systematic review. Clin Toxicol (Phila). 2011;49(1):2-12.

26. Vale JG, Krenzelok EP, Barceloux VD. Position statement and practice guidelines on the use of multi-dose activated charcoal in the treatment of acute poisoning. American Academy of Clinical Toxicology; European Association of Poisons Centres and Clinical Toxicologists. J Toxicol Clin Toxicol. 1999;37(6):731-51.

27. Schmidt S, Schmitz-Buhl M. Signs and symptoms of carbamazepine overdose. J Neurol. 1995;242:169-73.

28. Brahmi N, Kouraichi N, Thabet H, et al. Influence of activated charcoal on the pharmacokinetics and the clinical features of carbamazepine poisoning. Am J Emerg Med. 2006;24:440-3.

29. Graudins A, Peden G, Dowsett RP. Massive overdose with controlled-release carbamazepine resulting in delayed peak serum concentrations and life-threatening toxicity. Emerg Med (Fremantle). 2002;14:89-94.

30. Askenazi DJ, Goldstein SL, Chang IF, et al. Management of a severe carbamazepine overdose using albumin enhanced continuous venovenous hemodialysis. Pediatrics. 2004;113:406-9.

31. Ghannoum M, Bouchard J, Nolin TD, et al. Hemoperfusion for the treatment of poisoning: technology, determinants of poison clearance, and application in clinical practice. Semin Dial. 2014;27:350-61.

32. Ghannoum M, Roberts DM, Hoffman RS, et al. A stepwise approach for the management of poisoning with extracorporeal treatments. Semin Dial. 2014;27:362-70.

33. Bouchard J, Roberts DM, Roy L, et al. Principles and operational parameters to optimize poison removal with extracorporeal treatments. Semin Dial. 2014;27:371-80.

34. Meltzer H. Antipsychotic agents and lithium. In: Katsung BG, Masters SB, Trevor AJ (Eds). Basic and Clinical Pharmacology, 12th edition. New York: McGraw-Hill Medical; 2012. pp. 501-20.

35. Okusa MD, Crystal LJ. Clinical manifestations and management of acute lithium intoxication. Am J Med. 1994;97:383-9.

36. Unei H, Ikeda H, Murakami T, et al. Detoxication treatment for carbamazepine and lithium overdose. Yakugaku Zasshi. 2008;128:165-70.

37. Favin FD, Klein-Schwartz W, Oderda GM, et al. In vitro study of lithium carbonate adsorption by activated charcoal. J Toxicol Clin Toxicol. 1988;26:443-50.

38. Sirtori CR, Franceschini G, Galli-Kienle M, et al. Disposition of metformin (N,N-dimethylbiguanide) in man. Clin Pharmacol Ther. 1978;24:683-93.

39. Luft D, Deichsel G, Schmülling RM, et al. Definition of clinically relevant lactic acidosis in patients with internal diseases. Am J Clin Pathol. 1983;80:484-9.

40. Vecchio S, Protti A. Metformin-induced lactic acidosis: No one left behind. Crit Care. 2011;15:107.

41. Arroyo AM, Walroth TA, Mowry JB, et al. The MALAdy of metformin poisoning: Is CVVH the cure? Am J Ther. 2010;17:96-100.

42. Aghabiklooei A, Mostafazadeh B, Shiva H. A fatal case of metformin intoxication. Pak J Med Sci. 2011;27:943-4.

43. Peters N, Jay N, Barraud D, et al. Metformin-associated lactic acidosis in an intensive care unit. Crit Care. 2008;12:R149.

44. Biradar V, Moran JL, Peake SL, et al. Metformin-associated lactic acidosis (MALA): Clinical profile and outcomes in patients admitted to the intensive care unit. Crit Care Resusc. 2010;12:191-5.

45. Liu Y, Ouyang B, Chen J, et al. Effects of different doses in continuous veno-venous hemofiltration on plasma lactate in critically ill patients. Chin Med J (Engl). 2014;127: 1827-32.

46. Akoglu H, Akan B, Piskinpasa S, et al. Metformin-associated lactic acidosis treated with prolonged hemodialysis. Am J Emerg Med. 2011;29:575.e3-575.e5.

47. Guo PY, Storsley LJ, Finkle SN. Severe lactic acidosis treated with prolonged hemodialysis: Recovery after massive overdoses of metformin. Semin Dial. 2006;19:80-3.

48. Turkcuer I, Erdur B, Sari I, et al. Severe metformin intoxication treated with prolonged haemodialyses and plasma exchange. Eur J Emerg Med. 2009;16:11-3.

49. Ouellet G, Bouchard J, Ghannoum M, et al. Available extracorporeal treatments for poisoning: Overview and limitations. Semin Dial. 2014;27:342-9.

50. Bronstein AC, Spyker DA, Cantilena LR Jr, et al. 2011 Annual report of the American Association of Poison Control Centers' National Poison Data System (NPDS): 29th Annual Report. Clin Toxicol (Phila). 2012;50:911-1164.

51. Paasma R, Hovda KE, Hassanian-Moghaddam H, et al. Risk factors related to poor outcome after methanol poisoning and the relation between outcome and antidotes—A multicenter study. Clin Toxicol (Phila). 2012;50:823-31.

52. Paasma R, Hovda KE, Tikkerberi A, et al. Methanol mass poisoning in Estonia: Outbreak in 154 patients. Clin Toxicol (Phila). 2007;45:152-7.

53. Hovda KE, Hunderi OH, Tafjord AB, et al. Methanol outbreak in Norway 2002-2004: Epidemiology, clinical features and prognostic signs. J Intern Med. 2005;258: 181-90.

54. Graw M, Haffner HT, Althaus L, et al. Invasion and distribution of methanol. Arch Toxicol. 2000;74:313-21.

55. Gonda A, Gault H, Churchill D, et al. Hemodialysis for methanol intoxication. Am J Med. 1978;64:749-58.

56. Jacobsen D, McMartin KE. Methanol and ethylene glycol poisonings. Mechanism of toxicity, clinical course, diagnosis and treatment. Med Toxicol. 1986;1:309-34.

57. Kostic MA, Dart RC. Rethinking the toxic methanol level. J Toxicol Clin Toxicol. 2003;41:793-800.

58. Hovda KE, Jacobsen D. Expert opinion: Fomepizole may ameliorate the need for hemodialysis in methanol poisoning. Hum Exp Toxicol. 2008;27:539-46.

59. Mégarbane B, Borron SW, Trout H, et al. Treatment of acute methanol poisoning with fomepizole. Intensive Care Med. 2001;27:1370-8.

60. Kute VB, Godara SM, Shah PR, et al. Hemodialysis for methyl alcohol poisoning: A single-center experience. Saudi J Kidney Dis Transpl. 2012;23:37-43.

61. Liu JJ, Daya MR, Carrasquillo O, et al. Prognostic factors in patients with methanol poisoning. J Toxicol Clin Toxicol. 1998;36:175-81.

62. Bennett IL Jr, Cary FH, Mitchell GL Jr, et al. Acute methyl alcohol poisoning: A review based on experiences in an outbreak of 323 cases. Medicine (Baltimore). 1953;32: 431-63.

63. Waring WS, Ho C, Warner M. Significance of the osmolal gap in suspected ethylene glycol poisoning. Clin Toxicol. 2010;48(5):401-6.

64. Krasowski MD, Wilcoxon RM, Miron J. A retrospective analysis of glycol and toxic alcohol ingestion: Utility of anion and osmolal gaps. BMC Clin Pathol. 2012;12:1.

65. In: Nelson LS, Lewin NA, Howland MA, et al (Eds). Goldfrank's Toxicologic Emergencies, 9th Edition. New York: McGraw-Hill; 2010.

66. Hunderi OH, Hovda KE, Jacobsen D. Use of the osmolal gap to guide the start and duration of dialysis in methanol poisoning. Scand J Urol Nephrol. 2006;40:70-4.

67. Woodbury DM, Kemp JW. Pharmacology and mechanisms of action of diphenylhydantoin. Psychiatr Neurol Neurochir. 1971;74(2):91-115.

68. Case log counts (generic). Enterprise Reports, National Poison Data System, American Association of Poison Control Centers. Available from http://www.aapcc.org/data-system/. [Accessed October, 2018].

69. Kutt H, Winters W, Kokenge R, et al. Diphenylhydantoin metabolism, blood levels, and toxicity. Arch Neurol. 1964;11:642-8.

70. Narcy P, Zorza G, Taburet AM, et al. Severe poisoning with intravenous phenytoin in the newborn. Value of peritoneal dialysis [in French]. Arch Fr Pediatr. 1990;47(8):591-3.

71. Pillai U, Hothi J, Bhat Z. Severe propylene glycol toxicity secondary to use of anti-epileptics. Am J Ther. 2014;21(4):e106-e109.

72. Watson WA, Litovitz TL, Rodgers GC Jr, et al. 2002 Annual report of the American Association of Poison Control Centers Toxic Exposure Surveillance System. Am J Emerg Med. 2003;21(5):353-421.

73. Kawasaki C, Nishi R, Uekihara S, et al. Charcoal hemoperfusion in the treatment of phenytoin overdose. Am J Kidney Dis. 2000;35(2):323-6.

74. Brandolese R, Scordo MG, Spina E, et al. Severe phenytoin intoxication in a subject homozygous for CYP2C9*3. Clin Pharmacol Ther. 2001;70(4):391-4.

75. Rubinger D, Levy M, Roll D, et al. Inefficiency of haemodialysis in acute phenytoin intoxication. Br J Clin Pharmacol. 1979;7(4):405-7.

76. Adler DS, Martin E, Gambertoglio JG, et al. Hemodialysis of phenytoin in a uremic patient. Clin Pharmacol Ther. 1975;18(1):65-9.

77. Churchwell MD, Pasko DA, Smoyer WE, et al. Enhanced clearance of highly protein-bound drugs by albumin supplemented dialysate during modeled continuous hemodialysis. Nephrol Dial Transplant. 2009;24(1):231-8.

78. De Schoenmakere G, De Waele J, Terryn W, et al. Phenytoin intoxication in critically ill patients. Am J Kidney Dis. 2005;45(1):189-92.

79. Mowry JB, Spyker DA, Cantilena LR Jr, et al. 2013 Annual report of the American Association of Poison Control Centers' National Poison Data System (NPDS): 31st annual report. Clin Toxicol (Phila). 2014;52:1032-283.

80. Levy G. Pharmacokinetics of salicylate elimination in man. J Pharm Sci. 1965;54:959-67.

81. Hollister L, Levy G. Some aspects of salicylate distribution and metabolism in man. J Pharm Sci. 1965;54:1126-9.

82. Hill JB. Experimental salicylate poisoning: observations on the effects of altering blood pH on tissue and plasma salicylate concentrations. Pediatrics. 1971;47:658-65.

83. Hill JB. Salicylate intoxication. N Engl J Med. 1973;288:1110-3.

84. Temple AR. Acute and chronic effects of aspirin toxicity and their treatment. Arch Intern Med. 1981;141:364-9.

85. Jacobsen D, Wiik-Larsen E, Bredesen JE. Haemodialysis or haemoperfusion in severe salicylate poisoning? Hum Toxicol. 1988;7:161-3.

86. French LK, McKeown NJ, Hendrickson RG. Continuous renal replacement therapy for salicylate overdose in a patient with multisystem trauma. Clin Toxicol. 2011;49:515-627.

87. Munch JC, Ginsburg HM, Nixon C. The 1932 thallotoxicosis outbreak in California. J Am Med Assoc. 1933;100:1315-9.

88. Chamberlain PH, Stavinoha WB, Davis H, et al. Thallium poisoning. Pediatrics. 1958;22:1170-82.

89. Saha A, Sadhu HG, Karnik AB, et al. Erosion of nails following thallium poisoning: A case report. Occup Environ Med. 2004;61:640-2.

90. de Groot G, van Heijst AN. Toxicokinetic aspects of thallium poisoning. Methods of treatment by toxin elimination. Sci Total Environ. 1988;71:411-8.

91. Atkins HL, Budinger TF, Lebowitz E, et al. Thallium-201 for medical use. Part 3: Human distribution and physical imaging properties. J Nucl Med. 1977;18:133-40.

92. Sharma AN, Nelson LS, Hoffman RS. Cerebrospinal fluid analysis in fatal thallium poisoning: Evidence for delayed distribution into the central nervous system. Am J Forensic Med Pathol. 2004;25:156-8.

93. Hoffman RS, Stringer JA, Feinberg RS, et al. Comparative efficacy of thallium adsorption by activated charcoal, Prussian blue, and sodium polystyrene sulfonate. J Toxicol Clin Toxicol. 1999;37:833-7.

94. Suwelack B, Muller C, Welling U, et al. A case of potentially lethal thallium intoxication. Comparison of various elimination procedures. Trace Elem Electrolytes. 1994;11:51-4.

95. Blouin RA, Bauer LA, Bustrack JA, et al. Theophylline hemodialysis clearance. Ther Drug Monit. 1980;2:221-3.

96. Antoniou T, Gomes T, Mamdani MM, et al. Ciprofloxacin induced theophylline toxicity: a population-based study. Eur J Clin Pharmacol. 2011;67:521-6.

97. Gaudreault P, Guay J. Theophylline poisoning. Pharmacological considerations and clinical management. Med Toxicol. 1986;1:169-91.

98. Levy G, Koysooko R. Renal clearance of theophylline in man. J Clin Pharmacol. 1976;16:329-32.

99. Sessler CN. Theophylline toxicity: clinical features of 116 consecutive cases. Am J Med. 1990;88:567-76.

100. Hall KW, Dobson KE, Dalton JG, et al. Metabolic abnormalities associated with intentional theophylline overdose. Ann Intern Med. 1984;101:457-62.

101. Aitken ML, Martin TR. Life-threatening theophylline toxicity is not predictable by serum levels. Chest. 1987;91:10-4.

102. Olson KR, Benowitz NL, Woo OF, et al. Theophylline overdose: acute single ingestion versus chronic repeated overmedication. Am J Emerg Med. 1985;3:386-94.

103. Amitai Y, Lovejoy FH, Jr. Characteristics of vomiting associated with acute sustained release theophylline poisoning: Implications for management with oral activated charcoal. J Toxicol Clin Toxicol. 1987;25:539-54.

104. Sessler CN, Glauser FL, Cooper KR. Treatment of theophylline toxicity with oral activated charcoal. Chest. 1985;87:325-9.

105. Park GD, Spector R, Roberts RJ, et al. Use of hemoperfusion for treatment of theophylline intoxication. Am J Med. 1983;74:961-6.

106. Shannon M. Predictors of major toxicity after theophylline overdose. Ann Intern Med. 1993;119:1161-7.

107. Perrin C, Debruyne D, Lacotte J, et al. Treatment of caffeine intoxication by exchange transfusion in a newborn. Acta Paediatr Scand. 1987;76:679-81.

108. Hootkins R, Lerman MJ, Thompson JR. Sequential and simultaneous "in series" hemodialysis and hemoperfusion in the management of theophylline intoxication. J Am Soc Nephrol. 1990;1:923-6.

109. Thanacoody RH. Extracorporeal elimination in acute valproic acid poisoning. Clin Toxicol (Phila). 2009;47:609-16.

110. Franssen EJ, van Essen GG, Portman AT, et al. Valproic acid toxicokinetics: Serial hemodialysis and hemoperfusion. Ther Drug Monit. 1999;21:289-92.

111. Isbister GK, Balit CR, Whyte IM, et al. Valproate overdose: A comparative cohort study of self-poisonings. Br J Clin Pharmacol. 2003;55:398-404.

112. Perrott J, Murphy NG, Zed PJ. L-carnitine for acute valproic acid overdose: a systematic review of published cases. Ann Pharmacother. 2010;44:1287-93.

113. Farrar HC, Herold DA, Reed MD. Acute valproic acid intoxication: enhanced drug clearance with oral-activated charcoal. Crit Care Med. 1993;21:299-301.

114. Richardson D, Bellamy M. Intracranial hypertension in acute liver failure. Nephrol Dial Transplant. 2002;17:23-7.

115. Gubensek J, Buturovic-Ponikvar J, Ponikvar R, et al. Hemodiafiltration and high-flux hemodialysis significantly reduce serum valproate levels inducing epileptic seizures: case report. Blood Purif. 2008;26:379-80.

116. Lin CM, Lin JW, Tsai JT, et al. Intracranial pressure fluctuation during hemodialysis in renal failure patients with intracranial hemorrhage. Acta Neurochir Suppl. 2008;101:141-4.

32
CHAPTER

Extracorporeal Membrane Oxygenation

Anna L Condella, Edward W Boyer

INTRODUCTION

Extracorporeal membrane oxygenation (ECMO) is an advanced supportive therapy for patients experiencing or in imminent danger of cardiopulmonary collapse. Though ECMO has been used in cases of poisoning for over 20 years,[1] it remains a rare therapy relative to the number of poisoned patients.[2] In this chapter, we will review the use of ECMO as a therapy including its history and mechanics, as well as complications, and then discuss its application in poisoned patients.

BRIEF HISTORY

Extracorporeal membrane oxygenation, also referred to as extracorporeal life support (ECLS), is the process of cannulating a patient's vasculature, circulating the patient's blood outside of the body through artificial membranes that allow for gas exchange, and finally returning the patient's now-oxygenated blood to the body. In some cases, circulatory support (mechanical assistance of blood flow) is also provided. As a therapy, ECMO has been used in clinical practice since the 1970s and was developed from short-term cardiopulmonary bypass commonly used during cardiac surgery. In its early years, ECMO had high complication rates and showed no significant survival benefit over conventional

therapy.[3] Its use remained largely in neonatal and pediatric patients, including those with poisoning.[4-6] As technology improved, however, there was renewed interest in using ECMO as a supportive therapy outside the surgical or perisurgical adult patient, especially in patients with acute respiratory distress syndrome (ARDS).[7]

A landmark clinical trial in 2009, known as the CESAR (Conventional ventilatory support vs ECMO for Severe Adult Respiratory failure) trial, showed that patients with ARDS randomized to consideration of ECMO rather than conventional mechanical ventilation had improved survival without severe disability at 6 months. In addition, it provided data which suggested that choosing ECMO for these patients would even be cost-effective.[8] Since this study, ECMO has continued to gain traction as a viable supportive therapy in a variety of life-threatening illnesses, including those which cause circulatory collapse such as cardiac arrest or cardiogenic shock.[9] The Extracorporeal Life Support Organization (ELSO) is an international organization that was created with a goal of maintaining comprehensive data on the use of ECMO and providing clinical guidelines for this complex, resource-intensive therapy (Extracorporeal Life Support: The ELSO Red Book).[10]

MECHANICS OF EXTRACORPOREAL MEMBRANE OXYGENATION

Modalities

Extracorporeal membrane oxygenation has two modalities, veno venous (VV) or veno arterial (VA). VV-ECMO draws blood from a patient's venous system for extracorporeal oxygenation and removal of carbon dioxide, and then reintroduces it into the venous system. VV-ECMO is optimally used in patients who have pulmonary failure but still maintain adequate cardiac function to support circulation independent of mechanical assistance. In contrast, VA-ECMO removes blood from a patient's venous system and returns it to the arterial system, bypassing the heart and directly supporting circulation with a mechanical pump as well as oxygenation and carbon dioxide removal. VA-ECMO is used in patients with cardiac FAILURE that leads to an inability to support circulation independent of the ECMO circuit. Since most poisoned patients who receive ECMO do so for cardiac arrest or cardiogenic shock, VA-ECMO is the more common modality in poisoned patients.

Cannulation

The process of initiating ECMO is often referred to as "cannulation," but that is only part of the process. At a minimum, the team consists of an ECMO surgeon who will perform cannulation and a perfusionist who will manage the circuit. The circuit itself consists of the extracorporeal oxygenation membrane system (which both filters and pumps the blood), specialized cannulae between the unit and the patient, and the patient's vasculature itself. While technique can vary, in all cases the surgeons place the cannulae through femoral and/or internal jugular access and confirm with radiographs their positions in the venous and arterial system, respectively. The circuit is filled with normal saline and the patient placed on heparin to prevent clotting. Once the circuit is complete, a perfusionist monitors its parameters to ensure there is adequate flow of blood oxygenation, and ventilation.[11]

Complications

Both forms of ECMO are associated with complications including renal failure, limb ischemia, intracranial hemorrhage, bleeding at the cannula site and mechanical breakdowns of the circuit itself. In VV-ECMO, complications are less common, and have a lower effect on overall mortality.[12] VA-ECMO carries a higher rate of complications, in part due to the potential for arterial ischemia. One weighted meta-analysis found a pooled rate of kidney injury requiring renal replacement therapy higher than 40%.[13,14] Complications resulting in permanent disability were less common but still significant, with recent estimates of patients on VA-ECMO having a 15.2% rate of neurologic sequelae and 3.12% rate of lower extremity amputation.[13] It is important to consider these complications in context. Patients on VA-ECMO by definition have severe underlying illness, which independent of VA-ECMO may result in permanent disability. As with any intervention, the potential risks of VA-ECMO are relative to the likely sequelae of the patient's disease process.

INDICATIONS FOR EXTRACORPOREAL MEMBRANE OXYGENATION

For most practice environments, the decision to involve ECMO is both clinically and logistically challenging. This decision is made more difficult by the evolving availability and cost-effectiveness of ECMO. Institution-specific protocols for ECMO initiation are important guidelines for any provider.

From a clinical standpoint, the broad consensus is that ECMO is indicated in patients who have or are threatened with cardiopulmonary collapse, but for whom the underlying disease process is likely reversible. For example, guidelines published by ELSO suggest ECMO is indicated in any patient with "acute severe heart or lung failure with high mortality risk despite optimal therapy,"[10] where the risk of mortality is 80% or higher. The guidelines also caution that ECMO is relatively contraindicated in patients for whom there is no reasonable chance of survival (futility), or in patients who are likely to have severe disability. Due to the need for anticoagulation, for example, patients with intracranial hemorrhage are like to have far worse outcomes if placed on ECMO. Poisoned patients, as we will discuss further, have a favorable condition in this respect; they are limited only by the extent of the damage the toxin has caused prior to reversal or removal.[2,15]

From a logistical standpoint, ECMO is highly resource-intensive, requiring a team of specialists and equipment to rapidly intervene in a coordinated manner. Even if the patient is already in an ECMO-capable hospital, establishing a circuit requires either an operating room or a hospital room large enough to establish multiple sterile fields and maneuver large appliances around the patient's bed. Furthermore, once the circuit is established, the team may have to contend with the need to transfer the patient to an appropriate intensive care unit for continued management. Despite these difficulties, ECMO has been successfully applied in many challenging practice environments.[16] Recent trends have seen ECMO in a growing number of settings, including outside the hospital, as associated mortality for patients on ECMO decreases.[17,18]

Even when clinically indicated and logistically feasible, ECMO may not be possible for reasons of resource allocation or institutional exclusion. Some patient factors that are correlated with poor outcomes such as advanced age, severe sepsis, or severe brain injury, e.g, might be considered relative contraindications.[15] Furthermore, the associated cost of ECMO—and discussion over the appropriate allocation of this resource—continues to evolve.

PHARMACEUTICAL OVERDOSES

Many cases reported in medical literature for poisoned patients treated with ECMO are now adult intentional pharmaceutical overdoses, primarily of cardiac or psychiatric drugs and frequently involving multiple drugs.[11,19,20] A relatively early study of poisoned adults on ECMO reviewed all patients from 1997 to 2007 at a single center who were placed on ECMO for drug overdose. Most patients had ingested cardiotoxic drugs. Seven were cannulated following refractory cardiac arrest, and ten for refractory cardiogenic shock. This amounted to 17 patients, 13 of whom survived to hospital discharge (survival rate 76%) and 11 who had no significant cerebral performance deficits.[11] A larger 2012 retrospective cohort analysis of poisoned patients at two academic institutions where one center preferentially performed ECMO (referred to as ECLS). A comparison of patients treated with ECMO versus conventional therapies found significantly improved survival rate in ECMO (86% compared to 48% in conventional therapies).[20]

A literature review by Johnson et al. in 2013 identified 30 published cases patients with cardiotoxic drug poisoning treated with ECMO. Of these, 66% (20) patients survived without any serious sequelae. A striking feature of this review is the variety of drugs in the literature— single-agent poisonings included verapamil, flecainide, diltiazem, ibuprofen and bupropion, with each of the patients with these overdoses survived to full recovery.[19]

Overall, while randomized clinical trials or meta-analyses for ECMO in patients with pharmaceutical poisoning have not been performed, a growing body of evidence exists that ECMO has an important role in the critically ill overdose patient. Just as intensivists learned to consider mechanical ventilation for patients in imminent respiratory failure, and emergency physicians have learned to consider the need for cardiac catheterization in patients with a ST-elevation myocardial infarction, so may more and more toxicologists learn to consider the need for ECMO early in the course of massive cardiotoxic ingestion.

Some complications of ECMO must be considered especially in poisoned patients. One of these is the administration of intravenous lipid emulsion, a treatment often given to patients with ingestion of cardiogenic drugs. Evidence suggests that patients on intralipid and VA-ECMO have high rates of blood clot formation and fat deposition in the circuit;[21] this evidence, however, is limited by the small number of overall cases where the two have intersected.[9]

NONPHARMACEUTICAL POISONING

Extracorporeal membrane oxygenation for patients with nonpharmaceutical poisoning has been described in even fewer case reports. This should not, however, be considered a suggestion that ECMO would be less effective in nonpharmaceutical poisoning. In fact, this application of ECMO may have even more robust evidence because many nonpharmaceutically poisoned patients suffer isolated respiratory failure and may require only VV-ECMO. As detailed above, this form of ECMO carries lower complication rates and has randomized clinical data supporting its use in patients with respiratory failure.

Carbon monoxide poisoning is one form of common nonpharmaceutical poisoning now with multiple case reports of survival to full recovery.[22-24] Another recent case report detailed the survival of a patient with inhalation injury from zinc chloride (a common ingredient in smoke bombs), following VV-ECMO.[25] VV-ECMO was also successfully used as a bridge to lung transplant for a patient poisoned with paraquat, a common herbicide with high mortality in cases of inhalation injury and no antidote.[26,27] Patients with other toxic inhalations which lead to inhalation injury and respiratory failure have the potential to benefit from VV-ECMO (Table 1).[28-30]

Table 1: Summary of poisoning agents and their likely extracorporeal membrane oxygenation modality, with potential duration of treatment based on limited available evidence.

Agent	Symptoms of poisoning	Likely ECMO modality	Potential duration of treatment
Calcium channel blocking agents	Cardiovascular collapse	VA-ECMO	4–6 days[31]
Beta-adrenergic blocking agents	Cardiovascular collapse	VA-ECMO	4–6 days[20]
Tricyclic antidepressants	Cardiovascular collapse	VA-ECMO	1–4 days[32,33]
Colchicine ingestion	Cardiovascular collapse	VA-ECMO	4–14 days[34,35]
Paraquat inhalation	Respiratory failure	VV-ECMO	7–14 days[26,27]
Carbon monoxide inhalation	Respiratory failure and cardiovascular collapse	VV-ECMO or VA-ECMO	7–10 days[22,36]
Cyanide/undifferentiated smoke inhalation	Respiratory failure	VV-ECMO	10–14 days[37,38]

(ECMO: extracorporeal membrane oxygenation; VA: venoarterial; VV: venovenous)

PEDIATRIC CONSIDERATIONS

As with many medications, devices, and interventions, ECMO has not been thoroughly tested in pediatric patients. Although its utility remains unclear, a 2016 review of all ECMO cases in patients reported to the American College of Medical Toxicology Investigators Consortium (ACMT-ToxIC) registry found two children were placed on VA-ECMO for carbon monoxide poisoning and survived.[2] ECMO has also been used unsuccessfully in the treatment of arsenic poisoning in a 4-month-old infant, demonstrating the range of patient ages in which ECMO may be applied.[5]

CONCLUSION

Extracorporeal membrane oxygenation has been used as a supportive therapy in poisoned patients for many years and has good outcomes for the majority of patients. Although it remains a relatively rare intervention with limited evidence, all clinicians with a poisoned patient in high probability of cardiopulmonary collapse should consider ECMO as a matter of course. Poisoned patients have higher recoverability and are often younger in age, representing a favorable population for aggressive intervention with ECMO. As ECMO continues to evolve in technology and availability, so the number of poisoned patients who receive this intervention should increase.

KEY POINTS

- Extracorporeal membrane oxygenation is an advanced resource-intensive therapy indicated in patients with cardiopulmonary collapse due to a reversible cause
- Case reports and series have shown positive outcomes in the use of ECMO for poisoned patients who are threatened with or experience cardiopulmonary collapse
- Venoarterial–ECMO is most commonly used in pharmaceutical overdoses, while VV-ECMO is more appropriate in inhalation injury
- Extracorporeal membrane oxygenation continues to develop as a technology and should be considered early in the course of any poisoned patient requiring aggressive supportive therapy.

REFERENCES

1. Holzer M, Sterz F, Schoerkhuber W, et al. Successful resuscitation of a verapamil-intoxicated patient with percutaneous cardiopulmonary bypass. Crit Care Med. 1999;27(12):2818-23.
2. Wang GS, Levitan R, Wiegand TJ, et al. Extracorporeal membrane oxygenation (ECMO) for severe toxicological exposures: Review of the Toxicology Investigators Consortium (ToxIC). J Med Toxicol. 2016;12(1):95-9.
3. Morris AH, Wallace CJ, Menlove RL, et al. Randomized clinical trial of pressure-controlled inverse ratio ventilation and extracorporeal CO2 removal for adult respiratory distress syndrome. Am J Respir Crit Care Med. 1994;149(2 Pt 1):295-305.
4. Chyka PA. Benefits of extracorporeal membrane oxygenation for hydrocarbon pneumonitis. J Toxicol Clin Toxicol. 1996;34(4):357-63.
5. Lai MW, Boyer EW, Kleinman ME, et al. Acute arsenic poisoning in two siblings. Pediatrics. 2005;116(1):249-57.
6. Marciniak KE, Thomas IH, Brogan TV, et al. Massive ibuprofen overdose requiring extracorporeal membrane

oxygenation for cardiovascular support. Pediatr Crit Care Med. 2007;8(2):180-2.

7. Cavarocchi NC. Introduction to extracorporeal membrane oxygenation. Crit Care Clin. 2017;33(4):763-6.

8. Peek GJ, Mugford M, Tiruvoipati R, et al. Efficacy and economic assessment of conventional ventilatory support versus extracorporeal membrane oxygenation for severe adult respiratory failure (CESAR): a multicentre randomised controlled trial. Lancet. 2009;374(9698): 1351-63.

9. Tramm R, Ilic D, Davies AR, et al. Extracorporeal membrane oxygenation for critically ill adults. Cochrane Database Syst Rev. 2015;1:CD010381.

10. Extracorporeal Life Support Organization. ELSO Guidelines for Cardiopulmonary Extracorporeal Life Support(Version 1.3 edition). Ann Arbor: ELSO; 2013.

11. Daubin C, Lehoux P, Ivascau C, et al. Extracorporeal life support in severe drug intoxication: a retrospective cohort study of seventeen cases. Crit Care. 2009;13(4):R138.

12. Vaquer S, de Haro C, Peruga P, et al. Systematic review and meta-analysis of complications and mortality of veno-venous extracorporeal membrane oxygenation for refractory acute respiratory distress syndrome. Ann Intensive Care. 2017;7(1):51.

13. Cheng R, Hachamovitch R, Kittleson M, et al. Complications of extracorporeal membrane oxygenation for treatment of cardiogenic shock and cardiac arrest: a meta-analysis of 1,866 adult patients. Ann Thorac Surg. 2014;97(2):610-6.

14. Zangrillo A, Landoni G, Biondi-Zoccai G, et al. A meta-analysis of complications and mortality of extracorporeal membrane oxygenation. Crit Care Resusc. 2013;15(3): 172-8.

15. de Lange DW, Sikma MA, Meulenbelt J. Extracorporeal membrane oxygenation in the treatment of poisoned patients. Clin Toxicol (Phila). 2013;51(5):385-93.

16. Fagnoul D, Combes A, De Backer D. Extracorporeal cardiopulmonary resuscitation. Curr Opin Crit Care. 2014;20(3):259-65.

17. Karagiannidis C, Brodie D, Strassmann S, et al. Extracorporeal membrane oxygenation: evolving epidemiology and mortality. Intensive Care Med. 2016;42(5):889-96.

18. Reynolds JC, Grunau BE, Elmer J, et al. Prevalence, natural history, and time-dependent outcomes of a multi-center North American cohort of out-of-hospital cardiac arrest extracorporeal CPR candidates. Resuscitation. 2017;117:24-31.

19. Johnson NJ, Gaieski DF, Allen SR, et al. A review of emergency cardiopulmonary bypass for severe poisoning by cardiotoxic drugs. J Med Toxicol. 2013;9(1):54-60.

20. Masson R, Colas V, Parienti JJ, et al. A comparison of survival with and without extracorporeal life support treatment for severe poisoning due to drug intoxication. Resuscitation. 2012;83(11):1413-7.

21. Buck ML, Ksenich RA, Wooldridge P. Effect of infusing fat emulsion into extracorporeal membrane oxygenation circuits. Pharmacotherapy. 1997;17(6):1292-5.

22. McCunn M, Reynolds HN, Cottingham CA, et al. Extracorporeal support in an adult with severe carbon monoxide poisoning and shock following smoke inhalation: a case report. Perfusion. 2000;15(2):169-73.

23. Teerapuncharoen K, Sharma NS, Barker AB, et al. Successful treatment of severe carbon monoxide poisoning and refractory shock using extracorporeal membrane oxygenation. Respir Care. 2015;60(9):e155-60.

24. Baran DA, Stelling K, McQueen D, et al. Pediatric veno-veno extracorporeal membrane oxygenation rescue from carbon monoxide poisoning. Pediatr Emerg Care. 2018.

25. Chian CF, Wu CP, Chen CW, et al. Acute respiratory distress syndrome after zinc chloride inhalation: survival after extracorporeal life support and corticosteroid treatment. Am J Crit Care. 2010;19(1):86-90.

26. Kumar H, Singh VB, Meena BL, et al. Paraquat poisoning: A case report. J Clin Diagn Res. 2016;10(2):OD10-1.

27. Tang X, Sun B, He H, et al. Successful extracorporeal membrane oxygenation therapy as a bridge to sequential bilateral lung transplantation for a patient after severe paraquat poisoning. Clin Toxicol (Phila). 2015;53(9): 908-13.

28. Walker PF, Buehner MF, Wood LA, et al. Diagnosis and management of inhalation injury: an updated review. Crit Care. 2015;19:351.

29. Chacko J, Jahan N, Brar G, et al. Isolated inhalational injury: Clinical course and outcomes in a multidisciplinary intensive care unit. Indian J Crit Care Med. 2012;16(2): 93-9.

30. Kumar A, Chaudhari S, Kush L, et al. Accidental inhalation injury of phosgene gas leading to acute respiratory distress syndrome. Indian J Occup Environ Med. 2012;16(2):88-9.

31. St-Onge M, Dube PA, Gosselin S, et al. Treatment for calcium channel blocker poisoning: a systematic review. Clin Toxicol (Phila). 2014;52(9):926-44.

32. Kerr GW, McGuffie AC, Wilkie S. Tricyclic antidepressant overdose: a review. Emerg Med J. 2001;18(4):236-41.

33. Williams JM, Hollingshed MJ, Vasilakis A, et al. Extracorporeal circulation in the management of severe tricyclic antidepressant overdose. Am J Emerg Med. 1994;12(4):456-8.

34. Finkelstein Y, Aks SE, Hutson JR, et al. Colchicine poisoning: the dark side of an ancient drug. Clin Toxicol (Phila). 2010;48(5):407-14.

35. Boisrame-Helms J, Rahmani H, Stiel L, et al. Extracorporeal life support in the treatment of colchicine poisoning. Clin Toxicol (Phila). 2015;53(8):827-9.

36. Rose JJ, Wang L, Xu Q, et al. Carbon monoxide poisoning: Pathogenesis, management, and future directions of therapy. Am J Respir Crit Care Med. 2017;195(5):596-606.

37. Dries DJ, Endorf FW. Inhalation injury: epidemiology, pathology, treatment strategies. Scand J Trauma Resusc Emerg Med. 2013;21:31.

38. Thompson JT, Molnar JA, Hines MH, et al. Successful management of adult smoke inhalation with extracorporeal membrane oxygenation. J Burn Care Rehabil. 2005;26(1):62-6.

SECTION 9

Pesticides and Rodenticides

33. **Organophosphorus**
    JV Peter

34. **Carbamates and Newer Insecticides**
    Vijay Kumar Agarwal, Prakash K Khernar, Amit Goel

35. **Herbicides Poisoning: Paraquat and Diquat**
    Amit Goel, Omender Singh

36. **Organochlorines**
    Ravi Jain, Omender Singh

37. **Rodenticides**
    Sanjay V Patne, Subramanian Senthilkumaran

33
CHAPTER

Organophosphorus

JV Peter

INTRODUCTION

Organophosphate (OP) poisoning continues to be a major problem in developing countries, particularly in India. It is reported that there is one farmer suicide in India every 35 minutes and that the suicide rates are grossly under-reported.[1] This alarming trend has continued for several years despite many welfare measures initiated by the Government of India. On the other hand, in the hospital setting, better understanding of the clinical features and management of poisoned patients, particularly OP poisoning, has resulted in a reduction in the mortality of OP poisoning from over 50% in the 1980s (personal communication) to less than 5% recently.[2] This article will focus mainly on the management of OP poisoning.

CLINICAL PRESENTATION

Patients with OP or organocarbamate poisoning present with the cholinergic toxidrome.[3] The cholinergic toxidrome is summarized by the acronym *SLUDGE* which denotes *S*alivation, *L*acrimation, *U*rination, *D*efecation, *G*astrointestinal dysfunction and *E*mesis.[3,4] Clinically, it is impossible to distinguish between OP and organocarbamate poisoning or between different types of OP compounds, although certain compounds with certain properties tend to have slightly different courses in hospital. A suppressed cholinesterase activity

(butyryl—cholinesterase, pseudocholinesterase and red cell cholinesterase) of less than 25% is taken as supportive evidence of significant poisoning with an OP or carbamate compound.[5]

DETERMINANTS OF TOXICITY OF ORGANOPHOSPHATE COMPOUNDS

Broadly, OP compounds are classified as dimethyl and diethyl OPs.[6] Recently, other classes such as S-alkyl OPs have been described in human poisoning.[7] Various characteristics determine toxicity in OP poisoning. This includes the volume of poison ingested, the class of the compound (dimethyl, diethyl and S-alkyl), the World Health Organization (WHO) pesticide hazard class (class I, II or III), solubility characteristics (fat soluble and water soluble), chemical nature (thion and oxon) and possibly other yet undetermined patient factors that dictate distribution and elimination of the pesticide following ingestion.[6] The common OP compounds implicated in deliberate self harm (DSH) in India are summarized in Table 1 and classified based on the type of compound, WHO class of the compound[8] and chemical nature of the OP compounds.

Classification is based on the class of compound (dimethyl, diethyl, or S-alkyl), the WHO pesticide hazard classification (I, II or III) as well as the chemical nature of the compound (oxon and thion).

Pesticides and Rodenticides

Table 1: Classification of the common organophosphate compounds implicated in deliberate self harm in India.

WHO classification	Class of compound			Chemical nature
	Dimethyl	Diethyl	S-alkyl	
Class I	• Monocrotophos • Phosphamidon • Oxydemeton-methyl • Dichlorvos	–	–	Oxon
	• Methyl Parathion	• Phorate • Triazophos • Parathion	–	Thion
Class II			• Profenofos	Oxon
	• Dimethoate • Fenthion • Phenthoate	• Quinalphos • Chlorpyrifos • Ethion	–	Thion
Class III	• Acephate	–	–	Oxon
	• Malathion	–	–	Thion

(WHO: World Health Organization)

MANAGEMENT OF POISONING

The management of OP poisoning can be broadly classified as supportive therapy and specific therapy. The components of supportive and specific therapy are summarized in Table 2.

Supportive Therapy

Airway, Breathing and Circulation of a Critically Ill Patient

- *Airway:* Patients with OP poisoning often present with the inability to protect the airway. This is due to reduced consciousness which may be due to the poison, coingestion of other neurodepressive substances such as alcohol or secondary to cortical dysfunction due to trauma (as a result of a fall), hypoxia, hypotension and other metabolic effects of the poison. The airway may be compromised by aspiration of vomitus and secretions, foreign body,[9] oral structures (tongue falling back) or traumatic intubation, further compounding the problem. It is important that the airway is secured in this situation. The airway is cleared of secretions by suctioning. An oral airway may be inserted to keep the airway open, if the cause of the obstructed airway is the tongue falling back. Maneuvers such as the triple maneuver,[10] which involves chin-lift, jaw thrust and head-tilt may be deployed while preparing to secure the airway. The patient is preoxygenated during this

Table 2: Components of supportive and specific therapy in acute organophosphate poisoning.

Supportive therapy	Specific therapy
ABC—support of airway, breathing and circulation	Reduction of poison load
Management of complications related to poison	Antidotal therapy
Management of complications related to hospitalization*	Countering the clinical effect of poison on organ systems
	Measures to eliminate or enhance elimination of the poison

* Would include ventilator related complications, nosocomial infections.
(ABC: airway, breathing and circulation)

time with bag and mask ventilation and an assessment of the anticipated difficulty of the airway is undertaken simultaneously.[11] If difficult airway is anticipated, it may be prudent to get the anesthetist to be on standby. A rapid sequence induction (RSI) for intubation is preferred in these patients. Succinylcholine is generally avoided for neuromuscular blockade for intubation since clearance of this drug may be delayed due to acetylcholinesterase inhibition by the OP compound.[12] Nondepolarizing neuromuscular blocking drugs such as rocuronium may be used for intubation.

- *Breathing*: The breathing compound is also impaired in acute OP poisoning. Both type I and type II respiratory failure are observed in OP poisoning. Type I respiratory failure is contributed by V/Q mismatch as a result of shunting or dead space and type II respiratory failure due to hypoventilation as a result of central effects (neurodepressive effect of the poison, hypoxia and metabolic) compounded by peripheral effects (neuromuscular dysfunction) and increased work of breathing and resultant fatigue due to increase in airway resistance (compromised airway) and reduced compliance (bronchorrhea and aspiration). In a patient whose breathing is severely compromised, intubation and ventilation needs to be done immediately. However, in borderline patients, support of oxygenation, atropinization and measures to open airway may help prevent intubation. Atropine helps by drying the respiratory secretions, clearing the airway, improving the Glasgow Coma Scale (GCS) by its central effects on the brain and improving respiratory function by its effect on the neuromuscular junction.[13] There is no evidence to suggest that atropine should be withheld till the hypoxia is corrected.[14] Noninvasive ventilation may be tried in the subset of patients who are able to protect their airway. However, there are no studies on the role of noninvasive ventilation in OP poisoning. Often airway compromise and reduced GCS preclude the use of noninvasive ventilation in this setting.
- *Circulation*: Patients with OP poisoning present with bradycardia and hypotension. These respond well to rapid atropinization.[15] Hypotension is also managed with fluid resuscitation and if refractory, vasoactive agents may be used judicially. Atropinization and targets will be discussed in the specific therapy section below. In a subset of patients who are refractory to high dose atropine therapy (target heart rate not achieved), our experience (personal communication) suggests that a small dose of adrenaline as an infusion (1–2 μg/min) improves hemodynamics with a reduction in the dose of atropine required to maintain heart rate.

Management of Complications Related to the Poison

- *Intermediate syndrome:* About one-fifth to one-half of patients with OP poisoning develop profound neuromuscular weakness within 48–72 hours of DSH, termed as intermediate syndrome. These patients manifest weakness of proximal muscles, neck muscles and respiratory muscles[13] requiring intubation at the onset of weakness or continue to require mechanical ventilation following resolution of the cholinergic phase and the onset of intermediate syndrome. Treatment is supportive with mechanical ventilatory support and the muscle weakness is self-limiting lasting for 1–2 weeks with complete resolution usually.

  Electromyography (EMG) is characterized typically by neuromuscular transmission defects.[16,17] Patients with moderate muscle weakness have an initial decrement-increment pattern at high rates of stimulation, which progresses to decrement-increment patterns at intermediate and low frequency.[17] Further progression of muscle weakness results in decrement-increment response and repetitive fade patterns.[17]

- *Organophosphate coma*: Coma is seen in the acute phase of OP poisoning.[4] Altered conscious state is multifactorial as described earlier. Delayed OP encephalopathy and coma occur in some patients between 4 and 7 days after poisoning.[18,19] Patient may either develop an encephalopathy like picture or go into profound coma with clinical features consistent with brain death. The clinical clue to this brain death mimic is pin-point pupils as opposed to fixed dilated pupils in brain death. A computed tomography (CT) scan or magnetic resonance imaging (MRI) may be done to rule out structural changes in the brain; however, these are often negative and do not contribute to the management, unless there was profound hypoxia or hypotension at any time that could contribute to hypoxic brain injury. Electroencephalography shows bihemispheric slowing[18] implying that the patient is not brain dead. This phenomenon lasts 3–5 days and spontaneously resolves. The coma is thought to be due to saturation of central receptors by the OP compound over time and the delay is attributed to redistribution of the compound from the lipid tissue.[18,19] Clinicians should be aware of this problem and manage appropriately and counsel the patient's family that this is generally a transient phenomenon. No specific treatment is required. However, some patients may need increased atropine dose during this period due to resurgence of cholinergic symptoms.

Pesticides and Rodenticides

- *Extrapyramidal manifestations*: Some patients with severe OP poisoning develop discomforting extrapyramidal manifestations during the second week of hospitalization.[20-23] The manifestations include dystonia, rigidity and tremors.[20] These symptoms are self-limiting and resolve within 1–2 weeks of occurrence.[20] The extrapyramidal manifestations may be managed with the use of centrally acting anticholinergics such as trihexyphenidyl,[24] amantadine,[25] and dopamine agonists such as bromocriptine.[24]
- *Other complications*: Other complications related to the poison per se include cerebellar manifestations,[26] diaphragmatic paralysis[27] and late onset laryngeal dysfunction resulting in failed extubation.[28]

Management of Complications Related to Hospitalization

Patients with OP poisoning appear to be more prone for infection (personal communication). There is some evidence that OP compounds may interfere with leukocyte function,[29] which may explain the increased propensity to develop infections when compared with other agents of DSH. The need for prolonged mechanical ventilation as well as the need for organ support also predisposes the patient to ventilator-associated pneumonia (VAP), catheter-associated blood stream infections (CRBSI) as well as catheter-associated urinary tract infection (CAUTI), although the latter is not as frequently seen. These are managed as per standard protocols of management of infections, keeping in mind the need to look at local antimicrobial sensitivity patterns to guide antibiotic therapy.

Ventilator associated complications such as barotrauma are managed as per standard guidelines. Patients requiring renal replacement therapy (RRT) are supported by dialysis.

Specific Therapy

Reduction of Poison Load

This involves skin and gut decontamination. Skin decontamination is an important aspect and should not be neglected. The contaminated clothes are removed and the patient washed with soap and water. Care should be taken by the health personnel to avoid contamination as there are reports of healthcare providers developing cholinergic symptoms as a result of such exposure.[30]

Cholinesterase sponges have been applied on the skin in experimental animals; however, they have not been shown to be of benefit.

Gut decontamination is undertaken by forced emesis, if the patient is awake. Gastric lavage and activated charcoal along with a cathartic (e.g. sorbitol) may be used if the patient presents early in the course of poisoning. Studies on gastric lavage are limited and the position paper on gastric lavage suggests that the risk and harm may outweigh the benefits.[31] In OP poisoning, where there is increased gastric motility, the gastric residue may not be sufficiently high, particularly if the time interval between ingestion and lavage exceeds 2 hours. In those patients who have a compromised airway, lavage should only be done (if contemplated) after securing the airway. Activated charcoal has been assessed in a large randomized trial from Sri Lanka.[32] The study did not show any benefit of multidose activated charcoal on outcomes in acute OP poisoning.[32]

Antidotal Therapy

Atropine is the mainstay of antidotal therapy in acute OP poisoning. Rapid atropinization is recommended with an initial dose of 2-mg bolus with doubling of atropine dose every 2–5 minutes till atropinization.[15] Mandatory atropine targets that should be achieved are heart rate more than 100/min, systolic blood pressure (BP) more than 90 mm Hg and clear lung fields.[6] The heart rate targets may be lowered on subsequent days. Since a low heart rate, low BP and flooded lungs are potentially life-threatening, rapid atropinization is recommended. Other targets of atropinization that are monitored in clinical practice include pupil size (mid-position pupils) and bowel sounds (which should just be present). Once atropinization is achieved, target heart rate and BP may be maintained with atropine infusion. There is some evidence that atropine administration as an infusion may be preferred over bolus doses.[33] In patients who have atropine toxicity or are allergic to atropine, glycopyrrolate may be used. One study showed that both these drugs are equivalent although glycopyrrolate is more expensive than atropine.[34] Atropine may also have beneficial effects in reversing the central neurological manifestations seen early in the course of poisoning.[4]

Oximes are nucleophilic agents that have the ability to bind to OP compound and lift them off from the OP-cholinesterase site. However, several clinical trials[35-42] and meta-analyses[43-45] have failed to show a convincing

Organophosphorus

benefit of oximes in acute OP poisoning in humans. Although one study from Pune[46] showed benefit of pralidoxime in acute poisoning of moderate severity who presented to hospital within 2 hours of poisoning, these results have not been replicated in other studies. Some methodological problems (exclusion of sick patient in the Pune study) and ground level realities in DSH (late presenters) suggest that oximes may not be beneficial in human OP poisoning. Reasons for failure of oximes in OP poisoning include mega-dose intoxications, late administration of the antidote, aging characteristics and potential toxicity of the antidote.[43] In the absence of evidence, the use of oximes may be restricted to very early presenters (<2 h) with diethyl OP poisoning of moderate toxicity; even in this group, the evidence is not strong and consistent.

Another antidotal therapy that has been investigated is bioscavenger therapy. Bioscavenger therapy involves the use of enzymes such as cholinesterases to sequester highly toxic OP compounds. They are viewed as "anti-OP" agents rather than the OP compound being viewed as anticholinergic agents.[47,48] Purified human butyryl-cholinesterase is an attractive possibility since it has a long shelf life of more than 2 years in the lyophilized form. Studies suggest that a single dose in mice achieves therapeutic concentration for 4 days.[47,48] In the meantime studies have used fresh frozen plasma (FFP) as a source of cholinesterase. Although it appears that cholinesterase levels improve with FFP therapy,[49] this has not translated to meaningful improvements in clinical outcome in the trials that have used this therapy.[49,50] Albumin has also been tried as a bioscavenger in one trial.[49] There was no significant clinical benefit. However, the trials were underpowered to detect a clinically significant effect.

Countering the Effects of the Poison

Atropine successfully counters the cardiovascular effects of the poison by reversing the bradycardia and hypotension. Atropine, as mentioned earlier, is also able to counteract some of the central and peripheral neurological effects of the poison. Several other adjuncts have been used in clinical trials to try and reverse the clinical effects of the poison.[51] They include magnesium,[52] calcium channel blockers,[52] diazepam,[51] clonidine[51,53] and N-acetyl cysteine.[51,54] The various studies on these agents and the recommendations are summarized in Table 3. Of the agents, only magnesium

Table 3: Therapies used to counteract the effects of the poison.

Therapy	Physiological basis	Human studies	Recommendations
Magnesium	Potential for reversing neuromuscular junction effects; improve skeletal muscle CMAP; cardio-protective effect[51]	Eight comparative studies summarized in a meta-analysis;[52] reasonably well tolerated; some studies showed clinical benefit, some no benefit; pooled odds ratio benefit for mortality and ventilation	Methodological weakness and risk of bias are limitations; magnesium could be considered as an adjunct; more trials required
Calcium channel blocker	Blocking calcium channels thereby reducing acetylcholine release[52]	No human studies; studies on rats[52] reduced lethality (nimodipine) and protection against muscle fasciculation and convulsions (verapamil)	Need more animal studies before human studies are planned; potential to reduce blood pressure may be a limitation
Diazepam	Used for control of seizures and beneficial when given early[51]	No human studies; pretreatment with diazepam in animal models decrease toxicity[51]	Use diazepam or other newer benzodiazepines (e.g. midazolam) for control of seizures
Clonidine	Dose-related inhibition of soman induced cardiovascular channels[51]	One phase II trial of 48 patients;[53]; drop in blood pressure after third dose in 42%; no difference in mortality	Side effects preclude use
N-acetyl cysteine	Attenuation of generation of free radicals and alterations in antioxidant status[51]	One trial in humans involving 46 patients; less atropine requirements; no other outcome benefits; no major adverse effects[54]	Need further trials before routine use in humans OP poisoning

Note: In addition to the above agents, adenosine agonist[51] have been tried in animal models; however, there are no studies in humans. (CMAP: compound muscle action potential; OP: organophosphorus)
Source: : Reproduced in modified form from a table that will be published in "Case-based Review in Critical Care Medicine: A comprehensive preparatory book for the examinee."

appears promising in human OP poisoning. Eight studies have been summarized in a meta-analysis.[51] Pooled results suggest benefit for mortality and ventilation.[51] Larger randomized trials on magnesium are required for confirmation. However, there does not appear to be a major limitation to its use in patients since the dose used in these studies are replacement doses usually used in the critically ill on a routine basis. A dose effect may also need to be studied keeping in mind that higher doses of magnesium may by itself worsen muscle weakness.

Enhancing Elimination

Two methods of enhancing elimination of the poison have been employed and include alkalinization[51,55] and hemoperfusion.[56-58] The possible beneficial effects of alkalinization are enhanced pesticide clearance, volume expansion, improved tissue perfusion and effect on neuromuscular function.[51] Five studies have explored the role of alkalinization and this has been summarized in a meta-analysis.[55] There was marked heterogeneity in the included studies and a trend toward lower dose of atropine requirement was observed in the study. The evidence is, however, insufficient for recommendation for routine use in human OP poisoning.

Hemoperfusion has also been tried in OP poisoning, the basis being the extracorporeal removal of toxins. There have been three recent trials[56-58] on this topic. The results have been variable with use of less atropine, shorter time to improve GCS, and mortality improvement in some studies.[56-58] Cost and resource availability preclude widespread use of this treatment. The absence of properly conducted randomized trials also limits the recommendation of hemoperfusion for routine use in OP poisoning.

CONCLUSION

The morbidity and mortality due to OP poisoning can only be reduced by a multipronged strategy. This would involve the participation of various stakeholders from the government (to bring out legislation to ban the more toxic pesticides), the industry (pesticide manufacturer, to bring out formulations that are less harmful to humans), and healthcare professionals (to reduce the mortality when patients present with DSH). Such a strategy implemented well is likely to result in societal benefits (lives saved), economic benefits (increased productivity of the individual; cost of treatment) and healthcare benefits (reduced suicide burden; better utilization of healthcare resources). As we wait for that to happen, it is important that clinicians have adequate knowledge on the clinical presentation and management of OP poisoning so that the outcome of patients presenting to hospital with DSH will be improved.

KEY POINTS

- The main components of management of a patient with poisoning are supportive treatment (airway, breathing and circulation) and specific antidotal therapy (atropine)
- Multiple factors contribute to compromised airway and breathing in OP poisoning; intubation and ventilation may be required
- The circulatory component is best managed with atropine therapy, fluid resuscitation and judicious use of vasoactive agents, if the patient is refractory to atropine and fluids
- The role of adjuncts in OP poisoning requires further study.

REFERENCES

1. Rediff.com. (2018). Sainath P: How states fudge the data on declining farmer suicides. [online] Available from: http://www.rediff.com/news/column/p-sainath-how-states-fudge-the-data-on-farmer-suicides/20140801.htm [Accessed October, 2018]
2. Peter JV, John G. Management of acute organophosphorus pesticide poisoning. Lancet. 2008;371:2170.
3. Holstege CP, Borek HA. Toxidromes. Crit Care Clin. 2012;28:479-98.
4. Peter JV, Sudarsan TI, Moran JL. Clinical features of organophosphate poisoning: a review of different classification systems and approaches. Indian J Crit Care Med. 2014;18:735-45.
5. Peter JV, Cherian AM. Organic insecticides. Anaesth Intensive Care. 2000;28:11-21.
6. Peter JV, Jerobin J, Nair A, et al. Clinical profile and outcome of patients hospitalized with dimethyl and diethyl organophosphate poisoning. Clin Toxicol (Phila). 2010;48:916-23.
7. Eddleston M, Worek F, Eyer P, et al. Poisoning with the S-alkyl organophosphorus insecticides profenofos and prothiofos. QJM. 2009;102:785-92.
8. Peter JV. Author response to Letter to the Editor entitled, "Is there a relationship between the WHO hazard classification of organophosphate pesticide and outcomes in suicidal human poisoning with commercial organophosphate formulations?" Regul Toxicol Pharmacol. 2010;57:339-40.

9. Jose R, Chacko B, Iyyadurai R, et al. Polythene predicament. J Emerg Med. 2012;43:e31-3.
10. Matten EC, Shear T, Vender JS. Nonintubation management of the airway: airway maneuvers and mask ventilation. In: Hagberg CA (Ed). Benumof and Hagberg's Airway Management, 3rd Edition. Philadelphia; Elsevier; 2013. pp. 324-39.
11. El-Ganzouri AR, McCarthy RJ, Tuman KJ, et al. Preoperative airway assessment: predictive value of a multivariate risk index. Anesth Analg. 1996;82:1197-204.
12. Sener EB, Ustun E, Kocamanoglu S, et al. Prolonged apnea following succinylcholine administration in undiagnosed acute organophosphate poisoning; Acta Anaesthesiol Scand. 2002;46:1046-8.
13. Wadia RS, Sadagopan C, Amin RB, et al. Neurological manifestations of organophosphorus insecticide poisoning. J Neurol Neurosurg Psychiatry. 1974;37:841-7.
14. Konickx LA, Bingham K, Eddleston M. Is oxygen required before atropine administration in organophosphorus or carbamate pesticide poisoning?–A cohort study. Clin Toxicol (Phila). 2014;52:531-7.
15. Eddleston M, Buckley NA, Checketts H, et al. Speed of initial atropinisation in significant organophosphorus pesticide poisoning–a systematic comparison of recommended regimens. J Toxicol Clin Toxicol. 2004;42:865-75.
16. Jayawardane P, Senanayake N, Buckley NA, et al. Electrophysiological correlates of respiratory failure in acute organophosphate poisoning: Evidence for different roles of muscarinic and nicotinic stimulation. Clin Toxicol (Phila). 2012;50:250-3.
17. Jayawardane P, Senanayake N, Dawson A. Electro-physiological correlates of intermediate syndrome following acute organophosphate poisoning. Clin Toxicol (Phila). 2009;47:193-205.
18. Peter JV, Prabhakar AT, Pichamuthu K. Delayed-onset encephalopathy and coma in acute organophosphate poisoning in humans. Neurotoxicology. 2008;29:335-42.
19. Peter JV, Prabhakar AT, Pichamuthu K. In-laws, insecticide--and a mimic of brain death. Lancet. 2008;371(9612):22.
20. Kuzhiyelil KR, Mathew V, Zachariah A, et al. Extrapyramidal effects of acute organophosphate poisoning. Clin Toxicol. 2016;54:259-65.
21. Senanayake N, Sanmuganathan PS. Extrapyramidal man-ifestations complicating organophosphorus insecticide poisoning. Hum Exp Toxicol. 1995;14:600-4.
22. Hsieh BH, Deng JF, Ger J, et al. Acetylcholinesterase inhibition and the extrapyramidal syndrome: a review of the neurotoxicity of organophosphate. Neurotoxicology. 2001;22:423-7.
23. Brahmi N, Gueye PN, Thabet H, et al. Extrapyramidal syndrome as a delayed and reversible complication of acute dichlorvos organophosphate poisoning. Vet Hum Toxicol. 2004;46:187-9.
24. Goel D, Singhal A, Srivastav RK, et al. Magnetic resonance imaging changes in a case of extra-pyramidal syndrome after acute organophosphate poisoning. Neurol India. 2006;54:207-9.
25. Kalyanam B, Narayana S, Kamarthy P. A rare neurological complication of acute organophosphorous poisoning. Toxicol Int. 2013;20:189-91.
26. Fonseka MM, Medagoda K, Tillakaratna Y, et al. Self-limiting cerebellar ataxia following organophosphate poisoning. Hum Exp Toxicol. 2003;22:107-9.
27. Rivett K, Potgieter PD. Diaphragmatic paralysis after organophosphate poisoning. A case report. S Afr Med J. 1987;72:881-2.
28. Indudharan R, Win MN, Noor AR. Laryngeal paralysis in organophosphorous poisoning. J Laryngol Otol. 1998;112:81-2.
29. Hermanowicz A, Kossman S. Neutrophil function and infectious disease in workers occupationally exposed to phophoorganic pesticides: role of mononuclear-derived chemotactic factor for neutrophils. Clin Immunol Immunopathol. 1984:33:13-22.
30. Geller RJ, Singleton KL, Tarantino ML, et al. Nosocomial poisoning associated with emergency department treatment of organophosphate toxicity–Georgia 2000. J Toxicol Clin Toxicol. 2001;39:109-11.
31. Benson BE, Hoppu K, Troutman WG, et al. Position paper update: gastric lavage for gastrointestinal decontamination. Clin Toxicol. 2013;51:140-6.
32. Eddleston M, Juszczak E, Buckley NA, et al. Multiple-dose activated charcoal in acute self-poisoning: a randomised controlled trial. Lancet. 2008;371:579-87.
33. Abedin MJ, Sayeed AA, Basher A, et al. Open label randomized clinical trial of atropine bolus injection versus incremental boluses plus infusion for organophosphate poisoning in Bangladesh. J Med Toxicol. 2012:8:108-17.
34. Bardin PG, Van Eeden SF. Organophosphate poisoning. Grading the severity and comparing treatment between atropine and glycopyrrolate. Crit Care Med. 1990;18:956-60.
35. Cherian AM, Peter JV, Samuel J, et al. Effectiveness of P2AM (PAM–Pralidoxime) in the treatment of organophosphate poisoning (OPP). A randomized, double-blind placebo-controlled clinical trial. J Assoc Physicians India. 1997;45:22-4.
36. Johnson S, Peter JV, Thomas K, et al. Evaluation of two treatment regimens of pralidoxime (1 gm single bolus vs. 12 gm infusion) in the management of organophosphorus poisoning. A randomized double-blind controlled clinical trial. J Assoc Physicians India. 1996;44:529-31.
37. Cherian MA, Roshini C, Visalakshi J, et al. Biochemical and clinical profile after organophosphate poisoning–a placebo-controlled trial using pralidoxime. J Assoc. Physicians India. 2005;53:427-31.
38. De Silva HJ, Wijewickrema A, Senanayake N. Does pralidoxime affect outcome of management in acute organophosphate poisoning? Lancet. 1992;339:1136-8.
39. Abdollahi M, Jafaria A, Jalali N, et al. A new approach to the efficacy of oximes in the management of acute organophosphorus poisoning. Ir J Med Sci. 1995;20:105-9.

40. Chugh SN, Aggarwal N, Dabla S, et al. Comparative evaluation of atropine alone and atropine with pralidoxime (PAM) in the management of organophosphorus poisoning. JIACM. 2005;6:33-7.

41. Balali-Mood M, Shariat M. Treatment of organophosphate poisoning. Experience of nerve agents and acute pesticide poisoning on the effect of oximes. J Physiol Paris. 1998;92:375-8.

42. Eddleston M, Eyer P, Worek F, et al. Pralidoxime in acute organophosphorus insecticide poisoning –a randomized controlled trial. PLoS Med. 2009;6:e1000104.

43. Peter JV, Moran JL, Graham PL. Advances in the management of organophosphate poisoning. Expert Opin Pharmacother. 2007;8:1451-64.

44. Peter JV, Moran JL, Graham P. Oxime therapy and outcome in human organophosphate poisoning: an evaluation using meta-analytic techniques. Crit Care Med. 2006;34:502-10.

45. Buckley NA, Eddleston M, Li Y, et al. Oximes for acute organophosphate pesticide poisoning. Cochrane Database Syst Rev. 2011;16:CD005085.

46. Pawar KS, Bhoite RR, Pillay CP, et al. Continuous pralidoxime infusion versus repeated bolus injection to treat organophosphorus insecticide poisoning: a randomized controlled trial. Lancet. 2006;368: 2136-41.

47. Doctor BP, Saxena A. Bioscavengers for the protection of humans against organophosphate toxicity. Chem Biol Interact. 2005;157–158:167-71.

48. Saxena A, Sun W, Luo C, et al. Human serum butyrylcholinesterase: in vitro and in vivo stability, pharmacokinetics, and safety in mice. Chem Biol Interact. 2005;157–158:199-203.

49. Pichamuthu K, Jerobin J, Nair A, et al. Bioscavenger therapy for organophosphate poisoning–an open labelled pilot randomized trial comparing fresh frozen plasma or albumin with saline in acute organophosphate

poisoning in humans. Clin Toxicol (Phila). 2010;48: 813-9.

50. Guven M, Sungur M, Eser B, et al. The effects of fresh frozen plasma on cholinesterase levels and outcomes in patients with organophosphate poisoning. J Toxicol Clin Toxicol. 2004;42:617-23.

51. Peter JV, Moran JL, Pichamuthu K, et al. Adjuncts and alternatives to oxime therapy in organophosphate poisoning–is there evidence of benefit in human poisoning? A review. Anaesth Intensive Care. 2008;36:339-50.

52. Brvar M, Chan MY, Dawson AH, et al. Magnesium sulfate and calcium channel blocking drugs as antidotes for acute organophosphorus insecticide poisoning–a systematic review and meta-analysis. Clin Toxicol (Phila). 2018;56:725-36.

53. Perera PM, Jayamanna SF, Hettiarachchi R, et al. A phase II clinical trial to assess the safety of clonidine in acute organophosphorus pesticide poisoning. Trials. 2009;10:73.

54. El-Ebiary AA, Elsharkawy RE, Soliman NA, et al. N-acetylcysteine in acute organophosphorous pesticide poisoning; a randomized, clinical trial. Basic Clin Pharmacol Toxicol. 2016;119:222-7.

55. Roberts D, Buckley NA. Alkalinisation for organophosphorus pesticide poisoning. Cochrane Database Syst Rev. 2005;1:CD004897

56. Liang MJ, Zhang Y. Clinical analysis of penehyclidine hydrochloride combined with hemoperfusion in the treatment of acute severe organophosphorus pesticide poisoning. Genet Mol Res. 2015;14:4914-9.

57. Dong H, Weng YB, Zhen GS, et al. Clinical emergency treatment of 68 patients with severe organophosphorus poisoning and prognosis analysis after rescue. Medicine (Baltimore). 2017;96:e7237.

58. Bo L. Therapeutic efficacies of different hemoperfusion frequencies in patients with organophosphate poisoning. Eur Rev Med Pharmacol Sci. 2014;18:3521-3.

34
CHAPTER

Carbamates and Newer Insecticides

Vijay Kumar Agarwal, Prakash K Khernar, Amit Goel

INTRODUCTION

In the developing world, the toxins that are most commonly consumed are insecticides and a pesticide—aluminum phosphide.[1,2] Pesticides are classified by chemical type into various categories: organochlorines, organophosphates, carbamates, and pyrethroids. Their designated use further classifies them into herbicides, insecticides, fungicides, rodenticides, and fumigants. Carbamates are a recent addition to the insecticide family, and are relatively less toxic to humans because they reversibly inhibit the enzyme acetylcholinesterase (AChE), unlike irreversible inhibitors such as organochlorines and organophosphates. Carbamates—although similar in action to organophosphate compounds—reversibly inhibit AChE to cause a severe cholinergic crisis, albeit for a shorter duration, and their enzyme inhibition is rapidly reversed compared to that by organophosphate compounds.[1,2]

CARBAMATES

Epidemiology

The annual incidence of acute pesticide poisoning in developed countries is approximately 18/100,000,[3] and the numbers are ten times higher in the developing world.[4] In the Indian scenario, pesticides containing aluminum phosphide are the major cause of self-ingested poisoning.[5] Rural populations, which are predominantly agrarian, have easy access to these toxins and bear the major burnt of toxicity. The unavailability of especialty services such as securing emergency airway access as well as inadequately trained staff and equipment to deal with these very sick patients complicate the clinical resolution of carbamate toxicity. In addition, the lack of appropriate government guidelines to ban these highly toxic compounds (WHO Class I toxins) further constitute major reasons for the very high mortality rates associated with carbamate toxicity in India. A cross-sectional survey of 631 farmers from southern India showed that approximately 70% of farmers who apply pesticides do so by themselves, and 75% of these apply highly hazardous chemicals; moreover, 88% do not use any form of protection when applying pesticides.[6]

Pharmacokinetics

Carbamates are chemical esters of *N*-methylcarbamic acid, with variable toxicity based on whether the attached group is a phenol or an alcohol. Pesticide and insecticide compounds such as Baygon (propoxur), Sevin (carbaryl), Furadan (carbofuran), and Posse (carbosulfan) are the major agents causing clinical toxicity.[7] Moreover, depending on toxicity, concentration, and designated use, carbamates can be classified as suitable for "general" or "restricted" use. Various commercially available carbamate compounds, are presented in Table 1.

All carbamates are well absorbed through all primary routes of exposure, including contact with intact skin and mucosa, inhalation, and ingestion. Being lipophilic, they are usually evenly distributed throughout the body and have a high volume of distribution. Delayed effects of toxicity are not uncommon in obese patients because of the tendency of carbamates to undergo fat deposition. Carbamates undergo first-pass metabolism. Following exposure to large doses of carbamates, this effect is overwhelmed with resultant hepatotoxicity. In experimental animals, subchronic and chronic exposure typically resulted in greater hepatic involvement. Hepatic conjugation with sulfur and glucuronidation forms the major pathway of metabolism for carbamates, and the nontoxic, water-soluble metabolites of carbamates then undergo renal excretion. Carbamates, especially carbaryl insecticides, are hepatic enzyme inducers through phase-I isoforms of CYP2C9. They have been shown to reduce the effect of pentobarbital in experimental animals. In addition, inhibition of human hepatic phase-I metabolism through hepatic microsomal enzymes and CYP1A2 has been reported.[8]

Mechanism of Action

Carbamates and organophosphates share a single mechanism of action. Carbamates are reversible AChE inhibitors that act by carbamylating the esteratic site of the enzyme AChE, which is responsible for the breakdown of endogenous acetylcholine (ACh) secreted at the postsynaptic junction following nerve stimulation. Inhibition of AChE leads to the accumulation of ACh at the postsynaptic junction, causing excess stimulatory activity at muscarinic, ganglionic, skeletal muscle, and central nervous system (CNS) sites with exaggeration of their respective effects.[7] The AChE present in plasma and red blood cells (RBCs) is inhibited too, although related symptoms remain largely unknown. However, there are fewer CNS symptoms with carbamates because of their lower ability to permeate through the blood-brain barrier (BBB).[9] Symptoms and signs of carbamate toxicity vary based on their site of stimulation (Table 2).

Despite carbamates being classically described as reversible AChE inhibitors, a compound such as aldicarb [2-methyl-2-(methylthio) propionaldehyde] can have extreme toxicity because its reported LD is much smaller—an oral LD50 of 1.0 mg/kg in rat and a dermal LD50 of 20 mg/kg in rabbits.[10]

Aldicarb

Aldicarb, a white crystalline powder, may be dispersed thorough contaminated food or water although occupational exposure is not uncommon. Exposure via oral or dermal routes can produce extreme toxicity,

Table 1: Carbamate compounds, brands, and lethal doses—generic name.

	Brand names	LD50 (mg/kg)
Aldicarb	Temik, Sanacarb	0.5–1.5
Bendiocarb	Ficam, Garvox, Seedox, Dycarb, Multamat	34–156
Carbaryl	Sevin, Cabramec, Efaryl, Karl	250–850
Carbofuran	Furadan, Agrofuran, Carbodan, Carbosip, Cekufuran, Chinufur, Furacarb, Terrafuran	~8
Methomyl	Lannate, Dunet, Methavin, Methomex, Methosan, Nudrin, Pilarmate, Sathomin	17–24
Propoxur	Baygon, Unden, Mitoxur, Proper	40–50
Aminocarb	Matacil	50
Isoprocarb	Etrofolan, Isso, Mipcin	450
Pirimicarb	Aphox, Pirimor, Pilly, Pirimisct	100–200

Table 2: Characteristics of carbamate poisoning by site of stimulation.

Muscarinic features	• Bronchospasm • Bronchorrhea • Miosis • Lacrimation • Urination • Diarrhea • Hypotension • Bradycardia • Vomiting • Salivation
Nicotinic features	• Tachycardia • Mydriasis • Hypertension • Sweating
CNS features	• Confusion • Agitation • Coma • Respiratory failure
Neuromuscular features	• Muscle weakness • Paralysis • Fasciculation

with rapid symptom onset (≤15 minutes) followed by reduction of symptom intensity by 12 hours. Very high doses can cause respiratory paralysis and, consequently, death. Long-term low-level exposure to aldicarb may cause immunosuppression, but does not have significant adverse effects.[11]

Bendiocarb

An odorless, solid, white crystal with moderate toxicity, bendiocarb is absorbed through all normal routes, although dermal absorption constitutes the most rapid route causing toxicity. Without persistent exposure, symptoms usually reverse within 24 hours. CNS symptoms of headache, blurred vision, twitching, giddiness, and confusion are most common, besides characteristic features of a typical cholinergic crisis. Severe poisoning can lead to bronchospasm, respiratory arrest, and, sometimes, death.[11]

Carbaryl

Carbaryl is a moderate-to-severe toxicity general-use pesticide. Odorless, and available as a grayish-white powdered compound, it is absorbed though the oral, dermal, and inhalational routes. Toxicity symptoms resemble those of other carbamates. Intentional ingestion may cause death. Long-term high-dose exposure can cause neurological toxicity and, in a few cases, immunological abnormalities.[11]

Carbofuran

Carbofuran is available as an odorless, white, crystalline powder; the granular form was banned to protect birds because it resembles food grains, and ingestion by small birds can kill them. A liquid form is in use as a restricted-use pesticide formulation. Carbofuran's ChE-inhibiting effect is short-term and reversible. Death may result due to respiratory failure following high-dose intentional self-ingestion of carbofuran.[11]

Methomyl

A white, crystalline solid with a slight sulfurous odor, methomyl can produce severe toxicity if ingested orally. Toxicity symptoms and clinical management is the same as for other carbamates. Long-term exposure to methomyl may lead to covert inhibition of AChE which then results in flu-like symptoms, reversible on discontinuation of exposure. Individuals with prior long-term exposure to methomyl and suppressed AChE levels although asymptomatic may manifest signs of severe toxicity on acute exposure to low doses of methomyl.[11]

Propoxur

Propoxur—a white to cream-colored crystalline solid—is a highly toxic compound that is commonly marketed in combination with other organophosphates. Propoxur is routinely used in antimalarial mass fumigation. Personnel involved in propoxur dissemination exhibit a significant decrease in AChE levels, and marked recovery is noted on cessation of exposure. Thus far, no adverse cumulative toxicity effect has been reported.[11]

Clinical Features

Clinically, acute toxicity from carbamates cannot be differentiated from that caused by organophosphates. The acute cholinergic phase is characterized by a typical cholinergic toxidrome—diarrhea, urination, miosis/muscle weakness, bronchorrhea, bradycardia, emesis, lacrimation, and salivation/sweating (Dumbbells)—which results from overstimulation caused by ACh accumulation at synapses of the CNS and autonomic nervous system as well as at neurosynaptic junctions in skeletal muscles.[12,13] Plasma cholinesterase is simultaneously inhibited, although it has no clinical significance beyond the diagnosis of carbamate poisoning. The resolution of the cholinergic crisis is usually followed by an intermediate syndrome presenting within 24–96 hours of carbamates exposure or, at times, as a mixed "overlap syndrome". A new-onset muscle weakness involving respiratory muscles, signs of bulbar paralysis, and proximal limb weakness involving the neck muscles may be seen. This intermediate syndrome and delayed neuropathy is rarely observed with carbamate toxicity.[12,13]

Diagnosis

A diagnosis of carbamate toxicity is mainly based on clinical findings and a history of exposure to a toxic compound. The characteristic petroleum-like odor of carbamate compounds, together with signs of a cholinergic toxidrome, is enough for one to initiate immediate therapy. In cases where there is some ambiguity, an atropine challenge is intravenously administered with 0.6–1.2 mg atropine (in children

<12 years, 0.01 mg/kg); a resultant increase in the heart rate by 20–25 beats per minute usually rules out poisoning or may be indicative of mild toxicity.[14]

Laboratory evaluation of serum samples may not generate very reliable results, because the carbamate-inhibited AChE may recover spontaneously both in vitro and in vivo. Therefore, blood sampling to check for possibly lower levels of AChE activity should be done early, within 2–3 hours of carbamate intoxication.

Another method to confirm carbamate toxicity, which may sometimes be required for medicolegal purposes, is testing of urine samples. A carefully preserved urine sample can be tested for unique metabolites of carbamates even later. Although facilities for such a complex analysis may not be widely available, such testing may be of value for determining alpha-naphthol from carbaryl, isopropoxyphenol from propoxur, carbofuran phenol from carbofuran, and aldicarb sulfone, sulfoxide, and nitrile from aldicarb.

Management

The basic principles for the management of all pesticide intoxications are the same. The primary goal of management is to reduce the toxin load in the body by reducing its absorption, enhancing elimination, and neutralizing retained toxins.[13-15]

An early priority is the management of ABC's—the protection of airways, breathing, and circulation in all severely intoxicated patients. Patients who seem obtunded, delirious, with altered mentation, and/or any respiratory compromise should be considered for early airway management. Endotracheal intubation is undertaken with rapid sequential induction and applied Sellick's maneuver. Succinylcholine can be used for rapid induction of paralysis; however, it can prolong the neuromuscular blocking effect. Nondepolarizing agents are safe for use. Patients with carbamate toxicity may pose challenges to adequate ventilation secondary to complications such as bronchorrhea, bronchospasm, or aspiration of gastric content. In all such cases, atropine dosing, or dose escalation, is necessary to dry up respiratory secretions. High ventilatory pressure with high positive end-expiratory pressure (PEEP), limiting the plateau pressure to 30 cm H_2O, is needed for adequate oxygenation. Ventilated patients should receive appropriate sedation and adequate analgesia.

Furthermore, organ-supportive therapy—that is, management of seizures with benzodiazepines such as diazepam, midazolam, or lorazepam; therapy for hypotension or hypertension; avoidance of hepatotoxic medications in cases with hepatic enzyme dysfunction; and, rarely, support for acute pancreatitis—may be required. Lorazepam (adults, 2–4 mg IV and, children <12 years, 0.05–0.1 mg/kg IV, respectively over 2–5 minutes; maximum ≤8 mg for 12 hours) is increasingly used as a first-line agent for seizure control.

Given the ability of carbamates to permeate intact skin, individuals involved in direct care of patients with carbamate toxicity should use rubber gloves as latex/vinyl gloves are ineffective against this agent. Universal precautions of wearing cap, mask, protective goggles, rubber gloves, and rubber gown during initial handling of such patients are mandatory.

To minimize carbamate absorption, the patient should be distanced from the source of the toxin. This includes removal, bagging, and eventual discarding of any clothing as well as bathing and shampooing of the patient, with particular attention to skin folds, fingernails, postauricular regions, and the eyes where there may be remnants of toxic substances. Soap with 30% ethanol helps to hydrolyze carbamate compounds in an alkaline environment. The eyes should be washed with copious amounts of clean water for at least 15 minutes; in case of persistent irritation, refer for an ophthalmic examination.

Gastric lavage is the most controversial therapy in carbamate poisoning. A secured airway and stability of vital parameters constitute a priority before lavage, especially in patients at risk of respiratory distress. A few studies from Asia,[16] especially China, recommend repeated and extended lavage with saline or water for 48–72 hours because the aspirated fluid had significant traces of toxic material; however, these studies had significant methodological flaws, and meta-analysis that included these studies were inconclusive.[5] Activated charcoal may be used in patients presenting within an hour of exposure.

Antidote

Atropine is a time-tested, lifesaving antidote in pesticide poisoning. It provides symptomatic relief by acting as an antagonist at muscarinic receptors against the excess ACh at end-organ plates. A reversible ACh inhibitor, multiple dosing may be required until tissue concentrations of toxicants that inhibit AChE are reduced. However, atropine has adverse effects because, being a tertiary amine, it can achieve significant concentration in the

CNS, whereas carbamates, being quaternary compounds, penetrate poorly into the BBB. In severe toxicity, atropine could cause greater CNS effects before it adequately neutralizes the peripheral actions of carbamates.

Glycopyrrolate, a quaternary ammonium compound, does not pass through the BBB and, therefore, has fewer CNS side effects;[17] moreover, it has better control of secretions and less tachycardia.[18] An initial dose of 1.8–3.0 mg (children <12 years, 0.02 mg/kg) atropine as an intravenous (IV) bolus is followed by repeated dosing every 3–5 minutes until signs of atropinization (clear breath sounds, dry mouth, and absence of pulmonary secretions) appear; then, a last bolus of atropine is administered, followed by an hourly infusion comprising 10–20% of the total dose required for atropinization.[19]

Tachycardia, dilated pupils, sweating, flushing, and blood pressure changes may be unreliable as signs of atropinization because they may be caused by simultaneously ongoing pathology. Oral secretions may be unreliable in patients who are intubated, unconscious, or with an oropharyngeal airway. In recovering, stable patients, chest secretions are a reliable guide for tapering the atropine dose. Oral ingestion of liquid carbamates may induce early signs of pulmonary edema from aspiration of hydrocarbon fumes that is unresponsive to atropine therapy; this should be treated as an acute respiratory syndrome. Patients on atropine infusion should be monitored for signs for atropine toxicity such as absence of bowel sounds, fever, and confusion. The infusion should be stopped, and only restarted at 80% of the earlier infusion dose after the fever subsides.

The second-line antidotes are oximes, including pralidoxime (PAM), diacetylmonoxime (DAM), obidoxime, and others. Recommendations for oxime use are controversial; however, their unique mode of action—the reactivation of inhibited AChE—validates their continued use. AChE has two binding sites—the esteratic site occupied by carbamate compounds and the anionic site that binds oximes. Oximes thus attached form a new bond with the carbamyl atom of carbamates and diffuse away as oxime-carbamyl, leaving behind active AChE. With extended duration of the AChE and carbamyl complex, the carbamyl of carbamates loses the alkyl group, incapacitating it from binding with oximes—a process known as "aging". Considerable individual variation exists in the intoxicant aging process, with resultant concerns on oxime effectiveness. Most carbamate compounds are reversible, short-acting AChE

inhibitors that lead to spontaneous restoration of AChE activity; aging is an unlikely phenomenon for them.

The WHO-recommended PAM dose[20] for organophosphate intoxication is 30–45 mg/kg IV bolus over 20–30 minutes followed by an 8–12 mg/kg/hour infusion. However, a Cochrane review[21] found insufficient evidence to justify this recommendation.

Oxime use in carbamate poisoning remains controversial for a few reasons: carbamates have shorter duration of activity; reversible AChE inhibitors allow spontaneous regeneration of AChE activity; and oximes have variable affinity for the organophosphate-AChE complex. This does not, however, mean carbamate toxicity is nonfatal. Carbamates, in large doses, can cause prolonged inhibition and significant reduction in AChE levels. Oxime use in this scenario is justifiable. Moreover, oximes are recommended in mixed organophosphate-carbamate poisoning, or in poisoning with unknown pesticides presenting with initial muscarinic symptoms.[13]

Obidoxime is administered as a 250-mg loading dose, followed by a 750-mg infusion every 24 hours. Therapy can be continued until 12–24 hours after clinical recovery or absence of atropine requirement or ventilatory support for 7 days, whichever is later.

Some reasons for failure of oxime therapy are: inadequacy of fixed-dose regimens to neutralize supralethal doses; different half-lives of aging processes in different insecticides; and limited spectrum of oxime activity. Until there is more concrete evidence, oxime use in carbamate poisoning should be continued when clinical dilemma exists as to the specific insecticide causing toxicity, to derive benefits of early therapy initiation. The isolated use of PAM without atropine is unjustified.

PYRETHROIDS

The chemical substances used to reduce, stop, kill or repel any pest including insects, rodents and weeds to microorganisms are known as pesticide. Among the pesticides, pyrethroids are relatively less toxic to mammals in contrast to organophosphorus insecticides. This property has led to their increased used around the world.

We have staked our health by increasing the concentration of these pesticides in our food and environment indirectly by using them more in modern agriculture for increasing the productivity. Further they are being combined with other pesticides especially organophosphorus to overcome emerging pyrethroid resistance in agricultural pests, but they end up potentiating the detrimental toxic effects of each other for human lives.

Pyrethrins are found in the flower heads of *Chrysanthemum cinerariaefolium*. This is a natural insecticide and gets rapidly decomposed by sunlight. In 1949, first synthetic analogue allethrin was produced and they were named as pyrethroids. On the basis of structure and efficacy, they are further divided into type I and II. The common pyrethroids are as listed in Table 3.

They are widely used both commercially—for grain storage, in poultry pens, on dogs and cats to control lice and fleas[22] and against household pests like mosquitoes, houseflies, and cockroaches.[23]

Mechanism of Action

Pyrethroids are about 2,250 times more toxic to insects compared to mammals because insects have more sensitive sodium channel, smaller body size and lower body temperature.[24] Moreover, mammals have tough skin with less absorption and swift metabolism to nontoxic metabolites.[25,26] Rapid detoxification occurs by ester hydrolysis.

Piperonyl butoxide, a component of sesame oil is added to pyrethroids as it is synergist, prevents development of resistance and inhibits its degradation.

The main effects of pyrethroids are on sodium and chloride channels. Nerve and muscle are the principal targets of pyrethroid toxicity. Pyrethroids delay the closure of voltage-sensitive sodium channels in mammalian and invertebrate neuronal membranes. This permits prolong sodium influx, a so-called sodium "tail current"[27] and repetitive train of action potentials leading finally to conduction block. The "amplitude" of the tail current depends on number of sodium channels that have been modified by the pyrethroid concentration.

Especially type II pyrethroids have an action on voltage-dependent chloride channels, they decrease chloride channel current in nerves, muscles and salivary glands leading to salivation and myotonia.[28] Both type I and type II pyrethroids have been proposed to have proconvulsant action via benzodiazepine receptors.

Toxicokinetics

Absorption of pyrethroids depends on the exposure site—transdermally—1.2–1.5%, Orally—20–60%. The half-life is 8–10 hours,[29] due to distribution to fat. They are metabolized rapidly in the liver by oxidation and are excreted mainly as metabolites in urine but a proportion is excreted unchanged in feces.

Clinical Features[24]

Pyrethroids are mostly available commercially mixed with organic solvents and variable mix of other pesticides. Signs and symptoms of toxicities depend on route of exposure of toxin.

Skin

Most common adverse effect on the skin is paresthesia, as the cutaneous sensory nerve fibers are hyperactive even to the very low concentration of pyrethroids. Other complaints can be pruritus, tingling or pricking, erythema, burning and blisters formation.

Table 3: Commonly used pyrethroids.		
Type I	*Type II*	
Cyclopropanecarboxylic ester structure	Alpha-cyano-cyano group at the benzylic carbon atom	Alpha-cyano-phenylacetic 3-phenoxybenzyl esters
• Allethrin • Bioallethrin • Bifenthrin • Permethrin • d-Phenothrin • Prallethrin • Resmethrin • Bioresmethrin • Tefluthrin • Tetramethrin	• Cyfluthrin • Cyhalothrin • λ-Cyhalothrin • Cypermethrin • α-Cypermethrin • Deltamethrin • Fenpropathrin	• Fenvalerate • Esfenvalerate • Flucythrinate • Flumethrin • Tau-fluvalinate

Inhalational

Dust or aerosol droplets of pyrethroids are inhaled. Inhalation may result in nasal and respiratory irritation manifesting with cough, dyspnea, increased nasal secretions and sneezing.

Ingestion

Their ingestion can lead to nausea, vomiting, sore throat, mouth ulceration, dysphagia, and abdominal pain.

Injection

Necrotizing fasciitis develops at the site of subcutaneous injection.

Systemic

Systemic manifestations are less common and occur only after ingestion. They may present with nausea, vomiting, dizziness, headache, fatigue, palpitations, chest tightness and blurred vision.[30]

Convulsions and coma[30] may be the main life-threatening property of pyrethroid poisoning. They may develop within few minutes after ingestion of considerable amount and continue for days to weeks.

Alveolar dysfunction occurs via disruption of epithelium and spreading of infiltrates manifesting as acute respiratory distress syndrome (ARDS).

Cardiotoxicity manifests with electrocardiography (ECG) changes—ST and T wave changes, arrhythmias-tachycardia, ventricular ectopics and rarely sinus bradycardia.[30] These may persist for days to week depending on the amount of ingested poison.

Management

Systemic toxicity is less common but would require intensive care admission, mechanical ventilation and other life-supporting treatment for ARDS, status epilepticus and multiorgan dysfunction. Most of the patients exposed to pyrethroids require only skin or eye decontamination and symptomatic and supportive measures.

As most of these preparations have solvents which may increase the risk of aspiration pneumonia, gastric lavage is better avoided. Administration of active charcoal 50–100 g within 1 hour of ingestion of potentially toxic amount in an adult may be considered.

For paresthesias, topical application of dl-α-tocopherol acetate (vitamin E) reduced the severity of skin reactions by blockade of the pyrethroid-induced sodium tail current.[31]

Benzodiazepines should be considered for status epilepticus as most of the conventional antiepileptics are inferior in controlling seizures. Muscle fasciculations are also better treated with diazepam. Anticholinergic can be used for hypersalivation.[32] Beta-blocker—propranolol has been used for toxic tremors.

Ivermectin increases chloride currents and pentobarbital acts centrally as a membrane stabilizer as well as on chloride channels and helps in reducing choreoathetosis.

ORGANOPHOSPHATE-PYRETHROID COMBINATION

Organophosphate-pyrethroid combinations like cypermethrin-ethion, deltamethrin-triazophos, and deltamethrin-chlorpyrifos are being used to overcome emerging pyrethroid resistance in agricultural pests.[22]

Pyrethroids are usually safe, however in combination with organophosphate which themselves have very high mortality, toxicity is increased due to inhibition of detoxification of pyrethroid by organophosphate.[26] Though final adverse effect profile—organophosphate toxicity versus pyrethroid toxicity depends on the mix ratio of the two components.[33-35]

CONCLUSION

Characteristics signs and symptoms of cholinergic toxidromes facilitate easy diagnosis in cases of toxicity. The availability of the specific antidotes atropine and PAM adds to the therapeutic success rate following carbamate poisoning. Carbamates, less toxic than their predecessor organophosphates, have been recently introduced into the market with an aim to reduce the use of organophosphates and minimize overall animal toxicity. However, this aim has not been met because the majority of toxicity is reported from rural, undeveloped parts of the world where the availability of these highly toxic compounds is common. Several pesticides banned in other countries are still being used in India and are sold at higher-than-recommended concentrations. Furthermore, the changing socioeconomic equation has resulted in an increase in cases of self-ingestion. In carbamate poisoning, initial airway management plays a

Pesticides and Rodenticides

crucial role; but unfortunately, the lack of this facility in this part of the world apparently contributes to the high mortality rates associated with organophosphate and carbamate toxicities.

KEY POINTS

- Carbamate toxicity is easily diagnosed from clinical presentation because of its similarity with the toxicity caused by organophosphate compounds and the signs and symptoms of cholinergic toxidromes (Dumbbells)
- Ineffective early airway management and late nosocomial infection are the major factors contributing to mortality
- Atropine is the first-line therapeutic agent; however, excessive use and possible toxicity should be avoided; oximes, as part of early therapy, should be used until there is more specific research evidence
- Most of the mechanisms of pyrethroids toxicity are clear, but management of patients who are severely intoxicated is poorly understood. Most common complaint is paresthesia after dermal exposure and systemic manifestations are less common and only occur after ingestion.

REFERENCES

1. Gupta S, Ahlawat SK. Aluminum phosphide poisoning—a review. J Toxicol Clin Toxicol. 1995;33:19-24.
2. Eddleston M. Patterns and problems of deliberate self-poisoning in the developing world. Q J Med. 2000;93: 715-31.
3. Calvert GM, Plate DK, Das R, et al. Acute occupational pesticide-related illness in the US, 1998–1999: surveillance findings from the SENSOR-pesticides program. Am J Ind Med. 2004;45:14-23.
4. Eddleston M, Sudarshan K, Senthilkumaran M, et al. Patterns of hospital transfer for self-poisoned patients in rural Sri Lanka? Implications for estimating the incidence of self-poisoning acts in the developing world. Bull World Health Organ. 2006;84:276-82.
5. Li Y, Tse ML, Gawarammana I, et al. Systematic review of controlled clinical trials of gastric lavage in acute organophosphorus pesticide poisoning. Clin Toxicol. 2009;47:179-92.
6. Chitra GA, Muraleedharan VR, Swaminathan T, et al. Use of pesticides and its impact on health of farmers in south India. Int J Occup Environ Health. 2006;12:228-3.
7. Erdman AR. Pesticides—insecticides. In: Dart RC (Ed). Medical Toxicology, 3rd edition. Philadelphia: Lippincott Williams and Wilkins; 2003. pp. 1487-92.

8. Hodgson E, Levi PE. Metabolism of pesticides. In: Krieger RI, Hayes WJ, Laws ER (Eds). Handbook of Pesticide Toxicology. San Diego: Academic Press; 2001. pp. 531-62.
9. Saadeh AM, al-Ali MK, Farsakh NA, et al. Clinical and sociodemographic features of acute carbamate and organophosphate poisoning: a study of 70 adult patients in North Jordan. J Toxicol Clin Toxicol. 1996;34(1):45-51.
10. Dikshith TS, Diwan PV. Industrial Guide to Chemical and Drug Safety. Philadelphia: Wiley-IEEE; 2003. p. 185.
11. Dikshith TS, Diwan PV. Industrial Guide to Chemical and Drug Safety. Philadelphia: Wiley-IEEE; 2003. pp. 184-97.
12. Eddleston M, Buckley NA, Dawson AH. Management of acute organophosphorus pesticide poisoning. Lancet. 2008;371:597-607.
13. Rosman Y, Makarovsky I, Bentur Y, et al. Carbamate poisoning: treatment recommendations in the setting of a mass casualties event. Am J Emerg Med. 2009;27(9): 1117-24.
14. Eddleston M, Dawson A, Karalliedde L, et al. Early management after self-poisoning with organophosphorus or carbamate pesticide: a treatment protocol for junior doctors. Crit Care. 2004;8(6):R391-7.
15. Kalantri SP, Jajoo S. Protocol for management of pesticide poisoning. J Occup Environ Med. 2012;16:93-8.
16. Wadia RS. Treatment of organophosphate poisoning. Indian J Crit Care Med. 2003,7:85-7.
17. Brown JH, Taylor P. Muscarinic receptor agonists and antagonists. In: Hardman JG, Limbird LE (Eds). Goodman and Gilman's the Pharmacological Basis of Therapeutics, 10th edition. New York: McGraw-Hill; 2001. pp. 155-73.
18. Mirakhur RK, Dundee JW. Glycopyrrolate: pharmacology and clinical uses. Anaesthesia. 1983;38:1195-203.
19. Aaron CK. Organophosphates and carbamates. In: Ford MD, Delaney KA, Ling LJ, Erickson T (Eds). Clinical Toxicology. Philadelphia: WB Saunders Company; 2001. pp. 819-28.
20. WHO International Programme on Chemical Safety. Poisons information monograph G001. Organophosphorus pesticides. Geneva: World Health Organization; 1999.
21. Buckley NA, Eddleston M, Li Y, et al. Oximes for acute organophosphate pesticide poisoning. Cochrane Database Syst Rev. 2011;2:CD005085.
22. International Programme on Chemical Safety (IPCS). Environmental Health Criteria 97, Deltamethrin. Geneva: World Health Organization; 1990.
23. Matsunaga T, Makita TM, Higo A, et al. Studies on prallethrin, a new synthetic pyrethroid for indoor applications. I. The insecticidal activities of prallethrin. Jpn J Sanit Zool. 1987;38:219-23.
24. Bradberry SM, Cage SA, Proudfoot AT, et al. Poisoning due to pyrethroids. Toxicol Rev. 2005;24:93-106.
25. Narahashi T. Neuronal ion channels as the target sites of insecticides. Pharmacol Toxicol. 1996;78:1-14.
26. Bradbury SP, Coats JR. Comparative toxicology of the pyrethroid insecticides. Rev Environ Contam Toxicol. 1989;108:133-77.

Carbamates and Newer Insecticides

27. Miyamoto J, Kaneko H, Tsuji R, et al. Pyrethroids, nerve poisons: how their risks to human health should be assessed. Toxicol Lett. 1995;82-83:933-40.
28. Ray DE, Sutharsan S, Forshaw PJ. Actions of pyrethroid insecticides on voltage-gated chloride channels in neuroblastoma cells. Neurotoxicology. 1997;18:755-60.
29. Anadón A, Martinez-Larrañaga MR, Fernandez-Cruz ML, et al. Toxicokinetics of deltamethrin and its 4′-HO-metabolite in the rat. Toxicol Appl Pharmacol. 1996;141:8-16.
30. He F, Wang S, Liu L, et al. Clinical manifestations and diagnosis of acute pyrethroid poisoning. Arch Toxicol. 1989;63:54-8.
31. Song JH, Narahashi T. Selective block of tetramethrin-modified sodium channels by (+/-)-alpha-tocopherol (vitamin E). J Pharmacol Exp Ther. 1995;275:1402-11.
32. Ram JS, Kumar SS, Jayarajan A, Kuppuswamy G. Continuous infusion of high doses of atropine in the management of organophosphorus compound poisoning. J Assoc Physicians India. 1991;39:190-3.
33. Tripathi M, Pandey R, Ambesh SP, et al. A mixture of organophosphate and pyrethroid intoxication requiring intensive care unit admission: a diagnostic dilemma and therapeutic approach. Anaesth Analg. 2006;103:410-2.
34. Iyyadurai R, Peter JV, Immanuel S, et al. Organophosphate-pyrethroid combination pesticides may be associated with increased toxicity in human poisoning compared to either pesticide alone. Clin Toxicol (Phila). 2014;52(5):538-41.
35. Gupta B, Kerai S, Khan I. Organophosphate-pyrethroid combined poisoning may be associated with prolonged cholinergic symptoms compared to either poison alone. Indian J Anaesth. 2018;62:903-5.

35
CHAPTER

Herbicides Poisoning: Paraquat and Diquat

Amit Goel, Omender Singh

INTRODUCTION

Developing countries have many major public health issues including pesticides poisoning. The approximate estimate death in Asia pacific region is about 280,000–320,000 per year.[1,2]

Paraquat is most widely used bipyridyl agent and is an essential component of weed control in many agricultural regions, horticulture and forestry. India like many other countries reports this as leading pesticide killer.[3,4]

Paraquat poisoning is a global problem. Trinidad, Tobago and Samoa reported 63–76% suicide death in late nineties all attributed to paraquat self-poisoning.[5-8] Even developed countries like England and Wales have reported 56% deaths due to paraquat out of all pesticides ingestion between 1945 and 1989.[7,8]

As per the American Association of Poison Control Centers' National Poison Data System, paraquat was responsible for greater number of deaths than any other pesticide in 2008.[9] Almost all European countries have banned paraquat because of high mortality associated with it.

Paraquat is inherently toxic and there is no accepted and effective treatment guidelines for the poisoning. Most of the treatment options are extrapolated from small, uncontrolled animal studies. The treatment given is either supportive care alone or combinations of various supportive therapies. These supportive therapies include hemoperfusion (HP) and hemodialysis (HD), immunomodulation and antioxidant therapy. However, even the best of centers have the overall mortality greater than 50%.

CHEMISTRY

Paraquat (1,1'-dimethyl-4,4'-bipyridylium) is bis-quaternary ammonium compound with a molecular formula $C_{12}H_{14}N_2$.[10] It is usually synthesized as dichloride salt which is colorless hygroscopic, nonvolatile freely water soluble crystalline solid. Clay soil and anionic surfactants adsorb it strongly and rapidly inactivate it.

Diquat (1,1'-ethylene-2,2'-bipyridylium) is related structurally to paraquat. Both consists of a bipyridyl ring structure and are found as divalent cation linked with anions such as bromide and chloride.[1]

MECHANISM OF TOXICITY

Paraquat

Oxidative Stress and Generation of Free Radicals

Paraquat undergoes redox cycling by many enzymes systems and generates reactive oxygen species (ROS).

These include nicotinamide adenine dinucleotide phosphate (NADPH), NADH-ubiquinone oxidoreductase, cytochrome P450 reductase, nitric oxide (NO) synthase and xanthine oxidase.[10-13] Monocation radical (PQ+) is generated when paraquat undergoes metabolism via above, which rapidly reoxidized to bis-cation radical (PQ2+) and further generates superoxide (O_2^-) inside the cell. NADP donates while O_2 accepts electron in this reaction. Further, hydroxyl free radical (OH) is generated via Fenton reaction in the presence of iron.

Paraquat induces Nitric Oxide (NO) production from L-arginine by NO synthase enzyme system. When NO combines with superoxide, peroxynitrite ($ONOO^-$) is generated which is a nitrating intermediate and a very strong oxidant. These strongly active oxygen and nitrite species are highly toxic to most of the organs. Lungs have strong affinity to paraquat and show very severe toxicity as they take it up against a concentration gradient.[14]

Oxidative Stress and its Effects

Lipid peroxidation: Paraquat causes lipid peroxidation via free radicals. They oxidize polyunsaturated fatty acids via extracting hydrogen atoms from them. Widespread lipid peroxidation is the key initial pathophysiological process that affects cell functions and may also activate apoptosis, following paraquat poisoning.[15,16]

Mitochondrial toxicity: Mitochondria have complex I (NADH-ubiquinone oxidoreductase) which reduces paraquat and forms superoxide. Paraquat causes membrane depolarization, uncoupling and matrix swelling via Ca^{2+}-dependent transport systems.[17]

Oxidation of NADPH: Cellular defense against oxidative stress is impaired in response to paraquat-induced oxidized NADPH (e.g. reduction in glutathione production).

Activation of nuclear factor-kappa B (NF-kB): Normal cells have NF-kB in dormant stage attached to an inhibitory protein [inhibitor kBa (I-kBa)]. Reactive oxygen free radicals stimulate NF-kB by phosphorylating I-kBa. Activated NF-kB sets up inflammatory reaction in the cells by inducing target genes in the nucleus. This leads to attraction of inflammatory cells, platelet aggregation and fibrogenesis.[18]

Apoptosis: Paraquat induced generation of ROS and stimulation of NF-kB leads to apoptosis by deoxyribonucleic acid (DNA) and nuclear damage.[19]

Pathological Processes

The above explained multiple mechanisms are synergistic and usually occur simultaneously. The most likely explanation why no targeted therapy works when given after poisoning is this multiplicity of pathways.

Most of the other modalities of treatment target other less specific and more common unreasonable processes like inflammation.

Lungs: Paraquat toxicity has its major impact over lungs. Alveolar epithelium remains the most affected part in the lungs. The manifestations are acute alveolitis, diffuse alveolar collapse, congested vessels, apoptosis, attachment of polymorphonuclear leukocytes and activated platelets to the vascular endothelium.[20]

Paraquat toxicity to lungs manifests into three overlapping phases. In the acute "destructive phase," both type I and type II pneumocytes develop swelling, vacuolation and disruption of the endoplasmic reticulum and mitochondria. Sloughing of the alveoli leads to pulmonary edema. This initial phase is followed by proliferative phase wherein the mononuclear profibroblasts fill the alveolar space and mature into fibroblasts in next 7–10 days. Lung fibrosis finally ensues.[21]

Kidneys: The proximal convoluted tubules develop large vacuolation resulting in to necrosis.[22]

Liver: Paraquat poisoning can lead to mitochondrial damage and degeneration of rough and smooth endoplasmic reticulum in liver. These signs of hepatocellular injury may manifest within few days.

Toxicokinetics of Paraquat

Paraquat has rapid but incomplete absorption in gut upon ingestion. It is rapidly distributed to highly vascular organs, e.g. lung, liver, kidney, muscle. Within 12–24 hours after ingestion, kidneys excrete most of the absorbed paraquat rapidly. Paraquat has a high volume of distribution. Two-compartment model can be used to understand plasma paraquat concentration. Central compartment shows time-dependent elimination.[23,24] As the organs that are responsible for bioavailability and elimination shows toxic effects of poisoning, the kinetic parameters become nonlinear. With increasing dose, gut and liver develop toxicity.

In severe poisoning, renal clearance declines rapidly after a few hours. This leads to slow clearance of paraquat distributed to the deeper compartments over days

Pesticides and Rodenticides

to weeks. Based upon days of ingestion, the elimination half-life varies from hours to days. Type II pneumocyte actively takes up paraquat against a concentration gradient[24] which behaves like a third "toxic effect" compartment which has even slower elimination rate than the other deep compartments.

Diquat

It is a strong oxidizing agent, and exerts its poisonous effects by forming free radicals via a single electron addition. NADPH and cytochrome P450 catalyze this process. In contrast to paraquat, lungs do not uptake it actively and it has five times shorter half-life in lung than that of paraquat.

CLINICAL PRESENTATION

Paraquat

Skin

Normally external epithelium of the skin is a strong barricade. Excessive inhalation of aerosolized paraquat may cause stomatitis, epistaxis, sore throat and headache. Erythema, eruptions, boil and ulceration of skin may occur.[25]

Eyes exposure to concentrated paraquat may cause inflammation, ulceration to conjunctiva and cornea and diminution of vision. Although healing is slow but recovery is complete.[26]

Gastrointestinal Tract

As a result of local irritation paraquat leads to nausea vomiting and diarrhea. Ulceration of tongue (paraquat tongue) and mouth, sloughing of oropharyngeal mucosa, dysphagia. Severe cases may lead to perforation of esophagus[27] and mediastinitis, surgical emphysema, pneumothorax, pleural effusion. Liver is often affected leading to icterus hepatomegaly. Paraquat induced pancreatitis and its complications may cause pain in abdomen.

Renal

Renal dysfunction manifests as oliguric or nonoliguric failure and is mostly attributed to acute tubular necrosis. It becomes evident in 1–2 days. In some cases, glomerular and tubular bleeding is seen and others may present with proximal tubular dysfunction. Renal failure mostly presents with microscopic hematuria, proteinuria, glycosuria, phosphaturia aminoaciduria, excessive leakage of sodium and urate.

Pulmonary

Most of the affected patients have cough, hemoptysis, dyspnea. Rarely pneumothorax, pleural effusion and pulmonary edema may occur. Ingestion of substantial amount of paraquat may lead to development of acute respiratory distress syndrome and its manifestations like decreased PaO_2, gas diffusion and vital capacity. Chest X-ray is normal initially but patchy infiltration occurs progressing to complete opacification of one or both the lungs. Paraquat survivors usually show restrictive type of pulmonary dysfunction.[28]

Cardiovascular

Initially they have sinus tachycardia. Ventricular tachycardia, nonspecific T wave changes, intraventricular conduction defects may be seen lately. Terminal event may be hypotension, sinus bradycardia and cardiac arrest.

Neurological

Paraquat poisoning leads to cerebral edema manifesting with ataxia, convulsion and facial paresis and finally comma.

Endocrine

Paraquat leads to adrenal cortical necrosis particularly in severely poisoned patient with multiorgan failure.

Hematological

Polymorphonuclear leukocytosis is commonly seen with erythrocyte aplasia leading to normochromic anemia and hemolytic anemia. Metabolic derangements like raised creatine phosphokinase, hypocalcemia, metabolic acidosis are also commonly seen.

The clinical symptoms of paraquat ingestion rely upon the ingested quantity[29] and patients can be categorized into three classes:[30]

1. *Mild poisoning*: About 20 mg paraquat ion per kilogram of body weight. These patients are usually asymptomatic or may have gastrointestinal

symptoms like vomiting and diarrhea, but usually fully recover.

2. *Moderate-to-severe poisoning*: About 20–40 mg paraquat ion per kilogram of body weight. These patients usually develop severe caustic lesions in the gastrointestinal tract, progressive pulmonary fibrosis and acute renal failure. Deaths occur in 2–3 weeks, from severe respiratory failure.

3. *Fulminant poisoning*: More than 40 mg paraquat ion per kilogram of body weight. Ingestion in large quantity (>50–100 mL of 20% ion w/v) leads to fulminant organ failure affecting all the vital organs. These patients usually present with desaturation, hypoperfusion and metabolic acidosis. Multiple organ failure resulting in death occurs in hours to days.

Two main organs (kidneys and lungs) are usually affected with ingestion of smaller quantities of paraquat. They develop toxicity over the next 2–6 days leading to "moderate-to-severe" poisoning. Renal failure develops quite rapidly. However, as lung accumulates paraquat, they suffer maximum cell damage. The lung involvement has two phases: inflammation leading to acute alveolitis in 1–3 days and subsequent to this is secondary fibrosis. Patient typically presents with worsening respiratory functions due to decreased gas exchange in next 3–7 days. Ultimately in next 4–5 weeks severe hypoxia occurs due to ongoing fibrosis, leading to death. Liver dysfunction occurs in most of these patients. Mortality in this group remains very high (>50%).

However, the usual mode of death is neither renal nor liver damage and survivors usually do not show any long-term dysfunctions of these organs.

Diquat

Skin

Intact skin is an effective barrier against damage and absorption. Corrosive injury leads to burning and hemorrhagic ulceration of oral mucosa. Inhalation of aerosolized diquat may cause epistaxis and throat irritation. Eyes exposure may lead to conjunctivitis and corneal scarring. Nails growth is affected following contact and shedding occurs on prolonged exposure.

Gastrointestinal Tract

Diquat may cause severe and extensive mucosal ulceration. It can lead to vomiting, diarrhea and pain abdomen, paralytic ileus. Mild self-resolving liver dysfunction has been reported.

Renal

Nephrotoxicity ranging from proteinuria to acute renal failure has been seen developing as early as 1-hour. Hypovolemia decreased renal perfusion and direct toxic effect of diquat leads to acute tubular necrosis.[31]

Pulmonary

Diquat leads to development of pneumonia, pulmonary edema. Respiratory failure requiring mechanical ventilation may be there but pulmonary fibrosis seen in paraquat poisoning is not reported.

Cardiovascular

Life-threatening cardiac arrhythmias may be precipitated recurrent attacks of ventricular fibrillation, ventricular tachycardia.[31]

Neurological

Diquat poisoning can lead to development of grand mal seizures, status epilepticus, pontine bleed and coma. The development of aggressive behavior accompanied the complication of intracerebral bleed.

Hematological

Pancytopenia, thrombocytopenia and leukopenia have been seen.

MANAGEMENT

Patient initially presents to the triage, and from there after quick resuscitation they should be shifted to critical care unit for further management and support.

Resuscitation

Standard guideline and protocols of resuscitation (assessment and management of airway, breathing and circulation) should be used. Vomiting can result in aspiration, metabolic acidosis and compromise the airway. Acute alveolitis may further lead to tachypnea and hypoxia. However, as oxygen supplementation may further worsen oxidative stress, so it should be avoided in mild to moderate hypoxia.[32] Accept peripheral oxygen saturation (SpO_2) approximately 88–92%. An arterial blood gas and chest X-ray should be done routinely for all the patients.

Hypotension is mostly because of hypovolemia in the beginning and should be managed with repeated fluid boluses as required. Initially good urine output is required. However, fluid balance monitoring should be done judiciously as urine output starts lowering in first 24 hours and finally renal failure develops.

Patients generally remain alert and awake. In case of impaired consciousness, a strong suspicion of abuse of additional drugs (e.g. alcohol) or severe toxicity should be ruled out. This is due to hypotension, hypoxia or severe acidosis. Moreover, most of the resuscitative measures are futile in case of severe poisoning.

Confirmation and Risk Assessment

Systemic paraquat toxicity can be established by doing a simple bedside test. It uses bicarbonate and sodium dithionite. In an alkaline medium, sodium dithionite reduces paraquat to a blue radical and diquat to blue-green radical.

A high urine paraquat concentration (>1 mg/L) which indirectly reflects plasma level is a marker of grave outcome. So for confirmation and prognostication plasma levels should be done.[33] Plasma samples can be subjected to similar colorimetric technique used for urine.

To offer prediction of outcome from as early as 4 hours till 200 hours after ingestion certain nomograms and formulae for plasma paraquat concentrations have been derived.[34,35] They all have been shown to perform well in predicting death.[36] Plasma concentrations help in decisions making and prognostication. They are useful but not urgent or essential as they do not direct management interventions.

Clinical and laboratory features may also be used for prognostication. Faster the systemic signs and symptoms of poisoning (e.g. hypotension, severe hypoxia, acidosis and low Glasgow Coma Scale) develop worse the prognosis is. Progressive worsening renal dysfunction, chest radiograph and gastrointestinal symptoms are all adverse prognostic signs. "Burning sensation" in the skin has also been observed as a very poor prognostic sign.

Investigations

Apart from paraquat concentrations, hematology (full blood count) and biochemical parameters including serum electrolytes and kidney and hepatic function tests should be done every day. A chest X-ray should be done to rule out pneumomediastinum, pneumothorax or lung fibrosis. To assess present (early lung fibrosis) and long-term lungs condition, a computed tomography (CT) scan chest is helpful. If patient has pain abdomen and hyperglycemia, rule out acute pancreatitis.

Gastrointestinal Decontamination

As paraquat is a lethal poison with no established antidote, a single dose of activated charcoal or Fuller's earth following gastric lavage is advocated for consenting patients after protecting the airway, within 1 hour of ingestion of paraquat.[37,38] Recommended dosage of Fuller's earth:

- Adults and children over 12 years: About 100–150 g
- Children under 12 years: About 2 g/kg body weight.

However, none of these procedures have established clinical benefit in paraquat poisoning.[39]

Clearance Enhancement: Hemodialysis/Hemoperfusion

Hemodialysis (HD) and hemoperfusion (HP) are being done as a routine treatment at several places.[40,41] However, advantage of it is short lived. Firstly, most paraquat is eliminated rapidly as the kidneys get rid of it with very high clearance rate in the first 6–12 hours and relatively modest additional amount will be cleared by using extracorporeal therapies. Secondly, there is very short period when the enhanced clearance will affect lung concentration. A swine model has shown, clinical benefit only when HP was initiated within 2 hours postingestion.[23] Initiating HD/HP 2–4 hours after ingestion can reduce plasma paraquat concentration but that taken up by the lungs is reduced negligibly and hence is unlikely to change overall outcome. The subsequent clearance of accumulated paraquat from the lung is minimally dependent on the plasma concentration. Subsequently performed clinical studies have supported these conclusions.

Case fatality rate reported after routinely doing HP/HD has not changed and is still reported to be over 50%.[40,41]

However, the most important decision in beginning the treatment is early initiation and the choice of technique is secondary. Experimental models have shown, clearance by HD is static but that of HP is high initially but falls rapidly after about 90 minutes.[42]

Other Treatment Options

As paraquat is a lethal poison with grave outcome having no established treatment guidelines, supportive treatment is done either alone or in combination as follows.

Immunosuppression

Paraquat initiates an acute inflammatory response leading to lung fibrosis and death. Interference of this with immunosuppressants may inhibit the processes. Study suggests that the repeated cyclophosphamide and methylprednisolone pulses when combined with continuous dexamethasone are found to have mortality benefit in treating severely paraquat-poisoned patients with predicted mortality 50–90%.[43-45] Dexamethasone has shown a significantly reduced paraquat accumulation in the lungs. The ultimate value of these agents is not known, although some degree of benefit has been observed when given early in the course of treatment.[34]

Antioxidants

There are no clear human studies and data to support their role. Following therapeutic preparations have been tried:

Vitamin E
Vitamin E works by membrane stabilization, oxygen free radical scavenging, inhibiting the activation of NF-kB.[46,47]

Vitamin C
Vitamin C is an antioxidant and works by neutralizing free radicals.[48,49] High doses of vitamin C have been used in paraquat poisoning and have been shown to enhance the total antioxidant status of patient.[50]

N-Acetylcysteine
N-acetylcysteine (NAC) has shown multiple beneficial mechanisms—scavenging of ROS, increasing glutathione and reducing inflammation, lipid peroxidation and apoptosis. NAC restores a critical antioxidant defense, glutathione.[51,52] Studies has shown NAC to increase glutathione in alveolar type II pneumocytes exposed to paraquat.[53]

Deferoxamine

Reactive oxygen species are generated through Fenton reaction in the presence of iron. Iron enhances toxicity of paraquat. Deferoxamine (DFO) has been shown to be protective experimentally;[54-56] however, human studies are lacking to support DFO in paraquat poisoning.

Salicylic Acid
Salicylic acid acts as anti-inflammatory, antioxidant, hydroxyl radical scavenger[55] inhibits the activation of NF-kB,[57] and lipid peroxidation.[58,59]

Salicylic acid has pleiotropic effects but human studies are lacking.

Novel Therapies

Anti-C5a antibodies (IFX-1) have also been used as effective therapy for inflammatory responses induced by paraquat.[60]

Other Therapies

Lung irradiation has been proposed for inhibiting fibroblastic proliferation, but clinical role of it is uncertain.[61] Lung transplantation is of theoretical interest to a few patients only.[30]

Clinical Monitoring and Ongoing Care

Treatment of paraquat intoxication is based on three main tenets: (1) some patients are treatable; (2) early treatment initiation is necessary; (3) renal protection is the cornerstone of early treatment. We recommend the following treatment modality: extracorporeal elimination (HP), intravenous antioxidant administration (NAC, glutathione), diuresis with fluid and short-term cytotoxic drug treatment (steroid pulse therapy, cyclophosphamide).

OUTCOME

The mortality rate varies according to the amount ingested: greater than 60 mL, about 100%; 40–50 mL, more than 90%; 20–40 mL, 50–60%; 10–20 mL, 10–20%; less than 10 mL, less than 1%. The cause of death also varies in accordance with the amount ingested. Individuals ingesting greater than 100 mL fall in to "sudden death" group (death within the first 24 h), and cardiac arrest is the most frequent cause of death. Individuals in the "rapid progress" group (death within 7 days) ingest 50–100 mL, and the most common cause of death is respiratory failure, with or without acute renal failure. And those in the "slow progress" group (death

Pesticides and Rodenticides

within 2–4 weeks) ingest 15–40 mL, and death occurs in all due to respiratory failure.[62]

A patient is defined as a "survivor" if he or she survives greater than 3 months after poison ingestion with stable vital signs and stable lung function. It is extremely rare for a patient to die 3 months later, secondary to paraquat- or diquat-related problems.

CONCLUSION

Paraquat (bipyridyl agent) is a leading cause of death from pesticide poisoning with a mortality >50%.

Lungs are affected the most as they take up poison against a concentration gradient. There are no proven treatment or antidote available. Oxygen supplementation may further worsen oxidative stress, so it should be avoided in mild to moderate hypoxia. Extracorporeal elimination hemodialysis (HD)/hemoperfusion (HP), should be considered early (within 1–2 hours)

KEY POINTS

- Bipyridyl agents are lethal poison with grave outcome
- Oxidative stress and generation of free radicals are the mainstay of toxicity
- There are no established treatment guidelines

REFERENCES

1. Jeyaratnam J. Acute pesticide poisoning: a major global health problem. World Health Stat Q. 1990;43:139-44.
2. Eddleston M, Phillips MR. Self-poisoning with pesticides. BMJ. 2004;328:42-4.
3. Eddleston M. Patterns and problems of deliberate self-poisoning in the developing world. QJM. 2000;93:715-31.
4. Dawson AH, Eddleston M, Senarathna L, et al. Acute human lethal toxicity of agricultural pesticides: a prospective cohort study. PLoS Med. 2010;7:e1000357.
5. Hutchinson G, Daisley H, Simeon D, et al. High rates of paraquat-induced suicide in southern Trinidad. Suicide Life Threat Behav. 1999;29:186-91.
6. Bourke T. Suicide in Samoa. Pac Health Dialog. 2001; 8:213-9.
7. Dargan P, Shiew C, Greene S, et al. Paraquat poisoning: caution in interpreting prognosis based on plasma paraquat concentration. Clin Toxicol. 2006;44:762.
8. Casey P, Vale JA. Deaths from pesticide poisoning in England and Wales: 1945–1989. Hum Exp Toxicol. 1994;13:95-101.
9. Bronstein AC, Spyker DA, Cantilena LR Jr, et al. 2008 annual report of the American Association of Poison Control Centers' National Poison Data System (NPDS): 26th annual report. Clin Toxicol (Phila). 2009;47:911-1084.

10. Yang W, Tiffany-Castiglioni E. The bipyridyl herbicide paraquat induces proteasome dysfunction in human neuroblastoma SH-SY5Y cells. J Toxicol Environ Health A. 2007;70:1849-57.
11. Castello PR, Drechsel DA, Patel M. Mitochondria are a major source of paraquat-induced reactive oxygen species production in the brain. J Biol Chem. 2007;282: 14186-93.
12. Bonneh-Barkay D, Reaney SH, Langston WJ, et al. Redox cycling of the herbicide paraquat in microglial cultures. Brain Res Mol Brain Res. 2005;134:52-6.
13. Adam A, Smith LL, Cohen GM. An assessment of the role of redox cycling in mediating the toxicity of paraquat and nitrofurantoin. Environ Health Perspect. 1990;85:113-7.
14. Rannels DE, Kameji R, Pegg AE, et al. Spermidine uptake by type II pneumocytes: interactions of amine uptake pathways. Am J Physiol. 1989;257 (Pt 1):L346-53.
15. Yasaka T, Okudaira K, Fujito H, et al. Further studies of lipid peroxidation in human paraquat poisoning. Arch Intern Med. 1986;146:681-5.
16. Kurisaki E. Lipid peroxidation in human paraquat poisoning. J Toxicol Sci. 1985;10:29-33.
17. Costantini P, Petronilli V, Colonna R, et al. On the effects of paraquat on isolated mitochondria. Evidence that paraquat causes opening of the cyclosporin A-sensitive permeability transition pore synergistically with nitric oxide. Toxicology. 1995;99:77-88.
18. Schoonbroodt S, Piette J. Oxidative stress interference with the nuclear factor-kappa B activation pathways. Biochem Pharmacol. 2000;60:1075-83.
19. Denicola A, Radi R. Peroxynitrite and drug-dependent toxicity. Toxicology. 2005;208:273-88.
20. Dinis-Oliveira RJ, Sousa C, Remiao F, et al. Sodium salicylate prevents paraquat-induced apoptosis in the rat lung. Free Radic Biol Med. 2007;43:48-61.
21. Smith P, Heath D, Kay JM. The pathogenesis and structure of paraquat-induced pulmonary fibrosis in rats. J Pathol. 1974;114:57-67.
22. Fowler BA, Brooks RE. Effects of the herbicide paraquat on the ultrastructure of mouse kidney. Am J Pathol. 1971;63:505-20.
23. Pond SM, Rivory LP, Hampson EC, et al. Kinetics of toxic doses of paraquat and the effects of hemoperfusion in the dog. J Toxicol Clin Toxicol. 1993;31:229-46.
24. Gaudreault P, Karl PI, Friedman PA. Paraquat and putrescine uptake by lung slices of fetal and newborn rats. Drug Metab Dispos. 1984;12:550-2.
25. Sagar GR. Uses and usefulness of Paraquat. Hum Toxicol. 1987;6:7-11.
26. Joyce M. Ocular damage caused by paraquat. Br J Ophthalmol. 1969;53:688-90.
27. Smith LL, Wright A. Effective treatment for paraquat poisoning for rat and its relevance to treatment of paraquat poisoning in man. BMJ. 1974;4:569-71.
28. Yamashita M, Ando Y. A long-term follow-up of lung functions in survivor of paraquat poisoning. Hum Exp Toxicol. 2000;19:99-103.

29. Bismuth C, Hall AH. Paraquat Poisoning: Mechanisms, Prevention, and Treatment. New York: Marcel Dekker Inc.; 1995.

30. Vale JA, Meredith TJ, Buckley BM. Paraquat poisoning: clinical features and immediate general management. Hum Toxicol. 1987;6(1):41-7.

31. Vanholder R, Colardyn F. Diquat intoxication: report of two cases and review of literature. Am J Med. 1981;70:1267-71.

32. Hoet PH, Demedts M, Nemery B. Effects of oxygen pressure and medium volume on the toxicity of paraquat in rat and human type II pneumocytes. Hum Exp Toxicol. 1997;16:305-10.

33. Koo JR, Yoon JW, Han SJ, et al. Rapid analysis of plasma paraquat using sodium dithionite as a predictor of outcome in acute paraquat poisoning. Am J Med Sci. 2009;338:373-7.

34. Proudfoot AT, Stewart MS, Levitt T, et al. Paraquat poisoning: significance of plasma paraquat concentrations. Lancet. 1979;2:330-2.

35. Hart TB, Nevitt A, Whitehead A. A new statistical approach to the prognostic significance of plasma paraquat concentrations. Lancet. 1984;2:1222-3.

36. Senarathna L, Eddleston M, Wilks MF, et al. Prediction of outcome after paraquat poisoning by measurement of the plasma paraquat concentration. QJM. 2009;102: 251-9.

37. Vale JA. Position statement: gastric lavage. American Academy of Clinical Toxicology; European Association of Poisons Centers and Clinical Toxicologists. J Toxicol Clin Toxicol. 1997;35:711-9.

38. Vale JA, Kulig K. Position paper: gastric lavage. J Toxicol Clin Toxicol. 2004;42:933-43.

39. Eddleston M, Juszczak E, Buckley NA, et al. Multiple-dose activated charcoal in acute self-poisoning: a randomised controlled trial. Lancet. 2008;371:579-87.

40. Koo JR, Kim JC, Yoon JW, et al. Failure of continuous venovenous hemofiltration to prevent death in paraquat poisoning. Am J Kidney Dis. 2002;39:55-9.

41. Hong SY, Yang JO, Lee EY, et al. Effect of haemoperfusion on plasma paraquat concentration in vitro and in vivo. Toxicol Ind Health. 2003;19:17-23.

42. Van de Vyver FL, Giuliano RA, Paulus GJ, et al. Hemoperfusion-hemodialysis ineffective for paraquat removal in life-threatening poisoning? J Toxicol Clin Toxicol. 1985;23:117-31.

43. Lin JL, Lin-Tan DT, Chen KH, et al. Repeated pulse of methylprednisolone and cyclophosphamide with continuous dexamethasone therapy for patients with severe paraquat poisoning. Crit Care Med. 2006;34(2): 368-73.

44. Lin JL, Leu ML, Liu YC, et al. A prospective clinical trial of pulse therapy with glucocorticoid and cyclophosphamide in moderate to severe paraquat-poisoned patients. Am J Respir Crit Care Med. 1999;159:357-60.

45. Dinis-Oliveira RJ, Remiao F, Duarte JA, et al. P-glycoprotein induction: an antidotal pathway for paraquat-induced lung toxicity. Free Radic Biol Med. 2006;41: 1213-24.

46. Suntres ZE, Shek PN. Liposomal alpha-tocopherol alleviates the progression of paraquat-induced lung damage. J Drug Target. 1995;2:493-500.

47. Suzuki YJ, Packer L. Inhibition of NF-kappa B DNA binding activity by alpha-tocopheryl succinate. Biochem Mol Biol Int. 1993;31:693-700.

48. Minakata K, Suzuki O, Saito S, et al. Effect of dietary paraquat on a rat mutant unable to synthesize ascorbic acid. Arch Toxicol. 1996;70:256-8.

49. Perla V, Perrin NA, Greenlee AR. Paraquat toxicity in a mouse embryonic stem cell model. Toxicol In Vitro. 2008;22:515-24.

50. Hong SY, Hwang KY, Lee EY, et al. Effect of vitamin C on plasma total antioxidant status in patients with paraquat intoxication. Toxicol Lett. 2002;126:51-9.

51. Yeh ST, Guo HR, Su YS, et al. Protective effects of N-acetylcysteine treatment post-acute paraquat intoxication in rats and in human lung epithelial cells. Toxicology. 2006;223:181-90.

52. Hoffer E, Shenker L, Baum Y, et al. Paraquat-induced formation of leukotriene B4 in rat lungs: modulation by N-acetylcysteine. Free Radic Biol Med. 1997;22:567-72.

53. Hoffer E, Baum Y, Tabak A, et al. N-acetylcysteine increases the glutathione content and protects rat alveolar type II cells against paraquat-induced cytotoxicity. Toxicol Lett. 1996;84:7-12.

54. Kohen R, Chevion M. Paraquat toxicity is enhanced by iron and reduced by desferrioxamine in laboratory mice. Biochem Pharmacol. 1985;34:1841-3.

55. Arouma O, Halliwell B. The iron-binding and hydroxyl radical scavenging action of anti-inflammatory drugs. Xenobiotica. 1988;18:459-70.

56. Silverman FP, Petracek PD, Fledderman CM, et al. Salicylate activity. 1. Protection of plants from paraquat injury. J Agric Food Chem. 2005;53:9764-8.

57. Katerinaki E, Haycock JW, Lalla R, et al. Sodium salicylate inhibits TNF-alpha-induced NF-kappa B activation, cell migration, invasion and ICAM-1 expression in human melanoma cells. Melanoma Res. 2006;16:11-22.

58. Maharaj DS, Saravanan KS, Maharaj H, et al. Acetaminophen and aspirin inhibit superoxide anion generation and lipid peroxidation, and protect against 1-methyl-4-phenyl pyridinium-induced dopaminergic neurotoxicity in rats. Neurochem Int. 2004;44:355-60.

59. Furst R, Blumenthal SB, Kiemer AK, et al. Nuclear factor-kappa B-independent anti-inflammatory action of salicylate in human endothelial cells: induction of heme oxygenase-1 by the c-jun N-terminal kinase/activator protein-1 pathway. J Pharmacol Exp Ther. 2006;318:389-94.

60. Sun S, Jiang Y, Wang R, et al. Treatment of paraquat-induced lung injury with an anti-C5a antibody: potential clinical application. Crit Care Med. 2018;46:e419-25.

61. Talbot AR, Barnes MR. Radiotherapy for the treatment of pulmonary complicationS of paraquat poisoning. Hum Toxicol. 1988;7:325-32.

62. Gil HW, Hong JR, Jang SH, et al. Diagnostic and therapeutic approach for acute paraquat intoxication. J Korean Med Sci. 2014;29:1441-9.

36

CHAPTER

Organochlorines

Ravi Jain, Omender Singh

INTRODUCTION

Agriculture is the most important economic activity in India and contributes to major amount of country's gross domestic product. Fertilizers, pesticides played an important role in the Green Revolution and their use is on continuous rise since last five decades. Key studies in late 1980s have suggested that developing countries consumes around 80% of all pesticides in world.[1] Several legal, regulatory, and public awareness issues persist in developing world societies that leads to high level of agricultural chemicals exposure, and their target population is usually the first degree users of these chemicals, the agriculturists.[2]

There are many types of pesticides in use but, organochlorines (OCs) forms a major chemical class of pesticide in developing countries in Asia as they have low cost with broad spectrum of activity. Organochlorine pesticides (OCPs) amount for approximately 40% of all pesticides in use.[3-5]

Organochlorine pesticides are multipurpose chlorinated hydrocarbon chemicals. OCPs slowly disintegrate and tend to accumulate in animals in form of fat components, and so OCPs were termed as long-range atmospheric transport (LRAT) organic compounds and listed as persistent organic pollutants (POPs) by the Stockholm Convention.[6]

Among OCPs, dichlorodiphenyltrichloroethane (DDT) and hexachlorocyclohexane (HCH) were widely used in India in both agriculture and community medicine for pest and vector control. But environmental concerns lead to cessation of their use in agriculture in late 1990s, and now it is restricted for community health use for vector control according to World Health Organization (WHO) guidelines.[7,8]

Although chronic exposure is a larger public health concern, however acute exposure is actually a matter of concern for critical care physicians. Toxic level exposure of pesticides is one of the primary occupational hazards among developing world farmers and related industry workers even nonoccupational exposure is also noticed to be of major concerns in nonrelated populations in developing world because of high level of environmental contamination.[9-11]

Pesticide poisoning amounted to around one million deaths per annum all across the world in late 1990s.[12] OCs are second most common agricultural pesticide agents after aluminum phosphide, which are responsible for human toxicities in India. Agricultural pesticides are responsible for total of 12.8% toxicity incidences in India.[13]

PHARMACOLOGY

Table 1 lists pharmacological classification of OCPs. Table 2 provides concise summary of commonly available OCPs, their toxic lethal dose, common use, WHO classification based on LD_{50} and half-life in environment.

Organochlorines

Table 1: Organochlorine pesticides can be separated in five groups of compounds.

S. No.	Compounds
1.	DDT and its congeners (e.g. dicofol, methoxychlor)
2.	Hexachlorocyclohexane (i.e. benzene hexachloride) and isomers (e.g. lindane, gamma-hexachlorocyclohexane)
3.	Cyclodienes (e.g. aldrin, chlordane, dieldrin, endosulfan, endrin, heptachlor, isobenzan)
4.	Chlordecone, kelevan and mirex
5.	Toxaphene

(DDT: dichlorodiphenyltrichloroethane)

Table 2: Major organochlorine pesticides, toxic dose*, main uses, WHO classification based on LD_{50},**, half-life in environment.[14]

S No.	Chemical name	Toxic dose LD_{50}	Use	WHO classification based on rat oral dose LD_{50}	Half-life in environment
1.	Aldrin	Rat Oral: 39–60 mg/kg Dermal: 100 mg/kg Mouse Oral: 44 mg/kg	Insecticide	Highly hazardous	Moderate persistence half-life: 4–7 years
2.	Chlordane	Rat Oral: 200–700 mg/kg Dermal: 530–690 mg/kg Mice Oral: 145–430 mg/kg Dermal: 153 mg/kg	Insecticide	Moderately hazardous	High persistence half-life: 10 years
3.	Dichlorodiphenyltrichloroethane (DDT)	Rat Oral: 113–130 mg/kg Dermal: 2,510 mg/kg Mice Oral: 150–300 mg/kg	Acaricide Insecticide	Moderately hazardous	High persistence half-life: 2–15 years
4.	1,1-dichloro-2,2 bis (p-chlorophenyl)ethane (DDD)	Rat Oral: 4,000 mg/kg	Insecticide	Acute hazard is unlikely	High persistence half-life: 5–10 years
5.	Dichloro-diphenyl dichloroethane (DDE)	Rat Oral: 800–1,240 mg/kg	Insecticide	Slightly hazardous	High persistence half-life: 10 years
6.	Dicofol	Rat Oral: 684–1,495 mg/kg Rabbit Oral: 1,810 mg/kg Dermal: 2.1 g/kg	Acaricide	Moderately hazardous	Moderate persistence Half-life: 60 days
7.	Dieldrin	Rat Oral: 46 mg/kg Dermal: 50–120 mg/kg Mouse Oral: 38–77 mg/kg	Insecticide	Highly hazardous	High persistence half-life: 9 months
8.	Endosulfan	Rat Oral: 18–220 mg/kg Dermal: 74 mg/kg Rabbits Dermal: 200–359 mg/kg	Insecticide	Highly hazardous	Moderate persistence half-life: 35–150 days

Contd...

Contd...

S No.	Chemical name	Toxic dose LD$_{50}$	Use	WHO classification based on rat oral dose LD$_{50}$	Half-life in environment
9.	Endrin	Rat Oral: 3 mg/kg Dermal: 15 mg/kg Mouse Oral: 1.37g/kg Intravenous: 2,300 g/kg	Avicide insecticide	Highly hazardous	Moderate persistence half-life: 1 Day to 12 Years
10.	Heptachlor	Rat Oral: 40–220 mg/kg Dermal: 119–320 mg/kg Mouse Oral: 30–68 mg/kg	Insecticide	Highly – Moderately hazardous	High persistence half-life: 2 years
11.	Lindane	Rat Oral: 88–270 mg/kg Mouse Oral: 59–246 mg/kg	Acaricide Insecticide Rodenticide	Moderately hazardous	High persistence half-life: 15 months
12.	Methoxychlor	Rat Oral: 5,000–6,000 mg/kg Mice Oral: 2,000 mg/kg	Insecticide	Hazard is unlikely	High persistence half-life: <120 days acute
13.	Mirex	Rat Oral: 600–740 mg/kg	Insecticide	Acute hazard is unlikely	High persistence half-life: 10 years
14.	Toxaphene (Camphechlor) $C_{10}H_{10}C_{l8}$	Rat Oral: 80–293 mg/kg Dogs: 25 mg/kg	Acaricide Insecticide	Slightly hazardous	Moderate persistence half-life 11 Years

*Lethal dose: Pesticides are toxic compounds that have killing activity against particular targeted pests, hence it becomes unethical to test their lethal dose in humans. They have been tested in various other test animals for calculation of lethal dose in humans and expressed as LD$_{50}$.

**LD$_{50}$: It is the dose of active compound needed to kill 50% of test animal population. Smaller LD$_{50}$ confers to more toxic compound.[15]

PATHOPHYSIOLOGY AND MECHANISM OF TOXICITY

Organochlorine pesticides can be toxic to humans if exposure is in from of ingestion, inhalation, and skin contact of agent directly or by food contaminated with them.[16] OCPs are well absorbed orally, whereas skin or inhalational absorption is variable. The toxic effect of these agents depends on molecular size, volatility, lipid solubility, and central nervous system (CNS) effects.[17]

Very high fat solubility of OCP can lead to their accumulation in brain, kidney and endocrinal glands, apart from liver and adipose tissue. OCPs distribution to adipose tissues can be considered as self-detoxification.

Occasionally fat mobilization because of internal metabolic processes can lead to release of significant concentration in blood circulation and produce toxicological CNS effects.[18]

Chlorinated hydrocarbon insecticides are metabolized mainly in liver by microsomal enzymes system. These can be hydroxylated, dehydrochlorinated (lindane) or can be converted to stable epoxides (dieldrin from endrin). Some of these agents are eliminated by glutathione conjugation or glucuronides formation.

Most of these agents are usually excreted in bile and through feces later on. Their metabolites can be eliminated through kidney, especially after glucuronidation.

Half-life of these agents remains very high and presented separately in Table 1. The fat solubility accounts for prolong systemic effects, longer half-life of OCPs in toxicity.[19] Due to property of bioaccumulation contaminated food items became an important source for chronic exposure and long-term complications.[20,21]

Mechanism of Toxicity

On the basis of mechanism of action and primary symptoms these agents can be divided in two groups—(1) the DDT like compounds and (2) the chlorinated alicyclics. Their mechanism of action is slightly different.[22]

- The DDT like compounds works on axonal membrane of nervous system. At axonal membrane they prevent voltage gated sodium channel gate closure after membrane depolarization, thus cause continuous sodium leak and leads to a more negative "after potential" with hyperexcitability of the nerve. This leakage causes repeated discharges in the neuron either spontaneously or after a single stimulus, thus explains hyperexcitability of neurons. Their cardiac toxicity is attributed to high levels of circulating catecholamines[23]

- Rest 3 groups of Chlorinated cyclodienes lead to depressed CNS activity after a prolong exposure of 2-8-hour, this is followed by hyperexcitability, tremors, and then seizures. They probably bind and block the gamma-aminobutyric acid (GABA) chloride ionophore complex, thus leading to reduced flow of chloride ions into the nerve, they can lead to intracellular calcium accumulation by inhibiting inward calcium ion flux, and may also inhibit calcium and magnesium adenosine triphosphatase (ATPase) this further lead to sustained release of excitatory neurotransmitters[24-31]

  ○ Some different preparations of these agents like inhalational vapours, liquid forms can be rapidly absorbed from gastrointestinal (GI) tract, skin, and alveolar mucosa, these can lead to hypoxia atelectasis, chemical pneumonitis and in severe cases may lead to acute respiratory distress syndrome (ARDS), lung tissue necrosis, etc.

APPROACH TO PATIENT

History

As for any poison's exposure, poison exposure history is the most vital information and has a pivotal role in patient's management with OCPs poisoning. But history is not very clear in many intentional poisoning cases and every effort to identify the poison should be made, like wise retrieval of empty packets.

A comprehensive history and clinical examination is very helpful in managing various aspects of patient's management. One should try to obtain original containers and empty packets to review the poison and save samples for testing.

Package details varies by local laws of every country, as in India it is mandatory to display the actual content with strength on package and sign/symptoms related to exposure, followed by first aid and antidotes for that particular agent.

For further details and help one can contact regional poison information center.

BIOCHEMICAL EFFECTS OF TOXINS

Major biological effects of common OCPs have described in Table 3. Onset of symptoms is usually abrupt after acute exposure, can involve various organ systems as follows.

Neurological Effects

As aforementioned in "mechanism section", OCPs cause CNS depression followed by excitation, lead to confusion, delirium, hallucinations especially visual or auditory, lower seizure threshold.

These patient can have seizures with trivial stimulus, muscle spasms, fasciculation are common after exposure.[32,33,35-38,43,45]

Some of the OCPs (endosulfan, etc.) have been reported to precipitate refractory and super refractory status epilepticus that customarily have fatal outcome.[47]

Cardiovascular Effects

Arrhythmias, and acute cardiovascular symptoms predominates acute DDT exposure due to high level of circulatory catecholamine.[35]

Gastrointestinal Effects

Nausea, vomiting, abdominal pain, diarrhea may present with ingestion of OCP toxins.

Respiratory Effects

Acute respiratory distress and shortness of breath are the initial symptoms, this further lead to hypoxia, tachypnea, ARDS like illness after inhalational exposure.[46]

Pesticides and Rodenticides

Table 3: Biological effects of organochlorine pesticides.[14]

S No.	Chemical name	Biochemical effect in humans	References
1.	Aldrin and Dieldrin	Nervous system injury, reproductive, immunity deficits, carcinogenic effects, musculoskeletal and hematological effects (muscular twitching and tremors, aplastic anemia)	(32)
2.	Chlordane	Neuromuscular effects (ike tremors, in coordination) confusion and convulsions	(33)
3.	DDE/BHC	Dermatological symptoms to exposed surfaces Itching, eczema, psoriasis, skin rashes, leucoderma	(34)
4.	DDT	Oral irritation, neuromuscular and neuropsychiatric symptoms (e.g. fatigue, tremors, muscular weakness, in coordination, hyper excitability, anorexia, dizziness, headache, confusion, convulsion)	(35)
5.	Diazinon	Blurring of vision, neuropsychiatric symptoms (e.g. anxiety and restlessness, memory and affect disorders, and delirium) and acute pancreatitis	(36-38)
6.	Endosulfan	Neuropsychiatric symptoms (e.g. tremors, confusion, convulsion) and leukopenia, adverse effects on immune system Affects male reproductive system (like as, sperm count, semen quality, altered sperm morphology) and defects in male sex hormones, nucleic acid damages and mutation	(39-41)
7.	Lindane	Injury to renal, hepatic, nervous and reproductive system and decreased immunity, and also have teratogenic and carcinogenic effect	(42-45)
8.	Polychlorinated biphenyls (PCB)	Memory and neurological deficits	(45)
9.	Pentachlorophenol	Oral cavity and upper airway inflammation and tracheobronchitis, hematological effects (aplastic anemia), injury to renal and hepatic systems, immunity-related disorder, topical irritation to eye, oropharyngeal mucosa and exposed skin	(46)

(BHC: benzene hexachloride; DDE: dichlorodiphenyldichloroethylene; DDT: dichlorodiphenyltrichloroethane)

Secondary lung injury may occur after aspiration of vomited contents or gustatory secretion pooling during neurological compromise.

Dermatologic Effects

Itching, psoriasis, eczema, leucoderma, skin rashes, excoriation after skin exposure.[34]

Hematologic Effects

Anemia, neutropenia, immunodeficiency have been reported with certain specific agents exposure. They may be related to development of blood dyscrasias, aplastic anemia, neutropenia, leukemia.[35,40,42,46]

Other

Chronic long-term exposure of OCPs have been linked to nausea, anorexia, headaches visual disturbances, fatigue, muscle fasciculation/twitching.

Organochlorine pesticides have xenoestrogen like effect on thyroxin, to reduced synthesis and increased degradation in humans and animal models. Some researchers have found strong dose-response relationship between OCPs and diabetes prevalence. Male hormonal disturbances, defective spermatogenesis and reproductive toxicities have been reported with selected agents.[48,49]

Long-term nephrotoxicity, hepatotoxicity, and increased propensity to have breast and prostate cancers were also linked to exposure of OCPs.[50]

Negative effect of long-term exposure is also observed in the form of child developmental abnormalities, learning disabilities.[51]

DIFFERENTIAL DIAGNOSIS

A broad differential diagnosis from the following list should always be considered whenever there is lack of clear history of exposure of OCP. Relative poisoning toxidrome helps in identifying other intoxications.

List of Differentials

- Central nervous system stimulant poisoning
- Camphor toxicity
- Strychnine toxicity
- Picrotoxin toxicity
- Hypoxemia

- Idiopathic epilepsy
- Arsenic toxicity
- Hydrocarbon toxicity
- Toluene toxicity
- Toxicity, organophosphate and carbamate.

Work-up and Diagnostic Consideration

Exposure history is the most important information during work up of suspected toxicity patient.

Laboratory Studies

Patient should be evaluated for routine laboratory test that include rapid bedside glucose testing, Electrolytes (hyperkalemia), Complete blood counts (leukocytosis, pancytopenia), kidney function tests (azotemia, raised creatinine levels), liver function tests (Transaminitis and hyperbilirubinemia), coagulation profile (prolong coagulation tests) creatine phosphokinase (CPK), arterial or venous blood gas analysis, (pulmonary increased Aa gradient, hypoxemia, metabolic acidosis), serum lactate measurements, urine pregnancy testing, urinalysis, etc.

Screening for toxicology panels in serum and urine for common toxicants, particularly testing for paracetamol and acetyl-salicylic acid levels, if intentional coexposure is suspected.

Electrocardiography (sinus rhythm disturbances, QTc prolongation, ST segment changes) should be done. Chest radiography indicated in aspiration and lung injury cases.

Neuroimaging/diagnostic lumbar puncture/electro-encephalography (EEG) should be considered to rule out specific nervous system causes of seizures and altered sensorium.

One should always investigate other possible toxicants in unreliable history or possibility of coexposure with other pesticides (e.g. organophosphorus pesticides: identified by cholinergic toxidrome and plasma and red cell cholinesterase activity testing).

Chlorinated hydrocarbon levels can be identified in blood by gas-liquid chromatographic examination (can be measured, but not clinically helpful and it is not routinely available).

Gas chromatography and analytical studies of adipose tissues, breast milk, serum and urine can be considered for documentation of exposure only, they do not have any significant clinical implication. Blood levels correlate more with acute toxicity, while levels found in adipose tissue and breast milk reflect long-term and historic exposure.[52]

Chromatography method can detect much lower concentration, that may be present in general population because of long-term accumulation of OCP in food chain. These positive results cannot be linked with acute toxicity in humans, therefore raised blood OCP levels does not justify diagnosis of acute toxicity. In United States general population tissues concentration data is available with Centre for Disease Control Biomonitoring Program and can be used to interpret chromatography results.[53]

Forensic Examination

Chromatographic brain analytical studies are warranted for postmortem evaluation for suspected deaths due to acute exposure or chronic environmental pollution, because severity of toxicity correlates with brain concentration of these insecticides.

TREATMENT OF ORGANOCHLORINE PESTICIDE POISONING

Prehospital/Emergency Room Care

Safety of emergency medical service (EMS) provider/emergency room (ER) staff is to be ensured at all times. Patient and EMS personal may be at high risk of continuous and concomitant exposure of toxins so early environmental control is necessary in all cases.

Immediate removal of clothing and body wash with soap and water limits exposure through contact skin, and prevent continued absorption. For massive exposure and multiple cases help from HAZMAT (hazardous materials) team should be taken.

Induction of emesis is not recommended in case of ingestion of OCPs because patient may aspirate vomitus if develop drowsiness or depressed sensorium.

Assessment and maintenance of ABC (airway, breathing and circulation) with other vital signs during prehospital EMS care can save many lives.

Rapid sequence intubation is usually a practice standard while managing a toxicology case in EMS and ER.

Control of airway and breathing gives liberty for use of sedative and anticonvulsant medication in future course of hospital stay.

Pesticides and Rodenticides

After acute exposure patient may have cardiac dysrhythmia as a result of high circulating levels of catecholamine. Beta-blockers can be used to blunt this response. For hypotension phenylephrine is suggested vasopressor.

Other arrhythmias should be managed according to uniform cardiac arrhythmia management protocols (American or European Cardiac Life Support Algorithms).

For neurologic symptoms in prehospital phase, traditional protocol for seizure control is to be followed as such—first line: benzodiazepine, second line: antiepileptic medicines and third line: anesthetic agents. If patient is already intubated and paralyzed then frequent EEG monitoring to be done as soon as possible after intensive care unit (ICU) admission.

Hospital Specific Care

Every patient with OCPs exposure should be monitored/observed in hospital for sufficient lengths, as delayed development of signs and symptoms may be there, attributed to long $t_{1/2}$ of OCP compounds.

After adequate environmental control and ABC management, further specific management is started.

Digestive decontamination: Induction of emesis is not recommended as chances of aspiration are very high, and so role of naso-/orogastric tube is also controversial, as it may induce vomiting. Any lavage should be carried out with utmost care especially in case of liquid poison ingestion. Airway should always be secured before lavage.

Antidotes: No specific antidotes are available for OCPs poisoning.

Use of activated charcoal is recommended to absorb toxin present in the gut and also to enhances their fecal elimination and to minimizes systemic absorption.

Activated charcoal has been used as an emergency measure when toxin is not known. Drug absorption efficacy is 100–1,000 mg/g of activated charcoal. Usual dose is 0.5–1.0 g/kg enterally one time only within 30 minutes of intake, but it can be used up to 1–2 hours of chemical intake.

Multiple dose activated charcoal (MDAC) used in 10–20 g/ q2-4 hours enterally can exert "sink effect" regardless of route of exposure by creating a concentration gradient in GI circulation.

Activated charcoal use should be individualized and risk to benefit should be titrated in each case, as risk of aspiration is very high if patient develops any seizures. Aqueous preparation is usually preferred as sorbitol based charcoal can cause more nausea, vomiting, diarrhea.[54]

Cholestyramine is a nonabsorbable anion exchange resin and can be used for binding and to reduce reabsorption of bound drugs in GI tract, thus it can enhance elimination of toxicant in body.[55] Cholestyramine interferes with enterohepatic circulation of lipophilic chemicals. About 4 g of cholestyramine enterally every 6–12 hours to be taken with feeds only.[56]

Other methods to reduce absorption have also been tried with limited success, sucrose polymer (olestra), whole bowel irrigation were tried, but their use should be individualized to patients need.[57]

Forced dieresis, dialysis hemoperfusion or filtration is not very useful for toxin elimination.

Seizures are the main neurological symptom and sign of toxicity with OCP poisoning.

These patients can have status epilepticus very commonly (~33% reported in retrospective studies), thus continuous EEG monitoring is recommended for sedated and paralyzed patient on ventilator. Refractory seizures carries poor neurological prognosis with fatal outcome, hence termination of seizure should be attempted with standard treatment algorithms for status epilepticus. Although standard epilepsy medications are not seen to be working well in retrospective studies, these seizures can be controlled with drugs acting on GABA chloride ionophore complex (e.g. benzodiazepines, barbiturates, intravenous anesthetic agents).[47]

Other supportive care should be started as and when required during the course of treatment.

Lung protective ventilation strategy as per ARDS net trial protocols and latest evidence based practice is recommended for patients on ventilator.

For arrhythmias beta-blockers (propranolol/esmolol) remain the mainstay of therapy. Phenylephrine (pure alpha adrenergic agonist) can be used for fluid refractory hypotension. Phenylephrine has an advantage of having low myocardium stimulatory properties.

Like as, for any liver necrosis or elevated liver enzymes N-acetylcysteine can be tried for prevention of irreversible drug-induced liver injury (DILI).

Avoid nephrotoxic agents and dehydration to prevent any kidney injury, seizure episodes will lead to raised CPK levels and it should be treated with optimum hydration and monitoring strategy.

Prophylactic antibiotic use for aspiration pneumonia is not recommended and remains controversial.

After stabilization in hospital and control of immediate issues, follow-up care should be explained and arranged for possible long-term sequelae.

A psychiatrist consultation should always be taken for intentional/suicidal poisoning episodes, and patient health education session should be arranged as required.

For every toxicity case local guidelines for legal information and notification to regional poison information center should be followed.

CONCLUSION

Organochlorine compounds are among the most widely used pesticide chemicals, out of which DDT and HCH are banned for agricultural use and now used exclusively for public health purposes. Acute OCP toxicity usually manifest as CNS excitation and related neurological symptoms, whereas chronic exposure largely leads to chronic nonspecific general symptoms (nausea, headache, vomiting etc.), blood dyscrasias and malignancies. History of exposure is the most important tool for diagnosis as many other intoxicants share the similar toxicology profile. In every case of OCP toxicity the key of management remain decontamination, general supportive care and treatment of seizures.

Although epidemiologically acute OCP toxicity is not of that big magnitude but their tendency for slow degradation, long range atmospheric transport, bioaccumulation and subsequent chronic toxicity is major public health concern, and suitable stringent laws should be in place for their open use.

KEY POINTS

- Organochlorine pesticides are some of the most commonly used pesticide in developing countries, although their use is banned for agricultural use in most of the developed countries
- Organochlorine pesticides are metabolized slowly in body and in environment and have a very high $t_{1/2}$, thus have a property of bioaccumulation in food chain and long range atmospheric transport, and so these have been classified as POPs
- Other neurotoxin ingestion remains main differential diagnosis if exposure history is in doubt. Gas-liquid chromatography in the tissue samples, is rarely needed for clinical diagnosis of OCP toxicity, but

remains a valuable test for community or forensic medicine studies
- In absence of known antidote for OCPs, activated charcoal and cholestyramine remain the main stay of initial care to reduce absorption while other general supportive care remains the corner stone of therapy
- Although not reported well, seizures due to OCP ingestion is best controlled by drugs acting on GABA ionophore complex.

REFERENCES

1. WHO. Public health impact of pesticides used in agriculture. Geneva, Switzerland: World Health Organization; 1990.
2. Jong HK, Smith A. Distribution of organochlorine pesticides in soils from South Korea. Chemosphere. 2001;43(2):137-40.
3. FAO. Proceedings of the Asia Regional Workshop, Regional Office for Asia and the Pacific, Bangkok, Thailand. Rome: Food and Agriculture Organization of the United Nations (FAO); 2005.
4. Gupta PK. Pesticide exposure—Indian scene. Toxicology. 2004;198:83-90.
5. Lallas P. The Stockholm Convention on persistent organic pollutants. Am J Int Law. 2001;95:692-708.
6. United Nations Environment Programme. (2009). Report of the Conference of the Parties of the Stockholm Convention on Persistent Organic Pollutants on the Work of its Fourth Meeting UNEP/POPS/COP4/38. [online] Available from: http://chm.pops.int/TheConvention/ConferenceoftheParties/Meetings/COP4/COP4Documents/tabid/531/Default.aspx [Accessed October, 2018].
7. Jit S, Dadhwal M, Kumari H, et al. Evaluation of hexachlorocyclohexane contamination from the last lindane production plant operating in India. Environ Sci Poll Res. 2011;18(4):586-97.
8. UNEP. National Implementation Plans Stockholm Convention on Persistent Organic Pollutants (POPs) (Government of India), Secretariat of the Stockholm Convention. 2011.
9. Wasseling C, Aragon A, Castillo L, et al. Hazardous pesticides in Central America. Int J Occupat Environ Health. 2001;7(4):287-94.
10. Konradsen F, Van der Hoek, Cole W, et al. Reducing acute poisoning in developing countries—options for restricting the availability of pesticides. Toxicology. 2003;192:249-61.
11. Coronado GD, Thompson B, Strong L, et al. Agricultural task and exposure to organophosphate pesticides among farm workers. Environ Health Perspect. 2004;112:142-7.
12. Environews Forum. Killer environment. Environ Health Perspect. 1999;107:A62.
13. Srivastava A, Peshin SS, Kaleekal T et al. Human & Experimental. An epidemiological study of poisoning

cases reported to the National Poisons Information Centre, All India Institute of Medical Sciences, New Delhi. Toxicology. 2005;24:279-85.

14. Jayaraj R, Megha P, Sreedev P. Organochlorine pesticides, their toxic effects on living organisms and their fate in the environment. Interdiscip Toxicol. 2016;9(3-4):90-100.

15. Hock WK, Lorenz ES. (2006). Pesticide safety fact sheet: toxicity of pesticides. Penn State College of Agricultural Sciences Agricultural Research and Cooperative Extension Pesticide Education. [online] Available from: https://extension.psu.edu/downloadable/download/sample/sample_id/678/ [Accessed October, 2018].

16. Reigart JR, Roberts JR. Recognition and Management of Pesticide Poisonings, 5th edition. Washington DC: Environmental Protection Agency; 1999.

17. Bhalla M, Thami GP. Reversible neurotoxicity after an overdose of topical lindane in an infant. Pediatr Dermatol. 2004;(5):59-79.

18. COT. Committee on the Toxicity of Chemicals in Food, Consumer Products and the Environment. Risk Assessment of Mixtures of Pesticides and Similar Substances. Food Standards Agency, UK; 2002.

19. Mortensen ML. Management of acute childhood poisonings caused by selected insecticides and herbicides. Pediatr Clin North Am. 1986;33(2):421-45.

20. Nicolopoulou-Stamati P, Pitsos M. The impact of endocrine disrupters on the female reproductive system. Hum Reprod Update. 2001;7(3):323-30.

21. Hall RH. A new threat to public health: organochlorines and food. Nutr Health. 1992;8: 33-43.

22. Joy RM. The effects of neurotoxicants on kindling and kindled seizures. Fundament Appl Toxicol. 1985;5(1): 41-65.

23. Ishikawa Y, Charalambous P, Matsumura F. Modification by pyrethroids and DDT of phosphorylation activities of rat brain sodium channel. Biochem Pharmacol. 1989;38:2449-57.

24. Casida JE, Lawrence LJ. Structure–activity correlations for interactions of bicyclophosphorus esters and some polychlorocycloalkane and pyrethroid insecticides with brain-specific t-butyl bi cyclophosphorthionate receptor. Environ Health Perspect. 1985;61:123-32.

25. Cole LM, Casida JE. (1986). Polychlorocycloalkane insecticide-induced convulsions in mice in relation to disruption of the GABA-regulated chloride ionophore. Life Sci. 1986;39:1855-62.

26. Narahashi T. Neuronal Ion Channels as the Target Sites of Insecticides. Pharmacol Toxicol. 1996;18:1-14.

27. Huang J, and Casida JE. Role of cerebellar granule cell-specific GABA(A) receptor subtype in the differential sensitivity of [3H] ethynylbicycloorthobenzoate binding to GABA mimetics. Neurosci Lett. 1997;225:85-8.

28. Ratra GS, Kamita SG, Casida JE. Role of human GABA (A) receptor beta-3 subunit in insecticide toxicity. Toxicol Appl Pharmacol. 2001;172:233-40.

29. Ratra GS, Erkkila BE, Weiss DS, et al. Unique insecticide specificity of human homomeric [rho]1 GABAC receptor. Toxicol Lett. 2002;129:47-53.

30. Karatas AD, Aygun D, Baydin A. Characteristics of endosulfan poisoning: a study of 23 cases. Singapore Med J. 2006;47(12):1030-2.

31. Roberts DM, Dissanayake W, Rezvi Sheriff MH, et al. Refractory status epilepticus following self-poisoning with the organochlorine pesticide endosulfan. J Clin Neurosci. 2004;11(7):760-2.

32. USEPA. Health Effects Support Document for Aldrin/Dieldrin, U.S. Environmental Protection Agency, Office of Water (4304T). Washington, DC: Health and Ecological Criteria Division; 2003.

33. Agency for Toxic Substances and Disease Registry. Chlordane (1997). In: ATSDR Toxicological Profiles on CD-ROM. Boca Raton: Lewis Publishers; 1997.

34. Subramaniam K, Solomon Jebakumar RD. (2006). Organochlorine pesticides BHC and DDE in human blood in and around Madurai, India. Indian J Clin Biochem. 2006;21(2):169-72.

35. Klaassen CD, Amdur MO, Doull J. Casarett & Doull's Toxicology: The Basic Science of Poisons, 5th edition. New York: McGraw-Hill; 1996.

36. Reigert JR, Roberts JR. Organophosphate Insecticides. Recognition and Management of Pesticide Poisonings, 5th edition. U. S. Environmental Protection Agency, Office of Prevention, Pesticides and Toxic Substances, Office of Pesticide Programs, U.S. Government Printing Office. 1999;5:34-40.

37. Wagner SL. Diagnosis and treatment of organophosphate and carbamate intoxication. Hum Health Effects Pesticides 1997;12:239-49.

38. USEPA. Environmental Risk Assessment for Diazinon. Washington, DC:U.S. Environmental Protection Agency, Office of Prevention, Pesticides and Toxic Substances, Office of Pesticide Programs, U.S. Government Printing Office; 2000.

39. Pandey N, Gundevia F, Prem AS, et al. Studies on the genotoxicity of endosulfan, an organochlorine insecticide in mammalian germ cells. Mutat Res. 1990;242(1):1-7.

40. Susan S, Sania P. Endosulfan—a review of its toxicity and its effects on the endocrine system. Canada: World Wild Life Fund; 1999.

41. Singh N, Sharma A, Dwivedi P. Citrinin and endosulfan induced teratogenic effects in Wistar rats. J Appl Toxicol. 2007;27(2):143-51.

42. Sahoo DK, Roy A, Chainy GB. (2008). Protective effect of vitamin E and curcumin on L-thyroxine-induced rat testicular oxidative stress. Chem Biol Interact. 2008;176:21-8.

43. Bano M, Bhatt DK. Ameliorative effect of a combination of vitamin-E, vitamin-C α-lipoic acid and stilbene resveratrol on lindane induced toxicity in mice olfactory lobe and cerebrum. Indian J Exp Biol. 2010;8:48-150.

44. Vijaya Padma V, Sowmya P, Arun FT, et al. Protective effect of gallic acid against lindane induced toxicity in experimental rats. Food Chem Toxicol. 2011;49:991-8.

45. Jacobson JL, Jacobson SW. Intellectual Impairment in Children Exposed to Polychlorinated Biphenyls in Utero. N Engl J Med 1996;335(11):783-9.

46. Agency for Toxic Substances and Disease Registry (ATSDR). Toxicological Profile for Pentachlorophenol (Update) (Draft). Atlanta, GA: Public Health Service, U.S. Department of Health and Human Services; 1999.

47. Moon JM, Chun BJ. Acute endosulfan poisoning: a retrospective study. Hum Exp Toxicol. 2009;28(5):309-16.

48. Lee DH, Lee IK, Song K, et al. A strong dose-response relation between serum concentrations of persistent organic pollutants and diabetes: Results from the National Health and Examination Survey, 1999–2002. Diabetes Care. 2006;29:1638-44.

49. Mnif W, Hassine AI, Bouaziz A, et al. Effect of Endocrine Disruptor Pesticides: a Review. Int J Environ Res Public Health. 2011;8:2265-303.

50. Xu X, Dailey AB, Talbott EO, et al. Associations of serum concentrations of organochlorine pesticides with breast cancer and prostate cancer in U.S. adults. Environ Health Perspect. 2010;118:60-6.

51. Lee D, Jacobs DR, Porta M. Association of serum concentrations of persistent organic pollutants with the prevalence of learning disability and attention deficit disorder. J Epidemiol Community Health. 2007;61:591-6.

52. Frank R, Braun HE. Organochlorine residues in bird species collected dead in Ontario 1972-1988. Bull Environ Contam Toxicol. 1990;44(6):932-9.

53. Centers for Disease Control and Prevention. National Report on Human Exposure to Environmental Chemicals. [online] Available from: http://www.cdc.gov/exposurereport/ [Accessed October, 2018].

54. Morgan DP, Dotson TB, Lin LI. Effectiveness of activated charcoal, mineral oil, and castor oil in limiting gastrointestinal absorption of a chlorinated hydrocarbon pesticide. Clin Toxicol. 1977;11(1):61-70.

55. Kassner JT, Maher TJ, Hull KM, et al. Cholestyramine as an adsorbent in acute lindane poisoning: a murine model. Ann Emerg Med. 1993;22(9):1392-7.

56. Cohn WJ, Boylan JJ, Blanke RV, et al. Treatment of chlordecone (Kepone) toxicity with cholestyramine. Results of a controlled clinical trial. N Engl J Med. 1978;298(5):243-8.

57. Mutter LC, Blanke RV, Jandacek RJ, et al. Reduction in the body content of DDE in the Mongolian gerbil treated with sucrose polyester and caloric restriction. Toxicol Appl Pharmacol. 1988;92(3):4283-5.

37
CHAPTER

Rodenticides

Sanjay V Patne, Subramanian Senthilkumaran

INTRODUCTION

Rodenticides are the category of pest control chemicals intended to kill rodents. These are heterogeneous group of compounds that exhibit markedly different toxicities to humans and rodents. They are among the most toxic substances kept at homes. Even though, rodenticides are utilized worldwide. Specific types of rodenticide exposures critical care physicians commonly encounter vary regionally.

CLASSIFICATION OF RODENTICIDES

Rodenticides[1] are broadly classified into:
1. Non-anticoagulant compounds
2. Anticoagulant compounds.

The important classification of anticoagulant compound derivatives, and nature and toxicity of non-anticoagulant compounds is given in Tables 1 and 2, respectively.

BIOCHEMISTRY

- *Anticoagulants:* Anticoagulant rodenticides are tasteless, odorless or foul smelling pending upon the agent. Most exposures are oral; however, they have been reported through the dermal and inhalational routes. Specifically, brodifacoum is lipid soluble, concentrated in the liver, is approximately 100 times more potent than warfarin and long lasting with clinical effects that can range from days to months.
- *Barium:* Barium rodenticides no longer are available for sale in many countries but old product may remain. Barium carbonate as a powder may be inhaled and cause acute paralysis.

Table 1: Non-anticoagulant compounds: Nature and toxicity.

Nature of the compound	Nature of toxicity
• Arsenic • Barium carbonate • Strychnine • Thallium sulfate • Organic phosphorus compounds (OPC) • Yellow phosphorus • Zinc phosphide • Aluminum phosphide • Vacor • Tetramine	Highly toxic
• Cholecalciferol • α-Naphthylthiourea (ANTU)	Moderate toxicity

Table 2: Anticoagulant compound derivatives and generic name.

Derivative	Generic name
Coumarin derivatives	• First generation: Warfarin • Second generation: Brodifacoum, coumatetralyl, Difenacoum
Indandiones	• Diphacinone, Chlorophacinone

Rodenticides

- *Phosphides:* Zinc and aluminum phosphide are the most commonly available products. Usually are found as powders or pellets. In the presence of water and gastric acid, the metal is released and phosphine gas is produced. This gas may have a garlic odor.
- *Strychnine:* Strychnine is an extract from the seed of *Strychnos nux-vomica*. It is a bitter-tasting, odorless white powder. Most products contain 0.5% strychnine.
- *Tetramine:* The dose of tetramine which kills 50% of mammals (LD50) is 0.1–0.3 mg/kg and doses of 7.0–10.0 mg are considered lethal in humans. Tetramine is approximately 100 times more toxic to humans than potassium cyanide and might be a more powerful human convulsant than strychnine.
- *Yellow phosphorus:* It can get absorbed through skin, mucus membrane, respiratory and gastrointestinal epithelium. After absorption, it is distributed to all tissues, particularly the liver and the peak level is reached after 2–3 hours of toxic oral ingestion. Bile salts are important for absorption of phosphorus. Because of water content and low oxygen tension, phosphorus remains stable in gut for longer period.

PATHOPHYSIOLOGY

- *Anticoagulants:* Warfarin and warfarin-like anticoagulants disrupt enzymes in the liver. These rodenticides inhibit liver vitamin K reductases, which are essential to endogenous activation of hepatically synthesized clotting factors II, VII, IX and X and proteins C, S and Z. Bleeding from the coagulopathy may occur when factor concentrations decline to less than 25–30% of baseline levels.
- *ANTU:* The toxicity of ANTU results from its active metabolites. Lung reduced nicotinamide adenine dinucleotide phosphate-dependent cytochrome P450 enzymes seem to generate these injurious metabolites. Glutathione depletion seems to exacerbate the toxicity.
- *Bromethalin:* Bromethalin uncouples oxidative phosphorylation and interrupts nerve impulse conduction.
- *Barium:* After stimulating muscle, produces a depolarizing neuromuscular blockade. Potassium is shifted intracellularly along with blockage of cellular potassium channel efflux.[2]

- *Phosphine:* The mechanisms of phosphine toxicity are not completely understood; however, it may block cytochrome c and a oxidases. Free radical generation and lipid peroxidation also seem to have a role.
- *Strychnine:* Strychnine acts on the central nervous system as a competitive antagonist at glycine receptors. It also seems to block the action of GABA in spinal interneurons, although this inhibition is not as potent as that with glycine.
- *Yellow phosphorous:* It produces an exothermic reaction releasing phosphoric acid that causes direct tissue damage due to the production of free radicals against organic molecules. This, in turn, will bring about changes in ribosomal function and protein synthesis, failure of regulation of blood glucose and fatty degeneration of multiple organs. The reason for an increased predilection to cause liver toxicity is, however, not fully understood.

CLINICAL FEATURES

The important clinical manifestations of other *non-anticoagulant rodenticides* are as follows:

- *Arsenic:* Cardiovascular collapse (VT, Torsade de pointes), garlic odor, dysphagia, nausea vomiting, bloody diarrhea
- *Thallium sulfate:* Polyneuritis, alopecia, alteration in blood pressure
- *Organophosphate compounds:* "SLUDGE" (salivation, lacrimation, urination, defecation, gastrointestinal upset and emesis)
- *Yellow phosphorous:* Oral burns, abdominal pain, gastrointestinal (GI) bleed, hepatotoxicity and "smoking" luminescent stool
- *Vacor:* (yellow, yellow-green powder, peanut odor) Hyperglycemia, ketosis and neuropathies
- *Cholecalciferol:* Hypercalcemia, osteomalacia and calcifications
- *Red squill:* Digoxin-like action
- *Norbormide:* Vasoconstriction with ischemia
- *Strychnine:* Muscular spasms, twitches, hypersensitivity to stimuli and convulsions
- *Yellow phosphorus:* The clinical effects of acute poisoning are divided into three stages. *Stage 1*—the initial GI stage is characterized by vomiting, nausea, diarrhea, and abdominal pain, which occur within the first 24 hours after ingestion. Laboratory tests are almost normal during this period. During this

stage, sudden death may occur; it may be that the ingestion of a very large amount can directly result in cardiovascular arrhythmia and collapse within the first 24 hours. *Stage 2: (1–4 days)*—is essentially a symptom-free period, but liver enzyme levels are elevated and toxic hepatitis begins to spread. *Stage 3*—can end in acute liver failure and acute renal failure with metabolic derangements, encephalopathy, coagulopathy, arrhythmia, cardiogenic shock and abnormal liver tests. In short, this is a multiorgan failure; the third stage occurred between 4 days and 7 days. Patient's progress to the third stage because of the systemic effects of high-dose phosphorus after it has been absorbed[3]

- *Anticoagulant rodenticides:* They are toxic to virtually every organ/system in the body and the signs and symptoms may vary from asymptomatic to active bleeding.

Super Warfarin

The evolution of the warfarin resistance in rats has resulted in the development of a second-generation of anticoagulant rodenticides known as super warfarin. They have no role in human therapeutic anticoagulation.

Brodifacoum

It is the most common active ingredient in commercially available rodenticides usually found in a 0.005% concentration. It is used in agricultural and urban settings for rodent control and available in the forms such as solid, granular and pellet baits. It acts by blocking the activation of vitamin K. When vitamin K is not regenerated, the clotting factors II, VII, IX and X cannot be activated (extrinsic pathway) and coagulopathy develops.

CLINICAL MANIFESTATIONS

The clinical manifestations after ingestion range from being asymptomatic to active bleeding such as hematuria, vaginal bleeding, hematemesis, melena, soft tissue bruising, epistaxis, hemoptysis, hemarthrosis, retroperitoneal and intracranial hemorrhage. The coagulopathy may last weeks to months and can be associated with significant overall blood loss. Toxic hepatitis has been reported after 3–4 days even with single exposure.

WORKUP

Most patients seek medical attention many days after ingestion with evidence of coagulopathy. *In the acute phase,* the international normalized ratio (INR) and prothrombin time (PT) should be reassessed every 6 hours and repeated if prolongation is observed until the level plateaus. In suspected long-acting anticoagulation overdose, twice-daily INR evaluation for 2 days is essential to identify most patients at risk of coagulopathy. Assessment of glycemic status, electrolytes, liver function test and arterial blood gas analysis are warranted depending on the clinical picture. The presence of super warfarin can be estimated by special blood assays.

TREATMENT

- *Gastric lavage:* Gastric decontamination can be employed within 6 hours in cases of rodenticide poisoning but gastric lavage with water *is contraindicated in case of phosphide compound poisoning* because it liberates highly toxic phosphine gas when it comes in contact either with water or with hydrochloric acid in the stomach. The lavage can be done with Potassium permanganate (1:10,000) or with coconut oil. The exact mechanism by which coconut oil reduces the toxicity of phosphides is unknown but most probably it forms a protective layer around the gastric mucosa, thereby preventing the absorption of phosphine gas. Secondly, it helps in diluting the HCl and again inhibiting the breakdown of phosphide[4]
- *Role of blood transfusion in rodenticide poisoning:* In the case of hemorrhagic shock, active bleeding, impaired oxygen transport or emergency surgery, blood transfusion with fresh whole blood from related donor is indicated, as it contains both cellular components and coagulation factors. Fresh frozen plasma is used in life-threatening coagulopathy secondary to super warfarin toxicity as it immediately reverts by replacing active vitamin K-dependent coagulation factors.

Antidote for Super Warfarin Poisoning[5] (Flowchart 1)

Vitamin K

Vitamin K_1 (phytonadione) is the specific antidote for super warfarin poisoning. It helps in the hepatic

Flowchart 1: Algorithm for management of super warfarin poisoning.
(Used from Chapter Toxicity due to Anticoagulants with permission from the editor)

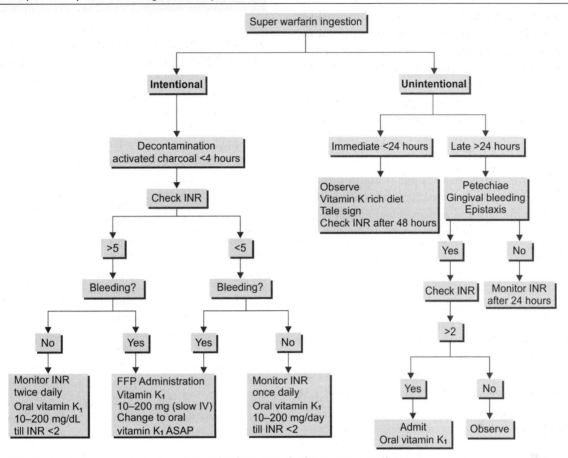

Source: Toxicity due to Anticoagulants. In: Suresh David (Ed). Text Book of Emergency Medicine.
(INR: international normalized ratio; FFP: fresh frozen plasma)

synthesis of coagulation factors II, VII, IX, and X. *Vitamin K2 (menaquinone) or Vitamin K3 (menadione)* are not effective and reliance on treatment with these or their analogs can lead to serious consequences.

Preferred route: Vitamin K$_1$ is available in several formulations such as oral, subcutaneous, intramuscular or intravenous. In super warfarin poisoning intravenous injection of vitamin K$_1$ is preferred, as it produces immediate response, but there is a risk of non-allergic, non-IgE mediated anaphylaxis. Early oral therapy is equally effective in patients with symptomatic coagulopathy and who is not on activated charcoal. Subcutaneous vitamin K$_1$ should be avoided as its absorption is unpredictable. Likewise, intramuscular vitamin K$_1$ may be discouraged as it may cause intramuscular hemorrhage.

Administering intravenous vitamin K$_1$: Vitamin K$_1$ injection (Phytonadione Injectable Emulsion, USP) is supplied as 1 mL ampoule at the concentration of 10 mg/mL. The required dose may be diluted with 100 mL of 0.9% sodium chloride injection or 5% dextrose injection and it's infused over 30–60 minutes, not exceeding 1 mg per minute.

- *Possible adverse reactions:* Rarely, intravenous administration of vitamin K can produce severe, shock-like reactions. Deaths have been reported after intravenous and intramuscular administration. These reactions are generally as a result of too rapid administration (> 1 mg/minute).

Optimum dose of vitamin K: A starting dose of 100 mg of vitamin K$_1$ may be given per day in four divided doses. The optimal dosage regimen thereafter remains unclear but should be titrated to correct the INR. The daily vitamin K dose required may be up to 600 mg depending on the severity of coagulopathy. The doses should aim to return INR to therapeutic, not normal concentrations.

Vitamin K_1 should be administered continuously at high doses and for prolonged periods of time; for example, 100 mg daily for many days, weeks and even months. This can vary from 2 months to a year depending on the half-life of the compound ingested and the severity. Initially parenteral vitamin K_1 is often indicated and oral route may be preferred if long-term administration is required.

Prophylactic vitamin K_1: The administration of prophylactic vitamin K_1 in an asymptomatic patient immediately after exposure to super warfarin with no laboratory evidence of coagulopathy is not indicated, as this may mask the onset of anticoagulant effects in the few patients who do require prolonged treatment and follow-up care.

In case of unintentional single ingestions of super warfarin: It is often seen in children who ingest a small dose of a warfarin-based rodenticide, INR prolongation is unusual. A diet rich in vitamin K such as spinach, Brussels sprouts and broccoli may be encouraged.

Guidelines do not exist regarding exact dose of N-Acetyl Cysteine (NAC) in yellow phosphorous so routinely intravenous NAC that was administered was according to the recommended clinical practice guidelines for the treatment of acetaminophen overdose— 150 mg/kg of NAC in 200 mL of 5% dextrose over 15–60 minutes and then 50 mg/kg in 500 mL of 5% dextrose over 4 hours followed by 100 mg/kg in 1000 mL of 5% dextrose over 16 hours. A cumulative dose of 300 mg/kg of injection NAC was administered over 21 hours.[6]

The indications for ICU admission in rodenticide poisoning are given in Table 3.

CONCLUSION

Rodenticide compounds are variable and hence, it becomes imperative to ensure the compound involved, before therapy is initiated. Baseline PT/INR must be obtained and FFP transfusion may be required in patients with serious bleeding. High dose vitamin K_1, remains the therapy of choice, which may be required for a prolonged period. However, patient must be observed for development of any allergic reaction. Recombinant factor VIIa (rFVIIa) or prothrombin complex concentrate (PCC), may also be used, if available. Associated co-ingestions and co-morbidities must be managed actively. Extracorporeal removal may enhance recovery

Table 3: Indications for ICU admission in rodenticide poisoning.

Agent	Indication
Long-acting anticoagulants	Life-threatening hemorrhage
ANTU	Pulmonary edema
Barium, Bromethalin	Ventilatory management, severe hypokalemia Refractory seizure
Phosphides	Hypotension, cardiac arrhythmias, coma, status epilepticus
PNU	Autonomic neuropathy with hypotension, encephalopathy, ketoacidosis
Fluoroacetates, fluoroacetamide	Cardiac dysrhythmias, coma, status epilepticus
Strychnine, Tetramine	Status epilepticus or severe muscle spasms with ventilator support, cardiac dysrhythmias, severe acidosis. Myocardial ischemia, status Seizure
Yellow phosphorus	Acidosis, Alerted sensorium, Elevated liver enzymes and cardiovascular instability

(ANTU: α-naphthylthiourea; PNU: N-3-pyridylmethyl-N′-p-nitrophenylurea)

from rodenticide poisoning. Patient should be evaluated for suicidal intent.

KEY POINTS

- Avoid drugs that may enhance bleeding or decrease metabolism of the anticoagulant
- Respiratory compromise can be multifactorial and may develop quickly or can be insidious for rodenticides
- Acidosis and cardiovascular instability are common after exposure to heavy doses of rodenticides
- Lack of data on transfer of super warfarin compounds across the placenta or excretion in breast milk
- Avoid the false reassurances of the asymptomatic phase in yellow phosphorus
- Early administration of intravenous NAC must be considered
- Potassium replacement alone reverses paralysis in barium poisoning.

REFERENCES

1. Flomenbaum NE, Frank G, Lewis R. Hoffman pesticides: an overview with a focus on principles and rodenticide. In: Gold frank (Ed). Text Book of Toxicological Emergencies, 8th edition. New York: McGraw-Hill; 2006. pp. 1470-9.
2. Rhyee SH, Heard K. Acute barium toxicity from ingestion of "snake" fireworks. J Med Toxicol. 2009;5(4):209-13.
3. Ravikanth R, Sandeep S, Philip B. Acute yellow phosphorus poisoning causing fulminant hepatic failure with parenchymal hemorrhages and contained duodenal perforation. Indian J Crit Care Med. 2017;21:238-42.
4. Senthilkumaran S, Ananth C, Menezes RG, et al. Aluminium phosphide poisoning: Need for revised treatment guidelines. Indian J Anaesth. 2015;59:831-2.
5. Senthilkumaran S. Toxicity due to anticoagulants. In: Suresh David (Ed). Text Book of Emergency Medicine, 1st edition. Philadelphia: Lippincott Williams & Wilkins; 2012. pp. 2053-66.
6. Kafeel SI, Chandrasekaran VP, Eswaran V. Role of N-acetyl cystine in outcome of patients with YP poisoning-An observational study. Natl J Emerg Med. 2012;1:35-40.

SECTION 10

Miscellaneous Toxicities

38. **Heavy Metal Poisoning**
   Prashant Nasa

39. **Envenomation: Snake, Scorpion, and Spider**
   Subramanian Senthilkumaran,
   Ponniah Thirumalai Kolundu Subramanian

40. **Plant Poisonings**
   Arvinth Soundarrajan, Subramanian Senthilkumaran,
   Ponniah Thirumalai Kolundu Subramanian

41. **Mushroom Poisoning**
   Nipun Verma, Ashish Bhalla, Shreya Singh

42. **Methotrexate and Other Chemotherapeutic Agents Toxicity**
   Akhilesh Singh, Omender Singh

43. **Metformin and Other Oral Hypoglycemic Agents**
   Prashant Singh, Omender Singh

44. **Chemical and Biological Warfare**
   Yash Javeri, Bharat Jagiasi, Gunjan Chanchalani

SECTION 10

Miscellaneous Toxicities

38 CHAPTER

Heavy Metal Poisoning

Prashant Nasa

INTRODUCTION

Heavy metals are ubiquitous in our environment and some of them are naturally occurring elements of earths' crust; they existed before any form of life on earth and expected to continue beyond humans' survival. In recent years, these have become increasing ecological and global public health concern because of environmental contamination through activities like use in industries, metal-mining and smelting, domestic use, and agricultural activities.[1,2] Heavy metal toxicity in acute medicine is an uncommon diagnosis, yet if remain undiagnosed may contribute to significant morbidity and mortality.[2,3] Which metals are considered as heavy metals? The definition of heavy metals used in literature varies. Heavy metals literally mean metals with density heavier than water. The two common criteria for classification of heavy metals are either based on atomic weight or on specific density (specific density of >5 g/cm³).[2] Some other manuscripts have used "heavy metal" as a general term comprising of all those metals and/or semimetals with linkage to environmental contamination and/or potential toxicity to human beings.[3-5] All heavy metals are toxic is not true, e.g. copper and selenium are pivotal in physiological and metabolic functions and commonly called as trace elements but are potentially toxic at high levels of exposure.[4] The International Union of Pure and Applied Chemistry in its report has recommended to stop using this terminology.[5] The human exposure to these metals is in different forms and may be some of this exposure is innocuous. The toxicity depends on factors like the type of metal, route, total dose, duration of exposure, chemical form of metal, and whether the exposure was acute or chronic.[6] There are patients related factors too which can influence toxicity like age, young children are more susceptible to lead toxicity; diet, heavy metals may be contaminants of dietary supplement; and lifestyle, cobalt toxicity related cardiomyopathy in alcoholics (Beers drinker's cardiomyopathy). The toxicity of these metals is commonly chronic and very rarely involves acute services of health care. The critical care or acute care physicians are involved in direct care of these patients only with either acute toxicity (iron or lead—intentional or unintentional ingestion) or less often in initial diagnosis of a patient presenting with multiorgan dysfunction where high index of suspicion based on previous experience or knowledge of the signs and symptoms may give a clue. These metals have also been implicated as potential carcinogenic by various international health agencies such as the World Health Organization, the Environmental Protection Agency of the United States, and the European Food Safety Authority.[4,7] In this chapter, we discussed arsenic, lead, mercury, cadmium, and chromium which are important to public health.

PATHOPHYSIOLOGY

Whatever the mode of entry of heavy metals to the body ingestion or inhalation of metallic dust and fumes, the blood is main medium of its initial action and transport to different organs in body.[8] The common mechanism proposed for heavy metal toxicity in blood is binding to oxygen, nitrogen, and sulfhydryl groups of proteins (Fig. 1). This result in alterations of enzymatic activity and induce synthesis of metal binding proteins, metalloproteinases. These molecules then bind to heavy metals using thiol-ligands and transport metals throughout the body and thus multiorgan toxicity.[6-8] Almost all organ systems are involved by the toxicity; however, there is predilection of certain organ systems like nervous system, liver, kidney, and hematopoietic system depending on pharmacokinetics of involved metal the duration (chronicity) and extent of the exposure, and the age of the patient.[4,6,8] The oxidative stress produced by these metals produce oxidation stress which may induce DNA damage, protein modification, lipid peroxidation, and others.

United States (US) Environmental Protection Agency (EPA) and International Agency for Research on Cancer has classified these metals either "known" or "probable" human carcinogens.[2,7,9]

GENERAL PRINCIPLES OF ASSESSMENT AND MANAGEMENT

The history of exposure where it is available is the most specific clue to diagnosis. The history should be detail in case of potential heavy metal toxicity and should include, but not limited to occupational exposures, dietary, lifestyle including recreational activities, and area of staying. However, in few cases it is very difficult to identify the source as symptoms are delayed after exposure.

The acute toxicity is mostly seen in case of occupational or accidental setting. The inhalational heavy metal toxicity called as "metal fume fever (MFF)" or "Monday morning fever" or, "Zinc shakes" is usually a self-limiting syndrome seen in industrial workers who are exposed to metal oxide fumes.[9,10] Though seen first with zinc oxide but may occur with other metals like magnesium, cobalt, and copper oxide too.[11] In acute heavy exposure, presentation may be like flu like with nausea, vomiting, cough, dyspnea, diarrhea, and abdominal pain with the symptoms starts as early as 3 hours.

The assessment of the patients includes evaluation of different organs for toxicity. The cardiac (cardiomyopathy, dysrhythmias), renal (acute tubular necrosis, acidosis), respiratory (acute interstitial pneumonia, bronchiolitis obliterans organizing pneumonia), and brain (encephalopathy) involvement may be seen in acute toxicity. The chronic toxicity, however, may involve any organ of body with predilection to nervous, hematopoietic, integumentary, and gastrointestinal (GI) system. The knowledge of toxidromes seen with heavy metal toxicity may raise an index of suspicion and clinical expert in toxicology should be involved for timely diagnosis and management (Table 1).

The specific laboratory testing for individual metal should be undertaken in case of suspicion after a liaison with laboratory staff. As these tests are infrequently ordered and/or mostly send to a nodal laboratory out of the hospital, the instructions on method of collection, type, and quantity of sample, precautions during transport, and time taken for reporting should be followed; the interpretation

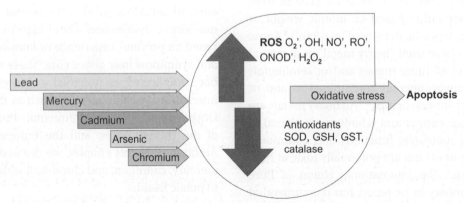

Fig. 1: Mechanism of heavy metal toxicity. (GSH: glutathione reductase; GST: glutathione S-transferase; H_2O_2: hydrogen peroxide; ROS: reactive oxygen species; SOD: superoxide dismutase)

Table 1: Clinical features and diagnosis of heavy metals toxicity.

Metal	Acute toxicity	Chronic toxicity	Diagnosis
Arsenic	Gastrointestinal: Nausea, vomiting, profound diarrhea Neurological: Encephalopathy, painful neuropathy Others: Hemolysis, acute kidney injury, mutisystem organ failure, prolonged QT syndrome	Skin: Hypopigmentation/hyperkeratosis Neurological: Encephalopathy, ascending peripheral neuropathy Cancer: Lung, urinary bladder, skin Diabetes	Arsenic concentration in 24-hour urine: • ≥ 50 µg/L urine • 100 µg/g creatinine
Lead	Gastrointestinal: Nausea, vomiting Neurological: Headache, seizures, ataxia, encephalopathy	Neurological: Encephalopathy, nephropathy, foot-drop/wrist-drop Hematological: Anemia Reproductive system: Decrease sperm count, infertility miscarriages, stillbirth	Blood lead level: For symptomatic patients • Children: Blood level >5 µg/dL, chelation therapy above 45 µg/dL • Adults : ≥70 µg/dL
Mercury	Elemental (vapor): Metal fume fever, erosive bronchitis, bronchiolitis Inorganic salts (ingestion): Caustic gastroenteritis	Acrodynia, tremors, erethism, behavioral changes, insomnia, amnesia	Blood levels more than for acute exposure 10 µg/L (whole blood); 20 µg/L (24-hour urine)
Cadmium	Metal fume fever—pneumonitis	Nephrotoxicity: Fanconi syndrome like presentation Bones: Osteomalacia, osteoporosis Cancer: Lung is the most definitively established site Others: Adrenals, testes, and the hemopoietic system	Blood level: ≥5 µg/L Urine: ≥15 µg/g creatinine
Chromium	Ingestion: GI ulcers hemorrhage, hemolysis, acute renal failure Inhalation: Rhinitis, rhinorrhea, asthma	Ingestion: Anemia, infertility, GI ulcers, dermatitis, skin ulcers Inhalation: Nasal ulcers, septal perforation, pulmonary fibrosis, lung cancer	No clear reference standard with urine and blood levels are send for diagnosis

(GI: gastrointestinal)

of results may also require help of a toxicology expert.[12] Hair analysis is usually unreliable and avoid for diagnosis. The interpretation of metal concentration in urine samples results should be done in relation to the timing of ingestion and collection of sample.

The important component of management for metal toxicity is the termination of source of exposure and if possible decontamination. Activated charcoal does not bind metals and thus is of limited usefulness in cases of metal ingestion. In case of acute exposure or in case of serious multiorgan failure, initial focus should be on good supportive care. General principles of toxicity should be applied like: airway patency and protection, mechanical ventilation in case of impending or overt respiratory failure, identify and treatment of cardiomyopathy and dysrhythmias, circulatory support with replacement of fluid and electrolytes, and monitor and support organ dysfunction. Chelating agents, if available, are definitive treatment for heavy metal toxicity which bind metals into stable compounds and either make them less toxic and/or enhance their excretion.[13-15] Chelation is rarely indicated in the acute poisoning except in lead encephalopathy. The chelation therapy for suspected or confirmed metal exposures should be made in consultation with a medical toxicologist or physician expert in toxicology. The use of chelating agents depends on the metal involved and the clinical circumstances. The most commonly used chelating agents are dimercaprol [British anti-Lewisite (BAL)], ethylenediamine tetraacetic acid (EDTA), succimer [dimercaptosuccinic acid (DMSA)], and penicillamine. These agents basically supply sulfhydryl groups which help in displacement of heavy metals from biological proteins and finally elimination from the body (Table 2).[14,15]

Miscellaneous Toxicities

Table 2: Chelating drugs.

Chemical name	Common name	Metabolism	Metal chelated
2,3-bis (sulfanyl) butanedioic acid	Dimercaptosuccinic acid (DMSA)	Urine (>90% as DMSA-cysteine disulfide conjugate)	Lead, arsenic, mercury, cadmium, silver, copper
Sodium 2,3-bis (sulfanyl) propane-1-sulfonate	Dimercaptopropane sulfonate (DMPS)	Urine (>84%)	Mercury, arsenic, copper, lead, cadmium, silver
2-[2-[bis(carboxymethyl)amino] ethyl-(carboxymethyl)amino] acetic acid	Ethylenediaminetetraacetic acid (EDTA)	Not metabolized, excreted unchanged	Lead, cadmium, zinc
(2S)-2-amino-3-methyl-3-sulfanylbutanoic acid	Penicillamine	Urine excretion as disulfides	Copper, arsenic, zinc, mercury, lead
2,3-bis(sulfanyl)propan-1-ol	Dimercaprol; British Anti-Lewisite (BAL)	Urine excretion unchanged	Arsenic, gold, mercury, lead (in combination with CaNa$_2$ EDTA)

SPECIFIC METALS

Arsenic

Arsenic is a lethal and ubiquitous heavy metal in our environment (20th most abundant element in earth's crust).[16] Arsenic toxicity is either accidental (industrial source, contaminated water, wine, pesticides) or from malicious source (suicidal or homicidal).[13,16] The dietary history especially herbal, Ayurvedic, and nutritional supplements is important because of potential contamination. Recently, arsenic is gaining interest for its medicinal interest in hematological malignancies (acute promyelocytic leukemias, multiple myeloma, myelodysplastic syndromes) and even some resistant solid blood tumors.[17,18]

Mechanism of Toxicity

Arsenic in inorganic form is potentially more toxic than its organic form. Trivalent inorganic arsenic binds the sulfydryl group of enzymes in citric acid cycle causing inhibition of pyruvate dehydrogenase and its conversion to acetyl coenzyme A, and hence affecting cell respiration (Fig. 1). It also blocks the production of glutathione and produces oxidative stress. Pentavalent forms are relatively less toxic and resemble inorganic phosphates which cause uncoupling of oxidative phosphorylation by forming dimercaptosuccinic acid adenosine diphosphate (ADP)-arsenate form instead of adenosine triphosphate (ATP).[19,20]

Clinical Features

Acute toxicity on ingestion present like infectious severe diarrhea, vomiting, and may complicate with cardiac dysrhythmias and shock. Inhalation route with gaseous form manifests as flu-like symptoms like headache, abdominal pain, nausea, vomiting, but can complicate with hemolysis, hemoglobinuria, acute kidney injury, and even death. Chronic exposure predominantly involves skin, hematological, and nervous system. "Mees" line (white bands on nails of fingers or toes), alopecia, hyperkeratotic dermatitis, peripheral neuropathy, ascending paralysis (like Guillain-Barré syndrome), and rarely liver and renal involvement is seen. Arsenic is potential carcinogenic as per US-EPA and associated with cancers of lung, urinary bladder and skin.[9,21]

Diagnosis

The hematological changes seen with chronic exposure are macrocytic anemia, elevated eosinophils, and basophilic stippling of red blood cell (RBC), while hemolytic anemia can be seen in acute exposure. The blood levels of arsenic may be false negative as arsenic is rapidly cleared from the blood. Arsenic is predominantly excreted in urine and 24-hour urine collection for total arsenic excretion can be diagnostic (Table 1). The urine levels can also be used to monitor the response to therapy.[22]

Treatment

In acute poisoning, the treatment is mainly supportive. The GI decontamination with activated charcoal has no role; whole bowel irrigation with polyethylene glycol, however, has shown to decrease absorption.[23] Hemodialysis is found to be useful in some cases and can be considered in acute course.[24] The dialysis, however,

Heavy Metal Poisoning 343

does not alter outcome and has no role in hemolysis. The chelation therapy is useful for acute toxicity with agents like BAL, DMSA and dimercaptopropane sulfonate (DMPS) with latter as drug of choice.[15,25]

Lead

Lead is another ubiquitous heavy metal in our environment with no biological role in humans. The human exposure is mainly occupational and rarely accidental: those living in certain developing countries, lower socio-economic strata, and those exposed to lower-grade gasoline, vehicles exhausts, paints, plumbing pipes, ceramic glazes, storage batteries, medical equipment, and lead faucets.[2,3,8] Children are more exposed to lead by hand-to-mouth activities in contaminated soils, paint chips, and toys made of lead.[8] Lead is most common environmental illness in children in United States. According to Centre of Disease Control and Prevention (CDC) surveillance, around half a million children aged 1–5 years have lead level above toxic range of 5 μg/dL (reference range by CDC).[26]

Mechanism

The lead toxicity is similar to other heavy metals, by causing increased production of reactive oxygen species (ROS) [hydroperoxide, hydrogen peroxide (H_2O_2), and singlet oxygen] and interference with generation of antioxidants. Lead inhibits glutathione and other antioxidants like superoxide dismutase and catalase. This causes intracellular oxidative stress which in turn causes cell membrane damage by lipid peroxidation. ROS may also cause damage to structural cellular proteins, nucleic acids, and eventually apoptosis (Fig. 1). There is another mechanism of lead toxicity by ability to replace biologicals ions like Ca^{2+}, Mg^{2+}, and Na^+ by lead ions. These important ions are involved in many physiological processes like intra- and intercellular signaling, protein folding, maturation, apoptosis, cellular transportation, enzyme regulation, and release of neurotransmitters.[27]

Clinical Features

The presentation of lead toxicity depends on form of lead (organic, inorganic, or metallic), age of exposure, duration, and time of exposure. As mentioned earlier, children are more susceptible to lead toxicity because of increased exposure and intestinal absorption in GI tract.

Acute exposure is mainly occupational at work place and involves predominantly GI and neurological systems with loss of appetite, nausea, colicky abdominal pain, headache, hallucinations, vertigo, fatigue, sleeplessness, and rarely renal dysfunction. Chronic exposure has mainly hematological and neurological manifestations. After absorption from GI tract, 99% of the lead is bound to the hemoglobin portion of RBCs and via the vascular system reaches and deposited into liver, kidney, bone, and hair. Microcytic anemia with basophilic stippling of RBCs is not characteristic but commonly seen.[2,3,8,27] Lead toxicity can cause tubular dysfunction and glomerular sclerosis.[28] Motor neuropathy (wrist or foot drop) with sensory sparing is seen in adults. Lead exposure during pregnancy can cross placental barrier and even found in breast milk. In children, lead exposure may cause mental retardation, birth defects, psychosis, autism, allergies and dyslexia.[8,27]

Diagnosis

Blood lead levels (BLL) more than 10 μg/dL is diagnostic. Symptoms, however, develop at higher exposure with pediatrics BLL more than or equal to 45 μg/dL and in adults more than or equal to 70 μg/dL.[29] Free erythrocyte protoporphyrin (FEP) level correlates with microcytic anemia. Liver and renal function tests to identify organ dysfunction are adjuvant tests.[13]

Treatment

The most effective treatment is to stop further exposure. As per US Occupational Safety and Health Administration (OSHA), the permissible exposure limit is 50 μg/m³ for an 8-hour shift. The employees should be mandatory abstained from work if the average of their last 3 BLLs is 50 μg/dL or higher. For children with BLL more than 10 μg/dL, community-based intervention involving nutritional, education, and environment modification should be undertaken. Chelation therapy is indicated for both acute and chronic exposure. Oral DMSA are first-line agents. Calcium disodium EDTA and BAL are parenteral chelating agents which can be used in cases of encephalopathy. With very high BLL (>100 μg/dL), combination of BAL and EDTA can be used.[15,30]

Mercury

Mercury is toxic to humans in any of its form—elemental, organic, or inorganic. Methyl mercury, organic form

Miscellaneous Toxicities

of mercury, with fish as major source is most deadly of all.

The mercury poisoning is usually through ingestion via contaminated food, injection seen in dental care procedures (using amalgams in endodontics), accidental (mercury thermometers, and sphygmomanometer), occupational— inhalational or absorption through skin (e.g. mining), and others (using fluorescent light bulbs and batteries).[2,3,8] The last century had seen at least two major public health disasters of mercury poisoning. The infamous Minamata Bay leak of mercury into water and other in Niigata, both in Japan, contaminating fish and other sea food with more than 2,000 and 700 victims, respectively.[31,32]

Pathophysiology

Mercury is potential toxic to any organ.

Organic mercury: Organic mercury which is available in three forms—aryl-, short-, and long-chain alkyl compounds, is readily absorbed from GI tract, because of high lipid solubility and corrosive properties. Noteworthy, methylmercury (an aryl form) is high lipid soluble, rapidly absorbed from GI tract (90–95%), and cross blood–brain barrier and placenta too. It freely distributes all over the body with deposition in brain, kidney, liver, hair, and skin. In blood, it gets oxidized to inorganic mercury which in turn bind to phosphoryl, carboxyl, and sulfhydryl groups interfering many cellular functional and metabolic pathways. Inorganic mercury results in oxidative stress, interference in DNA transcription, interference with heme synthesis, damages cell membrane integrity, and neurotransmitter disruption. The mechanism of mercury poisoning on the nervous system is by free radical production, inhibiting protein synthesis and repair and accumulation of neural excitotoxins (serotonin, aspartate, and glutamate).[2,3,8,33,34]

Inorganic mercury: It is also available in three forms— elemental or vapor, metallic, and mercurial. Elemental mercury (vapor) is available in liquid but easily vaporizes at room temperature and thus explains toxicity by inhalation (80% of cases). The inorganic mercury, as explained above, binds with sulfhydryl and selenohydryl, and damages the tertiary and quaternary structure of proteins.[8,33,34]

Other inorganic forms are available as mercuric salt with batteries as main source; skin is major port of entry, only 10% is absorbed enterally. The poor CNS penetration is attributed to its poor lipid solubility. The kidneys are the predominant site of accumulation and excretion and hence causing significant renal damage.[33,34]

Clinical Features

Acute elemental mercury (vapor) exposure via inhalation can lead to MFF and respiratory failure by causing erosive bronchitis and bronchiolitis. Low-grade chronic exposure causes neurological symptoms as vapor can cross blood–brain barrier and can cause tremors, erethism (irritability, excitability, anxiety, insomnia, and social withdrawal), personality and behavioral changes, insomnia, memory loss, and in severe cases even delirium and hallucinations. Dermal exposure by elemental mercury can cause allergic features known as acrodynia (pink disease). It causes erythema of the palms and soles, hands and feet, pruritus, desquamating rash, and even alopecia. The systemic manifestations can also be there which includes diaphoresis, tachycardia, hypertension, photophobia, irritability, anorexia, insomnia, constipation, or diarrhea by corrosive action on upper GI tract.[8,33,34]

Mercuric salts have mainly intestinal toxicity— abdominal pain, bloody diarrhea, and even shock. Acute renal injury develops in acute toxicity survivors. Subacute or chronic inorganic mercury intoxication has predominantly GI symptoms, and even neurologic and renal dysfunction. Chronic mercury toxicity promotes atherogenesis by lipid peroxidation and oxidative stress and is associated with coronary artery disease, stroke, and peripheral arterial disease.[35]

Organic mercury especially methylmercury after oxidation to inorganic mercury has neurotoxicity and dermal toxicity. The neurological features predominate with neuropsychiatric features, ataxia, visual loss, hearing loss, neuropathy, paralysis, and even death.[34]

Diagnosis

The blood, hair, and urine mercury levels are used for diagnosis of toxicity but none of them correlate with total body burden. Urine levels above 10–20 µg/L are significant. Urine levels are good indicator of inorganic and elemental mercury exposure, however, are unreliable for organic mercury (methylmercury) because of its elimination mainly in feces. Blood level are diagnostic for acute methylmercury exposure. It binds to erythrocytes with half-life of 44 days.[34] Hair and nail levels are used for both acute and chronic exposure

Heavy Metal Poisoning

especially methylmercury. A hair value of above 1.2 µg/g is diagnostic. Use of chelating agents for provocation in order to improve urine diagnostic levels is not routinely recommended and may be harmful.[13,36]

Treatment

In acute poisoning, emergency supportive care for airway, breathing, and circulation is standard especially with respiratory obstruction or failure seen with inhalation of elemental mercury and the ingestion of corrosive inorganic mercury. Activated charcoal can be used for GI decontamination for both organic and inorganic mercury. Gastric lavage can be considered for organic mercury. Chelating agents are indicated for symptomatic patients and/or positive blood or urine levels. BAL is traditionally recommended chelating agent and newer studies even support oral agents like DMSA.[34,35]

Cadmium

The cadmium exposure from environmental has increased over the years from burning of fossil fuel, metal mining and refining, use and development of phosphate fertilizers, food stocks from contaminated ground soil, and waste burning. Occupational exposure of cadmium is seen in industries involved in battery production, electroplating, and production of polyvinyl plastics and paints. Smoking is a major source of cadmium with levels in blood four to five times in smokers than in nonsmokers.

Mechanism of Toxicity

Cadmium is distributed all over the body after absorption. Around 60% is deposited in liver and kidney with very prolonged clearance half-life of over 25 years. Cadmium binds to sulfhydryl group-containing protein creating oxidative stress which affects cell proliferation, differentiation, and apoptosis (Fig. 1). The other mechanisms include competitive interference with zinc or magnesium causing interference in heme production, binds to mitochondrial, and inhibits cellular respiration and phosphorylation.[3,8,37,38]

Clinical Features

The manifestations of cadmium toxicity depend on route, quantity, and rate of exposure. Kidneys are the chief organ for toxicity owing to its deposition in proximal tubule followed by bone, liver, and placenta. Nephrotoxicity in seen mainly with occupational and environmental exposure of cadmium and produces a picture like Fanconi syndrome (glucosuria, aminoaciduria, phosphaturia, hypercalciuria, polyuria, and decreased buffering capacity).[37,38] Cadmium effects skeletal system by impairing vitamin D metabolism in kidney, decrease gut absorption of calcium, and direct effect of cadmium on bones and derangement of collagen metabolism, which can cause osteomalacia and/or osteoporosis.

Itai-itai disease (first seen in Japan) is most severe form of cadmium toxicity characterized by osteomalacia, osteoporosis, renal tubular dysfunction, and anemia.[39] Cadmium is linked epidemiologically to chronic vascular diseases like hypertension, coronary artery, peripheral vascular disease, and diabetes by its effect on vascular intima media thickness, oxidative stress, and increased lipid peroxidation.[37,38] Cadmium is also linked to male infertility by impairing spermatogenesis, sperm quality, and even decreases libido by decreasing testosterone level. In females, it inhibits the ovarian function and increases the rate of spontaneous abortions. Cadmium is carcinogenic, with lung being most established site and may be involved in lung, adrenals, testes, liver, hematopoietic system, bladder, and stomach malignancies.[4,8,37,38]

Diagnosis

Blood and urine levels are used to diagnose toxicity of cadmium level. The reference range for diagnosis in urine is 15 µg/g creatinine and blood 5 µg/L. Urine β_2-microglobulin is marker of nephrotoxicity.[13]

Treatment

Acute poisoning is rare and need similar approach as any other heavy metal. Activated charcoal cannot absorb cadmium and only GI irrigation may help. Among chelating agents, EDTA can significantly increase urinary elimination.[38] However, combination of chelating agents are more effective in cadmium toxicity with DMSA and *monoisoamyl-DMSA* is most optimal regimen.[2,37,38]

Chromium

Chromium in nature exists in its oxidation state (valence state) ranging chromium (II) to chromium (VI).[2] The two most stable state are chromium (III) (ferrochromite) and

Miscellaneous Toxicities

chromium (VI) while elemental chromium or chromium (0) is unstable and does not exist naturally.[2,3] The environmental contamination [predominant chromium (VI)] is mainly coming from industrial source (metal processing, leather tanning, stainless steel welding, and dyes and pigments especially ferrochrome and chrome pigment production).[2,40] Chromium (III) which is ubiquitous in environment are less toxic, because of no GI absorption and has a biological role in metabolism of glucose, fat, and protein metabolism by its effect on insulin action. Chromium (VI) is a major public health concern because of toxicity and mainly industrial exposure.[2,3,8] According to US-OSHA, maximum level of exposure for chromium in workplace is 5 $\mu g/m^3$, for an 8-hour time-weighted average.[41]

Mechanism and Clinical Features

Chromium (VI) is very powerful oxidizing agent. It is corrosive and inhalation is main port of entry followed by GI tract and skin, can easily pass through cell membranes and cause intracellular free radical production. Chromium (VI) after reaching its target cells is reduced by glutathione reductase (GSH), in presence of hydrogen peroxide and ascorbic acid, to produce unstable oxidative intermediates [chromium (V), (IV), hydroxyl radicals] and finally to chromium (III). As chromium III cannot enter target organs/cell, the amount and rate of entry of chromium IV into these cells/organs ultimately, decide its toxicity.[2] The corrosive nature causes nasal ulcers, rhinitis, rhinorrhea, asthma, nasopharyngeal pruritus, and on chronic exposure may cause perforation of nasal septa, pneumoconiosis, and restrictive lung disease. The ingestion and systemic absorption of chromium (VI) can cause GI ulcers, anemia, infertility (sperm damage), renal tubular damage, liver necrosis, and male reproductive system damage. The skin effect seen with dichromates and chromium (VI) includes dermatitis and ulcers seen mainly with occupational exposure. Intracellular oxidative stress can cause DNA damage, chromosomal abnormalities, DNA adducts, and alterations in replication and transcription of DNA. This explains its carcinogenic potential with increased risk of lung, nasal, and nasopharyngeal cancers.[2,3,8]

Diagnosis

Urine and blood levels are mainly send for diagnosis. Hair samples are not useful because of high risk of environmental contamination.

Treatment

In acute, high-level chromium exposure, the treatment is mainly supportive and symptomatic. In case of nephrotoxicity, urine alkalinization may help initially and gastric lavage in case of ingestion. Ten percent EDTA ointment is useful for dermatitis and might facilitate removal of chromate scabs. In case of chronic exposure, the main treatment is removal of patient from further exposure. Chelating agents are not useful in chromium toxicity.[2,14,15]

CONCLUSION

Heavy metal toxicity is increasingly becoming a major public health problem. The patients presenting in emergency with acute toxicity is uncommon; however, a focused history of exposure and knowledge of toxidromes seen with heavy metals and early expert consultation is key to their management. A close liaison with regional toxic center is pivotal in interpretation of laboratory results and recent evidence-based recommendations in management of such patients.

KEY POINTS

- Heavy metal poisoning is uncommon but incidence is increasing due to human-environmental interactions with urbanization and industrialization
- Diagnosis requires focused history of potential metal exposure and high index of suspicion in patients with abnormal multisystem presentations
- Acute management is mainly supportive, along with stopping further exposure, decontamination and elimination, if possible
- Long-term toxicity is multi-system and it varies as per the specifics of metal and management again is supportive with little role of chelating agents in few metals
- Many of the metals are potentially carcinogenic. Its knowledge, serial follow-up and close contact with the regional poison center is essential for proper management.

REFERENCES

1. Bradl H. Heavy Metals in the Environment: Origin, Interaction and Remediation, 6th volume. London: Academic Press; 2002.
2. Tchounwou PB, Yedjou CG, Patlolla AK, et al. Heavy metal toxicity and the environment. EXS. 2012;101:133-64.

3. Longo DL. Chapter e49: Heavy metal poisoning. In: Howard Hu (Ed). Harrison's Principles of Internal Medicine, 18th edition. New York: The McGraw-Hill; 2012.

4. Dorne JL, Kass GE, Bordajandi LR, et al. Human risk assessment of heavy metals: principles and applications. Met Ions Life Sci. 2011;8:27-60.

5. Duffus, JH. "Heavy metals"—a meaningless term? (IUPAC Technical Report). Pure Appl Chem. 2002;74:793-807.

6. Sue YJ. Mercury. In: Hoffman RS, Howland MA, Lewin NA, Nelson LS, Goldfrank LR (Eds). Goldfrank's Toxicologic Emergencies, 10th edition. New York, NY: McGraw-Hill Education; 2015. pp. 1334-44.

7. Koedrith P, Kim H, Weon JI, et al. Toxicogenomic approaches for understanding molecular mechanisms of heavy metal mutagenicity and carcinogenicity. Int J Hyg Environ Health. 2013;216(5):587-98.

8. Jaishankar M, Tseten T, Anbalagan N, et al. Toxicity, mechanism and health effects of some heavy metals. Interdiscip Toxicol. 2014;7(2):60-72.

9. Wu X, Cobbina SJ, Mao G, et al. Review of toxicity and mechanisms of individual and mixtures of heavy metals in the environment. Environ Sci Pollut Res Int. 2016;23(9):8244-59.

10. Malaguarnera M, Drago F, Malaguarnera G, et al. Metal fume fever. Lancet. 201329;381(9885):2298.

11. Greenberg MI, Vearrier D. Metal fume fever and polymer fume fever. Clin Toxicol (Phila). 2015;53(4):195-203.

12. Gordon T, Fine JM. Metal fume fever. Occup Med. 1993;8(3):504-17.

13. Keil DE, Berger-Ritchie J, McMillin GA. Testing for toxic elements: A focus on arsenic, cadmium, lead, and mercury. Lab Medicine. 2011;42:735-42.

14. Gummin DD, Mowry JB, Spyker DA, et al. 2016 Annual Report of the American Association of Poison Control Centers' National Poison Data System (NPDS): 34th Annual Report. Clin Toxicol (Phila). 2017;55(10):1072-252.

15. Sears ME. Chelation: Harnessing and enhancing heavy metal detoxification—a review. Sci World J. 2013;2013:219840.

16. Mandal BK, Suzuki KT. Arsenic round the world: a review. Talanta. 2002;58(1):201-35.

17. Emadi A, Gore SD. Arsenic trioxide-An old drug rediscovered. Blood Rev. 2010;24(4-5):191-9.

18. Lo-Coco F, Cicconi L, Breccia M. Current standard treatment of adult acute promyelocytic leukaemia. Br J Haematol. 2016;172(6):841-54.

19. Luna AL, Acosta-Saavedra LC, Lopez-Carrillo L, et al. Arsenic alters monocyte superoxide anion and nitric oxide production in environmentally exposed children. Toxicol Appl Pharmacol. 2010;245(2):244-51.

20. Balakumar P, Kaur J. Arsenic exposure and cardiovascular disorders: an overview. Cardiovasc Toxicol. 2009;9(4):169-76.

21. Cohen SM, Arnold LL, Beck BD, et al. Evaluation of the carcinogenicity of inorganic arsenic. Crit Rev Toxicol. 2013;43(9):711-52.

22. Hackenmueller SA, Strathmann FG. Total arsenic screening prior to fractionation enhances clinical utility and test utilization in the assessment of arsenic toxicity. Am J Clin Pathol. 2014;142(2):184-9.

23. Lech T, Trela F. Massive acute arsenic poisonings. Forensic Sci Int. 2005;151(2-3):273-7.

24. Duenas-Laita A, Perez-Miranda M, Gonzalez-Lopez MA, et al. Acute arsenic poisoning. Lancet. 2005;365(9475):1982.

25. Andersen O, Aaseth J. A review of pitfalls and progress in chelation treatment of metal poisonings. J Trace Elem Med Biol. 2016;38:74-80.

26. Betts KS. CDC Updates guidelines for children's lead exposure. Environ Health Perspect. 2012;120(7):a268.

27. Flora G, Gupta D, Tiwari A. Toxicity of lead: A review with recent updates. Interdiscip Toxicol. 2012;5(2):47-58.

28. Evans M, Fored CM, Nise G, et al. Occupational lead exposure and severe CKD: a population-based case-control and prospective observational cohort study in Sweden. Am J Kidney Dis. 2010;55(3):497-506.

29. CDC. US Department of Health and Human Services, National Institute for Occupational Safety and Health; 2013. Adult Blood Lead Epidemiology and Surveillance (ABLES). Available online as: https://www.cdc.gov/niosh/topics/ables/default.html

30. Lin JL, Ho HH, Yu CC. Chelation therapy for patients with elevated body lead burden and progressive renal insufficiency. A randomized, controlled trial. Ann Intern Med. 1999;130(1):7-13.

31. Mostafalou S, Abdollahi M. Environmental pollution by mercury and related health concerns: Renotice of a silent threat. Arh Hig Rada Toksikol. 2013;64:179-81.

32. Grandjean P, Satoh H, Murata K, et al. Adverse effects of methylmercury: environmental health research implication. Environ Health Perspect. 2010;118:1137-45.

33. Bernhoft RA. Mercury toxicity and treatment: a review of the literature. J Environ Public Health. 2012;2012:460508.

34. Rafati-Rahimzadeh M, Rafati-Rahimzadeh M, Kazemi S, et al. Current approaches of the management of mercury poisoning: need of the hour. Daru. 2014;22:46.

35. Park JD, Zheng W. Human exposure and health effects of inorganic and elemental mercury. J Prev Med Publ Health. 2012;45:344-52.

36. Risher JF, Amler SN. Mercury exposure: evaluation and intervention the inappropriate use of chelating agents in the diagnosis and treatment of putative mercury poisoning. Neurotoxicology. 2005;26(4):691-9.

37. Rafati Rahimzadeh M, Rafati Rahimzadeh M, Kazemi S, et al. Cadmium toxicity and treatment: An update. Caspian J Intern Med. 2017;8(3):135-45.

38. Bernhoft RA. Cadmium toxicity and treatment. Sci World J. 2013;2013:394652.

39. Umemura T, Wako Y. Pathogenesis of osteomalacia in Itai-itai Disease. J Toxicol Pathol. 2006;19:69-74.

40. Agency for Toxic Substances and Disease Registry (ATSDR). Toxicological Profile for Chromium. Atlanta, GA: U.S. Department of Health and Human Services, Public Health Service; 2008.

41. Occupational exposure to hexavalent chromium. Final rule. Occupational Safety and Health Administration (OSHA), Department of Labor. Fed Regist. 2006;71(39):10099-385.

39 CHAPTER

Envenomation: Snake, Scorpion, and Spider

Subramanian Senthilkumaran, Ponniah Thirumalai Kolundu Subramanian

INTRODUCTION

- There are about 3,000 species of snakes are found in the world and of them about 600 are venomous, mainly distributed in warm tropical regions[1]
- Global burden of snake bite is estimated to be about 421,000 envenomations and about 20,000 deaths each year.[2] About 50,000 people die of snake bite every year in India.[3]

TYPES OF SNAKES

Venomous snakes belong to two families—
1. *Family Elapidae*: Cobras, Kraits, and Coral Snakes. It has a subfamily:
   I. *Hydrophidae*: Sea snakes
2. *Family Viperidae*: The family of Viperidae has two subfamilies:
   I. Viperidae (Russell's viper, saw scaled viper)
   II. Crotalinae (Pit vipers, hump-nosed vipers and green pit vipers).

TOXIC EFFECTS OF SNAKE VENOM

- Snake venom is not a single component, but is highly complex mixture of a variety of components enzymatic and nonenzymatic proteins, and toxins with varying actions, which can work together having different toxicities; cytotoxic, neurotoxic, hemorrhagic, procoagulant and anticoagulant, nephrotoxicity and myotoxicity, etc.[4]
- Variation of venom composition of the same species may be due to geographical, seasonal or snake specific reasons, e.g. Russell's viper
- Quantity of venom injected at a bite is very variable, depending on the species and size of the snake and the mechanical efficiency of the bite
- For whatever the reason, a proportion of bites by venomous snakes do not result in envenoming, called dry bites.

PATHOPHYSIOLOGY

- Elapidae venom has predominately neurotoxins which causes paralysis of muscles by blocking the neuromuscular junction. These could be either postsynaptic (Elapidae) or presynaptic (Elapidae and some Viperidae)
- Some components of the neurotoxins have either direct or indirect action on the brain causing alteration of the level of consciousness
- Viperidae venom is rich in procoagulant enzymes and leads to coagulopathy. Hemorrhagins (zinc metalloproteinases) damage the endothelial lining of blood vessels causing spontaneous bleeding and direct red cell damage that produces intravascular hemolysis

CLINICAL FEATURES (TABLE 1)

- Hemolytic and myolytic phospholipase A2 produce rhabdomyolysis and myoglobinuria causing secondary renal failure and red cell membrane damage leading to hemolysis
- Local tissue injury occurs at the site of bite due to proteases, hyaluronidases and other enzymatic effects of the venom.

Russell's Viper

- Local swelling
- *Neurotoxicity*: Ptosis, external ophthalmoplegia, dysphagia, paralysis, etc.
- *Coagulopathy*: Incoagulable blood, hematuria, hematemesis, gum bleeding, etc.
- *Myotoxicity*: Myalgia, rhabdomyolysis
- Acute kidney injury.

Cobra

- Local swelling, blistering, tissue necrosis
- *Neurotoxicity*: Ptosis, external ophthalmoplegia, dysphagia, respiratory paralysis, limb and muscle weakness, etc.
- No coagulopathy.

Krait

- *Neurotoxicity*: Ptosis, external ophthalmoplegia, dysphagia, respiratory paralysis, limb muscle weakness, etc.
- No local effects/envenoming
- No coagulopathy.

Saw-scaled Viper

- Local bleeding and swelling

- *Coagulopathy*: Incoagulable blood and gum bleeding, etc.

Hump-nosed Viper

- Local swelling, hemorrhagic blisters, necrosis
- *Coagulopathy*: Incoagulable blood and gum bleeding, red urine, etc.
- Acute kidney injury.

Sea Snakes

- Acute rhabdomyolysis, trismus, myoglobinuria, hyperkalemia, acute kidney injury
- Neuromuscular paralysis, respiratory failure.

Green Pit Viper

Gross swelling and pain in the bitten limb and painful lymphadenopathy

DIAGNOSIS

- If the dead/live snake is brought, it can be identified
- Otherwise, the species responsible can be inferred from the clinical syndrome of symptoms and signs. Since we do not have any venom detections kits at the point of care so, the syndromic approach is useful[5]
- Circumstantial evidence is also help in krait bite—sleeping on the floor in a rural house, presenting with abdominal pain and neurotoxicity[6]
- It is supported by evidence of incoagulable blood detected by 20 minutes whole blood clotting test (20WBCT)—this is a very useful and informative bedside tests requires only a new, clean, dry, glass tube or bottle
- Point-of-care INR testing devices should not be used for snake bite cases to diagnose venom-induced consumption coagulopathy.[7]

Feature	Cobras	Kraits	Russell's viper	Saw scaled viper	Hump-nosed viper
Local pain/tissue damage	YES	NO	YES	YES	YES
Ptosis/neurological signs	YES	YES	YES	NO	NO
Hemostatic abnormalities	NO	NO	YES	YES	YES
Renal complications	NO	NO	YES	NO	YES
Response to neostigmine	YES	NO	NO	NO	NO
Response to ASV	YES	YES	YES	YES	NO

Table 1: Clinical aspects and therapeutic response of snake bite.

(ASV: antisnake venom)

INVESTIGATIONS

20-minute Whole Blood Clotting Test

- This is very useful bedside test to find out whether any evidence of coagulopathy
- In Southeast Asian region, incoagulable blood is diagnostic of a viper bite and rules out an elapid bite
- If there is any doubt, repeat the test in duplicate, including a "control" (blood from a healthy person)

Warning! If the tube or bottle used for the test is not made of ordinary glass, or if it has been used before and cleaned with detergent, its wall may not stimulate clotting of the blood sample in the usual way and test will be invalid.

- Depending on the availability, other investigations should include a full blood count with platelet, coagulation studies including d-dimer, FDP, PT, APTT and biochemical tests including creatine kinase. A urine analysis is helpful for detecting blood or myoglobin.

MANAGEMENT OF SNAKE BITE (FLOWCHART 1)

First Aid Treatment

- The four main steps involved in sequence in the correct first aid can be remembered by the mnemonic, Do it R.I.G.H.T.

  ○ *R = Reassure the patient.*
  (75% of snake bites are from a venomous species and that even if it is a venomous snake bite, on average only 50% of such bites actually envenomate, the rest are called "dry" bites)
  ○ *I = Immobilize without compression.*
  (Immobilize in the same way as a fractured limb. Do not allow the victim to walk, but should be carried. Do not apply any compression in the form of tight ligatures; their use can increase necrosis)
  ○ *G. H. = Get to Hospital fast.*
  (Traditional remedies have no proven benefit in treating snake bite).
  ○ *T= Tell the doctor.*
  (Any systemic symptoms such as drooping eyelids, double vision, dribbling and any taste of blood in the victim's mouth or developing bruising at the bite site that manifest on the way to hospital)

Most traditional first aid methods should be discouraged, they do more harm than good!

- Analgesia
- Antisnake venom
- Anticholinesterase therapy
- Tetanus prophylaxis if needed
- Local wound care
- Antibiotic should be considered in case of cellulitis or necrosis.

Flowchart 1: Clinical pathway: Snake bite management.

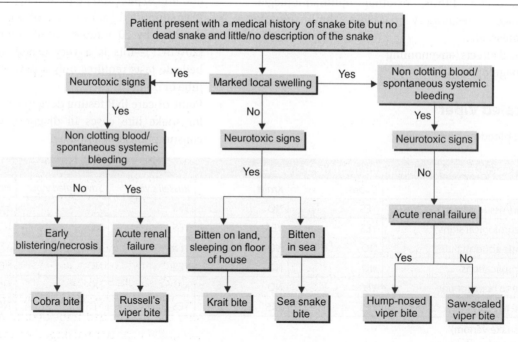

Envenomation: Snake, Scorpion, and Spider

Antisnake Venom Treatment

- Antivenom is the only specific antidote to snake venom
- The most important decision in the management of a snake bite victim is whether or not to give antivenom
- Antivenom treatment carries the risk of severe adverse reactions and in most countries it is costly and may be in limited supply
- Polyvalent antivenin manufactured in India will not neutralize venom of pit vipers.[8]

INDICATIONS FOR ANTIVENOM

Antivenom treatment is recommended if and when a patient with proven or suspected snake bite develops one or more of signs of systemic envenoming (Box 1).[9-11]

Box 1: Indications for antivenom.

Systemic envenoming
- Hemostatic abnormalities:
  - Spontaneous systemic bleeding (clinical)
  - Coagulopathy or thrombocytopenia (laboratory)
- Neurotoxic signs:
  - Ptosis
  - External ophthalmoplegia
  - Paralysis (clinical)
- Cardiovascular abnormalities:
  - Hypotension
  - Shock
  - Cardiac arrhythmia (clinical)
  - Abnormal ECG
- Acute renal failure:
  - Oliguria/anuria (clinical)
  - Rising blood creatinine/urea (laboratory)
- Hemoglobin-/myoglobinuria:
  - Dark brown urine (clinical)
  - Urine dipsticks, hyperkalemia (laboratory)

Local envenoming
- Local swelling involving more than half of the bitten limb (in the absence of a tourniquet)
- Swelling after bites on the digits (toes and especially fingers)
- Rapid extension of swelling (for example beyond the wrist or ankle within a few hours of bites on the hands or feet)
- Development of an enlarged tender lymph node draining the bitten limb

(ECG: electrocardiogram)

- Skin/conjunctival hypersensitivity testing does not reliably predict early or late antivenom reactions and is not recommended
- There is no absolute contraindication to antivenom treatment, but patients who have reacted to equine serum in the past and those with a strong history of atopic diseases should be given antivenom only if they have signs of systemic envenoming
- It may be monospecific or polyspecific antivenom should be given by the intravenous route only
- Intravenous infusion: Reconstituted freeze, dried or liquid antivenom is diluted in approximately 200–300 mL of isotonic saline and infused at a constant rate over a period of 1 hour and repeated as on need
- Snakes inject the same dose of venom into children and adults. Children must therefore be given the same dose of antivenin as adults. But, volume of the infusion should be adjusted according to the body weight and underlying diseases. Correct dose of antivenin, given promptly, is needed to save children
- Saving the mother's life is the priority in pregnancy. In this regard the mother should not be deprived of any treatment that is indicated.

ADVERSE REACTION TO ANTIVENOM

Anaphylaxis and anaphylactoid reaction is a major obstacle for the treatment of the antivenom and may be life threatening. In case of anaphylaxis, then:
- Stop antivenom
- About 0.5 mg of 1:1,000 adrenaline will be given IM for adults. Children are given 0.01 mg/kg body weight of adrenaline IM
- For long-term protection against anaphylactoid reaction, hydrocortisone, H1 and H2 blockers will be administered IV
- A second dose of 0.5 mg of adrenaline 1:1,000 IM is given after 10–15 minutes if the patient's condition has not improved or is worsening
- This can be repeated for a third and final occasion but in the vast majority of reactions, two doses of adrenaline will be sufficient
- If there is hypotension or hemodynamic instability, IV fluids should be given
- The ASV can be restarted slowly for 10–15 minutes after the patient had improved, under close monitoring. Then the normal drip rate should be resumed.

End Point for Antivenin

- Spontaneous systemic bleeding usually stops within 15–30 minutes
- Neurotoxic envenoming of the postsynaptic type will begin to improve as early as 30 minutes after antivenom, but usually takes several hours.

Criteria for Giving More Antivenom

- If the blood remains incoagulable as measured by 20WBCT 6 hours after the initial dose of antivenom, the same dose has to be repeated. It is based on the time taken for the liver to restore coagulable levels of fibrinogen and other clotting factors is 3–9, mean 6 hours
- In patients who continue to bleed briskly, the dose of antivenom should be repeated within 1–2 hours
- In case of deteriorating neurotoxicity or cardiovascular signs, the initial dose of antivenom should be repeated after 1–2 hours.

MANAGEMENT IN SPECIAL SITUATIONS

- *When no antivenom is available*: Conservative approach/plasmapheresis
- *Neurotoxic envenoming with respiratory paralysis*: Assisted ventilation
- *Hemostatic abnormalities*: Transfusion of clotting factors and platelets, fresh frozen plasma
- *Renal failure*: Dialysis
- *Dark brown urine (myoglobinuria or hemoglobinuria)*: Correct hypovolemia, and acidosis and consider a single early infusion of mannitol
- *Severe local envenoming*: Local necrosis, intracompartmental syndromes—surgical intervention may be needed but the risks of surgery in a patient with consumption coagulopathy, thrombocytopenia and enhanced fibrinolysis must be balanced against the life-threatening complications of local envenoming.

Disposition

- Patients without signs of envenomation should still be admitted for observation for 24 hours due to the potential delay in onset of findings of venom poisoning
- Any snake bite victim with signs or symptoms of envenomation should be admitted to the hospital.

Rehabilitation

Physical and psychological rehabilitation are needed for patients who have had complications and recovered following a long hospital stay.

SCORPION STINGS

Scorpion stings are acute life-threatening medical emergency which are common in rural areas of many tropical and subtropical regions of the world.

Epidemiology

- Out of 1,500 scorpion species known to exist, about 30 are of medical importance
- In India, 86 species of scorpions have been identified; *Mesobuthus tamulus* and *Palamneus gravimanus* are of medical importance[12]
- Even though millions of scorpion stings occur annually, most cases are minor, with localized pain and minimal systemic involvement. However, severe envenomation is a most important health issues in South Asia, Middle East and North Africa
- While the incidence of scorpion stings is higher in adults, the severity of envenomation is considerably greater in children, in whom the mortality is up to ten times higher than in adults.[13]

Toxicity of Venom

- Venom is deposited deep to subcutaneous tissue after sting and it is almost completely absorbed from sting site within 7–8 hours (70% of maximum concentration of venom in the blood reached within 15 min of sting)
- Several toxins have been identified in scorpion venoms, most of which are small peptide toxins that target voltage-dependent ion channels and toxins alter these channels, leading to prolonged depolarization and, hence, neuronal excitation[14]
- The toxins that have the greatest medical significance are the scorpion α-toxins which cause massive endogenous release of the catecholamines as well as other vasoactive peptide hormones.

Pathophysiology

- Scorpion venom delays the closing of neuronal sodium channels, resulting in "autonomic storm"

Envenomation: Snake, Scorpion, and Spider

owing to sudden outpouring of endogenous catecholamines into the circulation
- Parasympathetic effects are less severe compared to sympathetic effects
- The combination of sympathetic excitation and the release of catecholamine in plasma cause the majority of the severe systemic effects
- The severity of scorpion sting depends on the victim's age, the season, and the time between sting and treatment.

Clinical Manifestations

Despite the variety of different scorpion species exist, majority of them produce similar neurotoxic excitation. However, *Centruroides* and *Parabuthus* scorpions are associated primarily with neuromuscular toxicity, whereas severe envenomation from androctonus, buthus, and mesobuthus scorpions is associated with cardiovascular toxicity.

Local Manifestations

- Severe excruciating local pain
- Swelling, redness, local increase in temperature and regional lymph node involvement
- Local edema, urticaria, fasciculation, and spasm of underlying muscles are rarely seen due to serotonin
- Positive tap test is present (on tapping increase in paresthesia occurs) in some patients
- The stings from the *H. lepturus* scorpion of Iran do not cause immediate severe pain. The majority of cases are characterized by erythema, purpuric and bullous lesions that resolve, but in about 20% of cases there is delayed localized necrosis that develops over hours or days. The syndrome appears to be similar to that associated with bites by loxosceles spiders.

Systemic Manifestations

- Systemic symptoms may develop within minutes, but may be delayed as much as 24 hours. Features of autonomic nervous system excitation are transient cholinergic and prolonged adrenergic stimulation
- Hypertension is common and occurs early in response to sympathetic stimulation
- Prolonged massive release of catecholamines causes restlessness, piloerection, marked tachycardia, mydriasis, hyperglycemia, hypertension, toxic

myocarditis, cardiac failure and pulmonary edema
- All forms of electrocardiogram abnormalities are documented
- Priapism may occur secondary to cholinergic stimulation
- Vomiting and abdominal pain are common after scorpion stings
- Hemiplegia and other neurological lesions have been attributed to fibrin deposition resulting from disseminated intravascular coagulation
- Acute pancreatitis has been reported with *Leiurus quinquestriatus* and *Tityus* species
- Systematic features of *H. lepturus* scorpion sting are direct hemolysis with hemoglobinuria, and acute kidney injury that often warrants for dialysis.

On basis of clinical manifestations scorpion envenomation is graded into four grades.[15] Ideally, clinical grading should direct treatment.
- *Grade I*: Local pain and paresthesia without any systemic manifestation
- *Grade II*: Patient with pain and paresthesia distant from the site of sting with or without tachycardia and without cardiorespiratory signs
- *Grade III*: Patients with peripheral circulatory failure, cardiovascular and respiratory manifestations
- *Grade IV*: Patient with central nervous system manifestation and multisystem involvement.

Differential Diagnosis

Tachycardia, excessive secretions, wheezing, and respiratory distress accompanying serious scorpion stings may be mistaken for asthma, airway obstruction from a foreign body or poisoning with cholinergic agents such as organophosphate insecticides.

Investigations

There are no specific diagnostic investigations recommended for scorpion stings. Investigations should focus on potential complications of scorpion envenomation.

Treatment

- Mild pain can be alleviated by application of ice packs over the site of sting and with oral analgesics
- Severe excruciating local pain that does not respond to oral analgesia can be transiently relieved by ring block

Miscellaneous Toxicities

using combination of lignocaine and bupivacaine which can give prolonged relief from pain

- Prazosin is pharmacological and physiological antidote to scorpion venom actions. It totally reverses the metabolic and hormonal effects of alpha receptor stimulation[16]
- Prazosin (plain tablet not sustained release form) is administered orally as 1 mg in adults (children 30 μg/kg)
- Repeat prazosin in the same dose after 3 hours depending on the clinical response and later every 6 hours (not exceeding 5 mg total in a day) till the extremities are warm, dry and the peripheral veins are visible easily
- Prazosin can be given irrespective of blood pressure provided there is no hypovolemia
- Dobutamine is indicated for hypotension due to cardiogenic shock
- Nitroglycerin is used to treat pulmonary edema, where as other vasodilators like hydralazine, captopril, nifedipine, sodium nitroprusside, clonidine are not recommended because of potential adverse effects like sympathetic stimulation and reflex tachycardia
- Atropine used to reverse severe bradycardia associated with hypotension and excessive sweating or salivation can cause an autonomic storm with transient cholinergic stimulation followed by sustained adrenergic hyperactivity, hence it is contraindicated
- Neuromuscular incoordination, sympathetic agitation, and seizures are alleviated with administration of benzodiazepine
- The use of antivenom for scorpion stings remains controversial
- Commercially prepared antivenins are available in several countries for some of the most dangerous species. The dose is 5–25 mL of antivenom diluted in two to three volumes of isotonic saline to be given intravenously over an hour
- If there is no significant improvement, further doses of antivenom can be given[17] (total dose of antivenom required is 30–100 mL in severe envenomation).

Disposition

- Grade I and II envenomations after a short observation period (3–4 h after sting occurred) for progression of symptoms

- Grade III and IV envenomations require admission to ICU if they have not received antivenom, or have any evidence of a complication
- Encourage patient to return for progression of symptoms
- Patients suspected of severe envenomation should be hospitalized for at least 24 hours and closely observed for cardiovascular and neurological sequelae.

HYMENOPTERA STINGS

- Hymenoptera stings pose great hazards in tropics and it is the most important venomous insects known to humans
- More fatalities result from stings by these insects than by stings or bites by any other arthropod.

Entomology

- The Hymenoptera families of medical interest include: Apidae (honeybees), Bombidae (bumblebees), Vespidae (wasps, hornets and yellow jackets), and Formicidae (ants)
- The Bombidae and Vespidae have stingers that remain functionally intact after a sting, resulting in their ability to inflict multiple stings
- Yellow jackets may attack without provocation and are the most common cause of insect-induced anaphylactic reactions.

Toxicity of Venom

- Hymenoptera venom contains several components such as proteins, enzymes, and vasoactive amines
- Melittin is the major component of honeybee venom that can cause degranulation of basophils and mast cells
- Fire-ant venom is composed primarily of a transpiperidine alkaloid that causes tissue necrosis
- Honeybee venom is immunochemically distinct. However, yellow jacket and hornet venoms have a high degree of cross-reactivity
- The dose of venom delivered per sting may vary from none to the entire contents of the venom gland. It has been estimated that about 1,500 stings would be required to deliver a lethal dose of hymenoptera venom for a nonallergic adult who weighs 70 kg.[18]

Pathophysiology

- Hymenoptera venom contains different peptide antigens that all may trigger allergic reactions
- The most well-known allergic reaction is the type I anaphylactic or immediate hypersensitivity reaction and this is similar to immunoglobulin E (IgE) mediated allergic reactions
- Delayed reactions develop several days to a week after the sting and these reactions are non-IgE mediated
- Although most deaths result from immunologic mechanisms, some are from direct toxicity.

Clinical Manifestations

The patient may present with local or systemic signs of envenomation.

Local Manifestations

- Local reactions are common, resulting in swelling, erythema, and a burning sensation at the sting site, vesiculation and blisters, itching and a sensation of warmth
- These reactions are benign, resolve within hours to days, and are not predictive of systemic reactions to subsequent stings.

Systemic Manifestations

- There is no correlation between systemic reaction and the number of stings
- Vomiting, diarrhea, hypotension, syncope, angio-edema, bronchospasm, laryngospasm, rhabdomyolysis, coagulopathy and death
- The complications associated with severe hymenoptera envenomation include cerebral and myocardial infarction.

Delayed Reaction

It is believed to be immune complex mediated consists of serum sickness-like features appearing 5–14 days after a sting.

Differential Diagnosis

- Extensive local reactions must be differentiated from an infectious cellulitis
- Anaphylactic reactions may be due to variety of drugs, foods, and environmental allergens.

Investigations

- There are no specific diagnostic investigations recommended
- Creatine phosphokinase, coagulation profile, ECG and renal function should be checked in severe cases of multiple stings.

Treatment

- The single bee sting injury does not require any treatment
- The bee stingers often remain embedded in the patient's skin, and these have to be removed as soon as possible
- Rapid removal of the stinger by any means (the method is unimportant) is most effective in minimizing envenomation[19]
- Large local reactions usually respond well to a short course of antihistamines, analgesics, H2 blocker, and steroids
- Nebulized salbutamol may be considered for treatment of bronchospasm
- Renal function should be closely monitored and symptomatic treatment instituted[20]
- Provide tetanus prophylaxis if appropriate
- In cases of multiple wasp stings, secondary infections should be anticipated and appropriate antibiotic prophylaxis to cover skin flora
- Establish airway, breathing, and circulation to provide adequate airway, ventilation and perfusion
- Envenomated patients suffering anaphylaxis should receive an intramuscular epinephrine.

Disposition

- Minimal isolated local reaction can be discharged
- Life-threatening reaction requires 24 hours of observation
- Intensive care unit admission is required if there is worsening of symptoms, airway compromise and hemodynamic instability.
- Provide prescriptions for Epi-Pen to patients discharged after presenting with life-threatening reactions to bee stings.

CONCLUSION

- Differentiating between the biting species either as venomous or nonvenomous based on the bite marks is useless

Miscellaneous Toxicities

- If the captured or killed snake be brought to the ED with the victim, identification of the species should be carried out carefully as there is always an inherent danger in this practice as they can even envenomate when they are dead
- If patient received antivenom, monitor for delayed serum sickness
- Relying on the absence of a visible lesion at the site of the sting to rule out scorpion envenomation
- Patients experiencing a systemic reaction to wasp or bee stings should be referred to an allergy specialist
- Patient on beta-blockers who are resistant to epinephrine, glucagon can be administered.

KEY POINTS

- Antivenom is the mainstay of therapy for poisonous snake bite and there is no role for test dose
- The shorter the interval between envenomation and the onset of symptoms, the more severe is the morbidity and mortality

REFERENCES

1. Warrell DA. WHO/SEARO guidelines for the clinical management of snake bites in the Southeast Asian Region. Trop Med Pub Heath. 1999;30:1.
2. Warrell DA. Snake bite. Lancet. 2010;375:77-88.
3. Mohapatra B, Warrell DA, Suraveera W, et al. Snake bite mortality in India. A National representative mortality survey. PLoS Neglected Trop Dis. 2011;5(4):e1018.
4. Kasturiratne A1, Wickremasinghe AR, de Silva N, et al. The global burden of snake bite: a literature analysis and modeling based on regional estimates of envenoming and deaths. PLoS Med. 2008;5:e218.
5. Ariaratnam CA, Sheriff MH, Arambepola C, et al. Syndromic approach for treatment of snake bite in Sri Lanka: based on results of a prospective national hospital-based survey of patients envenomed by identified snakes. Am J Trop Med Hyg. 2009;81(4):725-31.
6. Ariaratnam CA, Sheriff MH, Theakston RD, et al. Distinctive Epidemiologic and Clinical Features of Common Krait (Bungarus caeruleus) Bites in Sri Lanka. Am J Trop Med Hyg. 2008;79(3);458-62.
7. Senthilkumaran S, David SS, Jena NN, et al. Limitations and consumer aspects of point-of-care in snake envenomation. Emerg Med Australas. 2014;26(2):208.
8. Ariaratnam CA, Thuraisingam V, Kularatne SA, et al. Frequent and potentially fatal envenoming by hump-nosed pit vipers (Hypnale hypnale and H. nepa) in Sri Lanka: lack of effective antivenom. Transac Royal Soc Trop Med Hyg. 2008;102:1120-6.
9. Senthilkumaran S, Khamis A, Manikam R, et al. Snakebite and severe hypertension: looking for the Holy Grail. Indian J Crit Care Med. 2014;18:186.
10. Senthilkumaran S, Meenakshisundaram R, Thirumalaikolundusubramanian P, et al. Cardiac toxicity following cobra envenomation. Clin Toxicol (Phila). 2012;50(9):862.
11. Senthilkumaran S, Balamurugan N, Menezes RG, et al. Snake bite and brain death—cause for caution? Am J Emerg Med. 2013;31:625-6.
12. Isbister GK, Bawaskar HS. Scorpion envenomation. N Engl J Med. 2014;371(5):457-63.
13. Mahadevan S, Rameshkumar R. Systemic manifestations in children with scorpion sting envenomation: how to manage? Indian J Pediatr.. 2015;82(6):497-8.
14. Chippaux JP. Emerging options for the management of scorpion stings. Drug Des Devel Ther. 2012;6:165-73.
15. Bawaskar HS, Bawaskar PH. Prazosin in management of cardiovascular manifestations of scorpion sting. Lancet. 1986;1(8479):510-1.
16. Bawaskar HS, Bawaskar PH. Prazosin therapy and scorpion envenomation. J Assoc Physicians India. 2000;48(12):1175-80.
17. Bawaskar HS, Bawaskar PH. Efficacy and safety of scorpion antivenom plus prazosin compared with prazosin alone for venomous scorpion (Mesobuthus tamulus sting: randomised open label clinical trial. BMJ. 2011;341:c7136.
18. Goddard J. Physician's guide to arthropods of medical importance, 4th edition. Boca Raton: CRC Press; 2003. pp. 4.
19. Balamurgan N, Senthilkumaran S, Thirumalaikolundu-subramanian P. Mass envenomation by honey bee-speed thrills. J Emerg Trauma Shock. 2010;3:420-1.
20. Senthilkumaran S, Ananth C, Benita F, et al. Acute kidney injury in wasp sting-do early bicarbonate and mannitol make a difference? Indian J Crit Care Med. 2014;18:701-2.

40
CHAPTER

Plant Poisonings

Arvinth Soundarrajan, Subramanian Senthilkumaran, Ponniah Thirumalai Kolundu Subramanian

INTRODUCTION

Plant kingdom is large and has many thousands of plants. India has a rich and varied flora. The rural community in general is dependent on their farms and gardens for food, and are occasionally get poisoned when they fail to identify toxic plants.

Children are especially at risk, as these are accessible and attractive, and consume plant materials without realizing its toxic effects.[1] Suicide using poisonous plants is fairly common in India, especially in rural areas, but homicide is rare.[2] Use of poisonous plants in herbal remedies, and "traditional medicines" are other causes of poisoning. Some of the more common poisonous plants in relation to its action along with examples seen in India are furnished in Table 1.[3-6]

INDIAN POISONOUS PLANTS

Some of the dangerously toxic plants most commonly implicated in poisoning in India are listed in Table 2.[7,8]

Abrus precatorius

The plant *A. precatorius* (Crab's eyes, Crow beards, jequirity bean, Rosary bean) grows in many parts of India and other tropical countries.

The seeds of the plant are colorful and attract children. Hence, they tend to eat crushed and broken ones accidently and are susceptible for this poisoning mostly.

The phytotoxin present in the seed is Abrin, a protein considered as deadliest poison colloquially known as ricin.[9]

Abrin inhibits elongation factors (EF) such as EF1 and EF2, and thereby prevents protein synthesis and leads to death. It also induces endothelial damage which increases capillary permeability and fluid leakage resulting in tissue edema. The parenteral form of the toxin is used for homicidal poisoning and inhalational

Table 1: Category of poisonous plants with examples.	
Category of poisonous plants	*Examples*
Irritant plants	Crab's eyes, castor, colocynth, croton, glory lily, marking nut, May apple, red pepper, rosary pea
Cardiotoxic plants	Aconite, autumn Crocus, common oleander, yellow oleander, suicide tree
Neurotoxic plants	Calotropis, cassava, chickling pea, datura, strychnos
Hepatotoxic plants	Neem
Miscellaneous toxic plants/plant products	Areca nut, *Cleistanthus collinus*, physic nut

Miscellaneous Toxicities

Table 2: Dangerously poisonous Indian plants most often implicated in poisoning.

Plant	Main toxic principle	Usual fatal dose
Ricinus communis (Castor)	Ricin	8–10 seeds
Abrus precatorius (Jequirity)	Abrin	1–3 seeds
Nerium oleander (Common oleander)	Oleandrin	5–15 leaves, 15 g root
Thevetia peruviana (Yellow oleander)	Thevetin	8–10 seeds, 15–20 g root
Cerbera odollam (Suicide tree)	Cerberin	1 kernel
Datura fastuosa (Thorn apple)	Atropine, hyoscine	50–100 seeds
Strychnos nuxvomica	Strychnine	1–3 g seeds
Cleistanthus collinus (Oduvan)	Cleistanthin A and B	A few leaves
Amanita phalloides (Death cap mushroom)	Amanitin, phalloidin	1 mushroom

form in bioterrorism.[10,11] The estimated fatal dose of abrin varies from species to species and for human being is 0.1–1 µg/kg body weight.

Clinical Features and Management

Ingestion of whole seed produces minimal or no symptoms due to protection by the hard outer layer. Any crack in the outer shell of the seeds leads to release of abrin which is poorly absorbed and presents with features of acute gastroenteritis. The symptoms and signs are nausea, vomiting, abdominal pain, diarrhea with or without blood, hypovolemia, hypotension, shock, and death.

Tachycardia, fever, headache, dilated pupils, irritability, hallucination, drowsiness, weakness, tetany, tremors, seizures, cerebral edema, dysrhythmias, flushing of skin, liver failure, and renal failure may manifest. Treatment is symptomatic and supportive.

Ricinus communis (Castor)

- The castor or castor oil plant *R. communis* (Euphorbiaceae: spurges) is also called mole bean, moy bean, or palma christi (Fig. 1)
- It is an ornamental plant found in many parts of India and the oil extracted from its seeds is also used medicinally as a purgative and as a lubricant for engines
- In India, castor seed extract is used systemically or topically in folk medicine to stimulate breast milk production
- Its main active principle is ricin, a toxalbumin, which is used in chemical warfare, as an experimental antitumor and immunosuppressive agent, and to poison moles
- Castor seeds (Fig. 2) are harmless when ingested whole, since their outer coating resists digestion, but if the seeds are crushed or chewed before being swallowed, ricin is released
- The pulp of the seed contains glycoproteins, which cause allergic dermatitis, rhinitis, and asthma in sensitized individuals.

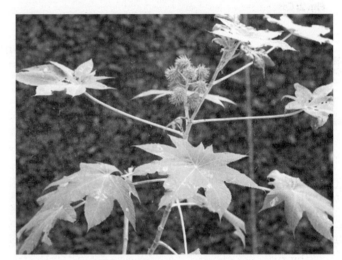

Fig. 1: *Ricinus communis* plant.

Clinical Features and Management

- Gastrointestinal (GI) symptoms like colicky abdominal pain, vomiting, and diarrhea
- Hemorrhagic gastritis and dehydration were seen in severe cases

Plant Poisonings

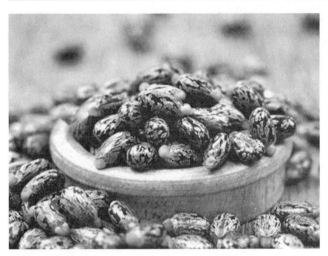

Fig. 2: Castor seeds.

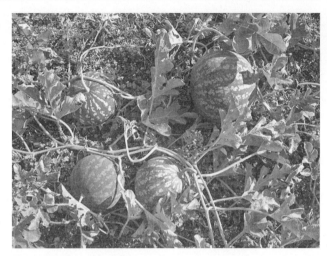

Fig. 3: *Citrullus colocynthis*.

- Delayed central nervous system toxicity may occur, especially involving the cranial nerves. Hematuria and acute renal and hepatic failure may develop
- Parenteral injection of ricin can be fatal in doses as low as 1 mg/kg body weight
- Treatment is symptomatic and supportive.

Citrullus colocynthis (Colocynth)

- The colocynth *C. colocynthis* (Cucurbitaceae: gourds or cucurbits) grows wild all over India (Fig. 3)
- The dried fruit pulp of colocynth is used as a purgative by rural people and the root is used in traditional system for jaundice, rheumatism, and constipation.

Clinical Features and Management

- Poisoning causes vomiting, diarrhea, hypotension, and shock
- Treatment is symptomatic and supportive.

Croton tiglium (Croton)

- *C. tiglium* (Euphorbiaceae: spurges) grows well in Assam, Bengal, and the Western Ghats (Fig. 4)
- Its seeds, oil, and root extract are used as a drastic purgative in folk medicine
- Plants of this family contain strongly irritant diterpene esters
- The stem, leaves, and seeds are mostly toxic, containing crotin (toxalbumin) and crotonoside (glycoside).

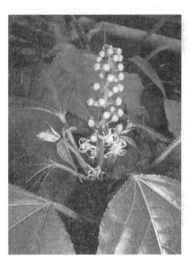

Fig. 4: *Croton tiglium*.

Clinical Features and Management

- Skin contact with the latex or chewing the stem causes erythema, swelling, and blistering after 2–8 hours
- Ingestion results in burning pain in the upper GI tract, vomiting, tenesmus, watery or blood-stained diarrhea, hypotension, collapse, coma, and death
- Drinking cold milk may alleviate the GI irritation
- Treatment is symptomatic and supportive.

Semecarpus anacardium (Marking Nut)

- The marking nut tree is a member of the Anacardiaceae, a family that includes cashew, mango, and poison ivy, and grows well in many parts of India (Fig. 5)

Miscellaneous Toxicities

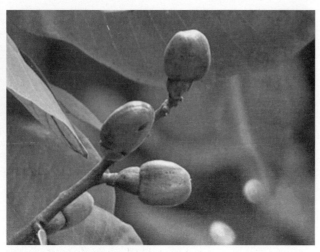

Fig. 5: *Semecarpus anacardium*.

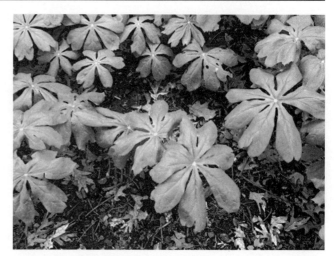

Fig. 6: *Podophyllum* species.

- The black, oily juice of the nut is used by dhobis (washermen) in India to make markings on the clothes before washing
- Extracts of the toxic nut, which contains semecarpol and bhilawanol, are used in folk medicine for various ailments, and the bruised nut is inserted into the vagina as an abortifacient
- The fatal dose ranges from 5–8 nuts.

Clinical Features and Management

- Skin contact with the acrid juice results in irritation, inflammation, vesication, and ulceration
- Ingestion causes blistering of the mouth and GI distress
- In severe cases, there is vomiting, abdominal pain, diarrhea, hypotension, tachycardia, delirium, and coma
- Pupils may be dilated
- Decontamination of skin with soap and water
- Milk may ameliorate GI symptoms
- Treatment is symptomatic and supportive.

Podophyllum Species (May Apple)

- *Podophyllum* spp. (Berberidaceae: barberries), including the May apple grow well in the hilly regions of Sikkim, Uttar Pradesh, Punjab, Himachal Pradesh, and Kashmir (Fig. 6)
- Resins of this plant are used as keratolytic agents, as topical treatment of condylomata acuminata (genital warts) and also in homoeopathy

- The most toxic parts are the leaves and rhizomes which contain at least 50% of podophyllotoxin (lignans and flavonols)
- Podophyllum and podophyllotoxin have effects similar to colchicine and vinblastine: antimitosis and inhibition of axoplasmic transport protein
- The toxins interfere with ribonucleic acid (RNA) and deoxyribonucleic acid (DNA) synthesis, and tricarboxylic acid cycle enzymes.

Clinical Features and Management

- Both ingestion and dermal application cause toxicity. About 30 minutes to several hours after ingestion patient develops nausea, vomiting, abdominal pain, and diarrhea, followed by fever, tachypnea, tachycardia, hypotension, ataxia, dizziness, lethargy, peripheral neuropathy, confusion, and altered sensorium
- Seizures may occur
- Thrombocytopenia and leukopenia are common
- Polyneuropathy generally appears in about a week and progresses for 2–3 months
- Consumption of Chinese herbal products containing extracts of podophyllum has caused neuropathies and encephalopathy[12]
- Treatment is symptomatic and supportive.

Capsicum Species (Red Pepper)

- Common Indian species include *Capsicum annuum* and *C. frutescens* (Solanaceae: nightshades) (Fig. 7).

- It is also known as chilly, chilli pepper, cayenne pepper, cherry pepper, cluster pepper, Christmas pepper, and cone pepper
- Its long tapering fruits, which become red when ripe, contain small, flat yellowish seeds which can be mistaken for datura seeds. Serious poisoning can result from mistaken identity. The differences between chilli and datura seeds are provided in Table 3
- Capsicum fruit and seeds are very popular in Indian cuisine
- In traditional medicine, it is used as an appetite stimulant and carminative
- The active principle is capsaicin, which is used in the treatment of neuralgia and diabetic neuropathy
- Capsicum vanillyl acids are irritants which deplete substance P from nerve terminals resulting in local swelling and pain due to dilatation of blood vessels, and intense excitation of sensory nerve endings, followed by relative insensitivity, the basis for the use of capsaicin in analgesic creams
- Accidental aspiration of pepper can be fatal. Inhalation has been used as a method of homicide.

Clinical Features and Management

- Cutaneous exposure causes a burning, stinging, pain, and occupational handling of chillies causes "chilli burns" or "Hunan hand"
- Ocular exposure causes intense pain, lacrimation, conjunctivitis, and blepharospasm, while inhalation or aspiration of chilli powder causes "chilli workers' cough"
- Ingestion results in nausea, vomiting, burning pain, salivation, abdominal cramps, and "burning" diarrhea
- Topical decontamination is carried out with liberal amounts of water and application of local and systemic analgesics
- Symptoms resulting from ingestion are relieved by sips of cool water or crushed ice
- Treatment is symptomatic and supportive.

Cerbera odollam (Suicide Tree)

- The suicide tree *C. odollam* (Apocynaceae: dogbanes), also known as the Kerala suicide nut, ordeal tree, pong-pong, or othalanga (Fig. 8), is endemic to South Asia, growing well in South India, especially in Kerala
- In Kerala, it is said to be responsible for about 50% of plant poisoning and 10% of all cases of poisoning
- Its fruits resemble unripe (green) mangoes
- The seeds are used in folk medicine as emeto-cathartics and the kernel of the fruit contains the cardiac glycoside cerberin, which blocks cardiac calcium ion channels.

Table 3: Differences between chilli and datura seeds.

Chilli seed	Datura seed
Small	Large
Yellow	Brown
Rounded and smooth	Reniform and pitted
Pungent odor	Odorless
Pungent taste	Bitter taste

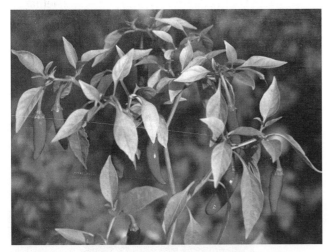

Fig. 7: *Capsicum* species.

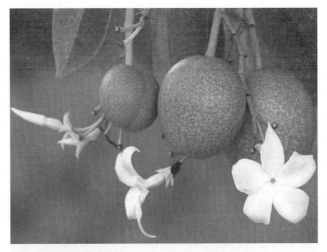

Fig. 8: *Cerbera odollam*.

Clinical Features and Management

- Manifestations of poisoning and treatment are the same as for oleanders
- Since it is difficult to detect at autopsy, and its flavor can be masked with strong spices, this is a fairly common agent of homicide and suicide in some parts of South India
- Accidental poisoning may result from confusion with unripe mango
- Treatment is symptomatic and supportive.

Calotropis Species

- The calotropis, madar, crown flower, giant milkweed, swallow wort, or Sodom apple (*Calotropis procera, C. gigantea*—Apocynaceae, Asclepiadoideae: milkweeds) grows wild throughout India (Fig. 9)
- It is used by rural practitioners to treat many ailments
- The milky juice of the plant was referred to as "vegetable mercury", as it was said to be effective in the treatment of syphilis
- According to Ayurveda, the dried whole plant is a good tonic, expectorant, and anthelmintic
- The powdered root is used in asthma, bronchitis, and dyspepsia
- The leaves are said to be useful in the treatment of arthralgia, swellings, and intermittent fevers
- The flowers are bitter, and are used as a digestive, astringent, and anthelmintic
- Calotropis is also used in homoeopathic medicines
- All parts of the plant, especially leaves and juice, contain calotoxin, calotropin, and uscharin.

Clinical Features and Management

- Contact of the juice with the skin results in intense irritation with redness, swelling, and vesication, and contact with eyes results in severe conjunctivitis
- It has been used by malingerers to simulate skin injury or conjunctivitis
- Ingestion of leaves or juice causes burning pain and vomiting
- Treatment is symptomatic and supportive.

Lathyrus sativus (Chickling Pea)

- The chickling pea, bluesweet pea, grass pea, or Indian pea *L. sativus* (Fabaceae/Leguminosae: legumes, peas, beans, pulses) grows well in Madhya Pradesh, Bihar, Uttar Pradesh, West Bengal, and Punjab (Fig. 10)
- The seeds ("kesari dal" in Hindi) are used as a cheap substitute for costlier lentils by the rural people in these states
- The toxic principle is β-N-oxalyl-L-α,β-diaminopropionic acid (ODAP).[13]

Clinical Features and Management

- Chronic intake of kesari dal leads to the development of lathyrism, characterized by gradually progressive bilateral spastic paraparesis
- Prodromal symptoms include cramps, prickling sensation, and nocturnal calf pain
- There are exaggerated tendon reflexes and extensor plantar responses
- Complete spastic paraplegia may result eventually

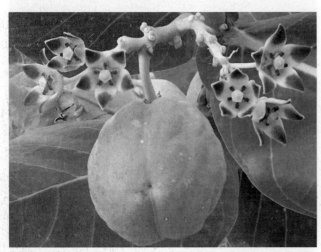

Fig. 9: *Calotropis* species.

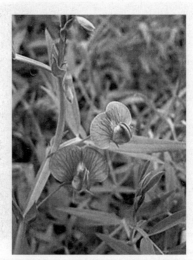

Fig. 10: *Lathyrus sativus.*

- There is no specific treatment. Once it develops, analgesics, generous diet, and large doses of vitamin B complex may help.

Azadirachta indica (Neem)

- The neem or margosa tree *A. indica* (Meliaceae: mahoganies) grows well in most parts of India and has been introduced into Africa and other tropical countries (Fig. 11)
- Various parts of the tree as well as the oil have been used in the treatment of a wide variety of ailments
- Seed oil (margosa oil) contains aflatoxins and leaves contain stearic, oleic, palmitic, and linoleic acids.

Clinical Features and Management

- Ingestion of neem leaf extract or an excess of margosa oil results in hepatotoxicity with vomiting, drowsiness, and encephalopathy
- Metabolic acidosis is often present
- Convulsions, myocarditis (with ventricular fibrillation), and pancreatitis have occurred
- There is no specific antidote available, and gastric lavage is not recommended for neem oil poisoning. The management is primarily symptomatic and supportive.

Areca catechu (Areca or Betel Nut)

- The areca or betel nut *A. catechu* (Arecaceae/Palmae: palms) grows well in Kerala, Karnataka, Goa, Assam, and West Bengal (Fig. 12)
- In India it is called "supari" and is chewed alone or as pan, a mixture of supari, lime, and other ingredients (with or without tobacco) wrapped in betel leaf (*Piper betel*)
- Of the toxic principles in leaf and nut, arecoline is cholinergic and arecaidine is probably carcinogenic.

Clinical Features and Management

- Arecoline is a bronchoconstrictor and can cause exacerbation of bronchospasm in asthmatic patients who chew betel nut
- The phenolic volatile oil present in betel nut is an alkaloid which produces cocaine-like reactions
- Treatment is symptomatic and supportive.

Cleistanthus collinus (Oduvan)

- *C. collinus* (Phyllanthaceae, formerly Euphorbiaceae) grows wild in dry hills of various parts of India from Himachal Pradesh to Bihar and southwards into Peninsular India (Fig. 13)[14]
- There are many names for this plant in different Indian languages such as Oduvanthalai/Nillipalai (Tamil Nadu and Puducherry); Kadishe (Andhra Pradesh); Karlajuri (West Bengal); and Garari (Hindi-speaking states of India)
- All parts of the plant contain a multitude of toxic glycosides and arylnaphthalene lignan lactones—cleistanthin A and B, collinusin, and diphyllin ("oduvin").

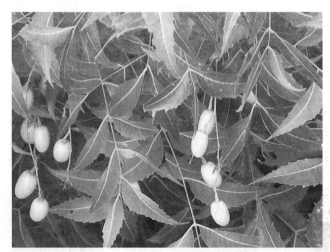

Fig. 11: *Azadirachta indica.*

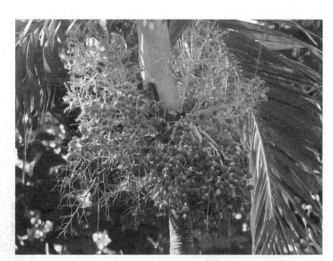

Fig. 12: *Areca catechu.*

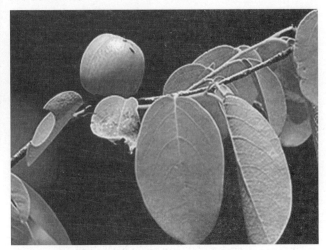

Fig. 13: *Cleistanthus collinus.*

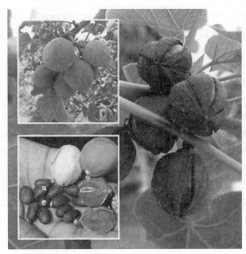

Fig. 14: *Jatropha curcas.*

Clinical Features and Management

- Vomiting, epigastric pain, breathlessness, visual disturbances (clouding/blurring/colored vision), giddiness, drowsiness, fever, tachycardia, hypotension, and/or respiratory arrest
- Adult respiratory distress syndrome, distal renal tubular acidosis, and shock secondary to inappropriate vasodilatation may also occur
- Electrocardiogram (ECG) changes may include QTc prolongation and nonspecific ST-T changes
- Rarely, a myasthenic crisis-like syndrome requiring assisted ventilation can occur due to *C. collinus* poisoning, which is said to respond to treatment with neostigmine
- Gastric lavage before 2 hours is beneficial
- The mainstay of *C. collinus* poisoning management is monitoring and correction of electrolyte imbalance, namely hypokalemia and metabolic acidosis as well as supportive
- The precise role of cardiac pacing in the setting of *C. collinus* poisoning is a matter of conjecture as the evidence for preventing deaths through its use is inadequate
- N-acetylcysteine, L-cysteine, melatonin, and thiol-containing compounds have all been suggested as possible antidotes for management of *C. collinus* toxicity.

Jatropha curcas (Physic Nut)

- The black seed of *J. curcas* (Euphorbiaceae: spurges) is known as "physic nut" or "purging nut" (Fig. 14)
- It contains curcan oleic acid. Apart from its use as a laxative, the seed oil is applied to painful joints
- The seeds possess the toxalbumin curcin.

Clinical Features and Management

- The crude oil of the plant when applied externally causes irritation, and when ingested causes severe diarrhea
- Ingestion of the seeds results in salivation, sweating, abdominal pain, diarrhea, weakness, and muscle twitching. Jatropha poisoning is generally not fatal in humans, although it may be so in animals
- Treatment is symptomatic and supportive.

Yellow Oleander

Poisoning due to deliberate self-harm with the seeds of yellow oleander (*Thevetia peruviana*) results in significant morbidity and mortality each year in South Asia (Fig. 15).[15]

Yellow oleander seeds contain highly toxic cardiac glycosides including thevetins A and B and neriifolin. Important epidemiological and clinical differences exist between poisoning due to yellow oleander and digoxin.[16]

Clinical Features and Management

Presents with wide variety of bradyarrhythmias and tachyarrhythmias following ingestion.

- Continuous ECG monitoring for at least 24 hours is necessary to detect arrhythmias

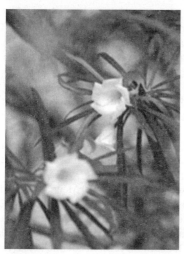

Fig. 15: Yellow oleander.

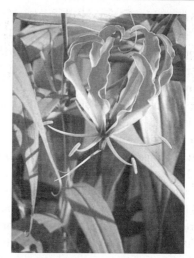

Fig. 16: *Gloriosa superba*.

- Correction of dehydration with normal saline is necessary, and antiemetics are used rarely to control severe vomiting
- Hypokalemia worsens toxicity due to cardiac glycosides, and hyperkalemia is life threatening. Both must be corrected
- Intravenous (IV) calcium increases the risk of cardiac arrhythmias and is not recommended in treating hyperkalemia
- Lidocaine is the preferred antiarrhythmic in the management of tachyarrhythmia
- Digoxin-specific antibody fragments remain the only proven therapy for yellow oleander poisoning.

Gloriosa superba

Gloriosa superba is a plant of the family Colchicaceae (Fig. 16) and that grows wild in several parts of South India. It is recognized as state flower of Tamil Nadu. This plant commonly called as flame lily, climbing lily, creeping lily, glory lily, gloriosa lily, tiger claw, and fire lily. It is called as kalihari (Hindi) and nabhi and nagati gadda (Telugu). The tubers of this plant have been found to contain several alkaloids such as colchicine, gloriosine, superbine, and salicylic acid and used in traditional medicine. Acute intoxication associated with the ingestion of this plant is indistinguishable from colchicine toxicity.[17]

Clinical Features and Management

- There are three progressive phases of poisoning:
  1. 10–24 hours after ingestion—GI phase mimicking gastroenteritis
  2. 24 hours to 7 days after ingestion—phase of multiorgan dysfunction
  3. In untreated patients, death results from rapidly progressive multiorgan failure, involving bone marrow suppression, kidney and liver failure, acute respiratory distress syndrome, arrhythmias and cardiovascular collapse, and neuromuscular involvement.
- Recovery typically occurs within a few weeks of ingestion, but with rebound leukocytosis and alopecia
- The first step of treatment is timely GI decontamination with activated charcoal for massive and recent ingestions may warrant gastric lavage
- Administration of granulocyte colony-stimulating factor might help in combating hematological cell deficiency
- Fab fragment antibodies for colchicine poisoning have been used; it is not commercially available.

CONCLUSION

Accidental poisoning with some of these plants or plant products may occur among inhabitants of rural areas, dependent on their farms and gardens for food, due to mistakes in identifying toxic plants, with children being at particular risk. Contamination of foodstuffs and the use of poisonous plants in traditional or folk medicine are other causes of poisoning. In the present context, recognition and management of few plant poisoning seen in India are described.

Some of the plant sap material causes allergic dermatitis in some susceptible individuals in 10–30 minutes and gets cleared within 10 days invariably. It is characterized by redness, papules, vesicles, bullae, or linear streaking. Skin decontamination is carried out by pouring liberal amounts of water and washing the patient. This shall be carried out immediately so as to avoid entry of toxins into the system. Always check the undersurface of finger nails and clean them with soap and water in order to prevent the entry of left out materials in the finger nails, which continue to spread the antigen to other parts of the body. Check for mild dermatitis which may require external steroid cream and antihistamine tablets. If the skin lesions are more and severe or delayed onset of skin reactions require oral steroids which shall be tapered of over 2–3 weeks.

Supportive treatment includes gut decontamination if arrives within 30–60 minutes, oral administration of charcoal, IV fluids, vasopressors, antiarrhythmic agents, and benzodiazepines and/or barbiturates for control of seizures, and urine alkalization by IV soda-bicarbonate. Overall, it is worth to identify the plant or get information from poison control centers. Monitor airway, breathing, and circulation Also, watch for metabolic parameters and provide appropriate care. If patients do not develop any symptoms and/or signs within 6 hours after exposure to plant toxins, toxicity is unlikely.

KEY POINTS

- Plant poisoning may be accidental, suicidal or homicidal
- Apart from systemic toxicity, patients may also develop local allergic skin reactions
- It may be useful to identify the plant or get information from poison control centers
- If patients do not develop any signs or symptoms within 6 hours after exposure, toxicity is unlikely.

REFERENCES

1. Ghorani-Azam A, Sepahi S, Riahi-Zanjam B, et al. Plant toxins and acute medicinal plant poisoning in children: a systematic literature review. J Res Med Sci. 2018;23:26.
2. Nagesh KR, Menezes RG, Rastogi P, et al Suicidal plant poisoning with Colchicum autumnale. J Forensic Leg Med. 2011;18(6):285-7.
3. Farthing K. Poisonous plants. Lab Medicine. 1996;22(4):200-3.
4. Welch KD, Panter KE, Gardner DR, et al. The good and the bad of poisonous plants: an introduction to the USDA-ARS poisonous plant research laboratory. J Med Toxicol. 2012;8:153-9.
5. Diaz JH. Poisoning by herbs and plants: rapid toxidromic classification and diagnosis. Wilderness Environ Med. 2016;27:136-52.
6. Senthilkumaran S, Meenakshisundaram R, Thirumalaikolundusubramanian P. Chapter 5: Plant toxins and the heart. In: Ramachandran R, Thirumalaikolundusubramanian P (Eds). The Heart and Toxins, 1st edition. USA: Academic Press (Elsevier); 2016. pp. 151-9.
7. Pillay VV. Common Indian poisonous plants. In: Warrell DA, Cox TM, Firth JD (Eds). Oxford Textbook of Medicine. United Kingdom: Oxford University Press; 2010. Chapter re-evaluated on July 20th 2015.
8. Poisonous plants. [online] Available from: https://www.emedmd.com/content/common-indian-poisonous-plants. [Accessed August, 2018].
9. Dickers KJ, Bradberry SM, Rice P, et al. Abrin poisoning. Toxicol Rev. 2003;22(3):137-42.
10. Roxas-Duncan VI, Smith LA. Of beans and beads: ricin and abrin in bioterrorism and biodefense. J Bioterr Biodef. 2012;S2:002. [online] Available from: http://dx.doi.org/10.4172/2157-2526.S2-002. [Accessed October, 2018].
11. Krenzelok EP, Mrvos R. Friends and foes in the plant world: A profile of plant ingestions and fatalities. Clin Toxicol (Phila). 2011;49(3):142-9.
12. Lee BK, Kim JH, Jung JW, et al. Myristicin-induced neurotoxicity in human neuroblastoma SK-N-SH cells. Toxicol Lett. 2005;157(1):49-56.
13. Rao SL, Adiga PR, Sarma PS. The isolation and characterization of β-N-Oxalyl-L-α,β-diaminopropionic acid: A neurotoxin from the seeds of Lathyrus sativus. Biochemistry. 1964;3:432-6.
14. Chrispai A. Cleistanthus collinus poisoning. J Emerg Trauma Shock. 2012;5(2):160-6.
15. Rajapake S. Management of yellow oleander poisoning. Clin Toxicol (Phila). 2009;47(3):206-12.
16. Senthilkumaran S, Saravanakumar S, Thirumalaikolundusubramanian P. Cutaneous absorption of oleander: Fact or fiction. J Emerg Trauma Shock. 2009;2:43-5.
17. Senthilkumaran S, Balamurugan N, Rajesh N, et al. Hard facts about loose stools-Massive alopecia in Gloriosa superba poisoning. Int J Trichology. 2011;3:126-7.

41 CHAPTER

Mushroom Poisoning

Nipun Verma, Ashish Bhalla, Shreya Singh

BACKGROUND

Fleshy fruiting bodies of certain higher fungi are commonly denoted as mushrooms.[1] Mushrooms are the source of food and article of trade across many cultures throughout the globe.[1] Thousands of species of mushrooms have been identified worldwide and around 100 of which are poisonous and 15–20 are fatal to humans.[2] People in India are known to consume nearly 283 species of wild mushrooms[3] and around 100 of such species are poisonous to humans.[4] Accidental consumption of poisonous mushrooms belonging to specific genera may lead to fatal outcomes including liver, renal and multiorgan failures.[4]

The first record of fatal poisoning was described in a family consisting of mother, daughter and two sons in Euripides (456–450 BC).[5] Majority cases (95%) of mushroom poisoning occur due to misidentification and accidental consumption of poisonous mushrooms. In around 5% cases, the poisoning results from intentional use of mushrooms for their mind-altering properties.[4] Severity of mushroom poisoning varies from mild gastrointestinal (GI) illness to severe liver or multiorgan failure(s) and death.[1,4] The severity depends on the type of mushroom consumed, quantity of toxin delivered, delay in treatment, genetic makeup of mushroom and host susceptibility. Processing, storing, boiling, freezing the food does not seem to affect the toxicity of poisonous mushrooms.[4]

PATHOPHYSIOLOGY

The reported poisonous species of mushroom in India includes *Amanita* species, and some members of the *Galerina*, *Lepiota*, and *Conocybe* genera[6,7] and *Omphalotus olivascens*, *Mycena pura* and *Chlorophyllum molybdites*.[3,8,9] *Amanita phalloides* forms the dominant cause of mushroom poisoning worldwide and as well as in India.[1,2] The toxins[10,11] incriminating the damage include cyclopeptides (i.e. amatoxins, phallotoxins, virotoxins), gyromitrins, orellanine, muscarine, psilocybin, muscimol/ibotenic acid, coprine, direct central neurotoxins, nephrotoxins, myotoxins, immunoactive toxins, hemolytic toxins and GI irritants.

The amatoxins, gyromitrins are hepatotoxic, orellanine is nephrotoxic, gyromitrins are epileptogenic, muscarine, psilocybin, muscimol, and ibotenic acid are neurotoxic and coprine induces the disulfiram-like reaction when combined with alcohol.

- *Cyclopeptides* include amatoxins[12] (high toxicity), phallotoxins (medium toxicity), and virotoxins (no toxicity). Amatoxins are the most common cause of hepatotoxicity related to mushroom poisoning. *Amanita*, *Galerina*, *Lepiota*, and *Conocybe* genera of mushrooms produce these toxins. Five types of amatoxins are known, the two most important ones include alpha-amanitin and beta-amanitin. Amanitins are heat resistant, water soluble and

Miscellaneous Toxicities

alcohol soluble. They are rapidly absorbed in enterohepatic circulation, have limited protein binding. They inhibit eukaryotic RNA polymerase II and protein synthesis, thus interrupting transcription in humans resulting in decreased mRNA, leading eventually to cell death. The effects are maximum metabolically active organs like liver and kidney. These are excreted in the urine and may be detected in the vomitus and feces. Hepatocellular damage is presumably caused by the formation of free radical intermediates. Examples of amatoxins containing mushrooms include *A. phalloides* (death cap), *Amanita virosa* (destroying angel), *Amanita verna* (fool's mushroom), and *Galerina autumnalis* (autumn skullcap). Phallotoxins are not absorbed and are toxic to cell membrane of enterocytes leading to initial diarrhea like illness.

- *Gyromitrins* are the toxins released by *Gyromitra esculenta*, *Gyromitra ambigua*, *Gyromitra gigas*, *Gyromitra infula* and *Verpa bohemica* genera of mushrooms. The route of intoxication may be oral or inhalation. These are metabolized to hepatotoxic hydrazine, a derivative, which inhibits cytochrome enzymes, induces oxidative damage, and depletes glutathione stores. It reduces γ-aminobutyric acid (GABA)-mediated neurotransmission and may lead to neurotoxicity resulting in seizures, hemolysis, methemoglobinemia and renal failure.
- *Orellanine* is the toxin released by *Cortinarius* mushroom (webcap). These are widely distributed across the globe including Europe, Japan and North America. The toxin is colorless, crystalline and causes nephrotoxicity (tubulotoxic) by itself or after conversion into orelline. These mushrooms also contain cortinarin A, B, and C which are nephrotoxic.
  Affected liver and intestines show fatty degeneration and/or severe inflammation.
- *Psilocybin* and psilocin are the toxins released by *Psilocybe, Panaeolus, Gymnopilus, Copelandia, Conocybe, Psathyrella,* and *Pluteus* genera of mushrooms. The toxins are serotoninergic and cause psychedelic effects analogous to lysergic acid.
- *Ibotenic acid and muscimol* are released by *Amanita muscaria* (fly agaric) and *Amanita pantherina* (panther cap) mushrooms. Ibotenic acid is a glutamate agonist in the central nervous system (CNS) and causes hallucinations. It may be metabolized to muscimol which is GABA agonist. There may be anticholinergic and muscarinic symptoms due to potent substances in these mushrooms.
- *Muscarines* are released by *Inocybe* and *Clitocybe* mushrooms. The action of muscarine is peripheral nervous system and results in typical symptoms of muscarine poisoning.
- *Coprine* is the toxin released by *Coprinus atramentarius* (inky cap) mushroom. Its metabolite (1-aminocyclopropanol) may block acetaldehyde dehydrogenase, and, results in accumulation of acetaldehyde upon consuming alcohol, therefore resulting in a reaction analogous to disulfiram. The effect may persist up to 72 hours after consumption.
- *Involutin* is released by *Paxillus involutus* mushrooms. It is GI toxic and leads to pain abdomen, nausea, vomiting, diarrhea followed by immune complex-mediated reactions like hemolytic anemia with hemoglobinuria, oliguria, anuria, and acute renal failure.
- *Lycoperdons* are released in the spores of puffball mushrooms, which upon inhalation may lead to allergic response and pneumonitis.
- *Gastrointestinal toxins* are there in the variety of mushrooms like *C. molybdites* (green gill), *Omphalotus illudens* (jack-o'-lantern), *Boletus piperatus* (peppery bolete), and *Agaricus arvensis* (horse mushroom), among many others.

EPIDEMIOLOGY

The fruiting stage of mushrooms tends to occur in the spring and fall of winters and the cases of poisoning tends to rise during this time.[1,13] These tend to occur in epidemics or sporadically and hence the exact incidence is unknown. The ingestion of poisonous mushrooms is accidental in 95% cases and intentional cases represent less than 5%.[4,6,14,15] Accidental cases arise due to misidentification of poisonous mushrooms.[14] Many outbreaks have been reported from various parts of India and abroad.[16-18]

Mortality/Morbidity

People in extremes of ages and poor baseline health are prone to high morbidity and mortality. Early diagnosis and treatment may alter the natural history of intoxication. Severe liver injury due to *Amanita* has variable spontaneous survival. Majority patients with mild toxicity survive but some series have quoted mortality of 40-60% with amatoxins related acute liver failure (ALF).[17]

CLINICAL PRESENTATION

History of consumption of mushrooms is paramount importance while eliciting the history of GI intoxication along with multiorgan involvements.[4] Since, the removal of toxins may alter the course and identification of ingested mushroom may help target-specific therapies. Time of ingestion, duration elapsed past symptoms, amount of mushroom consumed, the intake by other members of society and their symptoms must be looked very carefully.

Mushrooms are best classified by the physiologic and clinical effects of their poisons.[1,4,13] The traditional time-based classification of mushrooms into an early/low toxicity group and a delayed/high toxicity group may be inadequate. Additionally, many mushroom syndromes develop soon after ingestion. Out of these, *Amanita* poisoning forms the most common form of toxicity and cause of concern.

Amanita Poisoning[12]

Classically, clinical manifestations occur in four stages as described in Table 1. After initial lag phase ranging from 0 hour to 24 hours after ingestion, patients may develop GI symptoms which may last 6-24 hours and then a phase of convalescence is followed by hepatic and renal failures. Finally, patient lands up in multiorgan failures and death in 50-90% cases. However, sometimes GI symptoms may present earlier than 6 hours, making the differentiation between amatoxin poisoning and other benign mushroom exposure difficult.[14]

Adequate history is often clue to diagnosis and may be confirmed by an experienced mycologist and toxicological analysis. In the absence of mushroom for analysis, the diagnosis is largely clinical and can best be probable.[4,6]

The third phase of *Amanita* poisoning (i.e. the hepatorenal syndrome) is characterized by jaundice, hypoglycemia, coma, and multiorgan and system failure followed by death in 50-90% of patients. With therapy, mortality may be well below 10%.[1] The course of amatoxin poisoning typically lasts 6-8 days in adults and 4-6 days in children.[18]

Gyromitrin Poisoning

The clinical presentation often mimics *Amanita* poisoning.[6] After an initial lag phase of 6-10 hours, patient develops headache, abdominal pain, vomiting and diarrhea. Young and elderly patients and especially those on isoniazid develop hydrazine metabolites related neurotoxicity manifested as dizziness, confusion, seizures or coma. After inhalation, the symptoms of neurotoxicity may arise as early as 2 hours. Other manifestations include hemolysis, renal failure and rarely liver failure. Generally, recovery starts 2 days after symptom onset and may be delayed for 5-6 days. The course may be fatal in 2-4% cases.

Orellanine Poisoning[19]

The clinical symptoms start with minor GI symptoms lasting 24-48 hours after ingestion. Thereafter, a convalescent phase develops ranging from 3 days to 3 weeks. Then, patient develops polyuria with intense thirst leading on to renal failure. Renal replacement therapy is required in up to half the patients. Other symptoms include myalgias, muscle cramps, headache and seizures. Overall, the course may be fatal in 15% cases.

Psilocybin Poisoning[20]

The symptoms starts rapidly with hallucinations and generally subside within 2 hours. The course is generally benign and there is preserved consciousness, which is in contrast to ibotenic acid poisoning. Case reports of

Table 1: Clinical manifestations—four stages of Amanita poisoning.		
Phases	*Onset from ingestion*	*Symptoms and signs*
Stage 1	Lag phase 0–24 hours	Asymptomatic
Stage 2	Gastrointestinal phase 6–24 hours	Nausea, vomiting, crampy abdominal pain, and severe secretory diarrhea
Stage 3	Apparent convalescence 24–72 hours	Asymptomatic, worsening of hepatic and renal function indices
Stage 4	Acute liver failure 4–9 days	Hepatic and renal failure → multiorgan failure → death

Miscellaneous Toxicities

fatal poisoning have been described in small children after massive consumption in whom hallucinations are followed by fever, seizures, coma and death.

Muscarine Poisoning[21]

The symptoms arise typically 15–30 minutes of ingestion and include hypersalivation, hyperperspiration, and hyperlacrimation. Patients may develop abdominal pain, nausea, diarrhea, blurred vision, and labored breathing after large consumption. The course is generally benign and self-limiting in 2–3 hours and fatal in rarity.

Ibotenic Acid/Muscimol Poisoning[22]

The symptoms arise 1–2 hours of ingestion. Children present with glutaminergic symptoms in the form of illusions, delirium, hyperactivity, excitability, and seizures. Adults, usually present with GABAergic/muscimol effects in the form of dizziness, increased sleepiness and dysphoria. Adults may have fluctuating sensorium with periods of drowsiness and hyperactive delirium. The course is fatal in children with large amounts of intoxication within 12 hours. On the other hand, the course in adults is generally benign and rarely fatal.

Coprine Poisoning[23]

The symptoms usually arise similar to disulfiram reaction if the patient consumes alcohol within 2 hours of consumption of mushroom. Typically symptoms include nausea, vomiting, headache, chest pain, flushing, and diaphoresis. These may last for 2–3 hours and fatality is extremely rare.

Miscellaneous Gastrointestinal Poisons

Nonspecific GI symptoms including diarrhea, vomiting and nausea may occur after consuming poisonous mushrooms. The associated electrolyte and metabolic derangements that may rarely result in mortality.

DIFFERENTIAL DIAGNOSES

The common differentials include ALF due to viral hepatitis, acute renal failure due to any reason, adrenal crisis, encephalopathy due to sepsis or liver failure, food poisoning, acute bacterial or viral gastroenteritis, isoniazid toxicity, disulfiram toxicity, ALF, hallucinogens and septic/hemorrhagic shock. Again, the correct and adequate history is often clue to diagnosis.

LABORATORY STUDIES

Complete hemogram specifically looking for hemolysis as in gyromitrin poisoning, anemia due to renal failure in orellanine, leukocytosis due to sepsis. Serum electrolyte imbalances, acid-base disorders and dehydration may arise due to massive diarrhea, vomiting, renal failure, and sepsis. Arterial blood gas analysis may demonstrate hypoxia and metabolic acidosis. Hypocalcemia is seen in orellanine-induced renal failure, gyromitrin and amatoxin poisoning. Hypophosphatemia may occur with amatoxin and gyromitrin poisoning, especially in children. Hypoglycemia may occur in severe diarrhea or liver failure, e.g. *Amanita* and gyromitrin poisoning, electrolytes: electrolyte disturbances, such as hypokalemia, may occur in patients with severe gastroenteritis. Renal failure may arise due to multifactorial reasons and amatoxin and gyromitrin toxicity itself. Higher serum creatinine levels are associated with poor prognosis in *Amanita* poisoning. Liver function tests will reveal elevated bilirubin, alanine aminotransferase (ALT), lactate dehydrogenase, albumin and international normalized ratio (INR) especially in amatoxin and gyromitrin ingestions. Elevated serum ammonia is seen cases with ALF and fatal in 60%. Methemoglobinemia may be seen in gyromitrin poisoning and psilocybin poisoning. Elevated creatine phosphokinase (CPK) levels are a manifestation of rhabdomyolysis and may be diagnosed with elevated CPK levels as in with *Tricholoma* and *Russula* species. Toxicological analysis to rule out paracetamol, benzodiazepines, opiates, barbiturates and alcohol poisoning is generally required. Electrocardiogram may be required to identify cardiac rhythm abnormalities, electrolyte imbalances and orellanine poisoning.

Imaging Studies

Chest X-ray may reveal bilateral reticulonodular infiltrates as seen in puffball-induced allergic bronchoalveolitis. A computed tomography (CT) scan of the brain is indicated in all patients with encephalopathy in order to rule out structural disease or a bleed.

Renal ultrasound may show enlarged kidneys in orellanine poisoning.

Mushroom identification: Botanical identification of fungus is the most reliable confirmatory data required for diagnosis. However, according to a report, mushroom could not be identified in 82.7% cases.[24] This should not be insisted upon to make a diagnosis.

Liver biopsy may be done in patients, if transplant is contemplated. It may reveal diffuse hepatocellular necrosis in gyromitrin toxicity and fatty degeneration of the liver, with extensive central zone necrosis and centrilobular hemorrhage in *Amanita* poisoning.[25]

Renal biopsy may reveal interstitial nephritis in gyromitrin poisoning and loss of brush border, tubular vacuolization, necrosis, dedifferentiation of proximal tubules and binding in orellanine poisoning.[26]

TREATMENT OF MUSHROOM POISONING

Supportive treatment forms the backbone of management of mushroom poisoning with multiorgan involvement.[4,27] The approach needs to be aggressive, rapid and accurate. The most important step after maintaining circulation, airway and breathing is GI decontamination. The efficacy of lavage is maximum in initial 1 hour of ingestion beyond which the role is controversial. Multiple doses of activated charcoal should be administered daily for 3-4 days by oral route regardless of the time of presentation. It aims to inhibit the absorption of existing toxins in GI tract and blocks the enterohepatic circulation of toxins. Endotracheal intubation is required for patients in grade III–IV hepatic encephalopathy, hypoxia, hypercarbia, acidosis, shock. Blood transfusions may be required for blood loss with target hemoglobin of 7-9 g/dL. Circulatory support may be required with intravenous crystalloids and colloids with vasopressors in order to maintain mean arterial pressures above 70 mm Hg. Frequent blood sugar monitoring and correction is necessary. Cerebral edema associated with ALF should be managed with head end elevation to 30°, hyperventilation with target PCO_2 25–35 mm Hg, mannitol boluses, 3% hypertonic saline to maintain serum sodium up to 145–155 mEq/L, osmolality below 450 mOsm/kg. Finally, propofol and anticonvulsants may be necessary to bring down intracranial pressure (ICP) and prevent seizures.[27] Methemoglobinemia, after gyromitrin or psilocybin poisoning is treated with intravenous methylene blue. Hemolysis and hemoglobinuria associated with gyromitrin toxicity requires aggressive intravenous hydration and adequate urine output to prevent renal failure. Agitation and hyperactive delirium is treated with benzodiazepines. The correctable etiologies of agitation like hypoxia, hypovolemia, and shock should be correctly identified and corrected. Anticholinergic symptoms should be treated with benzodiazepines and rarely require physostigmine. Muscarinic symptoms may be treated with atropine infusions. Severe disulfiram-like reactions can be treated with fomepizole (4-methylpyrazole), if available. Renal failure, refractory electrolyte abnormalities, volume overload and metabolic derangements may require hemodialysis. Early hemoperfusion may prevent renal failure in patients with orellanine poisoning. Fulminant hepatic failure should be treated aggressively. The decision for liver transplantation[28] should be taken early in the course of disease within 3–4 days of admission. King's College Hospital,[29] Ganzert's criteria[30] (prothrombin index ≤25% with serum creatinine ≥106 µmol/L between day 3–10 of ingestion) and symptom onset within 8 hours or prothrombin index (PTI) at day 4 of ingestion below 10% or INR greater than 6.0[28] may guide the decision for liver transplantation. Patients with severe liver injury (ALT >10 times and INR >2.0 without encephalopathy) should be referred immediately to a center with a facility of liver transplantation.

Specific Therapies

Amatoxin Poisoning[7]

In addition to supportive treatment with airway, breathing and circulation, GI decontamination, the following modalities have been shown to improve outcomes in amatoxin poisoning.

Intravenous benzylpenicillin[31] *and silibinin*[32] *(extract of milk thistle)*: Both acts to reduce the uptake of amatoxins by hepatocytes. Silibinin has been shown to improve survival in patients with *Amanita* poisoning especially given within 48 hours of symptoms.[33,34]

Cimetidine: It inhibits cytochrome P-450 enzyme and may prevent the uptake of amatoxins by the oxidase system. *N*-acetylcysteine:[35] it repletes the glutathione stores and helps scavenge the free radical damage induced by amatoxins.

Plasma exchange with molecular absorbent regenerating system (MARS)[36,37] and Prometheus[38] has recently shown survival benefit in patients with *Amanita*-associated liver failure.

Gyromitrin Poisoning[6]

Seizures are generally controlled by antiepileptics like benzodiazepines. Pyridoxine supplementation that replete the GABA in brain; usually reduces the occurrence of seizures.

PROGNOSIS

The prognosis depends on the amount consumed, age of the patient, time of presentation and severity at presentation. Generally, with adequate and timely supportive and specific care, the survival has improved.[39] In amatoxin poisoning, the survival has risen from 40% to 80–90%.[40,41] In gyromitrin poisoning, course is generally benign and death is rare. In orellanine poisoning, a short time to symptom onset portends poor prognosis. Generally, the course is self-limiting and improves with supportive care. Fatality is reported in up to 15% cases. In psilocybin poisoning, prognosis is generally good.

CONCLUSION

Mushroom poisoning may occur due to consumption on nonedible toxic mushrooms. The type, amount and the interval between ingestion and onset of symptoms are important parameters for management. Identification of mushrooms may be difficult and should not delay management. Treatment is generally supportive. Follow the principles of Airway, Breathing, Circulation and Decontamination (ABCD). Multidose-activated charcoal and GI purging may help in reducing toxicity and hence, may be attempted. Education regarding the poisonous nature of wild mushrooms may act as a deterrent to mushroom foraging and ingestion.

KEY POINTS

- Mushroom poisoning occurs due to consumption on nonedible toxic mushrooms
- Most benign exposures have early-onset GI symptoms whereas *Amanita* toxicity generally has a lag period
- The type, amount and the interval between ingestion and onset of symptoms are important parameters for management
- Identification of mushrooms may be difficult and should not delay management
- Multidose-activated charcoal and GI purging help reduce toxicity but care must be taken to avoid dyselectrolytemia

- Patients ingesting coprine-containing mushrooms should be educated regarding the interaction with alcohol.

REFERENCES

1. Diaz JH. Amatoxin-containing mushroom poisonings: species, toxidromes, treatments, and outcomes. Wilderness Environ Med. 2018;29(1):111-8.
2. Verma N, Bhalla A, Kumar S, et al. Wild mushroom poisoning in North India: case series with review of literature. J Clin Exp Hepatol. 2014;4:361-5.
3. Datta A, Choudhary M, Devi R, et al. Diversity of wild edible mushrooms in Indian subcontinent and its neighboring countries. Rec Adv Biol Med. 2015;1: 69-79..
4. Diaz JH. Syndromic diagnosis and management of confirmed mushroom poisonings. Crit Care Med. 2005;33:427-36.
5. Jha S. (2012). Recent scenario in diversity, distribution and applied value of macrofungi: a review. [online] Available from https://www.researchgate.net/publication/221947197_Recent_scenario_in_diversity_distribution_and_applied_value_of_macrofungi_a_review. [Accessed November, 2018].
6. Karlson-Stiber C, Persson H. Cytotoxic fungi: an overview. Toxicon. 2003;42:339-49.
7. Enjalbert F, Rapior S, Nouguier-Soule J, et al. Treatment of amatoxin poisoning: 20-year retrospective analysis. J Toxicol Clin Toxicol. 2002;40:715-57.
8. Kumar M, Kaviyarasan V. Few common poisonous mushrooms of Kolli hills, South India. Mycotaxon. 1976;3:363.
9. Sarma TC, Sarma I, Patiri BN. Wild edible mushrooms used by some ethnic tribes of Western Assam. The Bioscan. 2010;3:613-25.
10. Berger KJ, Guss DA. Mycotoxins revisited: Part I. J Emerg Med. 2005;28:53-62.
11. Berger KJ, Guss DA. Mycotoxins revisited: Part II. J Emerg Med. 2005;28:175-83.
12. Mas A. Mushrooms, amatoxins and the liver. J Hepatol. 2005;42:166-9.
13. Diaz JH. Evolving global epidemiology, syndromic classification, general management, and prevention of unknown mushroom poisonings. Crit Care Med. 2005;33:419-26.
14. Colak S, Kandis H, Afacan MA, et al. Assessment of patients who presented to the emergency department with mushroom poisoning. Hum Exp Toxicol. 2015;34:725-31.
15. Trabulus S, Altiparmak MR. Clinical features and outcome of patients with amatoxin-containing mushroom poisoning. Clin Toxicol (Phila). 2011;49:303-10.
16. Sharma J, Malakar M. (2013). An expressive study of mushroom poisoning cases in Lakhimpur district of Assam. [online] Available from https://www.researchgate.net/publication/280642953_An_expressive_study_of_

Mushroom_poisoning_cases_in_Lakhimpur_district_of_ Assam. [Accessed November, 2018].

17. Bronstein AC, Spyker DA, Cantilena LR Jr, et al. 2009 annual report of the American Association of Poison Control Centers' National Poison Data System (NPDS): 27th annual report. Clin Toxicol (Phila). 2010;48: 979-1178.

18. Jan MA, Siddiqui TS, Ahmed N, et al. Mushroom poisoning in children: clinical presentation and outcome. J Ayub Med Coll Abbottabad. 2008;20:99-101.

19. Danel VC, Saviuc PF, Garon D. Main features of Cortinarius spp. poisoning: a literature review. Toxicon. 2001;39:1053-60.

20. Peden NR, Bissett AF, Macaulay KE, et al. Clinical toxicology of "magic mushroom" ingestion. Postgrad Med J. 1981;57:543-5.

21. George P, Hegde N. Muscarinic toxicity among family members after consumption of mushrooms. Toxicol Int. 2013;20:113-5.

22. Moss MJ, Hendrickson RG. Toxicity of muscimol and ibotenic acid containing mushrooms reported to a regional poison control center from 2002-2016. Clin Toxicol (Phila). 2018:1-5.

23. Haberl B, Pfab R, Berndt S, et al. Case series: alcohol intolerance with coprine-like syndrome after consumption of the mushroom Lepiota aspera (Pers.:Fr.) Quel., 1886 (Freckled Dapperling). Clin Toxicol (Phila). 2011;49: 113-4.

24. Mowry JB, Spyker DA, Cantilena LR Jr, et al. 2012 annual report of the American Association of Poison Control Centers' National Poison Data System (NPDS): 30th annual report. Clin Toxicol (Phila). 2013;51:949-1229.

25. Bartoloni St Omer F, Giannini A, Botti P, et al. Amanita poisoning: a clinical-histopathological study of 64 cases of intoxication. Hepatogastroenterology. 1985;32: 229-31.

26. Myler RK, Lee JC, Hopper J Jr. Renal tubular necrosis caused by mushroom poisoning. Renal biopsy findings by electron microscopy and use of peritoneal dialysis in treatment. Arch Intern Med. 1964;114:196-204.

27. Wendon J, Cordoba J, Dhawan A, et al. EASL Clinical Practical Guidelines on the management of acute (fulminant) liver failure. J Hepatol. 2017;66:1047-81.

28. Escudie L, Francoz C, Vinel JP, et al. Amanita phalloides poisoning: reassessment of prognostic factors and indications for emergency liver transplantation. J Hepatol. 2007;46:466-73.

29. O'Grady JG, Alexander GJ, Hayllar KM, et al. Early indicators of prognosis in fulminant hepatic failure. Gastroenterology. 1989;97:439-45.

30. Ganzert M, Felgenhauer N, Zilker T. Indication of liver transplantation following amatoxin intoxication. J Hepatol. 2005;42:202-9.

31. Ganzert M, Felgenhauer N, Schuster T, et al. Amanita poisoning—comparison of silibinin with a combination of silibinin and penicillin. Dtsch Med Wochenschr. 2008;133:2261-7.

32. Lacombe G, St-Onge M. Towards evidence-based emergency medicine: best BETs from the Manchester Royal Infirmary. BET 1: Silibinin in suspected amatoxin-containing mushroom poisoning. Emerg Med J. 2016;33:76-7.

33. Abenavoli L, Izzo AA, Milic N, et al. Milk thistle (Silybum marianum): a concise overview on its chemistry, pharmacological, and nutraceutical uses in liver diseases. Phytother Res. 2018;32:2202-13.

34. Hruby K, Csomos G, Fuhrmann M, et al. Chemotherapy of Amanita phalloides poisoning with intravenous silibinin. Hum Toxicol. 1983;2:183-95.

35. Montanini S, Sinardi D, Pratico C, et al. Use of acetylcysteine as the life-saving antidote in Amanita phalloides (death cap) poisoning. Case report on 11 patients. Arzneimittelforschung. 1999;49:1044-7.

36. Pillukat MH, Schomacher T, Baier P, et al. Early initiation of MARS' dialysis in Amanita phalloides-induced acute liver injury prevents liver transplantation. Ann Hepatol. 2016;15:775-87.

37. Zhang J, Zhang Y, Peng Z, et al. Experience of treatments of Amanita phalloides-induced fulminant liver failure with molecular adsorbent recirculating system and therapeutic plasma exchange. ASAIO J. 2014;60:407-12.

38. Bergis D, Friedrich-Rust M, Zeuzem S, et al. Treatment of Amanita phalloides intoxication by fractionated plasma separation and adsorption (Prometheus'). J Gastrointestin Liver Dis. 2012;21:171-6.

39. Saviuc PF, Danel VC, Moreau PA, et al. Erythromelalgia and mushroom poisoning. J Toxicol Clin Toxicol. 2001;39:403-7.

40. Karvellas CJ, Tillman H, Leung AA, et al. Acute liver injury and acute liver failure from mushroom poisoning in North America. Liver Int. 2016;36:1043-50.

41. Giannini L, Vannacci A, Missanelli A, et al. Amatoxin poisoning: a 15-year retrospective analysis and follow-up evaluation of 105 patients. Clin Toxicol (Phila). 2007;45:539-42.

42
CHAPTER

Methotrexate and Other Chemotherapeutic Agents Toxicity

Akhilesh Singh, Omender Singh

INTRODUCTION

With rise in cancer over the last few decades, the probability to encounter patients with chemotherapeutic drug-induced toxicity has also increased.[1] Most chemotherapeutic drugs target cells which multiply rapidly and target nucleic acids as well as their precursors that synthesize rapidly during cell division. Apart from oncological indications chemotherapeutic agents are used for treatment of other disorders as well [e.g. uses of methotrexate (MTX)].

The properties which differentiate chemotherapeutic agents are the severity and incidence of toxic effects which may occur at therapeutic doses. Chemotherapeutic drugs have the lowest therapeutic indices, that may often lead to multisystem toxicity.[2] These toxicity can be acute and latent. These properties increase risk of morbidity and mortality associated with treatment.

The management of chemotherapy-induced toxicity consists of discontinuation and/or reduction in their dose, use of alternative drugs or their analogs, use of cytoprotective drugs, or growth factors.[2]

Methotrexate Toxicity

Methotrexate is an analog of folate, an antimetabolite chemotherapeutic drug exhibiting antiproliferative, anti-inflammatory, and immunomodulating properties. It is clinically used in treating malignancies, dermatological and rheumatic disorders, and also in termination of gestation.[3] It can be administered intravenously (IV), intramuscularly, intrathecally, and orally. Dosing of MTX is varied in view of its multiple indications.[4]

Methotrexate toxicity may be idiosyncratic and/or dose dependent. The toxic profile of MTX depends on the dose administered. MTX containing regimens may be categorized as low (<50 mg/m^2), intermediate (50–500 mg/m^2), or high-dose HD-MTX (>500 mg/m^2), depending on its dose.

Serious adverse events and high mortality have been reported with medical and patient errors.[5] Acute MTX toxicity may present as pancytopenia, gastrointestinal (GI), mucositis, hepatotoxicity, pulmonary toxicity, neurotoxicity, and acute renal failure.[6,7]

Methotrexate Metabolism

Methotrexate undergoes metabolism in the liver, intracellularly to polyglutamated forms.[8] Hydrolase enzymes convert the polyglutamated forms back to MTX, thereby increasing intracellular half-life of MTX, leading to increased MTX levels despite extracellular removal.[8]

Pharmacokinetics of Methotrexate

Regardless of serum concentration, about 50% MTX-protein binding occurs.[9] MTX kinetics depends

Methotrexate and Other Chemotherapeutic Agents Toxicity

significantly upon its dosage and route of administration. Absorption of MTX plateau is achieved between 25 mg and 50 mg on oral administration[10] and at doses less than 30 mg, almost complete intestinal uptake occurs, whereas plasma MTX concentration is less than 10% when MTX dose of approximately more than 80 mg is administered.[11] In the kidneys, elimination of MTX occurs by glomerular filtration, tubular reabsorption, and secretion.[11]

Certain drugs like sulfonamides, penicillin, non-steroidal anti-inflammatory drugs (NSIADs), salicylates, probenecid, benzimidazoles, and barbiturates may increase serum MTX concentration. Impairment of glomerular is the prime reason for increased MTX elimination filtration time.[11]

Exposure 1.7 times of an equivalent oral dose from bulk cerebrospinal fluid (CSF) absorption into systemic circulation, can result due to intrathecal administration of MTX.[12]

Methotrexate's Mechanism of Action

Methotrexate competitively inhibits *dihydrofolate reductase* so that FH_2 and active FH_4 cannot be generated from folate, neither existing FH_2 can be recycled. MTX metabolites inhibit *thymidylate synthase*, thus blocking thymidine synthesis. Hence, thymidylate and purine biosynthesis is reduced leading to halt in DNA synthesis and cells can no longer divide.

Rapidly proliferating cells depend on nucleotide creation for DNA replication and RNA synthesis are most affected by MTX (e.g. malignancies, lymphoblasts, GI tract, bone marrow, synovial macrophages, and epithelia).

Methotrexate Poisoning with "Therapeutic Dosing"

Patients with deranged kidney function are at highest risk of developing MTX toxicity, as MTX is mainly excreted by kidneys; however, increased concentrations are seen in the absence of preexisting renal disease. Administration of nephrotoxic agents, including IV contrast, can also induce MTX toxicity.[13] Acute renal failure and tubular necrosis may occur due to precipitation of the metabolites or MTX itself in the renal tubules.[14]

Clinical Manifestations

Signs and symptoms of acute MTX toxicity are based on extent and severity of organ involvement.

Hematologic Toxicity

High-dose MTX therapy is often associated with hematotoxicity.[15] It presents with thrombocytopenia followed by a rapidly progressive leukoneutropenia.[16] Leukopenia is observed after 1–3 weeks.[17]

With low-dose MTX, hematologic toxicity is low.[18] In patients with rheumatoid arthritis (RA) being treated with MTX, the prevalence of hematologic toxicity is about 3% and pancytopenia around 1.4%.[19] High incidence of pancytopenia is seen with advanced age, hypoalbuminemia, folic acid deficiency, concomitant infections, dehydration, and co-administration of drugs.[20,21]

Basis of therapy includes discontinuation of MTX, granulocyte colony-stimulating factor (G-CSF), and methylprednisolone.[22]

Nephrotoxicity

Acute renal failure is generally secondary to acute tubular necrosis caused by MTX (2–4%)[23] and may be severe and formidable. Precipitation of MTX or its metabolites in the renal tubules may lead to nephrotoxicity[24,25] due to obstruction and reduction in renal clearance and prolongation of MTX high levels. MTX may also affect tubular epithelium directly leading to vasoconstriction of the afferent arteriole.[16,26]

Methotrexate and its metabolites are not easily soluble in acidic urine.[27] Hence, increasing the urinary pH may result in greater solubility of the MTX and its metabolites, reducing their harmful effects. Clinically, patients with acute renal failure may be asymptomatic.[28]

Pulmonary Toxicity

Pulmonary toxicity may present with acute interstitial pneumonitis, interstitial fibrosis, pleuritis, pleural effusions, bronchiolitis obliterans organizing pneumonia (BOOP), noncardiogenic pulmonary edema, or pulmonary nodules and is seen in up to 10% of patients.[29] Tapering of steroids, use of chemotherapeutic agents (cyclophosphamide or bleomycin) increase the risk of pulmonary toxicity. Old age, diabetes, disease-modifying antirheumatic drugs (DMARDs), and hypoalbuminemia are few risk factors associated with pulmonary toxicity in oral low-dose MTX therapy.[30]

Neurotoxicity

Methotrexate therapy may cause acute, subacute, and chronic neurotoxicity and is associated with intrathecal or IV administration of MTX.[31] Leukoencephalopathy is

Miscellaneous Toxicities

the most common acute neurologic manifestation[27] that presents with insomnia, confusion, agitation, seizure, and coma and is diagnosed by magnetic resonance imaging.[32] Intrathecal administration of MTX may cause headache, nausea, vomiting, and aseptic meningitis.[33] Aminophylline or leucovorin is indicated for MTX neurotoxicity.[34,35]

Gastrointestinal Toxicity

Methotrexate causes variety of GI disorders. Patients may present with abdominal pain, vomiting, and diarrhea. Long-term MTX is associated with hepatotoxicity.[36] Supplementation of folic acid 1 mg/day or folinic acid 2.5 mg/week leads to decreased in incidence of aminotransferases elevation.[37]

Mucocutaneous Toxicity

High-dose MTX can manifest with cutaneous toxicity. Clinical manifestations may include oral mucosa ulcerations, photosensitivity, multiform erythema, urticaria, and vasculitis.[38,39] Low-dose MTX can also induce cutaneous small-vessel vasculitis in patients with collagen vascular disease.[40]

Diagnostic Evaluation

Patient presenting with suspected signs and symptoms of MTX toxicity must be admitted in a critical care units and reverse barrier nursing protocol should be instituted. Routine blood investigations—complete hemogram, renal function test liver function test, and serum MTX levels should be done. For patients with pulmonary and neurological symptoms, chest radiography and/or brain imaging is needed.

Renal Functions

As MTX is excreted mainly by the kidneys, it is necessary to assess kidney functions. MTX dose adjustment is necessary for patients with impaired renal functions.

For creatinine clearance (CrCl) between 30 mL/min and 60 mL/min, dose of MTX has to be reduced by 50% and for CrCl between 10 mL/min and 30 mL/min, dose has to be reduced by 75%.[23]

Monitoring Plasma Methotrexate Concentration

Methotrexate levels should be monitored for MTX-HD therapy. The aim is to identify patients who are at highest risk for MTX toxicity. Plasma MTX levels should be measured at 24 hours, 48 hours, and 72 hours after initiation of the infusion.

To avoid MTX toxicity, levels should be above 10 μM at 24 hours, 1 μM at 48 hours, and 0.15 μM at 72 hours.[23]

Management of Methotrexate Toxicity

Targets involved in managing acute MTX toxicity are broadly based on:

- Elimination of MTX from the body
- Antidotal strategies [folinic acid (leucovorin), thymidine, and glucarpidase]
- Organ-specific care.

Elimination of Methotrexate from Body (Hydration and Urine Alkalization)

Maintaining adequate hydration and urine alkalization: To prevent intratubular precipitation of MTX, aggressive hydration should be maintained. Brisk diuresis (>60 mL/h) by administration of IV saline is necessary for MTX elimination.[23,27]

Maintaining alkaline urine pH: MTX and its metabolite 7-OH-MTX, have 20 and 12-fold increased solubility, respectively when pH increases from 5 to 7.[23,41] Precipitation of MTX and 7-OH-MTX in renal tubules occurs when pH is lower than 5.0.[23] It is important to initiate MTX infusion when the urine pH is more than or equal to 7.0 and to maintain it, until plasma MTX levels are less than 0.1 μM.

Drainage of third-space fluids: Third-space fluids lead to a prolonged MTX plasma half-life leading to risk of toxicity, hence drainage of third-space fluid is recommended to prevent toxicity.[23]

Folinic Acid—Leucovorin Rescue Therapy

Folinic acid or leucovorin is antidote of choice for MTX toxicity. In 1948, leucovorin (5-formyl-FH4, folinic acid, citrovorum factor, calcium folinate) was first identified[42] and was reported to effectively reverse MTX toxicity, that was resistant to folate rescue.[43,44]

Administration of leucovorin is necessary to avoid the metabolic blockage imposed by MTX. Within 24–36 hours of initiation of, MD-MTX infusion, leucovorin rescue should be started. Commonly administered doses of leucovorin rescue varies between 10 mg/m^2 and 15 mg/m^2, 6 hourly until plasma MTX levels are below 0.2 μM.[23]

Oral dose of leucovorin is 20–40 mg and is bioequivalent to IV administration because of decreased absorption of the inactive form and presystemic intestinal metabolism. Active intestinal transport is saturated at doses more than 40 mg PO.[23]

Recommended doses of 100 mg/m² or 1,000 mg/m² every 6 hours and as high as 10 g/day are indicated for MTX toxicity. Reversal of toxicity is not seen in patients with MTX concentrations more than 100 µmol/L.[23,45]

In patients receiving MTX for nonmalignancy causes—leucovorin should be continued till the serum MTX concentration is 10 nmol/L (0.01 µmol/L). In patients receiving MTX as chemotherapy, leucovorin should be continued till MTX levels are 50–100 nmol/L (0.05–0.1 µmol/L).[23,46]

Leucovorin infusion must not exceed 160 mg/min because of high calcium content (0.004 mEq calcium per mg of leucovorin), intrathecal administration of leucovorin is contraindicated.[47] In case, more than 10 mg/m² is required to be administered, leucovorin should be dissolved in sterile water.

Thymidine was available as a rescue agent (*thymidylate salvage*) in the starting of year 1978.[48,49] Thymidine is no longer available as a therapy for MTX toxicity.

Glutamate carboxypeptidase (CPDG2, carboxypeptidase G2, and glucarpidase) is an antidote approved by the US Food and Drug Administration (USFDA) in 2012. It is indicated for patients who have delayed MTX elimination or acute kidney injury (AKI) and plasma MTX concentrations above 0.1 mmol/L.[50]

Recommended dose is 50 units/kg IV to be administered over 5 minutes. Within 15 minutes of its administration, serum MTX concentrations have been shown to get reduced by 95–99%.[2]

Methotrexate metabolites have a tendency to cross-react with mostly available MTX immunoassays, thus to determine actual serum MTX levels, high-performance liquid chromatography should be used. CPDG2 has a 15-fold higher affinity for MTX than for leucovorin although affinity for folate is similar.[51]

In cases of inadvertent IT-MTX administration, intrathecal CPDG2 has been administered with complete patient recovery.[52]

Role for Extracorporeal Drug Removal

Patients with worsening renal functions are at high risk of developing MTX toxicity and high-flux hemodialysis or charcoal hemoperfusion has been reported to be useful.[53,54] Repeat dialysis sessions may be required as MTX redistribution from the cellular compartment may result in a rebound increase in MTX levels.[2]

Peritoneal dialysis is not useful as it has minimal affect on serum MTX concentrations because its MTX clearance occurs only in the first hour of exchange.[55]

Avoiding Drug Interactions

Co-administration of drugs that may either displace MTX from serum proteins and/or reduce MTX clearance may lead to increased MTX toxicity. Interactions are commonly seen with trimethoprim and sulfamethoxazole and NSAIDs.[56,57] Alteration in elimination of MTX are also reported with pyrazoles, aminoglycosides, probenecid, some penicillin, macrolides, omeprazole,[58] piperacillin,[59] and amphotericin B.[60]

Role of Folate

As MTX blocks the enzyme responsible for folate utilization and activation, thus it is not an effective antidote.[23]

CHEMOTHERAPEUTIC DRUG-ASSOCIATED TOXICITY

Use and evolvement of chemotherapeutic drugs has significantly increased in past 2 decades and so has the toxicity associated with them. Due to disease complexity, a great majority of these patients[61] are on multidrug regimens. To manage severe toxicity, termination of exposure is often crucial. The toxicity onset depends on the dosage and the nature of the drug involved. Subsequently, these agents cause varied generalized as well as organ-specific toxicities.

Chemotherapeutic agents are categorized into various classes depending upon their chemical structure and mechanism of action (Table 1).[62]

Neurological Toxicity

Central and peripheral neurotoxicity are encountered with chemotherapeutic toxicity.[63] Common neurotoxic agents are vincristine, ifosfamide, and cisplatin.[64] Other agents are enlisted in the Table 2.

Ifosfamide and cisplatin toxicity may present as altered mental status due to nonconvulsive status epilepticus.[64,65]

Miscellaneous Toxicities

Table 1: Classification of chemotherapeutic agents.

Class	Commonly used agents
Alkylating agents	Busulfan, dacarbazine Nitrogen mustards: Chlorambucil, cyclophosphamide, ifosfamide, and melphalan Platinoids: Cisplatin, carboplatin, oxaliplatin, procarbazine, and temozolomide
Antimetabolites	Methotrexate Purine analogs: Fludarabine, mercaptopurine, and pentostatin Pyrimidine analogs: Capecitabine, cytarabine 5-Fluorouracil (5-FU), Gemcitabine
Antimitotics	Taxanes: Docetaxel, paclitaxel Vinca alkaloids: Vincristine, vindesine, and vinorelbine
Antibiotics	Anthracycline: Doxorubicin, daunorubicin, idarubicin, dactinomycin, and bleomycin
Monoclonal antibodies	L-asparaginase, rituximab, cetuximab, and trastuzumab
Protein kinase inhibitor	Erlotinib, gefitinib, and dasatinib
Selective estrogen receptor modulator	Tamoxifen
Topoisomerase inhibitors	Camptothecins: Irinotecan, topotecan
Epipodophyllotoxins	Etoposide, teniposide

Table 2: Chemotherapeutic neurotoxins.

Toxicity	Drugs
Cerebrovascular accident, TIA	Bevacizumab, cisplatin, and erlotinib
Acute cerebellar syndrome with ataxia	Cytarabine, 5-FU
Encephalopathy	Cisplatin, fludarabine, 5-FU, ifosfamide, methotrexate, and vincristine
Seizures	Busulfan, temozolomide, vinblastine, and chlorambucil
Sagittal sinus thrombosis	L-asparaginase
Hemiparesis	Methotrexate
Parkinsonism-like syndrome	L-asparaginase
Peripheral neuropathy	Fludarabine, vincristine, taxanes, and cisplatin
Reversible posterior leukoencephalopathy	Cytarabine, cisplatin, bevacizumab, and gemcitabine

(5-FU: 5-fluorouracil; TIA: transient ischemic attack)

Vincristine-associated neurotoxicity presents with diverse neurologic symptoms from peripheral neuropathy, focal cranial nerve palsies to encephalopathy. Route of drug administration is also determinants of neurologic complications. Accidental intrathecal administration can be lethal, although have delayed presentation.

Peripheral neuropathy is also seen with paclitaxel, cisplatin, and oxaliplatin.

Management

Supportive care is the mainstay in management of chemotherapy-induced neurologic toxicity after the exclusion of infectious causes.

Antidote for neurotoxicity: Methylene blue.[66,67]

Dose: Methylene blue 1% solution IV (initial dose of 50 mg in adults).

Cardiovascular Toxicity

Anthracyclines, specifically doxorubicin, cause cardiac toxicity in the acute, subacute, and chronic setting. DNA disruption and myocyte death due to generation of hydroxyl radicals are main cause of cardiotoxicity.[68]

Table 3 enlists the cardiovascular toxicities associated with chemotherapeutic drugs.[68-70]

Management

The management of cardiovascular toxicity is similar to the management from cardiogenic and vascular causes. Anthracycline exposure should be avoided with patients with anthracycline-associated cardiotoxicity.

Dexrazoxane is the antidote, which inhibits doxorubicin-induced generation of hydroxyl radicals.[71] Incidence of anthracycline-associated congestive heart failure (CHF) and left ventricular dysfunction is reduced in patients receiving co-administration of dexrazoxane with doxorubicin chemotherapy.[72,73]

Hematopoietic Toxicity

Bone marrow suppression is common side effect of chemotherapeutic agents and is associated with serious complications and may warrant early termination of chemotherapy (Table 4).

Methotrexate and Other Chemotherapeutic Agents Toxicity

Table 3: Cardiovascular toxicities.

Toxicity	Drugs
Hypotension	Etoposide, fludarabine, MTX, paclitaxel, and procarbazine
Myocarditis	Cyclophosphamide
Myocardial necrosis	Cyclophosphamide
Pericarditis/pericardial effusion	Bleomycin, busulfan, cyclophosphamide, cytarabine, MTX, and dasatinib
Pericardial fibrosis	Bleomycin
QT-prolongation	Dasatinib, sorafenib, and lapatinib
Sudden cardiac death	Cetuximab
Thromboembolic complications	Bevacizumab, cisplatin, gemcitabine, erlotinib, L-asparaginase, tamoxifen, MTX, and sunitinib
Cardiac ischemia	Bevacizumab, cisplatin, docetaxel, fludarabine, 5-FU, paclitaxel, rituximab, vincristine, and vinblastine
CHF, LV dysfunction	Anthracyclines (daunorubicin, doxorubicin, and epirubicin) Cisplatin, cyclophosphamide (high dose), cytarabine, and docetaxel Paclitaxel, mitomycin, and sunitinib
Dysrhythmias	Cisplatin, cyclophosphamide (high doses), and daunorubicin Doxorubicin, 5-FU, fludarabine, paclitaxel, and rituximab
Hypertension	Cisplatin, bevacizumab, etoposide, vincristine, vinblastine, and vinorelbine
Capillary leak syndrome	Gemcitabine

(CHF: congestive heart failure; 5-FU: 5-fluorouracil; MTX: methotrexate)

Neutropenia is single most important dose-limiting complications of chemotherapy. Vinorelbine administration may cause granulocytopenia.

Cyclophosphamide, MTX, and mitomycin C are frequently associated with leukopenia. Procarbazine and fludarabine toxicity may lead to hemolytic anemia.

Thrombotic angiopathy may manifest as thrombotic thrombocytopenic purpura (TTP) or hemolytic uremic syndrome (HUS). The drugs most commonly associated with causing HUS are mitomycin C and gemcitabine.[74,75] Other agents which have also been associated with causing thrombotic angiopathy include bleomycin, carboplatin, cisplatin, daunorubicin, tamoxifen, alemtuzumab, bevacizumab, erlotinib, sunitinib, and imatinib.[76,77]

L-asparaginase therapy may lead to depression of clotting factors. Dasatinib toxicity may cause thrombocytopenia and platelet dysfunction.[78]

Management

The management of hematopoietic toxicity is supportive. For stimulation of bone marrow cell lineage, recombinant hematopoietic growth factors, e.g. granulocyte-macrophage colony-stimulating factor (GM-CSF) are indicated.[79] Treatment may include transfusion of blood and blood products, factor repletion, and symptomatic care. Source of infection should be ruled out in febrile patients. In patients with severe hemolysis, hematologist consultation should be sought and plasma exchange should be considered.[79]

Pulmonary Toxicity

Pulmonary toxicity associated with chemotherapy has low incidence (<10%) and it is challenging as it mimics metastatic lung or infective manifestation.

Table 4: Hematopoietic toxicity.

Busulfan	Epirubicin	Pentostatin	
Capecitabine	Etoposide	Procarbazine	
Carboplatin	Fludarabine	Rituximab	
Chlorambucil	5-fluorouracil (5-FU)	Temozolomide	
Cisplatin	Gemcitabine	Thioguanine	
Dacarbazine	Idarubicin	Vinblastine	
Dasatinib	Methotrexate	Vinorelbine	
Daunorubicin	Paclitaxel	Docetaxel	Mercaptopurine

Miscellaneous Toxicities

Most common chemotherapeutic pulmonary toxin is bleomycin.[80] Patients with bleomycin toxicity may develop hypersensitivity reaction, nodular changes, interstitial pneumonitis, pleural effusion, pulmonary edema, BOOP, and progressive pulmonary fibrosis (Table 5).

Busulfan, melphalan, and chlorambucil toxicity are associated with high mortality. Common pulmonary toxicities and causative agents are enlisted in Table 6.

Management

The treatment involves discontinuation of the causative agent, steroids, antibiotics, and supportive care. Pulmonary fibrosis may have a prolonged course and may show a poor response to conventional treatment. Oxygen therapy may worsen bleomycin-associated pulmonary toxicity, and hence, it should be administered cautiously only during emergency management of patients with hypoxia.

Gastrointestinal and Hepatotoxicity

Mucositis, chemotherapy-induced nausea and vomiting (CINV), diarrhea and severe constipation, hemorrhagic pancreatitis, and hepatic fibrosis are few complications associated with chemotherapeutic toxicity.[81-84]

Common chemodrugs causing mucositis and hepatotoxicity are enlisted in Tables 6 and 7.

Table 6: Chemotherapeutic hepatotoxins.

Toxicity	Drugs
Biliary structure	Fluorodeoxyuridine (5-FU metabolite, intra-arterial)
Cholestasis	Cisplatin, gemcitabine, mercaptopurine
Granulomatous hepatitis	Procarbazine
Hepatocellular injury	L-asparaginase, busulfan, cisplatin, cytarabine, and 5-FU Erlotinib, gefitinib, gemcitabine, MTX, and paclitaxel Sunitinib, vinorelbine
Hepatorenal syndrome	Erlotinib

(5-FU: 5-fluorouracil; MTX: methotrexate)

Table 5: Chemotherapeutic pulmonary toxins.

Toxicity	Drugs
BOOP	Bleomycin, cetuximab, chlorambucil, cyclophosphamide, MTX, and mitomycin C
Bronchospasm	Vincristine, pentostatin
Hemoptysis	Bevacizumab
Hypersensitive pneumonitis	Cetuximab, fludarabine, MTX, paclitaxel, and vinblastine
Interstitial pneumonitis	Bleomycin, cetuximab, chlorambucil, and cyclophosphamide Dactinomycin, docetaxel, erlotinib, gefitinib, and gemcitabine Mitomycin C, MTX, paclitaxel, and vinorelbine
Noncardiogenic pulmonary edema	Docetaxel, dasatinib, imatinib, MTX, paclitaxel, and Procarbazine
Pulmonary arterial hypertension	Dasatinib
Pulmonary fibrosis	Azathioprine, bleomycin, busulfan, and chlorambucil Cyclophosphamide, erlotinib, gefitinib, and melphalan MTX, oxaliplatin, panitumumab, and procarbazine

(BOOP: bronchiolitis obliterans organizing pneumonia; MTX: methotrexate)

Table 7: Chemotherapeutic agents causing mucositis.

Classes	Agents
Alkylating agents	Carboplatin, chlorambucil, cisplatin, and cyclophosphamide
Antimetabolites	Dacarbazine, mechlorethamine, and melphalan Capecitabine, cytarabine, fludarabine, 5-FU, and gemcitabine Mercaptopurine, MTX, and pentostatin
Antibiotics	Dactinomycin, daunorubicin, epirubicin, and mitomycin C
Antimitotic agents	Docetaxel, paclitaxel
Topoisomerase inhibitors	Etoposide
Tyrosine kinase inhibitor	Dasatinib, sunitinib, and sorafenib

Management

Management of oral mucositis involves assessment of the airway. Topical viscous lidocaine, oral and IV opioids pain relief, proton pump inhibitors (PPIs) or H2-receptor blockers, antiemetics are recommended.[85]

Ondansetron, which is a first-generation 5-HT3 antagonist, is the drug of choice for managing of CINV. In patients with persistent emesis, dexamethasone should be considered. For intractable emesis, benzodiazepines, olanzapine, and metoclopramide, aprepitant, and fosaprepitant (NK-1 antagonists) are recommended in the consultation with oncologist.[86]

Volume and electrolyte repletion are cornerstone of chemotherapy-induced diarrhea treatment. In cases of infective diarrhea, antibiotics should be considered.

Loperamide is drug of choice in patients with noninfectious chemotherapy-induced diarrhea. For severe and refractory diarrhea, octreotide is recommended.[86]

Methylnaltrexone is recommended for opioid-induced constipation with poor response to laxatives.[87]

For management of chemotherapy-induced hepato-toxicity, removal of the causative agent and general supportive care are all that is required. Transplant consultation should be sought for severe hepatotoxicity.

Renal Toxicity

Cisplatin is a common chemotherapeutic nephrotoxin (Table 8). Drugs affecting the proximal tubule can cause Fanconi syndrome, characterized by wasting of glucose, phosphate, potassium, and bicarbonate by the kidneys.[88]

Thrombotic angiopathy may manifest as HUS, which is secondary to deposition of fibrin in afferent arterioles and glomeruli.[89]

Management

Supportive therapy is indicated for management of renal complications. Hemodialysis should be considered if indicated. Amifostine is indicated for treatment and prevention of cisplatin-induced nephrotoxicity.[90,91]

Genitourinary Toxicity

Hemorrhagic cystitis is the most common genitourinary chemotherapeutic toxicity. The causative agent is acrolein metabolite of cyclophosphamide and ifosfamide that leads to oxidative cellular damage of

Table 8: Chemotherapeutic nephrotoxins.

Toxicity	Drugs
Acute renal insufficiency	Carboplatin, erlotinib, and nitrosoureas (carmustine, streptozotocin) Oxaliplatin, pentostatin
Acute tubular necrosis	Cisplatin, ifosfamide, imatinib, and MTX
Chronic kidney disease	Cisplatin, ifosfamide, and nitrosoureas
Crystal nephropathy	MTX
HUS	Bleomycin, cisplatin, gemcitabine, and mitomycin C
Renal tubular acidosis	Streptozotocin
Tubulopathy	Cisplatin, ifosfamide

(HUS: hemolytic uremic syndrome; MTX: methotrexate)

the uroepithelium.[92,93] Vincristine chemotherapy causes urinary retention.

Management

Treatment for hemorrhagic cystitis is mainly supportive. Irrigation of bladder is indicated in the presence of urinary retention or obstructive hematuria. Antidote of choice is Mesna, that has been recommended for the prevention of hemorrhagic cystitis induced by ifosfamide and cyclophosphamide.

Dermatologic Toxicity

Dermatological toxicity may manifest as hypersensitivity reactions, erythema multiforme (EM), Stevens-Johnson syndrome (SJS), or toxic epidermal necrolysis (TEN).

Chemotherapeutic agents which are associated with EM/SJS/TEN include chlorambucil,[94] actinomycin,[95] MTX,[96] rituximab,[97] and sorafenib.[98]

Both immune and nonimmune mechanisms are concomitant in hypersensitivity reactions. Most of these reactions occur immediately, within several minutes to several hours, of administration of the offending drug. Anaphylactoid reactions are seen with paclitaxel and docetaxel administration.[99]

Management

The management of anaphylaxis involves airway assessment, management of shock, stopping of the offending

Miscellaneous Toxicities

drug, and treatment with histamine antagonists, epinephrine, and steroids. Immunoglobulin therapy may be helpful.

EXTRAVASATION OF CHEMOTHERAPEUTIC AGENTS

Extravasation of chemotherapeutic drugs may cause severe skin and soft tissue irritation, necrosis, and may even lead to compartment syndrome.[100]

Anthracyclines, vinca alkaloids, and nitrogen mustard are characterized as vesicants, and may cause an inflammatory response and have the potential to cause severe tissue damage.[99]

Clinical manifestations include local skin erythema, tenderness, edema, blisters, ulceration, and tissue necrosis.[99]

The management consists of immediately stopping of the infusion, aspiration of extravasated drug, and intermittent cooling.[101] Dexrazoxane, hyaluronidase, and sodium thiosulfate are indicated in extravasation of the earlier listed vesicants, respectively.[102]

CONCLUSION

With rise in cancer over the last few decades, the probability to encounter patients with chemotherapeutic drug-induced toxicity has also increased. Toxicity from these agents can also occur at therapeutic doses. Toxicity with these drugs can lead to significant mortality and morbidity and can worsen already poor outcomes. Early recognition is key in management of chemotherapeutic agents-induced toxicity. Although specific antidotes are available for certain agents, general supportive care remains the mainstay of the therapy.

KEY POINTS

- Early recognition is key in management of chemotherapeutic agents-induced toxicity.
- High-dose MTX may cause nephrotoxicity.
- Hydration, urine alkalization, leucovorin rescue, and high flux hemodialysis are recommended in management of MTX toxicity.
- Glucarpidase is emerging as an alternate to leucovorin therapy and hemodialysis.
- Knowledge of organ-specific chemotherapeutic drug-induced toxicity is vital in management.

- Specific antidotes are available for chemotherapeutic drug-induced toxicity though their role is limited.

REFERENCES

1. Devita VT, Hellman S, Rosenberg SA. Principles and Practice of Oncology, 6th edition. Lippincott: Williams and Wilkins; 2001. pp. 2256-315.
2. Rang HP, Dale MM, Ritter JM. Anticancer drugs. In: Rang HP, Ritter JM (Eds). Textbook of Pharmacology, 7th edition. New York: Elsevier; 2012. pp. 673-87.
3. Farber S, Diamond LK, Mercer RD, et al. Temporary remissions in acute leukemia in children produced by folic acid antagonist, 4-aminopteroyl-glutamic acid (aminopterin). N Engl J Med. 1948;238:787-93.
4. Widemann BC, Balis FM, Kempf-Bielack B, et al. High dose methotrexate-induced nephrotoxicity in patients with osteosarcoma. Cancer. 2004;100:2222-32.
5. Goldsmith P, Roach A. Methods to enhance the safety of methotrexate prescribing. J Clin Pharm Ther. 2007;32: 327-31.
6. Bhatnagar A, Verma R, Vasudevan B, et al. Acute methotrexate toxicity presenting as ulcers in plaques of psoriasis vulgaris. Indian Dermatol Online J. 2015;6: 232-3.
7. Fridlington JL, Tripple JW, Reichenberg JS, et al. Acute methotrexate toxicity seen as plaque psoriasis ulceration and necrosis: a diagnostic clue. Dermatol Online J. 2011;17:2.
8. Dervieux T, Furst D, Lein DO, et al. Polyglutamation of methotrexate with common polymorphisms in reduced folate carrier, aminoimidazole carboxamide ribonucleotide transformylase, and thymidylate synthase are associated with methotrexate effects in rheumatoid arthritis. Arthritis Rheum. 2004;50: 2766-74.
9. Treon SP, Chabner BA. Concepts in use of high-dose methotrexate therapy. Clin Chem. 1996;42:1322-9.
10. Roenigk HH, Auerbach R, Maibach H, et al. Methotrexate in psoriasis: Consensus conference. J Am Acad Dermatol. 1998;38:478-85.
11. Joerger, M, Huitema AD, van den Bongard HJ, et al. Determinants of the elimination of methotrexate and 7- hydroxy-methotrexate following high-dose infusional therapy to cancer patients. Br J Clin Pharmacol. 2006;62:71-80.
12. Bostrom BC, Erdmann GR, Kamen BA. Systemic methotrexate exposure is greater after intrathecal than after oral administration. J Pediatr Hematol Oncol. 2003;25:114-7.
13. Harned TM, Mascarenhas L. Severe methotrexate toxicity precipitated by intravenous radiographic contrast. J Pediatr Hematol Oncol. 2007;29:496-9.
14. Buchen S, Ngampolo D, Melton RG, et al. Carboxypeptidase G2 rescue in patients with methotrexate intoxication and renal failure. Br J Cancer. 2005;92: 480-7.

15. Isacoff WH, Townsend CM, Eiber FR, et al. High dose methotrexate therapy of solid tumors: observations relating to clinical toxicity. Med Pediatr Oncol. 1976;2:319-25.

16. Retenauer S, Chauveau D, Récher C. Surdsage au méthotrexate: complications, prise en charge et prevention. High-dose methotrexate: toxicity, management and prevention. Reanimation. 2009;18:654-8.

17. Bertino JR. Clinical pharmacology of methotrexate. Med Pediatr Oncol. 1982;10:401-11.

18. Agarwal V, Chauhan S, Singh R, et al. Pancytopenia with the first dose of methotrexate in a patient with psoriatic arthritis. J Indian Rheumatol Assoc. 2005;13:60-1.

19. Gutierrez-Ureña S, Molina JF, García CO, et al. Pancytopenia secondary to methotrexate therapy in rheumatoid arthritis. Arthritis Rheum. 1996;39:272-6.

20. Yang CP, Kuo MC, Guh JY, et al. Pancytopenia after low dose methotrexate therapy in a hemodialysis patient: case report and review of literature. Ren Fail. 2006;28:95-7.

21. Kuitunen T, Malmström J, Palva E, et al. Pancytopenia induced by low-dose methotrexate. A study of the cases reported to the Finnish Adverse Drug Reaction Register from 1991 to 1999. Scand J Rheumatol. 2005;34:238-41.

22. Kondo H, Date Y. Benefit of simultaneous rhG-CSF and Methylprednisolone 'pulse' therapy for methotrexate-induced bone marrow failure in rheumatoid arthritis. Int J Hematol. 1997;65:159-63.

23. Widemann BC, Adamson PC. Understanding and managing methotrexate nephrotoxicity. Oncologist. 2006;11:694-703.

24. Jacobs SA, Stoller RG, Chabner BA, et al. 7-Hydroxymethotrexate as a urinary metabolite in human subjects and rhesus monkeys receiving high dose methotrexate. J Clin Invest. 1976;57:534-8.

25. Smeland E, Fuskevåg OM, Nymann K, et al. High-dose 7-hydromethotrexate: acute toxicity and lethality in a rat model. Cancer Chemother Pharmacol. 1996;37:415-22.

26. Stark AN, Jackson G, Carey PJ, et al. Severe renal toxicity due to intermediate-dose methotrexate. Cancer Chemother Pharmacol. 1989;24:243-5.

27. Donehower RC, Hande KR, Drake JC, et al. Presence of 2,4-diamino-N10-methylpteroic acid after high-dose methotrexate. Clin Pharmacol Ther. 1979;26:63-72.

28. Widemann BC, Balis FM, Murphy RF, et al. Carboxypeptidase-G2, thymidine, and leucovorin rescue in cancer patients with methotrexate-induced renal dysfunction. J Clin Oncol. 1997;15:2125-34.

29. Erasmus JJ, McAdams HP, Rossi SE. Drug-induced lung injury. Semin Roentgenol. 2002;37:72-81.

30. Alarcon GS, Kremer JM, Macaluso M, et al. Risk factors for methotrexate-induced lung injury in patients with rheumatoid arthritis. A multicenter, case-control study. Methotrexate-Lung Study Group. Ann Intern Med. 1997;127:356-64.

31. Brugnoletti F, Morris EB, Laningham FH, et al. Recurrent intrathecal methotrexate-induced neurotoxicity in an adolescent with acute lymphoblastic leukemia: Serial clinical and radiologic findings. Pediatr Blood Cancer. 2009;52:293-5.

32. Shuper A, Stark B, Kornreich L, et al. Methotrexate treatment protocols and the central nervous system: significant cure with significant neurotoxicity. J Child Neurol. 2000;15:573-80.

33. Weiss HD, Walker MD, Wiernik PH. Neurotoxicity of commonly used antineoplastic agents (first of two parts). N Engl J Med. 1974;291:75-81.

34. Bernini JC, Fort DW, Griener JC, et al. Aminophylline for methotrexate-induced neurotoxicity. Lancet. 1995;345:544-7.

35. Winick NJ, Bowman WP, Kamen BA, et al. Unexpected acute neurologic toxicity in the treatment of children with acute lymphoblastic leukemia. J Natl Cancer Inst. 1992;84:252-6.

36. Sotoudehmanesh R, Anvari B, Akhlaghi M, et al. Methotrexate Hepatotoxicity in Patients with Rheumatoid Arthritis. Middle East J Dig Dis. 2010;2:104-9.

37. Prey S, Paul C. Effect of folic or folinic acid supplementation on methotrexate-associated safety and efficacy in inflammatory disease: a systematic review. Br J Dermatol. 2009;160:622-8.

38. Del Pozo J, Martínez W, García-Silva J, et al. Cutaneous ulceration as a sign of methotrexate toxicity. Eur J Dermatol. 2001;11:450-2.

39. Heenen M, Laporte M, Noel JC, et al. Methotrexate induces apoptotic cell death in human keratinocytes. Arch Dermatol Res. 1998;290:240-5.

40. Goerttler E, Kutzner H, Peter HH, et al. Methotrexate-induced papular eruption in patients with rheumatic diseases: a distinctive adverse cutaneous reaction produced by methotrexate in patients with collagen vascular diseases. J Am Acad Dermatol. 1999;40:702-7.

41. Fox RM. Methotrexate nephrotoxicity. Clin Exp Pharmacol Physiol. 1979;5:43-4.

42. Sauberlich HE, Baumann CA. A factor required for the growth of Leuconostoc citrovorum. J Biol Chem. 1948;176:165-73.

43. Schoenbach EB, Greenspan EM, Colsky J. Reversal of aminopterin and amethopterin toxicity by citrovorum factor. J Am Med Assoc. 1950;144:1558-60.

44. Jaffe N, Jorgensen K, Robertson R, et al. Substitution of l-leucovorin for d,l-leucovorin in the rescue from high-dose methotrexate treatment in patients with osteosarcoma. Anticancer Drugs. 1993;4:559-64.

45. Flombaum CD, Meyers, PA. High-dose leucovorin as sole therapy for methotrexate toxicity. J Clin Oncol. 1999;17:1589-94.

46. Bleyer WA. New vistas for leucovorin in cancer chemotherapy. Cancer. 1989;63:995-1007.

47. Trinkle R, Wu JK. Intrathecal leucovorin after intrathecal methotrexate overdose. J Pediatr Hematol Oncol. 1997;19:267-9.

48. Grem JL, King SA, Sorensen JM, et al. Clinical use of thymidine as a rescue agent from methotrexate toxicity. Invest New Drugs. 1991;9:281-90.

49. Graham-Cole CL, Thomas HD, Taylor GA, et al. An evaluation of thymidine phosphorylase as a means of preventing thymidine rescue from the thymidylate synthase inhibitor raltitrexed. Cancer Chemother Pharmacol. 2007;59:197-206.

50. Widemann BC, Schwartz S, Jayaprakash N, et al. Efficacy of glucarpidase (carboxypeptidase g2) in patients with acute kidney injury after high-dose methotrexate therapy. Pharmacotherapy. 2014;34:427-39.

51. Sherwood RF, Melton RG, Alwan SM, et al. Purification and properties of carboxypeptidase G2 from Pseudomonas spp. strain RS-16. Use of a novel triazine dye affinity method. Eur J Biochem. 1985;148:447-53.

52. Widemann BC, Balis FM, Shalabi A, et al. Treatment of accidental intrathecal methotrexate overdose with intrathecal carboxypeptidase G2. J Natl Cancer Inst. 2004;96:1557-9.

53. Saland JM, Leavey PJ, Bash RO, et al. Effective removal of methotrexate by high-flux hemodialysis. Pediatr Nephrol. 2002;17:825-9.

54. Wall SM, Johansen MJ, Molony DA, et al. Effective clearance of methotrexate using high-flux hemodialysis membranes. Am J Kidney Dis. 1996;28:846-54.

55. Diskin CJ, Stokes TJ, Dansby LM, et al. Removal of methotrexate by peritoneal dialysis and hemodialysis in a single patient with end-stage renal disease. Am J Med Sci. 2006;332:156-8.

56. Katchamart W, Bourré-Tessier J, Donka T, et al. Canadian recommendations for use of methotrexate in patients with rheumatoid arthritis. J Rheumatol. 2010;37:1422-30.

57. Franck H, Rau R, Herborn G. Thrombocytopenia in patients with rheumatoid arthritis on long-term treatment with low dose methotrexate. Clin Rheumatol. 1996;15:266-70.

58. Suzuki K, Doki K, Homma M, et al. Co-administration of proton pump inhibitors delays elimination of plasma methotrexate in high-dose methotrexate therapy. Br J Clin Pharmacol. 2009;67:44-9.

59. Najjar TA, Abou-Auda HS, Ghilzai NM. Influence of piperacillin on the pharmacokinetics of methotrexate and hydroxymethotrexate. Cancer Chemother Pharmacol. 1998;42:423-8.

60. Gaïes E, Trabelsi S, Sahnoun R, et al. Modification de la pharmacocinétique du méthotrexate suite à l'administration d'amphotéricine B : à propos d'un cas. J Afr Cancer. 2010;2:264-6.

61. World Health Organization. 2013. Available at: http://www.who.int/mediacentre/factsheets/fs297/en/index.html. Accessed April 15, 2013.

62. Wang RY. Antineoplastic overview. In: Nelson LS, Lewin NA, Howland MA (Eds). Goldfrank's Toxicologic Emergencies, 9th edition. New York: McGraw-Hill; 2011. pp. 770-7.

63. Hildebrand J. Neurological complications of cancer chemotherapy. Curr Opin Oncol. 2006;18:321-4.

64. Sioka C, Kyritsis AP. Central and peripheral nervous system toxicity of common chemotherapeutic agents. Cancer Chemother Pharmacol. 2009;63:761-7.

65. Lyass O, Lossos A, Hubert A, et al. Cisplatin-induced non-convulsive encephalopathy. Anticancer Drugs. 1998;9:100-4.

66. Patel PN. Methylene blue for management of ifosfamide-induced encephalopathy. Ann Pharmacother. 2006;40:299-303.

67. Ajithkumar T, Parkinson C, Shamshad F, et al. Ifosfamide encephalopathy. Clin Oncol. 2007;19:108-14.

68. Shaikh AY, Shih JA. Chemotherapy-induced cardiotoxicity. Curr Heart Fail Rep. 2012;9:117-27.

69. Outomoro D, Grana DR, Azzato F, et al. Adriamycin-induced myocardial toxicity: new solutions for an old problem? Int J Cardiol. 2007;117:6-15.

70. Senkus E, Jassem J. Cardiovascular effects of systemic cancer treatment. Cancer Treat Rev. 2011;37:300-11.

71. Jones RL, Swanton C, Ewer MS. Anthracycline cardiotoxicity. Expert Opin Drug Saf. 2006;5:791-809.

72. Swain SM, Whaley FS, Gerber MC, et al. Cardioprotection with dexrazoxane for doxorubicin-containing therapy in advanced breast cancer. J Clin Oncol. 1997;15:1318-32.

73. Marty M, Espie M, Lombart A, et al. Multicenter randomized phase III study of the cardioprotective effect of dexrazoxane (Cardioxane) in advanced/metastatic breast cancer patients treated with anthracycline-based chemotherapy. Ann Oncol. 2006;17:614-22.

74. Gemcitabine for injection. Indianapolis: Eli Lilly; 2013.

75. Mitomycin C for injection. Bedford: Ben Venue Laboratories Inc.; 2000.

76. Kwaan HC, Gordon LI. Thrombotic microangiopathy in the cancer patient. Acta Haematol. 2001;106:52-6.

77. Blake-Haskins JA, Lechleider RJ, Kreitman RJ. Thrombotic microangiopathy with targeted cancer agents. Clin Cancer Res. 2011;17:5858-66.

78. Dasatinib tablets. Princeton: Bristol-Myers Squibb Company; 2013.

79. Dale DC. Advances in the treatment of neutropenia. Curr Opin Support Palliat Care. 2009;3:207-12.

80. Fyfe AJ, McKay P. Toxicities associated with bleomycin. J R Coll Physicians (Edinb). 2010;40:213-5.

81. Mitchell EP. Gastrointestinal toxicity of chemotherapeutic agents. Semin Oncol. 2006;33:106-20.

82. Inrhaoun H, Kullman T, Elghissassi I, et al. Treatment of chemotherapy-induced nausea and vomiting. J Gastrointest Cancer. 2012;43:541-6.

83. Irinotecan injection. New York: Pfizer Inc.; 2011.

84. Fluorouracil injection. New York: Pfizer Inc.; 2012.

85. Keefe DM, Schubert MM, Elting LS, et al. Updated clinical practice guidelines for the prevention and treatment of mucositis. Cancer. 2007;109:820-31.

86. Benson AB, Ajani JA, Catalano RB, et al. Recommended guidelines for the treatment of cancer-treatment induced diarrhea. J Clin Oncol. 2004;22:2918-26.

87. Gatti A, Sabato AF. Management of opioid-induced constipation in cancer patients: focus

88. Perazella MA, Moeckel GW. Nephrotoxicity from chemotherapeutic agents: clinical manifestations, pathobiology, and prevention/therapy. Semin Nephrol. 2010;30:570–81.

89. Saif MW, McGee PJ. Hemolytic-uremic syndrome associated with gemcitabine: a case report and review of the literature. JOP. 2005;6:369-74.

90. Hensley ML, Hagerty KL, Kewalramani T, et al. American Society of Clinical Oncology 2008 Clinical practice guideline update: use of chemotherapy and radiation therapy protectants. J Clin Oncol. 2008;27: 127-45.

91. Santini V. Amifostine: chemotherapeutic and radiotherapeutic protective effects. Expert Opin Pharmacother. 2001;2:479-89.

92. Kintzel PE. Anticancer drug-induced kidney disorders. Drug Saf. 2001;24:19-38.

93. Korkmaz A, Topal T, Oter S. Pathophysiological aspects of cyclophosphamide and ifosfamide-induced hemorrhagic cystitis: implication of reactive oxygen species and nitrogen species as well as PARP activation. Cell Biol Toxicol. 2007;23:303-12.

94. Chlorambucil tablets. Research Triangle Park: Heumann Pharma GmbH for GlaxoSmithKline LLC; 2004.

95. Dactinomycin injection. Deerfield: Baxter Oncology GmbH for Lundbeck; 2012.

96. Methotrexate tablets. Fort Lee: Excella GmbH for DAVA Pharmaceuticals; 2010.

97. Rituximab injection. San Francisco: Genentech Inc.; 2010.

98. Sorafenib tablets. Wayne: Onyx Pharmaceuticals Inc. for Bayer HealthCare Pharmaceuticals Inc.; 2013.

99. Huang V, Anadkat M. Dermatologic manifestations of cytotoxic therapy. Dermatol Ther. 2011;24:401-10.

100. Wang RY. Special considerations: extravasation of xenobiotics. In: Nelson LS, Lewin NA, Howland MA (Eds). Goldfrank's Toxicologic Emergencies, 9th edition. New York: McGraw-Hill; 2011. pp. 793-5.

101. Mechlorethamine hydrochloride powder for solution. Deerfield: Baxter Oncology GmbH for Lundbeck LLC; 2012.

102. Dexrazoxane for injection. Bedford (OH): Ben Venue Laboratories for TopoTarget A/S; 2007.

CHAPTER 43

Metformin and Other Oral Hypoglycemic Agents

Prashant Singh, Omender Singh

INTRODUCTION

Several drugs, belonging to different classes, are used to treat diabetes mellitus (DM). Broadly, these drugs[1,2] can be studied under the heading of hypoglycemic agents, such as insulin and sulfonylureas and the other one being antihyperglycemic agents, such as biguanides, the alpha glucose inhibitors, and troglitazone.

Oral hypoglycemic agents (OHA), used to treat type 2 DM, are one of the most common drugs to treat diabetes.[3] Their easy accessibility, may lead to abuse, overdose or poisoning.[4] Hypoglycemia is the most frequent complication caused by accidental overdose or suicidal intake of oral hypoglycemic drugs.

The following are the commonly used OHAs used as single agent or in combinations (Table 1).[5,6]

Overdose of different OHA (Flowchart 1) can lead to hypoglycemia and other complications based on their mechanism of action and overdose. For example, metformin, a biguanide,[7] does not cause much decrease in serum glucose so it is not designated as hypoglycemic agent, rather it is labeled as antihyperglycemic agent. Overdose of antihyperglycemic agents can lead to life-threatening complications (e.g. lactic acidosis from metformin).[1] Drugs from sulfonylureas class mainly cause hypoglycemia. Poisoning with agents such as thiazolidinediones and alpha-glucosidase inhibitors, and have been reported. Newer agents like

Table 1: Classification of commonly used oral hypoglycemic agents.

1.	Sulfonylureas First generation: Tolbutamide, chlorpropamide Second generation: Glibenclamide, glipizide, gliclazide, glimepiride
2.	Biguanides: Metformin
3.	Thiazolidinediones: Rosiglitazone, pioglitazone
4.	Meglitinides: Repaglinide, nateglinide
5.	Alpha glucosidase inhibitors: acarbose, miglitol
6.	Dipeptidyl peptidase-4 (DPP-4) inhibitors: sitagliptin
7.	Glucagon-like peptide (GLP-1) analog: exenatide

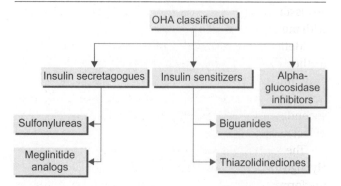

Flowchart 1: Classification of oral hypoglycemic agents (OHA).

BIGUANIDES (METFORMIN)

Biguanides were first formed in 1920s but introduced in 1950s. Out of metformin, phenformin and buformin, metformin is often used as monotherapy or in combination with other oral diabetic medications for treatment of both DM 1 and DM 2 either with insulin or sulfonylureas. Its main effect is expressed by the inhibition of hepatic gluconeogenesis.

When compared to other agents used in the treatment of type 2 DM, it decreases mortality particularly in obese patients, therefore prescribed in higher doses. It may lead to hyperlactatemia with metabolic acidosis which may be associated with high mortality rate of up to 50%. This potentially life-threatening condition not only occurs after an overdose, but may also occur at therapeutic doses especially in patients who have an underlying liver or kidney disorder.[8]

Metformin acts by different mechanisms such as decreasing lipid oxidation, free fatty acid concentration, delayed absorption of glucose, increased utilization of intestinal glucose, increased production of lactate, inhibition of hepatic gluconeogenesis, and increased uptake of peripheral insulin glucose.

Metformin is incompletely absorbed; it has 40–60% bioavailability, with 20–30% found in faeces. Absorption is slower than rate of elimination. In overdose situation absorption may be prolonged. The notable risk known with metformin overdose is that of metformin-associated lactic acidosis (MALA), which is defined as serum lactate levels above 5 mmol/L with arterial pH below 7.35 along with metformin exposure.

Metformin-associated lactic acidosis has been further classified into "incidental (or chronic) MALA" and "intentional or acute MALA". Chronic MALA may occur after prolonged metformin accumulation and is secondary to alterations in production and/or clearance of lactate.[9-11]

The incidence of MALA is still not clear.[12-16] Hypoglycemia is not supposed to be a major side effect of metformin overdose.[14,17-20] The pathophysiology of MALA in metformin poisoning is of complex nature and is still not fully comprehendible.[21,22] The accumulation of metformin, is in much higher concentrations in the intestines compared to other tissues. The production of lactate in the intestines is doubled.[21] It further increases portal lactate concentrations leading to decrease in the pH of the liver. It also impairs conversion of lactate to pyruvate via enzyme pyruvate carboxylase leading to lactate accumulation.[22] Also high concentration of metformin, causes significant drug accumulation due to renal failure, due to increase in lactate production by hepatocytes and decrease in glucose utilization.[21] Combination of these actions result in an accumulation of lactate in the blood.

Lactic acidosis is a known adverse complication of metformin overdose, with a reported mortality of up to 50%. Around 90% of the adsorbed metformin is eliminated through the kidneys within the first 24 hours in patients having normal renal functions and has no metabolites. Its side effects are varied gastrointestinal (GI) disturbances like abdominal pain, nausea, vomiting, gastritis to name a few. The clinical picture of MALA is nonspecific. However, a classical triad of acute kidney failure, along with severe lactic acidosis and increased serum metformin levels has been suggested. The diagnosis may be further complicated by the fact that metformin levels are not routinely available and acute metformin toxicity can also present without any renal dysfunction. Hence, high degree of suspicion is warranted to make timely diagnosis based on history, clinical picture, and surrogate markers like lactic acidosis.

Metformin assays are not routinely available; the clinical utility of metformin is also controversial. Toxicity from acute metformin overdose may present as abdominal pain, vomiting, and diarrhea.[19,23-25] The remaining clinical effects appear to be secondary to the resultant profound lactic acidosis. Altered mental status, including agitation, confusion, lethargy, and coma, may occur. Tachypnea, hypotension, hypothermia, ventricular dysrhythmia, decreased cardiac output, shock, and death may occur as acidosis progresses.[18,20,24,26]

Decreased peripheral circulation, hypotension, may lead to type A lactic acidosis in addition to the in addition to MALA.[24] Hypotension results from decreased systemic vascular resistance and may be resistant to standard vasopressor therapy until the acidosis is resolved.[24,27] Also, as the patient becomes hypotensive, decreased renal perfusion, increases the risk of renal failure and

Miscellaneous Toxicities

decreased metformin clearance, which prolongs the overdose.

Aggressive symptomatic management is recommended for metformin toxicity as there is no recommended antidote. Fluid resuscitation, treatment of acidemia, enhancement of lactate metabolism and removal of metformin through with dialysis form the cornerstone of therapy.

Patients who present within one hour of ingestion, after ensuring airway protection, activated charcoal should be given. Resuscitation of hypotensive patients should be done with intravenous (IV) crystalloids. Patients, who are unresponsive to aggressive fluid therapy using IV crystalloids, should be managed with vasopressor agents. In patients with persistent respiratory failure, endotracheal intubation and mechanical ventilation should be considered.[28-33]

Hypoglycemia if present should be treated with dextrose 0.5–1 g/kg. Metformin alone does not cause hypoglycemia, so other causes should be ruled out. Sodium bicarbonate can be used in severely acidemic patients that are not responsive to other supportive measures, but its use and efficacy is controversial.

Initial correction of acidosis with infusions of sodium bicarbonate should be done. A reasonable initial dose is 1–2 mEq/kg of sodium bicarbonate. The use of soda bicarbonate is still doubtful, as it may cause rebound metabolic alkalosis, leftward shift of hemoglobin dissociation curve and metabolic disturbances. Also, large infusions of sodium bicarbonate present a large sodium load which may worsen intracellular acidosis.[24,28,29] In addition, in a number of cases, sodium bicarbonate alone has not stopped the acidosis.[22,27,28]

As metformin is dialyzable, hemodialysis with a bicarbonate buffered solution is recommended in severe cases of MALA.[23-27,34-36] General indications for hemodialysis include lactate concentration more than 20 mmol/L, pH less than or equal to 7.03, shock, decreased level of consciousness and failure of other methods of supportive care. Intermittent hemodialysis (IHD) is the initial treatment option of choice. However, slow-low efficiency dialysis (SLED) or continuous renal replacement therapy (CRRT),[37] may be considered in hemodynamically unstable patients unable to withstand IHD. In addition to removal of metformin and lactates, hemodialysis may also aid in correction of acid-base disturbance, and help in maintaining fluid and electrolyte balance.

SULFONYLUREAS

First-generation sulfonylurea compounds came into existence way back in 1955. They were tolazamide, tolbutamide, and chlorpropamide (Flowchart 2). Drugs like chlorpropamide have long half-lives, 48 hours approximately. Second-generation sulfonylureas came into existence in 1984 which included drugs like glipizide, glibenclamide, glicazide, and glimepiride. They have shorter half-lives in comparison with first-generation sulfonylureas.[1,2]

Pharmacology and Toxicology

Sulfonylureas act by inhibiting adenosine triphosphate (ATP)-sensitive potassium channels in pancreatic beta cell membranes by allowing potassium efflux from the cell. Inhibition of these potassium channels causes increase in intracellular potassium levels, which result in depolarization. This causes calcium influx, which thereby activates the secretory system that releases insulin. Sulfonylureas also lead to hypoglycemia by increasing the release of endogenous insulin by promoting exocytosis of insulin.[38-40]

The toxicity of sulfonylurea agents is a direct extension of their normal pharmacology. When used inappropriately (in overdose or in patients without

Flowchart 2: Classification of sulfonylureas.

diabetes), hypoglycemia can result. Certain antibiotics and antifungals can lead to increased risk of hypoglycemia when taken with sulfonylureas.[41]

Hypoglycemia from sulfonylureas is common and can result from small doses or by delay or delay or missing a meal alcohol intake, exercising more than usual, poor oral intake, nausea or vomiting. Hypoglycemia can be continuous in nature or present with delayed onset. Prolonged observation is required particularly with long-acting drugs to maintain euglycemia.[1,7] Studies have indicated that glipizide can lead to hypoglycemia even within few minutes of intake. The complexity of symptoms may also depend upon the total time of hypoglycemia. In an individual, who is nondiabetic the signs and symptoms of hypoglycemia surface when serum glucose drops below 40 mg/dL. Signs may include the following (Table 2).[1,3]

Laboratory Studies

Different methods can be employed to investigate lab values for hypoglycemia. Tests for oral hypoglycemic overdose may include serum glucose test to detect hypoglycemia, complete blood count (CBC), baseline electrolytes especially potassium and urine toxicology screening.

Imaging Studies

Computed tomography (CT) head without, and then followed by IV contrast should be done in patients with altered mental status, focal neurological deficit or new onset of seizures.

In patients with severe electrolyte abnormalities, tests like electrocardiography (ECG) are recommended.

Table 2: Symptoms of oral hypoglycemic agents overdose.

Hyperadrenergic symptoms	*Neuroglycopenic symptoms*
• Anxiety • Nervousness • Irritability • Nausea and vomiting • Palpitations and tachycardia • Transient neurological deficit • Sweating • Pallor • Hypersalivation • Emesis • Papillary changes	• Decreased cognitive ability • Agitation and emotional liability • Sensations of warmth • Blurred vision • Slurred speech • Lethargy • Confusion • Unresponsiveness • Focal neurological deficits • Transient neurological deficits

Treatment

The main goal in OHA overdose is supportive care, which includes effective management of ABC that is primary intervention in controlling airway, breathing, and circulation followed by rapid correction of hypoglycemia. In case of overdose gastric decontamination should be done. Administration of activated charcoal is recommended at the earliest, desirably within 1 hour of ingestion.

Administration of IV glucose rapidly resolves the effects of hypoglycemia. It is safer in patients with altered sensorium due to hypoglycemia, where there is risk of aspiration involved too. The onset of IV route is quick and absolves the side effects of hypoglycemia. Its onset is quicker than compared with oral administration of sugar. Glucagon is also beneficial in the treatment and can be administered by different routes such as IV, intramuscular, or subcutaneous. Glucagon has great advantage that it can be given intramuscularly in situations where IV access cannot be obtained immediately.

Mostly all patients who present with hypoglycemia need monitoring. in case of accidental or suicidal ingestion of sulfonylurea, studies and data suggest that intensive monitoring for at least 16 hours is recommended as hypoglycemia sometimes can be delayed and prolonged and frequent glucose measurement may be required.[40]

Intravenous access should be secured. If the patient is drowsy, monitoring of cardiac parameters, and pulse oximetry are indicated. Until the patient becomes stable, oral glucose administration should be avoided.

Administration of IV glucose to patients with hypoglycemic symptoms is advocated. The requirement of IV glucose administration may persist for several hours to days depending upon the pharmacokinetics of the drug. Octreotide or diazoxide can also be administered to patients who do not respond to continuous glucose administration. Gluconeogenesis is accomplished with glucagon. Sudden low blood glucose levels require IV dextrose.

Dextrose (D-Glucose)

In emergent situations dextrose is used to immediately elevate serum glucose.[1,7,42] In patients who are drowsy and there is fear of risk of aspiration parenterally injected dextrose is helpful. The advantage of concentrated dextrose infusions is that in small volume it provides higher amounts of glucose and energy. Direct oral

Miscellaneous Toxicities

absorption results in a rapid increase in blood glucose concentrations. It is effective in small doses. Once clinical euglycemia is established based on clinical findings, and generally accompanied by a serum glucose more than or equal to 60 mg/dL (3.3 mmol/L), the patient should be given a calorie-rich meal. 50 mL of 50% dextrose in sterile water (D50W) contains only 25 g of dextrose or 100 calories, whereas food provides a calorie-rich and longer lasting source of glucose.[4,5]

Glucagon

Glucagon, is a polypeptide hormone[1,7] which is produced by pancreatic alpha cells of the islets of Langerhans. It is also extracted from beef and pork pancreas. Chemically unrelated to insulin. It is effective in small doses and with its usage no evidence of toxicity has been reported. The half-life of glucagon in plasma is around 3–6 minutes, which is similar to that of insulin. It is indicated for severe hypoglycemic reactions in patients with diabetes treated with insulin, but can be used also with oral hypoglycemic overdose. Dosage for glucagon is as follows; 0.5 mg subcutaneous/intramuscular/intravenous (SC/IM/IV); may be repeated in 15 minutes if necessary. Glucagon exerts opposite effects of insulin on blood glucose. It increases blood glucose levels by inhibiting glycogen synthesis and enhancing formation of glucose from noncarbohydrate sources, such as proteins and fats (gluconeogenesis). It also increases glycogenolysis in liver in addition to and lipolysis in adipose tissue and accelerated hepatic glycogenolysis. Parenteral administration[4,5] of glucagon produces relaxation of the smooth muscle of the stomach, duodenum and almost whole GI tract; it also increases force of contraction in the heart.

Different studies suggest that both IV dextrose and octreotide should be used for patients with a sulfonylurea overdose and hypoglycemia. IV dextrose is administered, to raise the blood glucose level acutely, thereby increasing glucose delivery to the brain. Octreotide is a somatostatin analog that inhibits insulin release from pancreatic beta-islet cells. IV dextrose, while crucial for resuscitation, should not be used as monotherapy for a sulfonylurea overdose. When given alone, IV dextrose may cause a transient hyperglycemia due to increased insulin release, causing recurrent episodes of hypoglycemia. This increase in insulin release can be minimized by octreotide.[43]

In adults, the dose of octreotide is 50–150 μg administered by IM, or SC injection 6 hourly. Octreotide may also be given as an IV bolus over several minutes or by continuous IV infusion.[41,44-48] In almost all cases, intermittent intramuscular and subcutaneous dosing is sufficient and IV infusion is unnecessary to maintain normoglycemia.

Serum glucose should be periodically monitored to identify any recurrence of hypoglycemia. The optimal interval is not known. Once the initial hypoglycemia is corrected, we suggest measuring blood glucose twice more at 30 minutes intervals. If the patient maintains euglycemia, serum glucose can be checked every 4–6 hours thereafter.

MEGLITINIDES

The meglitinides namely nateglinide and repaglinide are chemically distinct amino acid derivatives used for the treatment of type 2 DM. They increase release of insulin from the β-cells in the pancreas through closure of the ATP sensitive potassium channel in a manner similar to the sulfonylureas. They differ from the sulfonylureas in structure, binding profile, duration of action, and mode of excretion.[49-51] Of these, the most important from a toxicity perspective is the short time of action.

Overdose

Peak serum repaglinide and nateglinide concentrations occur in 30 minutes to one hour.[50] Onset of hypoglycemia after acute overdose occurs within 2 hours.[51] Both drugs are protein bound (>98%) and primarily metabolized in the liver, by cytochrome P450 isoenzyme (CYP) 3A4 and CYP2C9.[52,53] Nateglinide has a minor metabolite produced by the mixed function oxidase system. However, this metabolite does not significantly affect the prandial release of insulin. Onset and duration of clinical effects during therapeutic use are 30 minutes and less than 4 hours, respectively, for repaglinide and nateglinide. Both can be administered on a one-meal-one-tablet, no-meal-no-tablet basis.

Clinical Findings

The acute clinical effects from repaglinide and nateglinide overdose are similar to those of the sulfonylureas. There is a lowered risk of the potential prolonged hypoglycemic periods of these drugs when compared with sulfonylureas owing to their short duration of action. Initial symptoms may be varied including restlessness, sweating, drowsiness, aggressive behavior, tremors, and confusion. If the patient's blood glucose level continues to fall, these symptoms may be superseded by increase in central nervous system (CNS) depression, seizures, and coma. Onset of symptoms is expected to be rapid (under 30 minutes) and of short duration (less than 8 hours).

Treatment

The goal of management of repaglinide and nateglinide overdose is the return of euglycemia. Activated charcoal is expected to bind both repaglinide and nateglinide to prevent absorption if initiated early. It is recommended in large overdose situations especially associated with suicide attempts.

In the asymptomatic patient with acute ingestion, clinical observation and monitoring along with regular blood glucose measurement during initial 2–4 hours postingestion is advisable. If asymptomatic after 4 hours, the patient can be safely discharged. Serum concentrations of repaglinide and nateglinide are not widely available and generally not measured. In the case of unintentional ingestion in an adult or child, prompt feeding of the patient may be sufficient.[54,55]

For patients with documented hypoglycemia, infusion of 10% dextrose injection is required to achieve a blood glucose concentration of more than 80 mg/dL. Occasional supplemental bolus doses of 25% or 50% dextrose injection and oral dextrose supplementation may be needed. Because of the short time of action of nateglinide and repaglinide, it is unlikely that octreotide would be necessary to manage refractory hypoglycemia.

ALPHA-GLUCOSIDASE INHIBITORS

Acarbose and miglitol, the only α-glucosidase inhibitors that reversibly inhibit glucoamylase, sucrase, maltase, and isomaltase in the brush border of the small intestine. This causes delay in the hydrolysis of complex carbohydrates. Fermentation of the microorganism *Actinoplanes utahensis* leads to the formation of acarbose a complex pseudotetrasaccharide.[1,7,56,57] Owing to its large molecular size less than 2% of acarbose is absorbed as the parent drug.[56] Acarbose which remains unabsorbed is extensively metabolized in the gut, of which approximately half is excreted in the feces. Miglitol is absorbed in low doses, it does not bind to protein and is renally cleared without hepatic biotransformation.[57] Its half-life is approximately 0.4–1.8 hours. No reports

of overdose with α-glucosidase inhibitors could be found. However, different studies, clinical trials and pharmacokinetic data, indicate that α-glucosidase inhibitors may lead to significant injury in acute overdose conditions.[58-60] Diarrhea and abdominal discomfort have been reported as side effects with therapeutic usage and is commonly seen in the overdose situations. Acarbose does not stimulate the release of endogenous insulin, so apparently it is not expected to cause hypoglycemia in acute overdose.[58-60] Similar to other α-glucosidase inhibitors, miglitol does not have other clinically relevant extraintestinal effects only abdominal discomfort and diarrhea may occur.[60-62] The primary risk associated with acarbose appears to be hepatic injury from chronic therapy.[63-70] There does not appear to be a significant risk of hepatic injury from miglitol.[62,71] No specific therapy should be required with overdose of the α-glucosidase inhibitors.

DIPEPTIDYL PEPTIDASE-4 INHIBITORS

Sitagliptin, a new drug oral antidiabetic agent[1,7] belongs to the class of DPP-4 inhibitor (dipeptidyl peptidase-4) agents which act on the incretin axis, and is used either as, monotherapy or as combination therapy in patients intolerant to metformin. They reduce glycosylated as well as fasting and postprandial plasma glucose levels.[72-73] These drugs are essentially well-tolerated, and hypoglycemia is a rare complication of its overdose, and have affirmative acceptability for use in noninsulin-dependent diabetes mellitus (NIDDM).

A combination of sitagliptin and metformin is commonly prescribed compared to monotherapy due to these safety aspects and a better and sustained hemoglobin A1c (HbA1c) control and reduction. One case was reported with severe MALA which responded to treatment with hemodialysis and sodium bicarbonate.[74] Metformin is the second most commonly prescribed oral antidiabetic medication in both monotherapy and combination therapy.[1,7]

SERUM GLUCOSE TRANSPORTER-2 INHIBITORS

New class of drugs, serum glucose transporter 2 (SGLT2) inhibitors, as their name implies inhibits SGLT2 in the proximal nephron, it blocks glucose reabsorption in the kidney, increasing glucosuria.[75-77] Only oral medication available is empagliflozin, rest are parenteral or SC.

Miscellaneous Toxicities

Acute ingestions of SGLT2 inhibitors were well-tolerated with no hypoglycemia but only minor side effects. For patients with unintentional ingestions, a reasonable approach would include at least, mental status changes, polyuria, or tachypnea.[75-77] However, many combinations are available commercially and overdose of these drugs along with other OHAs may present with a complicated clinical picture, difficult to diagnose and manage.

CONCLUSIONS

The clinical manifestations and severity of OHA toxicity differs widely and depends on the agent involved and the dose ingested. The manifestations of metformin poisoning appear to be the most severe and life threatening and should be strongly suspected in patients presenting with high-anion gap metabolic acidosis and high blood lactate levels. In addition to early aggressive care to manage hyperlactatemia and metabolic acidosis, patients with severe toxicity may benefit with extra-corporeal toxin removal. With introduction of newer classes of OHAs, it becomes imperative for the intensivists to be aware of their toxicokinetics in order to manage their toxicities and overdoses, effectively.

KEY POINTS

- The toxicity of OHAs differs widely in clinical manifestations and severity
- Metformin-associated lactic acidosis is life-threatening and should be strongly suspected in patients presenting with high-anion gap metabolic acidosis and high blood lactate levels
- Metformin toxicity may also occur when metformin is consumed in therapeutic doses by patients with underlying liver or kidney disorder
- A combative management strategy for MALA is advocated
- The management of the OHAs like sulfonylureas and meglitinides focuses primarily on restoring and maintaining euglycemia
- In OHA-induced hypoglycemia supplemental dextrose may be sufficient therapy. However, for patients who do not respond to dextrose or who develop prolonged hypoglycemia, treatment with octreotide is recommended.

REFERENCES

1. Defronzo RA. Banting Lecture. From the triumvirate to the ominous octet: a new paradigm for the treatment of type 2 diabetes mellitus. Diabetes. 2009;58(4):773-95.
2. DeFronzo RA, Eldor R, Abdul-Ghani M. Pathophysiologic approach to therapy in patients with newly diagnosed type 2 diabetes. Diabetes Care. 2013;36 Suppl 2:S127-38.
3. Hanchard B, Boulouffe C, Vanpee D. Sulfonylurea-induced hypoglycaemia: use of octreotide. Acta Clin Belg. 2009;64(1):56-8.
4. Choudhry P, Amiel SA. Hypoglycemia: current management of controversies. Postgrad Med J. 2011;87(1026):298-306.
5. Lacherade JC, Jacqueminet S, Preiser JC. An overview of hypoglycemia in the critically ill. J Diabetes Sci Technol. 2009;3(6):1242-9.
6. Kane MP, Abu-Baker A, Busch RS. The utility of oral diabetes medications in type 2 diabetes of the young. Curr Diabetes Rev. 2005;1(1):83-92.
7. Oats JA, Wood AJ. Oral hypoglycemic agents. N Engl J Med. 1989;321(18):1231-45.
8. Blow O, Magliore L, Claridge JA, et al. The golden hour and the silver day: detection and correction of occult hypoperfusion within 24 hours improves outcome from major trauma. J Trauma. 1999;47(5):964-9.
9. Dell'Aglio D, Perino L, Kazzi Z, et al. Acute metformin overdose: examining serum pH lactate levels and metformin concentrations in survivors versus nonsurvivors: A systematic review of the literature. Ann Emerg Med. 2009;54(6):818-23.
10. Vecchio S, Protti A. Metformin-induced lactic acidosis: No one left behind. Crit Care. 2011;15(1):107-9.
11. Arroyo AM, Walroth TA, Mowry JB, et al. The MALAdy of metformin poisoning: Is CVVH the cure? Am J Ther. 2010;17(1):96-100.
12. Misbin RI, Green L, Stadel BV, et al. Lactic acidosis in patients with diabetes treated with metformin. N Engl J Med. 1998;338(4):265-6.
13. Chan NN, Brain HP, Feher MD. Metformin-associated lactic acidosis: a rare or very rare clinical entity? Diabet Med. 1999;16(4):273-81.
14. Crofford OB. Metformin. N Engl J Med. 1995;333(9):588-9.
15. Stang M, Wysowski DK, Butler-Jones D. Incidence of lactic acidosis in metformin users. Diabetes Care. 1999;22(6):925-7.
16. Stahl M, Berger W. Higher incidence of severe hypoglycaemia leading to hospital admission in type 2 diabetic patients treated with long-acting versus short acting sulphonylureas. Diabet Med. 1999;16(7):586-90.
17. Spiller HA. Management of antidiabetic medications in overdose. Drug Saf. 1998;19(5):411-24.
18. Spiller HA, Quadrani DA. Toxic effects from metformin exposure. Ann Pharmacother. 2004;38(5):776-80.

19. Spiller HA, Weber JA, Winter ML, et al. Multicenter case series of pediatric metformin ingestion. Ann Pharmacother. 2000;34(12):1385-8.

20. McLelland J. Recovery from metformin overdose. Diabet Med. 1985;2(5):410-1.

21. Misbin RI, Green L, Stadel BV, et al. Lactic acidosis in patients with diabetes treated with metformin. N Engl J Med. 1998;338(4):265-6.

22. Bailey CJ. Biguanides and NIDDM. Diabetes Care. 1992;15(6):755-72.

23. Jurovich MR, Wooldridge JD, Force RW. Metformin-associated nonketotic metabolic acidosis. Ann Pharmacother. 1997;31(1):53-5.

24. Teale KF, Devine A, Stewart H, et al. The management of metformin overdose. Anaethesia. 1998;53(7):698-701.

25. Heaney D, Majid A, Junor B. Bicarbonate haemodialysis as a treatment of metformin overdose. Nephrol Dial Transplant. 1997;12(5):1046-7.

26. Chang CT, Chen YC, Fang JT, et al. Metformin-associated lactic acidosis: case reports and literature review. J Nephrol. 2002;15(4):398-402.

27. Gjedde S, Christiansen A, Pedersen SB, et al. Survival following a metformin overdose of 63 g: a case report. Pharmacol Toxicol. 2003;93(2):98-9.

28. Ryder RE. The danger of high dose sodium bicarbonate in biguanide-induced lactic acidosis: the theory, the practice and alternate therapies. Br J Clin Pract. 1987;41(5): 730-7.

29. Lalau JD, Westeel PF, Debussche X, et al. Bicarbonate haemodialysis: an adequate treatment for lactic acidosis in diabetics treated by metformin. Intensive Care Med. 1987;13(6):383-7.

30. Chalopin JM, Tanter Y, Besancenot JF, et al. Treatment of metformin-associated lactic acidosis with closed recirculation bicarbonate-buffered hemodialysis. Arch Intern Med. 1984;144(1):203-5.

31. Lalau JD, Lacroix C, Compagnon P, et al. Role of metformin accumulation in metformin-associated lactic acidosis. Diabetes Care. 1995;18(6):779-84.

32. Teale KF, Devine A, Stewart H, et al. The management of metformin overdose. Anaesthesia. 1998;53(7):698-701.

33. Chang CT, Chen YC, Fang JT, et al. Metformin-associated lactic acidosis: case reports and literature review. J Nephrol. 2002;15(4):398-402.

34. Kruse JA. Metformin-associated lactic acidosis. J Emerg Med. 2001;20(3):267-72.

35. Lalau JD, Andrejak M, Moriniere P, et al. Hemodialysis in the treatment of lactic acidosis in diabetics treated by metformin: a study of metformin elimination. Int J Clin Pharmacol Ther Toxicol. 1989;27(6):285-8.

36. Barrueto F, Meggs WJ, Barchman MJ. Clearance of metformin by hemofiltration in overdose. J Toxicol Clin Toxicol. 2002;40(2):177-80.

37. Garg SK, Singh O, Deepak D, et al. Extracorporeal treatment with high-volume continuous venovenous hemodiafiltration and charcoal-based sorbent hemoperfusion for severe metformin-associated lactic acidosis. Indian J Crit Care Med. 2016;20(5):295-8.

38. American Diabetes Association. 8. Pharmacologic approaches to glycemic treatment. Diabetes Care. 2017;40(Suppl 1):S64-74.

39. American Diabetes Association. 6. Glycemic targets. Diabetes Care. 2017;40(Suppl 1):S48-56.

40. Gerich JE. Oral hypoglycemic agents. N Engl J Med. 1989;321(18):1231-45.

41. Spiller HA, Sawyer TS. Toxicology of oral antidiabetic medications. Am J Health Syst Pharm. 2006;63(10): 929-38.

42. Yamamoto W, Fukui T, Rahman M, et al. Estimation of the prevalence of noninsulin dependent diabetes mellitus in a rural area of Japan. J Epidemiol. 1996;6(3):114-9.

43. Garratt KN, Brady PA, Hassinger NL, et al. Sulfonylurea drugs increase early mortality in patients with diabetes mellitus after direct angioplasty for acute myocardial infarction. J Am Coll Cardiol. 1999;33(1):119-24.

44. Dougherty PP, Klein-Schwatz W. Octreotides role in management of sulfonylurea induced hypoglycemia. J Med Toxicol. 2010;6(2):199-206.

45. Eliasson L, Renström E, Ammälä C, et al. PKC-dependent stimulation of exocytosis by sulfonylureas in pancreatic beta cells. Science. 1996;271(5250):813-5.

46. McLaughlin SA, Crandall CS, McKinney PE. Octreotide: an antidote for sulfonylurea-induced hypoglycemia. Ann Emerg Med. 2000;36(2):133-8.

47. Braatvedt GD. Octreotide for the treatment of sulphonylurea induced hypoglycaemia in type 2 diabetes. N Z Med J. 1997;110(1044):189-90.

48. Carr R, Zed PJ. Octreotide for sulfonylurea-induced hypoglycemia following overdose. Ann Pharmacother. 2002;36(11):1727-32.

49. Culy CR, Jarvis B. Repaglinide: a review of its therapeutic use in type-2 diabetes mellitus. Drugs. 2001;61(11): 1625-60.

50. Keilson L, Mather S, Walter YH, et al. Synergistic effects of nateglinide and meal administration on insulin secretion in patients with type 2 diabetes mellitus. J Clin Endocrinol Metab. 2000;85(3):1081-6.

51. Moses RG, Gomis R, Frandsen KB, et al. Flexible meal-related dosing with repaglinide facilitates glycemic control in therapy-naïve type 2 diabetes. Diabetes Care. 2001;24(1):11-5.

52. Kikuchi M. Modulation of insulin secretion in non-insulin-dependent diabetes mellitus by two novel oral hypoglycaemic agents, NN623 and A4166. Diabet Med. 1996;13(9 Suppl 6):S151-5.

53. Nakayama S, Hirose T, Watada H, et al. Hypoglycemia following a nateglinide overdose in a suicide attempt. Diabetes Care. 2005;28(1):227-8.

54. Niemi M, Backman JT, Neuvonen M, et al. Rifampin decreases the plasma concentration and effects of repaglinide. Clin Pharmacol Ther. 2000;68(5): 495-500.

55. Karara AH, Dunning BE, McLeod JF. The effect of food on the oral bioavailability and the pharmacodynamic actions of the insulinotropic agent nateglinide in healthy subjects. J Clin Pharmacol. 1999;39(2):172-9.

56. Clissold SP, Edwards C. Acarbose. A preliminary review of its pharmacodynamic and pharmacokinetic properties, and therapeutic potential. Drugs. 1988;35(3):214-43.

57. Ahr HJ, Boberg M, Brendel E, et al. Pharmacokinetics of miglitol. Absorption, distribution, metabolism, and excretion following administration to rats, dogs, and man. Arzneimittelforschung. 1997;47(6):734-45.

58. Yee HS, Fong NT. A review of the safety and efficacy of acarbose in diabetes mellitus. Pharmacotherapy. 1996;16(5):792-805.

59. Hollander P, Pi-Sunyer X, Coniff RF. Acarbose in the treatment of type I diabetes. Diabetes Care. 1997;20(3):248-53.

60. Coniff R, Krol A. Acarbose: a review of US clinical experience. Clin Ther. 1997;19(1):16-26.

61. Martin AE, Montgomery PA. Acarbose: an alpha-glucosidase inhibitor. Amer J Health-Syst Pharm. 1996;53(19):2277-90.

62. Scott LJ, Spencer CM. Miglitol: a review of its therapeutic potential in type 2 diabetes mellitus. Drugs. 2000;59(3):521-49.

63. Sels JP, Nauta JJ, Menheere PP, et al. Miglitol (BAY m 1099) has no extraintestinal effects on glucose in healthy volunteers. Br J Clin Pharmacol. 1996;42:503-6.

64. Sels JP, Kingma PJ, Wolffenbuttel BH, et al. Effect of miglitol (BAY m 1099) on fasting blood glucose in type 2 diabetes mellitus. Neth J Med. 1994;44(6):198-201.

65. Andrade RJ, Lucena M, Vega JL, et al. Acarbose-associated hepatotoxicity. Diabetes Care. 1998;21(11):2029-30.

66. Andrade RJ, Lucena MI, Rodriguez-Mendizabal M. Hepatic injury caused by acarbose. Ann Intern Med. 1996;124(10):931.

67. Carrascosa M, Pascual F, Aresti S. Acarbose-induced acute severe hepatotoxicity. Lancet. 1997;349(9053):698-9.

68. Diaz-Guitierrez FL, Ladero JM, DiazRubio M. Acarbose-induced acute hepatitis. Am J Gastroenterol. 1998;93(3):481.

69. Fujimoto Y, Ohhira M, Miyokawa N, et al. Acarbose-induced hepatic injury. Lancet. 1998;351(9099):340.

70. De La Vega J, Crespo M, Escudero JM, et al. Acarbose-induced acute hepatitis. Report of two events in the same patient. Gastroenterol Hepatol. 2000;23:282-4.

71. Carlson RF. Miglitol and hepatotoxicity in type 2 diabetes mellitus. Am Fam Physician. 2000;62(2):315-8.

72. Furukawa S, Kumagi T, Miyake T, et al. Suicide attempt by an overdose of sitagliptin, an oral hypoglycemic agent. Endocr J. 2012:59(4):329-33.

73. IwamotoY, Tajiam N, Nonaka K, et al. Dose ranging efficacy of sitagliptin, a dipeptidyl peptidase inhibitor, in Japanese patients with type 2 diabetes mellitus. Endocr J. 2010;57(5):383-94.

74. Sehra S, Jaggi S, Sehra D, et al. Management of sitagliptin and metformin combination toxic overdose. J Assoc Phys India. 2016;64(11):80-1.

75. Schaeffer SE, DesLauriers C, Spiller HA, et al. Retrospective review of SGLT2 inhibitor exposures reported to 13 poison centers. Clin Toxicol. 2018;56(3):204-8.

76. Abdul-Ghani MA, DeFronzo RA. Inhibition of renal glucose reabsorption: a novel strategy for achieving glucose control in type 2 diabetes mellitus. Endocr Pract. 2008;14(6):782-90.

77. Abdul-Ghani MA, DeFronzo RA, Norton L. Novel hypothesis to explain why SGLT2 inhibitors inhibit only 30-50% of filtered glucose load in humans. Diabetes 2013;62(10):3324-8.

44 CHAPTER

Chemical and Biological Warfare

Yash Javeri, Bharat Jagiasi, Gunjan Chanchalani

INTRODUCTION

Ever since the dawn of civilization, humans have used toxins to cause assassination of armies. Initially, warfare with chemical and biological agents was considered purely an issue of nation security, but as more and more civilians were at risk, the role of medical fraternity in disaster management with use of such agents increased. Exposure to warfare agents may happen due to a military or terrorist attack, or secondary to an industrial accident. The role of emergency and prehospital care is currently well established in the management of these life-threatening emergencies, but the role of critical care is yet to be highlighted. The scientific research and evidence is also largely lacking. Recently, a series of consensus statements[1] for management of critically ill patients during disaster were published.

Management of patients of an incident involving chemical or biological weapons of destruction requires a multidisciplinary approach involving the emergency, critical care, toxicology, infectious diseases, and public health care. The role of emergency prehospital care is mainly triage of the victims and decontamination prior to safe transportation of the affected individuals. The role of critical care unit is mainly use of specific antidotes and anti-infectives with providing prolonged life-support measures, and appropriate isolation and cohorting.

Factors which affect the severity[2,3] of a biological and chemical warfare include:

- *Dispersal method*: Release of warfare agents via water or food supplies causes limited casualties as compared to the dispersal in the aerosolized form. Also for an air borne attack, "point dispersal" through a single source has a limited casualty rate, compared to "line dispersal" from a moving source.
- *Volatility*: Higher the volatility, faster the evaporation of liquid agent to the vapor form, thus faster the dispersal.
- *Persistence*: Higher the persistence of the agent, longer the agent remains in contact with the body surface thus causing more harmful effects. There is also a risk of contamination of the environment and secondary exposure to rescue medical personnel.
- *Toxicity*: The toxicity of the agents can be divided into either "lethal", causing immediate death or as "incapacitating" causing symptoms which are long lasting.
- *Latency*: The time delay between exposure to an agent and onset of clinical symptoms is called latency. Use of agents with longer latency may require more medical monitoring of exposed victims, and also may have difficulty in identifying the source of the agent.

CHEMICAL WARFARE

Chemical warfare agents include chemicals which are man-made to either kill or incapacitate the victim. They are mainly volatile agents and can also be absorbed through intact skin, to produce immediate effects.

History[4,5]

The use of poisoned arrows to hunt animals has been known since the prehistoric times. The preindustrial era, saw the use of artillery shells filled with cacodyl cyanide during the Crimean War. In the industrial era, with rapidly advancing technological development, the large-scale use of chemical ammunition was witnessed during the First World War—the German chlorine attack in 1915. Thereafter, more and more lethal chemical nerve agents were developed, during the Second World War, but fortunately never deployed. Later in the 1980s, the chemical warfare agents were used during the Iran-Iraq war, victimizing more than 1 lakh people.

The Regulatory Laws[5,6]

The law against the use of poisonous gas has been documented as early as 1899 in the Hague declaration. The Geneva protocol of 1925, and later the International Humanitarian Law, further continued the ban and prohibition of use of poisonous gas. In 1997, the Convention on the Prohibition of the Development, Production, Stockpiling and Use of Chemical Weapons and their Destruction (Chemical Weapons Convention, CWC) came into force. The convention has been signed by 192 states till January 2018. The Organisation for the Prohibition of Chemical Warfare, the implementing body of the convention, has declared that approximately 72,000 tons of chemical warfare agents have been destroyed. There still remain four states (Democratic People's Republic of Korea, Egypt, Israel, South Sudan) which have not yet signed the CWC.

Chemical Warfare Agents[2,7]

Novichok Agents[8]/"Newcomer" Class of Nerve Agents (Substance-33, A-230, A-232, A-234, Novichok-5, Novichok-7)

These are available in liquid form or as a dusty formulation. The three main advantages of Novichok agent as a military agent are it does not violate the Chemical Weapons Treaty based on the individual agent's chemical subgroup; it has a long shelf life; and it is highly potent. It produces the cholinergic or muscarinic toxidrome, by binding acetylcholinesterase. This may progress to prolonged neuroparalysis, causing respiratory failure. It also causes peripheral neuropathy by binding to the peripheral sensory nerves. Treatment involves mainly immediate decontamination use of intravenous (IV) atropine and pralidoxime or obidoxime as antidotes. Diazepam is used to control seizures. Use of IV lipid emulsion as an adjunctive therapy should be considered in the critically ill patients. Reactive oxime like potassium 2,3-butanedione monoximate as an antidote is used in Europe.

Nerve Agents (Sarin, Tabun, Soman, VX)

They are irreversible inhibitors of cholinesterase enzymes, usually used as vapor. They can cause toxicity by inhalation, absorption through skin and mucous membrane, or by ingestion. After exposure, the symptoms are triphasic—initial phase being a cholinergic crisis lasting 24–48 hours, followed by respiratory failure as in intermediate syndrome lasting 4–18 days, followed by a delayed polyneuropathy. Atropine and oximes can be used as antidotes during the first phase. Other adjunctive therapeutic agents are nebulized ipratropium bromide for bronchospasm and diazepam for seizures. Pyridostigmine[9] has been used for pre-exposure prophylaxis, by the military in case of anticipation of chemical warfare with a nerve agent.

Blistering Agents/Vesicants (Arsenicals and Mustards)

Mustard gas has a garlic or mustard odor. They cause chemical burns and lead to erythema, edema, and blistering of the epithelium. If ingested or inhaled, may have systemic symptoms like respiratory failure, blindness, vomiting, pancytopenia, and cancer. Mustard gas has a period of latency of 4–12 hours following exposure. Treatment of exposure to blistering agents involves following the burns protocol with hydration and prevention of secondary infection.

Choking Agents (Chlorine, Phosgene, and Chloropicrin)

These are highly volatile, causing respiratory distress on inhalation which is followed by a variable latency, and ultimately leading to inflammation of the distal

Chemical and Biological Warfare

respiratory tract, causing severe pulmonary edema, respiratory failure, and permanent lung damage. Chlorine has a distinctive odor. Treatment is mainly supportive, with use of high-dose steroids via IV or inhalation route. Oral zafirlukast and glutathione have been used after phosgene poisoning.

Blood Agents (Hydrocyanic Acid and Cyanogen Chloride)

They are lethal agents, usually deployed in a vapor form. Antidote is sodium thiosulfate with sodium nitrite and hydroxocobalamin.

Incapacitating and Harassing Agents [Vomiting Agents (Adamsite, Diphenylchloroarsine), Tear Gases (2-Chlorobenzalmalononitrile), Capsaicin Spray, Psychoactive Drugs (Lysergic Acid Diethylamide—LSD, Cannabinoids)]

These agents are used as sensory irritants and to temporarily incapacitate the victims, and usually do not require intensive care unit (ICU) treatment.

Pre-exposure Prophylaxis for Chemical Warfare

Serpacwa[9] (skin exposure reduction paste against chemical warfare agents) is a 50:50 mixture of perfluoroakylpolyether and polytetrafluoroethylene, used as a topical agent by the military to protect against chemical warfare. In animal studies, it has shown to be protective against sulfur mustard, VX, soman, T-2 mycotoxins, and CS. There is no systemic absorption or side-effects of the agent, but some may develop flu-like symptoms. Its duration of action is up to 6 hours.

Medical Management against Chemical Weapons

Quick Toxidrome Recognition[10]

Multiple victims at the scene with no signs of trauma, and clusters of them collapsing with similar complaints, should raise the suspicion of a chemical warfare attack and the scene should be analyzed to identify chemical agent. It is important to identify the chemical agent early,

as administration of the specific antidote significantly improves survival. Toxidrome recognition of specific patterns of signs and symptoms of the classes of chemical agents is the primary step of determining treatment protocol. Toxidromes matching most rapidly lethal agents, like nerve agents, cyanide should be considered first (Table 1). Thereafter, identifying toxidromes resembling agents which require decontamination, close monitoring, and supportive care should be done (e.g. pulmonary agents, vesicant, caustic, and riot-control agents, anesthetic agents, anticholinergic agents).

Decontamination

Decontamination is needed when the victim has been exposed to the liquid form of the agent. The scene should be divided into three zones:[10] hot zone, the contaminated area; cold zone, the uncontaminated area; and the warm zone, the area between the hot and cold zone where decontamination can be done. Ideally, decontamination should be rapid and should be done at the scene of exposure, before transportation. Decontamination can be done by showering, and by use of soap or hypochlorite solution. Use of dry bleach should be avoided[11] in decontamination of nerve agents, as their hydrolysis may produce toxic metabolites. For example, Novichok agents on hydrolysis with dry bleach produce hydrofluoric acid, hydrochloric acid, hydrogen cyanide, and oxime, which can produce cholinergic effects in the exposed individuals. Mustard gas has a prolonged persistence

Table 1: Initial toxidrome recognition.[10]

	Initial toxidrome	Agent class	Initial treatment
Urgently Identify Agent	Increased secretions or muscle effects (fasciculations, weekness, paralysis), with or without miosis	Nerve agent	Administer atropine and pralidoxime, provide urgent care and spot decontamination at the site
	Bradypnea or apnea, gasping, collapse, and seizures with or without cynaosis	Asphyxiant	Administer cyanide antidote, provide urgent care and spot decontamination at the site
	Bradypnea or apnea, sedation, miosis	Opioid agent	Administer naloxone, provide urgent care and spot decontamination at the site

Miscellaneous Toxicities

and hence decontamination of the victims is essential. Although decontamination is must to minimize exposure to the health care personnel, lifesaving treatment should not be delayed.

Treatment

Rapid identification of the causative agent will help in providing early specific treatment, and use of an antidote. Till definitive diagnosis is done, treatment is largely supportive. Specialized analytical laboratories play a major role in identification of the agent, by analyzing the victim's body fluids, as well as samples of air, water, and soil.

Protection

Emergency medical personnel involved in evacuation of the victims from the scene should use air purifying respirators, splash suits, and chemical resistant gloves. All medical personnel involved in the care of the patient should use protective clothing and face masks, and barrier precautions. Correct disposal of body fluids and clinical waste should be done to decrease secondary exposure rates.

Prevention

Prevention of further exposure into the community is mainly via public health interventions, to create widespread awareness of the warning signs and measures to protect themselves. Steps to expedite evacuation from the scene, sheltering, and distribution of gas masks, help reduce exposure of more individuals.

BIOLOGICAL WARFARE

Biological warfare can be caused by agents like bacteria, fungi, viruses, and toxins, which are added in water, air, or food (with an intent to cause disease and death). Fungi, though have the potential to be used as bioweapons, they have not been used till date. Some authors classify toxins as agents of chemical warfare, as they are nonliving. Bioterrorism can be achieved by aerosol spraying, or by ingestion through food and water, or by absorption or injection into the skin.

The key difference between chemical warfare and biological warfare is the longer incubation period with the use of weapons of biological warfare, compared to weapons of chemical warfare. Also, there is a possibility of secondary casualties with the use of bioweapons, as some agents may reproduce in the initial host.

The main points favoring occurrence of a bioterrorism,[12] versus the occurrence of a natural outbreak are:
- More clustering of cases, with similar incubation periods causing "explosion" of the disease in that community
- Nonseasonal, nonendemic occurrence
- Localization in a geographical location
- More respiratory symptoms as aerosol route is the mode of transmission.

History

The history of using biological weapons for warfare, dates back to the 14th century BC,[13] rams infected with tularemia were send to the enemies. In the premicrobiology era, biological warfare involved crude use of human cadavers, animal carcasses, and filth to contaminate air, food chains, or water resources.

With the concepts of microbiology explained by Louis Pasteur and Robert Kochs, it became easier to develop biological weapons for mass destruction. In the postmicrobiology era, the use of biowarfare to threaten humans was used during the First World War, when animal feed was infected with *Bacillus anthracis* or *Burkholderia mallei*. During the Second World War, Japan used biological weapons, against China. Thereafter, research involving aggressive development of bioweapons continued, and many allegations of biowarfare attack were made. The Soviet Union established a vast secret biowarfare project Biopreparat to promote biowarfare research and production. The recent attacks by bioweapons have been with the use of *Salmonella typhimurium* contaminated salad bars in Dalles in 1984, and use of anthrax letters in New York in 2001.

The Regulatory Laws[14]

After the development of bioweapons secretly during the First World War, it became an international political concern. Thus, in 1925 the Geneva protocol was signed which disallowed the use of chemical and biological weapons in war, but the research and production continued. Aggressive development of biological weapons continued, until World Health Organization (WHO) pressurized to abandon the offensive research and thus the Biological and Toxin Weapons Convention (BTWC) was signed by all governments in 1972. This law prohibited the research, development, production, stockpiling, and use of weapons of biological destruction.

Bioterrorism—Modern Concerns

Biological warfare agents are deadly as well as cheap and are thus considered as the poor man's nuclear bomb. With the development and easy availability of gene-editing technology, bioterrorism has the potential to turn more evil and disastrous.

Biological Warfare Agents[2]

The Centers for Disease Control and Prevention[15] (CDC) has classified biological warfare agents into three different categories according to their infectiousness, virulence, public perception, impact, and cost and sophistication of countermeasures (Table 2).[15]

Bacteria

Bacteria have been used as biowarfare agents as they can be easily cultured and have high secondary infectivity as well as rapid fatality.

Bacillus anthracis causes anthrax via the cutaneous route, via inhalation of the spores, and via ingestion of infected meat. Acquisition of inhalational anthrax (woolsorter disease) is highly lethal, causing initial prodromal respiratory symptoms, which rapidly progresses to necrotizing hemorrhagic mediastinitis, leading to multiorgan failure and rapid fatality. Ciprofloxacin is used for treatment and also as chemoprophylaxis.

Warfare use *Yersinia pestis* causes mainly pneumonic plague, with almost 100% fatality. Treatment of choice is streptomycin. Alternative drugs are gentamicin, doxycycline, and chloramphenicol.

Tularemia caused by *Francisella tularensis,* is mainly fatal, if acquired via aerosolized route. Treatment is with streptomycin or gentamicin. A live-attenuated vaccine is available.

Viruses

Viruses are highly infectious, as well as stable when weaponized, usually deployed through the aerosolized route.

Viral hemorrhagic fever can cause a range of symptoms, which can be rapidly fatal. Treatment is only supportive, and isolation and contact precautions are needed to prevent further spread.

Table 2: The Centers for Disease Control and Prevention (CDC) classification of agents of biological warfare.[15]

Category	Bacteria	Viruses	Toxins	Parasites
A	<ul><li>*Bacillus anthracis* (anthrax)</li><li>*Yersinia pestis* (plague)</li><li>*Francisella tularensis* (tularemia)</li><li>*Brucella* species (brucellosis)</li><li>Food safety threats (e.g. Salmonella species, *Escherichia coli* O157:H7, Shigella, *Staphylococcus aureus*)</li></ul>	<ul><li>Variola virus (smallpox)</li><li>Hemorrhagic fever viruses (Ebola, Marburg, Lassa and Machupo viruses)</li></ul>	<ul><li>*Clostridium botulinum* toxin</li></ul>	
B	<ul><li>Glanders (*Burkholderia mallei*)</li><li>Melioidosis (*Burkholderia pseudomallei*)</li><li>Psittacosis (*Chlamydia psittaci*)</li><li>Q-fever (*Coxiella burnetii*)</li><li>Typhus (*Rickettsia prowazekii*)</li><li>Cholera (*Vibrio cholerae*)</li></ul>	<ul><li>Viral encephalitis (alphaviruses, e.g. Venezuelan, eastern, or western equine encephalitis)</li></ul>	<ul><li>Epsilon toxin of *Clostridium perfringens*</li><li>Ricin toxin of *Ricinus communis*</li><li>Abrin toxin of *Abrus precatorius*</li><li>Staphylococcal enterotoxin B</li></ul>	<ul><li>*Cryptosporidium parvum*</li></ul>
C	<ul><li>Multidrug-resistant *Mycobacterium tuberculosis*</li></ul>	<ul><li>Nipah virus</li><li>Hantavirus</li><li>SARS</li><li>H1N1</li><li>HIV/AIDS</li><li>Encephalomyelitis viruses</li><li>(Tick borne encephalitis, others)</li></ul>	–	–

Miscellaneous Toxicities

Viruses causing viral encephalitis are highly infectious, causing a high fatality. Treatment is largely supportive.

Variola virus causing small pox has a high fatality rate of up to 70%. The population exposed is also highly susceptible as the herd immunity has dropped after the cessation of vaccination. Cidofovir has shown in vitro activity against the virus.

Toxins (Botulinum Toxin, Ricin Toxin)

Botulinum toxin is produced by *Clostridium botulinum*, and acts a neurotoxin, by permanently inhibiting the synthesis of acetylcholine. There are seven serotypes (A to G), of which type A is most potent and is usually deployed through the aerosol route and sometimes through the food. It causes neuromuscular blockade, which initially affects the ocular and bulbar muscles and further progresses over 1–4 days to involve the respiratory muscles. Decontamination to prevent exposure to health care workers and early ventilator support is usually needed. A trivalent antitoxin against serotypes A, B, and E may be effective, if used early after oral ingestion.

Ricin toxin is derived from castor seeds *Ricinus communis*. It acts by interrupting protein synthesis. Inhalation of toxin in high doses can be rapidly fatal, whereas low doses mainly cause neurological symptoms like confusion, seizures, and coma. Ingestion of the toxin causes abdominal pain and diarrhea. Treatment is mainly supportive.

Medical Management against Biological Weapons

Early Recognition

Recognition of a disease due to a biological warfare agent can be difficult due to a prolonged incubation period. An occurrence of an outbreak of an unusual disease can help the clinician suspect a biological disaster. The usual clinical presentation is of initial nonspecific symptoms, which progresses rapidly to shock. The suspicion of a biological threat is usually low in the early phase, as the presentation is similar to that of a case of septic shock. However, when more and more individuals, without major risk factors present in a similar way, a high suspicion should be raised.

Microbiological help may be limited, as most of the agents need special medium for culture (e.g. tularemia), and may at times be considered as a contaminant (e.g. *Bacillus*).

Decontamination

Usually limited role, as bioweapons are mostly used as aerosols. However, removal of clothing and cleaning with antiseptic soap and water helps reduce the skin organisms by 99.99%. If there is suspicion of use of bioweapon via skin route, then a sporicidal agent (like 0.5% sodium hypochlorite) should be used to disinfect the skin followed by irrigation with water.

Treatment[16]

Treatment is directed at the suspected disease. Consensus recommendation[17] for the treatment of anthrax, include high-dose penicillins, tetracycline, chloramphenicol, and erythromycin. Antitoxins, raxibacumab, and anthrax immune globulin may also be used. For plague, gentamicin, cefotaxime, and levofloxacin can be used. Streptomycin is the drug of choice for tularemia. Botulism immune globulin should be used on exposure to *C. botulinum*, to attenuate the symptoms. Only supportive treatment is helpful in the treatment of smallpox, as antivirals are still in development. Treatment of viral hemorrhagic fever also remains supportive, with volume correction and replacement of blood and blood products. Ribavirin has shown to be effective against Lassa fever and viruses of Hantavirus genus.

Protection

Protection of the health care workers and for the masses at risk may be considered with the use of chemoprophylaxis and vaccination. Chemoprophylaxis with doxycycline or a fluoroquinolone should be done for plague. Immediate vaccination for small pox should be done for all personnel taking care of the victims. Anthrax usually does not require any prophylaxis as it lacks person-to-person transmission. Botulinum toxoid is used for pre-exposure prophylaxis against botulism. For viral biowarfare attacks, no effective prophylaxis exists.

Prevention

Most of the disease of biowarfare have limited (e.g. viral hemorrhagic fevers) to no (e.g. anthrax) person-to-person transmission. To prevent the spread of the organisms, use of universal precautions, barrier isolation with high-efficiency particulate air (HEPA) air filtration, and use of masks is adequate. However, disease like smallpox has a high second infection rate and in such cases, cohorting and quarantine of patients should be done early. Suspected cases of pneumonic plague require strict isolation for the initial 4 days of antibiotics.

CONCLUSION

Chemical and biological warfare may put an unexpected, overwhelming burden on the intensive care. There may be need of unusual medications, antidotes, and vaccines, along with protection of the health care workers. Being aware of the possible signs and symptoms, along with adequate preparedness, will help overcome the disaster.

KEY POINTS

- Disaster planning and management of chemical and biological warfare attack requires a multidisciplinary approach
- Immediate availability of personal protective equipment for health care professionals and decontamination of the victims at the scene site are important steps in management of exposure to chemical warfare agent
- Early identification of the agent and use of specific antidote against the chemical warfare agent significantly improves survival
- Unusual infectious disease presentation in a large number of previously healthy individuals should raise a suspicion of a biological warfare
- Treatment and isolation or quarantine to prevent further spread is important
- Chemoprophylaxis and vaccination should be considered in health care workers and individuals both pre- and postexposure
- A rapid response and adequate preparedness by the medical community, public health, and the government is essential to combat the chemical and biological warfare attacks.

REFERENCES

1. Mangerich A, Esser C. Care of the critically Ill and injured during pandemics and disasters: CHEST consensus statement – introduction and executive summary. 2014;146(4 Suppl):8S-34S.
2. White SM. Chemicals and biological weapons: implications for anesthesia and intensive care. Br J Anesth. 2002;89:306-24.
3. Moles M. Mass casualties, traumatic and toxic injury and advanced life support. J Int Trauma Anesth Crit Care Soc. 1996;6:12-7.
4. Pitschmann V. Overall view of chemical and biochemical weapons. Toxins. 2014;6:1761-84.
5. Mangerich A, Esser C. Chemical warfare in the First World War: reactions 100 years later. Arch Toxicol. 2014;88: 1909-11.
6. Timperley CM, Forman JE, Abdollahi M, et al. Advice on chemical weapons sample stability and storage provided by the Scientific Advisory Board of the Organisation for the Prohibition of Chemical Weapons to increase investigative capabilities worldwide. Talanta. 2018;188:808-32.
7. Rogers GC, Condurache CT. Antidotes and treatments for chemical warfare/terrorism agents: an evidence-based review. Clin Pharmacol Ther. 2010;88(3):318-27.
8. Chai PR, Hayes BD, Erickson TB, et al. Novichok agents: a historical, current, and toxicological perspective. Toxicology Communications. 2018;2(1):45-8.
9. Leikin JB, Thomas RG, Walter FG, et al. A review of nerve agent exposure for the critical care physician. Crit Care Med. 2002;30:2346-54.
10. Ciottone GR. Toxidrome recognition in chemical weapons attacks. N Engl J Med. 2018;378:1611-20.
11. Ellison DH. Handbook of Chemical and Biological Warfare Agents, 2nd edition. Boca Raton, FL: Taylor and Francis Group; 2008.
12. Noah DL, Sobel AL, Ostroff SM, et al. Biological warfare training: Infectious disease outbreak differentiation criteria. Military Medicine. 1998;163(4):198-201.
13. Barras V, Greub G. History of biological warfare and bioterrorism. Clin Microbiol Infect. 2014;20:497-502.
14. Wheelis M, Dando M (Eds). Deadly Cultures: Biological Weapons Since 1945. Cambridge, MA: Harvard University Press; 2006.
15. Bossi P, Garin D, Guihot A et al. Bioterrorism: management of major biological agents. Cell Mol Life Sci. 2006;63: 2196-212.
16. Adalja AA, Toner E, Inglesby TV. Clinical management of potential bioterrorism-related conditions. N Engl J Med. 2015;372:954-62.
17. Stevens DL, Bisno AL, Chambers HF, et al. Practice guidelines for the diagnosis and management of skin and soft tissue infections: 2014 update by the Infectious Diseases Society of America. Clin Infect Dis. 2014;59 (2):147-59.

Index

Page numbers followed by *b* refer to box, *f* refer to figure, *fc* refer to flowchart, and *t* refer to table

A

Abrus precatorius 357, 358
Accidental poisoning 70
Acetaminophen 20, 23, 203, 208, 274
    concentration, serum 205
    metabolism of 204*fc*
    normal metabolism of 204*fc*
    poisoning 32*b*, 203
    toxicity, management of 275*t*
Acetazolamide 28, 215
Acetylcholine 110
Acetylcholinesterase 23
Acetylcysteine 16, 32, 33
Acetylene 152
Acid 4, 8, 218
    absorbable 28
    addition of 26
    adenosine diphosphate 342
    base
        abnormalities 211
        analysis 30
        disorders 26, 212, 370
        disturbances 26
        status 26
    ibotenic 368, 370
    injury 219
Acidosis 28, 124, 340
    acute respiratory 29
    dilutional 28
    intracellular 29
    lactic 27, 387
    respiratory 29
Acrylonitrile 152
Actinoplanes utahensis 391
Activated charcoal 7, 8*b*, 16, 36, 135, 232
    multiple dose 8, 36, 188, 196, 211, 232, 264, 276
Activated partial thromboplastin time 48, 49, 237
Acute respiratory distress syndrome 220, 251, 309
Adamsite 397
Adenosine
    antagonism 110
    monophosphate, cyclic 180
    triphosphate 243, 342, 388
        cardiac 61
Adnexa 219
Adult respiratory distress syndrome 115
Advanced cardiac life support 3, 16, 168, 251
Agitation 186

Agriculture fertilizers and industrial refrigerant 223
Air filtration 401
Airway 3, 61, 148, 214, 296
    management 86
    protection 220
Alanine aminotransferase 370
Albumin dialysis 9, 10
Albuminuria 163
Alcohol 4, 8, 93, 136
    dehydrogenase
        inhibitor 27
        hepatic 278
    intoxication, acute 229
    like ethanol 5
    use disorder 118
Aldehyde dehydrogenase 119
Aldicarb 304
Aldrin 321, 324
Alkalemia 215
Alkali 219
    ingestion 4
    injury 223
Alkalinization 214, 300
    therapy 215
Alkalosis
    acute respiratory 29
    metabolic 29
    prevents drug 52
    respiratory 29
Alkylating agents 378, 380
Allergic reactions 32, 62
Allergies 211
Allobarbital 275
Alpha-glucosidase inhibitors 386, 391
Alprazolam 81
Aluminum 174
    phosphide 5, 19, 27, 174, 330
        poisoning 174, 176
    toxicity 47, 50
Alveolitis, acute 315
Amanita 367, 368, 370, 371
    pantherina 368
    phalloides 52, 268, 358, 367
    poisoning 369
        stages of 369*t*
Amatoxin 367
    poisoning 371
American Academy of Clinical Toxicology 7, 36, 65
American College of Chest Physicians 47
American College of Medical Toxicology 61

Amino acids, excitatory 110
Aminocarb 304
Aminopyridine 110
Amiodarone 4, 10, 167, 227
Amitriptyline 6, 8, 186
Ammonia 151, 154
    anhydrous 223
Amoxapine 186
Amphetamine 5, 14, 20, 28, 81, 85, 257
Analgesics 248
Anaphylaxis 207
    management of 381
Anemia 50
    hemolytic 342
    severe 238
Angiotensin converting enzyme 146
Anion gap 12, 13, 27, 124
    metabolic acidosis, causes of 13*t*
Anorexia 344
Anthracyclines 382
Anthrax 400
    immune globulin 400
Antiarrhythmics 185
    beta-blockers 4
    treatment 188
Antibiotic 24, 380
Antibody fragments, digoxin-specific 40
Anticancer drug 24
Anticholinergic 5
    effects 186
    symptoms 371
Anticoagulants 4, 5, 148, 330, 331
    rodenticide 228, 330, 332
    rodenticide poisoning 46
Anticonvulsants 5, 133
    overdose 133
        management of 141
Antidepressants 5
    cyclic 5
Antidigoxin fab 197
Antidotal therapy 90, 298
Antidotes 3, 15, 15*t*, 31, 72, 74*t*, 206, 274, 306, 378
    for specific
        drug 148*t*
        poison 148*t*
    mechanism of action of 31*t*
    second-line 307
    universal 36
Antiepileptic drugs 24, 133
    classification of 133*t*
    intravenous 109
    overdose, management of 134

Index

Antifungal drugs 24
Antihistamines 5, 185, 190
Antihyperglycemic agents 386
Anti-infective agents 248
Antimetabolites 231, 378, 380
Antimicrobials drugs 231
Antimitotic agents 380
Antimycobacterial drugs 248
Antioxidants 317
Antiplatelets 148
Antipsychotics 185, 257
Antisnake venom 56, 57b, 148, 349
   indications of 56b
   treatment 351
Antitoxins 400
Antivenom 352
   indications of 351b
Apamin 110
Apixaban 238, 239
Apoptosis 313
Areca catechu 363, 363f
Argatroban 236
Argon 152
Argyreia nervosa 104
Arrhythmias 33, 178, 188, 279
   beta-blockers 326
   cardiac 15, 326
   management of 96
   ventricular 52
Arsenic 5, 112, 258, 260, 330, 331, 342
   poisoning 39b
Arterial blood gas 14, 112, 130, 175, 246, 249, 370
   analysis 187
Artery catheter, pulmonary 180
Ascites 222
Asphyxiants, simple 152t, 154
Aspiration 297
   pneumonia 4
Aspirin 27, 212, 280
Asthma 4, 46
Ataxia 50
Atomic absorption spectrophotometer 21
Atrial fibrillation 94, 194
   chronic non-valvular 236
Atrial tachycardia, paroxysmal 94
Atropine 16, 33, 33b, 112, 160, 196, 298, 306
   indications of 33t
Atropinization, signs of 307
Attention deficit hyperactivity disorder 186
Autonomic nervous system 129
Azadirachta indica 363, 363f

B

Bacillus 400
   anthracis 398, 399
Bacteria 399
Barbiturate 4, 14, 20, 77, 114, 134, 136, 138, 259, 262, 266, 274, 275
   toxicity, management of 276t
Barium 9, 110, 330, 331
   bromethalin 334
   carbonate 330

Bee venom 110
Beers drinker's cardiomyopathy 339
Bendiocarb 304, 305
Bentonite 36
Benzene hexachloride 324
Benzodiazepines 4, 20, 77, 78, 93, 96, 114, 134, 138, 148, 211, 257, 371
   ingestion 258
   poisoning 41
Benzyl alcohol 47
Benzylpenicillin, intravenous 371
Benzylpiperazines 102
Beta-adrenergic blocking agents 291
Beta-blocker 34, 110, 178, 179, 257
   poisoning 37
   role of 96
   toxicity 179t
Beta-chain variant 247
Betamethasone 22
Bicarbonate 12
   administration of 29
   K 27
   level 14
   wasting of 26
Biguanides 387
Bilirubin 204
Biochemistry 179, 330
Biogenic amines 110
Biological warfare 398
   agents 399
   classification of agents of 399t
Bipyridyl agent 312
Bishydroxycoumarin 227
Bivalirudin 236
Biventricular devices 171
Bleeding 237, 258
   intracranial 237, 238
Bleomycin 375
Blood 71
   agents 397
   brain barrier 304
   carboxyhemoglobin levels 163t
   cyanide levels 251t
   flow, mechanical assistance of 288
   glucose 14
   lead levels 24, 38, 343
   methemoglobin levels 23
   pressure, systolic 15, 298
   stream infections, catheter-associated 298
   transfusion, role of 332
   urea 179
      nitrogen 14, 27, 120
Blurred vision 186
Body packer syndrome 94
Boric acid 10
Botulinum
   antitoxin-heptavalent 34
   immunoglobulin 35
      dose of 35b
   toxin 4, 400
Botulism 34, 128
   differential diagnosis of 130t
   signs of 129t
   symptoms of 129t

Bowel obstruction 8
Bowel perforations 8
Bradyarrhythmia 40, 169
   management of 196
Bradycardia 5, 5t, 167b, 250, 279, 305
   symptomatic 40
Brain
   ischemia, mechanism of 243
   syndrome, acute 91
Breathing 4, 61, 148, 214, 296, 297
British anti-lewisite 39, 112
   dosing regimens of 39b
Brodifacoum 227, 332
Bromadiolone 227
Bromethalin 331
Bromides 9
Bromine 151, 266
Bromocriptine 35
Bronchiolitis obliterans organizing pneumonia 340, 375, 380
Bronchorrhea 33, 297, 305
Bronchospasm 4, 33
Brugada pattern 187
Bupivacaine 185
Bupropion 27
Burkholderia mallei 398
Butane 152
Butyrylcholinesterase 23

C

Cadmium 258, 260, 341, 345
   poisoning 38
   treatment 345
Calcium 37, 174, 179, 182
   channel blocker 4, 5, 10, 37, 64, 73, 167, 178, 179, 179t, 265, 299
      overdose 178
      poisoning 34, 37
   chloride 16, 37, 180
   disodium 37
   gluconate 16, 37, 180
   intravenous 180
   oxalate crystals 122f
Camphechlor 322
Camphor 27, 266
Cannabinoids 78, 93
   synthetic 100, 101
   toxicity 80
Cannabis indica 77
Capillary blood glucose 179
Capsaicin spray 397
Carbamates 5, 8, 167, 303
   and newer insecticides 303
   compounds 304t
   poisoning 33, 48
      characteristics of 304t
   toxicity, diagnosis of 305
Carbamazepine 8, 10, 20, 24, 133, 134, 185, 266, 274, 276, 277
   toxicity, management of 276t

Index 405

Carbaryl 303-305
Carbofuran 304, 305
Carbon dioxide 4, 70, 152, 156, 246
  partial pressure of 147
Carbon monoxide 4, 5, 28, 112, 148, 152, 162,
    164, 242-245, 257
  poisoning 4, 43, 162, 242, 244-246, 290
Carbonate 27
Carbonic anhydrase 250
  inhibitor 28, 215
Carboxyhemoglobin 21, 43, 147, 162, 242, 245,
    246f
Carboxyhemoglobinemia 242
Carboxymethyl cellulose 36
Carcinoid 54
Cardiac arrest 189, 250
Cardiac glycosides 194, 198
  poisoning 34
Cardiotoxic plants 357
Cardiovascular abnormalities 351
Cardiovascular effects 187, 245
Cardiovascular system 186, 211, 219
Cardiovascular toxicity 95, 378, 379t
  management 378
Castor seeds 359f
Cathartics 7
Cathinones 28
  synthetic 100
Cavity, abdominal 222
Cellular hyoxia 4
Central nervous system 11, 19, 63, 73, 77, 82,
    85, 86, 93, 94, 100, 110, 119, 124, 133,
    186, 219, 232, 248, 270, 304, 391
  complications 189
  depressant 77, 81t
    overdose 78
  depression 124
  drugs 231
  effects 187
  mild 259
  stimulants 85
Cerbera manghas 194
Cerbera odollam 358, 361, 361f
Cerebellum 251
Cerebral edema 283
  development of 283
  risk of 283
Cerebrospinal fluid 130, 280
  exchange 9, 269
Chemical
  asphyxiants 152t
  warfare agents 148, 158, 159t, 396
  weapons convention 396
Chemotherapeutic agents 231, 380t
  classification of 378t
  extravasation of 382
  toxicity 374
Chemotherapeutic drug 374, 377
Cherry pepper 361
Chest pain 55, 96
Chloral hydrate 6
Chloramphenicol 400
Chlordane 321, 324

Chloride 12
  depletion alkalosis 29
  loss 29
Chlorine 27, 151, 155, 159, 396
Chlorophacinone 227
Chlorophyllum molybdites 367
Chloropicrin 396
Chloroquine 185
Chlorpropamide 9, 262
Choking agents 396
Cholecalciferol 330, 331
Cholestasis 380
Cholestyramine 28, 326
Cholinergic 5
  agents 167
  receptors, over stimulation of 112
  toxidrome 305
    symptoms of 309
Cholinesterase 20
  levels 15, 22
Christmas pepper 361
Chromatography
  mass spectrometry 95
  thin-layer 22, 102
Chromium 9, 341, 345
Chronic obstructive pulmonary disease 78, 282
Chrysanthemum cinerariaefolium 308
Cicuta douglasii 111
Ciguatoxin 110
Cimetidine 207, 371
Circulation 5, 61, 148, 214, 296
Cisplatin 9
  toxicity 377
Citrullus colocynthis 359, 359f
Cleistanthus collinus 358, 363, 364f
Clobazam 134
Clomipramine 186
Clonazepam 134
Clonidine 5, 167, 257, 299
Clostridium botulinum 34, 128, 400
Cluster pepper 361
Coagulopathy, absence of 232
Cobra 349
Cocaine 4, 5, 14, 20, 28, 81, 185
  intoxication 93
  poisoning 3
Colchicine ingestion 291
Collagen metabolism, derangement of 345
Coma 179, 186, 251, 283
  cocktail 6, 6t
Common organophosphate compounds,
    classification of 296t
Complete blood count 14, 135
Computed tomography 112, 130
Cone pepper 361
Conocybe genera 367
Consciousness, level of 3
Continuous positive airway
    pressure 164
Copelandia 368
Copper sulfate 258, 259
Coprine 368
  poisoning 370

Corrosive
  acids, ingestion of 218
  agents 222
    poisoning 220b
  ingestion 218
  injury 223
    management of 220
Cortical necrosis, acute 258
Coumarin derivatives 330
Crab's eyes 357
Crack lung 97
Cranial nerves 129
Creatinine 179
Croton tiglium 359, 359f
Crow beards 357
Crystal nephropathy 381
Crystalloids 211
  intravenous 388
Cyanide 4, 5, 28, 148, 152, 250t
  antidotes 251
  poisoning 5, 246
    signs of 251t
    symptoms of 250t, 251t
  toxicity 250
Cyanogen chloride 397
Cyanohemoglobin 147
Cyclooxygenase 211
Cyclopeptides 367
Cyclophosphamide 9, 375, 379
Cyclopropanecarboxylic ester structure 308
Cystitis, hemorrhagic 381
Cytochrome 247
  oxidase 250
Cytopathic hyoxia 4

D

Dabigatran 238
  etexilate 236
Dantrolene 38
Dapsone 8
Datura 258
  fastuosa 358
  seed 361t
Death cap mushroom 358
Deep tendon reflexes 130
Deferoxamine 39, 317
  dose modification of 39t
Delirium 186
Deoxybarbiturate 134
Depression
  myocardial 4
  respiratory 15, 186, 279, 283
Depressive disorder, major 186
Desipramine 186
Desirudin 236
Desomorphine 104
Dexamethasone 22
Dexmedetomidine 167
Dexrazoxane 378, 382
Dextromethorphan 88
  mechanism of toxicity of 89fc
  poisoning 88t
  toxicity 88

Principles and Practice of Critical Care Toxicology

Dextropropoxyphene 8, 185
Dextrose 6, 112, 180, 182, 389
D-glucose 389
Diabetes
   insipidus 258
   mellitus 386
      noninsulin dependent 277
Dialysis 32
   indications of 10t
   sustained low-efficiency 9, 265, 267
Diaphoresis 62, 344
Diarrhea 54, 261, 305
Diazepam 16, 81, 134, 266, 299
Diazinon 324
Dichlorodiphenyldichloroethylene 324
Dichlorodiphenyltrichloroethane 111, 112, 320, 321, 324
Dichloroethane 321
Dichlorophenoxyacetic acid 9
Dicofol 321
Dieldrin 321, 324
Diflunisal 9
Digitalis lanata 194
Digitalis purpurea 194
Digoxin 5, 20, 266, 270, 274, 284
   ingestion, chronic 40
Dihydropyridines 178
Diltiazem 185
Diluted thrombin time 237
Dimercaprol 39
Dimercaptopropane sulfonate 343
Dimercaptosuccinic acid 51, 341
Dimethyltryptamine 81
Diode array detector 21
Dipeptidyl peptidase-4 inhibitors 391
Diphenadione 227
Diphenhydramine 185, 190
Diphenylchloroarsine 397
Diquat 314, 315
   cardiovascular 315
   gastrointestinal tract 315
   hematological 315
   neurological 315
   pulmonary 315
   renal 315
   skin 315
Direct thrombin inhibitors 236
Disability-adjusted life-years 118
Disease-modifying antirheumatic drugs 375
Disopyramide 8
Dispersal method 395
Distress, respiratory 222
Disulfiram toxicity 370
Dithiobisnitrobenzoate 23
Divalproex 134
Dizziness 62
D-lactate 27
Dopamine 110
Dothiepin 186
Doxepin 186
Drugs 15t, 229
   abuse 4
   and cosmetics Act 68

and cosmetics Rules 69
   category of 115t
   induced liver injury, causes of 203
Dry flushed skin 186
Dry mouth 186
Dyshemoglobinemias 242
Dyspepsia 55
Dyspnea 62
Dysrhythmias 340
   life-threatening 282

E

Early end-organ damage 270
Echocardiography, two-dimensional 95
Edema
   cardiogenic pulmonary 4
   noncardiogenic pulmonary 4
Edetate calcium disodium, dosing regimen of 38t
Edoxaban 238
Elapid snakes 260
Electrocardiogram 63, 86, 101, 111, 175, 187
   toxidromes 12
Electrocardiography 95, 179, 187
Electroencephalograph 112
Electrolytes 179
   correction of 196
   serum 14, 213
Electromyogram 101
Electromyography 130
Electron impact mass spectrometry 101
Elemental mercury, acute 344
Emergency cardiopulmonary bypass 9
Emulsion therapy 135
Encainide 185
Encephalopathy 205, 340
   ifosfamide-induced 44
Endosulfan 321, 324
Endothelial cells 210
Endotracheal
   intubation 388
   tube administration 34
End-stage renal disease 266
Environmental protection agency 339
Enzyme
   acetylcholinesterase 303
   cyclooxygenase 210
   linked immunosorbent assay 101, 128, 196
Epipodophyllotoxins 378
Epsilon-aminocaproic acid 238
Erythema multiforme 381
Erythrocyte protoporphyrin 343
Erythromycin 28, 227, 400
Erythroxylum coca 93
Eslicarbazepine 133, 135
Ethane 152
Ethanol 4, 21, 28, 118
   metabolite 20
Ethosuximide 133, 134, 138
Ethyl dibromide 10
Ethyl glucuronide 20

Ethylene 124, 152
   glycol 4, 5, 10, 21, 26, 121, 122
      poisoning 27, 41, 49, 122f, 125
      toxicity 49, 55
Ethylenediaminetetraacetic acid 22, 71, 112, 341
Euglycemia 391
European Association of Poisons Centers and Clinical Toxicologists 7, 36
Extracellular fluid 29
Extracorporeal Life Support 168, 171, 183, 288
   organization 288
Extracorporeal liver assist devices 269
Extracorporeal membrane oxygenation 9, 10, 16, 170, 176, 288-291
   mechanics of 289
Extracorporeal therapy 9, 169, 180, 183, 189, 207, 255, 264, 265, 274
   role of 212
   selection of 9
Extracorporeal toxin removal 264, 269, 271, 271fc, 274, 275t, 276-284
   role of 274t, 275-278, 280-283
   techniques of 9b
   types of 265

F

False morel toxicity 49
Fanconi syndrome 259
Fast ventricular rate 195
Fat
   absorption of 55
   accumulation 62
Fatal poisoning 367
Fatty acid
   long-chain 54
   metabolism theory 61
Felbamate 133
Fentanyl 20, 81
Ferric chloride spot test 213
Fever 214
Fibrillation, ventricular 95, 186
Flecainide 185
Fluconazole 227
Fluid 215
   attenuation inversion recovery 246
   intravenous 215
   management 168
Flumazenil 6, 16, 40, 148
   role of 79
Fluoride 9, 262
   ions 222
Fluoroacetamide 334
Fluoroacetates 334
Fluorouracil 9, 379
Flurazepam 81
Flushing 251
Folate, role of 377
Folic acid 42
Folinic acid 148, 376
Fomepizole 41, 125
   dosing schedule of 41t
Foodborne botulism 128

Index | 407

Fool's mushroom 368
Forensic toxicology 68
Formaldehyde 151
Formic acid 122
Fosphenytoin 134
Francisella tularensis 399
Free radical generation 242
Fresh frozen plasma 148, 233, 239, 268, 299
Fumigants 303
Fungicides 303

G

Gaba receptor inhibition 112
Gabapentin 133, 134, 141, 257
Galerina 367
    autumnalis 368
Gamma-aminobutyric acid 11, 77, 110, 112, 133, 134, 138, 186, 250, 323
Gamma-chain variant 247
Gamma-glutamyl transferase 204
Gamma-hydroxybutyrate 14, 148
Gamma-hydroxybutyric acid 78
    overdose 80
Gangrene 46
Gas chromatography 21
    mass spectrometry 21, 100, 190
Gasping syndrome 47
Gastric
    decontamination 87, 175, 206
    lavage 7, 71, 232, 298
    mucosa 210
Gastrointestinal
    bleeding 238
    decontamination 7, 179, 214, 316
    distress 119
    disturbances 387
    dysfunction 295
    obstruction 46
    perforation 221
    system 211, 340
    toxicity 376
    toxins 368
    tract 26, 186, 219
Genitourinary obstruction 46
Genitourinary toxicity 381
    management 381
Glacial acetic acid 219
Glasgow coma scale 147, 297
    score 5, 15, 64
Glomerular filtration rate 8
Gloriosa superba 365, 365*f*
Glucagon 16, 42, 148, 169, 182, 390
    intravenous 180
Glucagonoma 42
Glucose
    6-phosphate dehydrogenase 44, 247
        deficiency 50
    insulin 176
    supplemental 214
    transporter-2 inhibitors, serum 391
Glutamate 109
    carboxypeptidase 377

    dehydrogenase 250
    receptor activation 112
Glutamic acid decarboxylase 138
Glutathione 31
    reductase 340*f*, 346
    S-transferase 340*f*
Glutethimide 10
Glyceryl trinitrate 16
Glycine 216
    receptor inhibition 112
Glycol 26, 124
Glycolate 28
Glycopyrrolate 298
Glycoside
    cardioactive 167
    poisoning, nonpharmacological cardiac 40
Glycosuria 163, 314
Gold poisoning 39*b*
Green pit viper 349
Guanosine monophosphate 182
    cyclic 171
Guillain-Barré syndrome 130
Gymnopilus 368
Gyromitra
    ambigua 368
    esculenta 111, 368
    gigas 368
    infula 368
    mushroom 112
Gyromitrin 368
    poisoning 369, 372

H

Hair 71
Haldane effect 242
Hallucinogenic intoxication, management of 89
Hallucinogens 87
Harassing agent 397
Headache 62, 327
Heart
    block 40, 186
    disease, ischemic 178
    failure, congestive 379
Heavy metal 10, 112
    poisoning 259, 339
    toxicity 339, 340
        diagnosis of 341*t*
        mechanism of 340*f*
Hematological system 211
Hematuria 314
Hemodiafiltration 9
Hemodialysis 10, 41, 112, 125, 215, 262, 264, 316
    advantages of 266*t*
    disadvantages of 266*t*
    indications of 215*b*
    intermittent 9, 266, 276, 278-284
    role of 42
Hemodynamic status, assessment of 232
Hemofiltration 10
Hemoglobin 242, 244, 351

    binding 242
    M disease 247
Hemoglobinuria 352
Hemolytic uremic syndrome 379, 381
Hemoperfusion 9, 10, 265, 266, 276, 280, 281, 284, 300, 316
    advantages of 267*t*
    disadvantages of 267*t*
    indications of 10*t*
Hemorrhage 4
    gastrointestinal 229
    intracerebral 237
    intracranial 3, 46, 49, 289
    subarachnoid 238
    subdural 238
Hemostatic abnormalities 351, 352
Heparin overdose 48
Hepatic failure 32, 47, 208
Hepatitis, granulomatous 380
Hepatocellular injury 380
Hepatorenal syndrome 369, 380
Hepatotoxic plants 357
Hepatotoxicity 324
    risk of 205
Hepatotoxins, chemotherapeutic 380*t*
Herbal
    ecstasy 102
    incense 101
    products 230
    smoking blends 101
Herbicides 64, 303
    poisoning 312
Heroin 5
Hexachlorocyclohexane 320
High performance liquid chromatography 230
High-dose insulin 171
    euglycemia
        regimen 169*b*
        therapy 169, 180, 181
    therapy 42, 43*b*, 171
High-performance liquid chromatography 21
His-Purkinje fibers 185
Histamine ethanol 110
Hornet bite 258, 261
Human carcinogens 340
Hump-nosed viper 349
Hurricanes 242
Hyaluronidase 382
Hydantoin 134
Hydralazine 5
Hydration 376
Hydrazines 112
Hydrocarbon 4, 8
    chlorinated 325
Hydrochloric acid 28, 222
Hydrocodone 81
Hydrocyanic acid 397
Hydrofluoric acid 222
    burns 37
Hydrogen
    chloride 151, 159
    fluoride 159
    peroxide 340*f*, 343
    sulphide 4, 5, 28, 70, 151, 152

Principles and Practice of Critical Care Toxicology

Hydroperoxide 343
Hydroxocobalamin 16, 43, 148
Hydroxychloroquine 185
Hymenoptera stings 354
Hyperammonemia 283
Hyperbaric oxygen 43, 112, 164
   therapy 43, 44t, 157
Hyperglycemia 179
Hyperkalemia 261, 325
Hyperphosphatemia 222
Hypersensitivity reactions 49, 50, 55
Hypertension 5, 5t, 96, 178, 237, 344
   abdominal 222
   control of 87
Hyperthermia 62, 87, 94, 97, 114, 186
   control of 90
   malignant 38
Hypertriglyceridemia 114
Hyperventilation 4, 30
Hypnotics, nonbenzodiazepine 78
Hypocalcemia 222
Hypofibrinogenemia 267
Hypoglycemia 119, 179, 205, 386, 388, 389
   sulfonylurea-induced 54
Hypokalemia 196
Hyponatremia 110
Hypoperfusion 27
Hypoprothrombinemia 46
Hypotension 5, 5t, 33, 52, 119, 124, 186, 188,
    189, 250, 261, 279
Hypothermia 119, 211
Hypothyroidism 55
Hypoventilation 4, 119
Hypoxemia 4t, 27
Hypoxia inducible factor 1-alpha 244

I

Idarucizumab 239
Ifosfamide 377
Iminostilbene 134
Imipramine 22, 186
Indian Evidence Act 70
Indian Penal Code 69
Indian poisonous plants 357
Indoxacarb 185
Infant botulism, adult-type 129
Infarction, myocardial 97, 242, 245
Inferior vena cava 176
Inhibiting cellular oxygen utilization 152
Initial toxidrome 397
   recognition 397t
Insecticide 5, 185, 303
Insulin 5, 112, 148, 182
   glucose, peripheral 387
   intravenous high-dose 180
Insulinoma 42
Intensive care unit 15, 64, 115, 131, 147, 187,
    196, 220
International Agency for Research on Cancer
    340
International normalized ratio 232, 237
Interstitial nephritis, chronic 258

Interstitial pneumonia, acute 340
Intestinal colonization botulism 129
Intoxication, features of 87
Intra-aortic balloon pump 170, 189
Intranasal spray 45
Intravenous lipid emulsion 170, 180-182
   therapy 171
Intubation 189
   emergency 15
Iodide 9
Ion
   channel modulation theory 61
   coupled plasma atomic emission
     spectrometry 21
   flux, disturbances of 110
Ipomoea violacea 104
Iron 8, 20
   enhances toxicity 317
   poisoning 39
Irritant gases, distribution of 152f
Ischemia, myocardial 94
Isoniazid 5, 9, 27, 110, 112
Isoprocarb 304
Isopropanol 123, 124
Isopropyl alcohol 123

J

Jatropha curcas 364, 364f

K

Kerosene 4, 7
Ketamine 20, 90
Ketoacidosis 27
   alcoholic 28
Ketones 26, 28, 124
Ketosis 28
Kidney 47, 210, 313
   disease, chronic 262, 381
   injury, acute 257-259
Kikendall and Zargar classification 219
Krait 349
Kratom 103
Kussmaul-Kien respirations 259

L

Labetalol 96
Lacosamide 133, 137
Lactate 26
   dehydrogenase 370
Lactic acidosis, metformin associated 278, 387
Lactose 28
Lambert-Eaton syndrome 130
Lamotrigine 133, 134, 137
Lathyrus sativus 362, 362f
Lead 5, 112, 343
   poisoning 37, 45, 258, 259
   toxicity 343
Leiurus quinquestriatus 353
Lepiota 367
Leucovorin 53, 376

administration of 376
   rescue therapy 376
Leukopenia 267
Levetiracetam 133, 134, 140
Levocarnitine 54
Levosimendan 181
Lidocaine 110
Lignocaine 189
Lindane 322, 324
Linezolid 88
Lipid emulsion
   infusion 169
   regimen 170b
   therapy 60, 64b
    initiation of 61
Lipid peroxidation 313, 340
Lipid sink theory 60
Liquid chromatography-mass spectrometry
    100
Lithium 5, 8-10, 20, 112, 258, 260, 274, 277
   toxicity, management of 277t
Liver 313
   biopsy 371
   cell failure 205
   disease 41
    chronic 54
    pre-existing 207
   failure
    acetaminophen-induced 207t
    acute 46, 203
   function
    abnormal 237
    tests 14, 204, 214
   parenchyma 229
   transplant 207
Local anesthetic 60, 64, 185
   eutectic mixture of 248
   systemic toxicity 60, 63
Loperamide 381
Lorazepam 134
Low glomerular filtration rate 261
Low molecular-weight heparin 48, 48b, 238
Lung 313
   fibrosis, early 316
   injury, acute 62
Lycoperdons 368
Lysergic acid diethylamide 20, 88, 103, 397

M

Magnesium 174, 299
   citrate 7, 28
   sulfate 7
Magnetic resonance imaging 130, 131
Maintenance therapy 61
Mannitol 28
Maprotiline 186
Marijuana, synthetic 20
Mean arterial pressure 42
Mechanical ventilation 189
Medicolegal case 68
Meglitinides 390
Membrane stabilizing activity 179

Menadione 232, 333
Mental disorders, statistical manual of 118
Meprobamate 9
Mercury 341, 343
    inorganic 344
    organic 344
    poisoning 39*b*
    tablets 22
    thermometers 344
Mesobuthus tamulus 352
Metabolic acidosis 13, 26-28, 30, 125, 222, 259, 261
    analysis of 26, 27*fc*
    etiology of 26
    high anion gap 26
    normal anion gap 28
Metaflumizone 185
Metals 5, 223
    fume fever 158, 340
Metamizole 266
Metformin 28, 274, 277, 386, 387
    overdose 387
    toxicity, management of 278*t*
Methadone 20, 45
    metabolite 20
Methamphetamine 20, 85, 86
Methane 4, 152
Methanol 4, 10, 21, 26, 27, 120, 124, 257, 258, 274, 278
    poisoning 9, 27, 41, 125
    toxicity 53
        management of 279*t*
Methaqualone 20, 266
Methemoglobin 21, 156, 242, 247*f*, 248
Methemoglobinemia 4, 5, 44, 147, 247, 248*t*, 249, 370
    signs of 248*t*
    symptoms of 248*t*
Methomyl 304, 305
Methotrexate 9, 24, 28, 148, 262, 374, 375, 379-381
    metabolism 374
    pharmacokinetics of 374
    poisoning 375
    toxicity 52, 53, 374
        management of 376
    uses of 374
Methoxetamine 91
Methoxychlor 322
Methoxyketamine 91
Methyl isocyanate 151, 155
Methyl mercury 343, 344
Methylene blue 16, 44, 171, 182
Methylenedioxy-3-methoxy-phenethylamine 102
Methylenedioxymethamphetamine 20, 85, 102, 110, 111, 115
Methylenedioxy-N-hydroxyamphetamine 102
Methylnaltrexone 381
Methylphenidate 20
    metabolite 20
Methylprednisolone 22
Methyltestosterone 231

Metoclopramide 5, 28
Microsomal ethanol oxidizing system 119
Midazolam 81
Minimum toxic dose 203
Mitochondrial dysfunction 242
Mitragyna speciosa 103
Molecular adsorbent recirculating system 10, 269
Monday morning fever 340
Monitoring plasma methotrexate concentration 376
Monoamine oxidase 85
    inhibitors 44
Monoclonal antibodies 378
Morphine 20, 81
Multiorgan system failure 125, 259
Munchausen syndrome 229
Muscarine 368
    poisoning 370
Muscimol poisoning 370
Mushroom
    identification 370
    management of 268
    poisoning 52, 367
        treatment of 371
Myasthenia gravis 48, 130
Mycena pura 367
Mydriasis 186
Myeloperoxidase 243, 244
Myoclonic twitching 186
Myoglobinuria 351, 352

N

N-acetylcysteine 31, 33, 176, 274, 317
    adverse effects of 32, 207
    dosage protocols of 32*b*
    therapy, indications of 206
N-acetyl-P-benzoquinone imine 31, 203, 275
Naloxone 6, 16, 44, 90, 148
Narcotic Drugs and Psychotropic Substances Act 69
National Academy of Clinical Biochemistry 20
National Institute Alcohol Abuse and Alcoholism 118
Nausea 32, 62, 327, 387
Necrosis, hepatic 222
Neon 152
Nephritis, interstitial 257
Nephrotoxic agents 326
Nephrotoxicity 345, 375
    long-term 324
Nephrotoxins, chemotherapeutic 381*t*
Nerium oleander 194, 358
Nerve agent 396
    class of 396
    poisoning 34
Nerve gas agents 112
Neurocritical Care Society 49
Neuroexcitation 114
Neuroglycopenic symptoms 389
Neuroleptic malignant syndrome 35
Neurological system 211

Neuromuscular dysfunction 297
Neuropathy, peripheral 50
Neurotoxic 348
    envenoming 352
    plants 357
    signs 351
Neurotoxicity 250, 375
    central 377
    peripheral 377
Neurotoxin
    chemotherapeutic 378*t*
    ingestion 327
Neutral protamine hagedorn 49
Neutropenia 379
Nicotinamide adenine dinucleotide 247*f*
    phosphate, oxidation of 313
Nitric oxide 181, 244
    synthase 244
        inhibition 61
Nitrites 148
Nitrofurantoin 4
Nitrogen 4, 152
    mustards 151
    oxides of 151, 152
Nitroglycerine 96
N-methyl-D-aspartate 88, 109, 244
Nondihydropyridines 178
Nonsteroidal anti-inflammatory drugs 27, 29, 210, 265
    adverse effects of 211*t*
    classification of 211*t*
    overdose 210
Norbormide 331
Norepinephrine 110
Normobaric oxygen therapy 164, 246
Nortriptyline 186
Novichok agents 396
Nucleophilic agents 298
Nystagmus, multidirectional 279

O

Obidoxime 307
Obsessive-compulsive disorders 186
Obsolete technology 270
Obtundation 251
O-cresol reagent 22
Octreotide 54, 112
Omeprazole 227
Omphalotus olivascens 367
Ophthalmoplegia 186
Opiates 5, 14, 20, 29, 93
Opioid 4, 5, 10, 78, 257
    long-acting 45
    overdose 80
Oral anticoagulants, direct acting 236, 237*t*-239*t*
Oral hypoglycemic agents 112, 386, 386*t*
    classification of 386*fc*
    overdose, symptoms of 389*t*
Oral mucositis, management of 381
Oral N-acetyl cysteine protocol 206
Orellanine 368

poisoning 369
Organic phosphorus compounds 330
Organochlorines 320
    pesticide 320, 321t, 324, 327
        biological effects of 324t
        poisoning, treatment of 325
Organophosphate 4, 5, 8, 33, 112, 257, 304
    coma 297
    compounds 167, 331
        toxicity of 295
    poisoning 33b, 47, 48t, 295, 296t
Organophosphorus 10, 23, 258, 295
    pesticides 325
    poisoning 15, 258
Osmolar gap 11, 28, 124
Oxalate 28
    crystals 124
Oxandrolone 231
Oxcarbazepine 133, 134
Oximetry 249
Oxoproline 26
Oxycodone 20, 81
Oxygen 6, 148
    saturation gap 15
    supplementation 315
    therapy 246, 246f
    utilization 28
Oxyhemoglobin 156, 162
    dissociation curve 242
Oxyphenbutazone 266
Ozone 151

P

Pacemaker 180, 182
Pain 62
    abdominal 55, 258, 387
    chronic 186
    neuropathic 186
    severe abdominal 222
Palamneus gravimanus 352
Pancreatitis 55, 62
Paracetamol 20, 22, 203
    metabolism of 204fc
    normal metabolism of 204fc
    poisoning 31, 203
    serum 23
Paraoxon 266
Paraphenylenediamine 257, 258
Paraquat 10, 258, 312, 314
    detection of 22
    induces nitric oxide 313
    poisoning 259, 312
Parasiticides 64
Parathion 266
Paresthesias 50
Partial thromboplastin time 48
Paxillus involutus 368
Penicillamine 4, 45
Penicillins 400
Pentachlorophenol 324
Pentohexital sodium 275
Perampanel 138

Peritoneal dialysis 9, 10, 269, 377
Pesticide 293, 303
    intoxications 306
    poisoning 320
    types of 320
Phallotoxins 367
Phencyclidine 5, 14, 20, 90
Phenethylamines 102
Phenformin 28
Phenobarbital 8-10, 20, 133
Phenobarbitone 24, 81, 134, 138
Phenol 222, 223
Phenothiazines 5, 22, 185
    pseudoephedrine 5
Phentolamine 96
Phenylbutazone 266
Phenyltriazine 134
Phenytoin 8, 10, 24, 110, 133-135, 274, 279,
        280, 282
    toxicity, management of 280t
Pheochromocytoma 42
Phosgene 151, 155, 159, 396
Phosphate 12
Phosphaturia aminoaciduria 314
Phosphides 174, 331, 334
Phosphine 152, 174, 331
Phosphodiesterase inhibitors 181
Photophobia 344
Physostigmine 5, 46
Phytomenadione 232
Phytonadione 46, 232, 332
Pink disease 344
Piperazines 102
Piperonyl butoxide 308
Pirimicarb 304
Piroxicam 227
Plant kingdom 357
Plasma acetaminophen levels versus time,
        semilogarithmic plot of 24f
Plasmapheresis 10, 268
Platelet 210
    activation 243
    transfusion 148
Pneumonia, ventilator-associated 115, 298
Pneumothorax 4
Podophyllum species 360
Poisoning 3, 19, 68, 72fc, 146fc
    acute 19, 162, 274, 342
    causes of 357
    chronic 21
    circumstances of 70
    fulminant 315
    homicidal 70
    inhalational 151
    management of 296
    mild 314
    moderate-to-severe 315
    nonanticholinesterase 48
    nonpharmaceutical 290
    organocarbamate 295
    plant 357
    severity score 147
    subacute 163
    suicidal 70

Poisonous mushrooms
    accidental consumption of 367
    toxicity of 367
Poisonous plants, category of 357, 357t
Poisons 4, 15t, 74t
    binding 265
    counteract effects of 299, 299t
    gastrointestinal 370
    load, reduction of 298
    neurodepressive effect of 297
Poliomyelitis 130
Polychlorinated biphenyls 324
Polyethylene glycol electrolyte solution 8
Polymerase chain reaction 128
Polyoxyethylated castor oil 47
Polysorbate 47
Posaconazole 24
Positive end-expiratory pressure 306
Potassium 8, 12, 27, 176
    channel
        blockers 110, 167
        openers 110
    chloride 215
    cyanide test 249
    iodide 55, 56b
    permanganate 175
Pralidoxime 16, 47, 112, 148, 160
Prednisolone 22
Pregabalin 133, 141
Pregnancy test 14
Primidone 133, 134
Procainamide 185, 266
Propane 4, 152
Propofol 28, 114
    infusion syndrome 114
Propoxur 303-305
Propoxyphene 14, 20
Propranolol 110, 179, 227
Propylene glycol 26, 28, 279
    toxicity 259
Propyphenazone 266
Protamine
    neutralization dose of 48b, 48t
    sulfate 48
Protein 265
    binding 265
        degree of 10
    bound toxins 269
    kinase inhibitor 378
    modification 340
Proteinuria 314
Prothrombin complex 148
    concentrate 233
Prothrombin time 232, 237
Proton pump inhibitors 20
Protriptyline 186
Proximal tubular cells 260
Prussian blue 112
Psathyrella 368
Psilocybe 368
Psilocybin 89, 368
    poisoning 369
Psychoactive drugs 397

Index **411**

Pulmonary edema 29, 250
    clinical features of 179
    signs of 307
Pulse
    contour cardiac output 180
    pressure variation 168
Pylorospasm 213
Pyramidal signs 186
Pyrethroids 110, 111, 307, 308, 308*t*
Pyridoxine 49, 112

Q

Quick toxidrome recognition 397
Quinidine 5, 110, 185
Quinine 8, 185

R

Randomized control trials 60, 168, 196
Raxibacumab 400
Reactive airway dysfunction syndrome 152
Reactive oxygen species 243, 312, 343
Real time mass spectrometry 100
Rebound toxicity 229
    risk of 233
Red blood cell 23, 304, 342
    cholinesterase 23
Rehabilitation 352
Renal biopsy 371
Renal dysfunction 39*t*, 48, 387
Renal failure 27, 124, 260, 351, 374
Renal function
    abnormal 237
    tests 213
Renal replacement therapy 261
    continuous 9, 215, 267, 276-279, 281-284
Renal tubular acidosis 26, 27, 260, 381
Renin angiotensin system 29
Respiratory 94
    failure 145, 146, 146*t*, 388
        pathogenesis of 145
    irritants 151*t*, 153
    rate 214
    system 211
    tract 219
Resuscitation 16
    cardiopulmonary 16, 63, 168
Retigabine 133
Rhabdomyolysis 257*t*
Ricin toxin 400
Ricinus communis 358
    plant 358*ff*
Rifampicin 136
Risperidone 5
Rivaroxaban 238, 239
Rodenticides 5, 258, 293, 303, 330
    classification of 330
    poisoning 332, 334*t*
Rohypnol 5
Ropivacaine 185
Rotenone 28
Rufinamide 133, 137

Rumack-Matthew nomogram 205*f*, 206
    drawbacks of 206
Russell's viper 349

S

Salicylate 4, 8-10, 12, 20, 22, 26, 30, 112, 212, 213, 216, 262
    levels, serum 23, 213
    overdose 281
    poisoning 52, 53
        management of 214
    toxicity, management of 281*t*
Salicylic acid 212, 274, 280, 317
Salmonella typhimurium 398
Salvia 103
Saw-scaled viper 349
Schilling's test, abnormal 55
Scorpion stings 352
Sea snakes 349
Sedation 87
Sedative
    hypnotic 4, 5, 78
        overdose, management of 79
    overdose of 29
Seizures 15, 179, 186, 188
    chemical agents causing 112*t*
    epileptic 109
    isoniazid-induced 49
    toxin-induced 109, 113*fc*
    treatment of 61
Selective serotonin reuptake inhibitor 44, 111
Selenium 266
Semecarpus anacardium 359, 360*f*
Serotonergic drugs 88
Serotonin 110
    and norepinephrine reuptake inhibitors 44
Serum lactate predict life-threatening poisoning 179
Sesame oil, component of 308
Shell fish poisoning 130
Shock 257
    cardiogenic 186
Silibinin 371
Silo Filler's disease 153
Silymarin 52
Single pass albumin dialysis 10
Sinoatrial node 188
Sinus bradycardia 55, 94, 186, 187, 195, 314
Skin 219
Slaughterhouse sledgehammer effect 153
Snake 258, 348
    bite 4, 260
        management of 260, 350, 350*fc*
        neuroparalytic 148
        therapeutic response of 349*t*
    types of 348
    venom 257
        toxic effects of 348
Society of Critical Care Medicine 49
Sodium 12, 27
    bicarbonate 16, 52, 188, 215
        hypertonic 170

channel
    blockers 110, 168, 185, 187*t*
    opener 110
    voltage-dependent 134
    voltage-gated 112, 185
nitrite 16, 50
    solution 50*t*
sulfate 7
thiosulfate 16, 51
valproate 138
Sorbitol 8, 298
Sotalol 167, 179
Stat quantitative serum toxicology assays 20
Status epilepticus 109, 115
    complications of 115
    nonconvulsive 115
    refractory 115, 116*fc*
    super-refractory 109
ST-elevation myocardial infarction 95
Steroids 22
Stevens-Johnson syndrome 381
Street pharmacists 99
Stroke 237
    syndromes 130
    volume variation 168
Strophanthus gratus 194
Strychnine 330, 331, 334
Strychnos nuxvomica 358
Succinimide 134
Succinylcholine 46
Suicide tree 358, 361, 361*f*
Sulfate 12
Sulfhemoglobinemia 251
Sulfmethemoglobin 73
Sulfonamides 9, 262
Sulfonylureas 112, 388
    agents, toxicity of 388
    classification of 388*fc*
Sulfur dioxide 151
Sulfuric acid 218
Superoxide dismutase 340*f*
Superwarfarin 232
    poisoning, management of 333*fc*
    toxicity 227
Sympathomimetics 5
    drugs 84
Syndrome of inappropriate antidiuretic hormone secretion 134
Systemic inflammatory response syndrome 162

T

Tachyarrhythmia 40, 170
    management of 197
Tachycardia 5, 5*t*, 168*b*, 186, 251, 261, 307, 344
    control of 87
    supraventricular 95
    ventricular 95, 186
Tachypnea 214, 257
Tear gases 397
Terlipressin 171
Testosterone 231
Tetanus 4

Tetracycline 400
Tetrahydrocannabinol 20
Tetrahydrofolate 120
Tetramine 330, 331, 334
Tetrodotoxin 185
Thaimine 6
Thallium 9, 112, 274, 281
  sulfate 330, 331
  toxicity, management of 282t
Theophylline 5, 8, 10, 20, 27, 112, 274, 282
  anhydrous 282
  toxicity 282, 283t
Therapeutic plasma 268
  exchange 9, 10, 268
Therapeutic serum levels 276
Thevetia peruviana 194, 358, 364
Thiamine 55
Thiopentone 81
Thioridazine 185
Thiosulfate 148
Thrombin time 237
Thrombocytopenia 47
Thrombolytics 4
Thrombotic thrombocytopenic purpura 379
Thymidine 377
Thymidylate
  salvage 377
  synthase 375
Thyroid stimulating hormone secretion 55
Thyroxine 10, 265
Tiagabine 133, 134
Tick paralysis 130
Tiletamine 91
Tissue
  hypoxemia 27
  necrosis of 219
Topiramate 28, 133, 134, 140
Topoisomerase inhibitors 378, 380
Toxaphene 322
Toxic agents 258
Toxic alcohol 28, 118, 259
  parameter, comparisons of 124t
  poisoning 42, 52, 53
Toxic dose 174, 210, 321t
  ingestion of 230
Toxic epidermal necrolysis 381
Toxic inhalation gases 4
Toxic manifestations 88, 212
Toxic megacolon 186
Toxic plants 357
Toxic substances 306
Toxicity 52, 64, 212, 327, 395
  acute 340, 342
  aspects of 227
  chemotherapy-induced 374
  hematopoietic 378, 379t
  mechanism of 89fc, 242, 312, 323, 342, 345
  mitochondrial 313
  mucocutaneous 376
  multiorgan 340
  neurological 377
  pulmonary 375, 379
  stages of 88t
  systemic 151

Toxicodynamics 174, 228
Toxicokinetics 186, 190, 228, 274-278, 280-283, 308
  considerations 9
Toxicological analysis, systematic 21
Toxicology 28, 68, 203
  tests 21
    advanced 21
Toxidromes 3, 9, 11t
  approach 72
Toxins 9t, 185, 229, 400
  biochemical effects of 323
  chemotherapeutic pulmonary 380t
  dialyzability of 264
  diarrhea-inducing 28
  direct metabolism of 28
  examples of 110t
  extracorporeal
    elimination of 9
    removal of 264
  hematological 225, 375
  induced acute renal failure 257
  renal 255
Tramadol 20, 88
Tranexamic acid 238
Transfusion reactions, risk of 233
Tricyclic antidepressant 4, 5, 10, 14, 20, 29, 64, 111, 168, 185, 186t, 257, 265, 274, 291
  poisoning 52
  toxicity, clinical features of 186t
Trimipramine 186
Troponins, cardiac 95
Tryptamines 103
Tubular necrosis, acute 258, 340, 381
Tyrosine kinase inhibitor 380

U

Unconsciousness 5b
Upper gastrointestinal endoscopy 221
  contraindications of 221t
  indications of 221t
Urinary
  acidification, role of 90
  alkalization 262
  retention 186
  toxicology panel 112
  tract infection, catheter-associated 298
Urine 71
  acidification 9, 87
  alkalization 9, 376
  drug screens 20
    limitations of 20

V

Valproate 138
Valproic acid 20, 133, 134, 136, 139, 274, 283
  toxicity 283
    management of 284t
Vancomycin 24
Vasoplegia 44
Vasopressors 168, 180, 182
  therapy 181

Venoarterial-extracorporeal membrane oxygenation 148, 183
Venovenous hemofiltration, continuous 176
Ventricular premature complexes 195
Verapamil 4, 185
Verpa bohemica 368
Vigabatrin 133, 134, 138
Viperid snakes 260
Vipomas 54
Viral hemorrhagic fevers 400
Virotoxins 367
Visual disturbance 125
Visual dysfunction 278
Vitamin
  B complex 363
  B_6 110
  B_9 42
  C 317
  E 317
  K 228, 229, 332
    antagonists 46
    optimum dose of 333
    serum levels of 230
    therapy 233
  K1 46, 148, 232, 233, 332
    prophylactic 334
  K3 232, 333
Vomiting 32, 62, 327, 397
Voriconazole 24
Warfarin 227-229
  ingestion, acute 233
  mechanism of action of 228ff
  serum levels of 230
  toxicity 46, 229, 233

W

Water hemlock 111
Wernicke's encephalopathy 55
White phosphorus 222
Whole blood clotting time 57
Whole bowel irrigation 8, 179
Woolsorter disease 399
Wound botulism 128

X

Xanthine oxidase 250
Ximelagatran 236

Y

Yellow oleander 358, 364, 365f
Yellow phosphorus 330, 331, 334
Yersinia pestis 399

Z

Zargar classification 220, 222t
Zinc 174
  chloride 290
  phosphide 330
  shakes 340
Zonisamide 133, 134, 137